Essentials of Geriatrics Medicine

Essentials of Geriatrics Medicine

Editor: Benjamin Thornberg

AMERICAN
MEDICAL PUBLISHERS
www.americanmedicalpublishers.com

AMERICAN
MEDICAL PUBLISHERS
www.americanmedicalpublishers.com

Cataloging-in-Publication Data

Essentials of geriatrics medicine / edited by Benjamin Thornberg.
p. cm.
Includes bibliographical references and index.
ISBN 978-1-63927-002-6
1. Geriatrics. 2. Older people--Diseases. 3. Older people--Health and hygiene. 4. Older people--Medical care.
5. Gerontology. 6. Aging. I. Thornberg, Benjamin.
RC952 .E87 2021
618.97--dc23

American Medical Publishers,
41 Flatbush Avenue,
1st Floor, New York,
NY 11217, USA

ISBN 978-1-63927-002-6 (Hardback)

Contents

Preface

Geriatrics medicine is a field of medicine that deals with the health care of elderly people. The main aim of geriatrics medicine is to promote health by preventing and treating diseases and disabilities in elderly people. Geriatrics medicine focuses on the distinctive need of elderly persons. It focuses on the unique needs of elderly people which makes it quite different from standard adult medicine. Geriatrics medicine aims to treat diseases that are present and achieve healthy aging. It focuses on achieving the patient's highest priorities in the context of multiple chronic conditions, and on preserving function. It deals with increasing complexity, geriatric giants, and practical concerns. Some sub-specialties of geriatrics medicine are geriatric anesthesia, geriatric nutrition, geriatric pharmacy, geriatric podiatry, geriatric audiology, etc. This book contains some path-breaking studies in the field of geriatrics medicine. It strives to provide a fair idea about this discipline and to help develop a better understanding of the latest advances within this field. Those in search of information to further their knowledge will be greatly assisted by this book.

After months of intensive research and writing, this book is the end result of all who devoted their time and efforts in the initiation and progress of this book. It will surely be a source of reference in enhancing the required knowledge of the new developments in the area. During the course of developing this book, certain measures such as accuracy, authenticity and research focused analytical studies were given preference in order to produce a comprehensive book in the area of study.

This book would not have been possible without the efforts of the authors and the publisher. I extend my sincere thanks to them. Secondly, I express my gratitude to my family and well-wishers. And most importantly, I thank my students for constantly expressing their willingness and curiosity in enhancing their knowledge in the field, which encourages me to take up further research projects for the advancement of the area.

Editor

1

Plantar Temperature Response to Walking in Diabetes with and without Acute Charcot: The Charcot Activity Response Test

Bijan Najafi,[1,2] James S. Wrobel,[3] Gurtej Grewal,[1] Robert A. Menzies,[4] Talal K. Talal,[4] Mahmoud Zirie,[4] and David G. Armstrong[1]

[1] *Southern Arizona Limb Salvage Alliance (SALSA), University of Arizona College of Medicine, Tucson, AZ, USA*
[2] *Arizona Center on Aging, University of Arizona, Tucson, AZ, USA*
[3] *University of Michigan, Medical School, Ann Arbor, MI, USA*
[4] *Diabetic Foot and Wound Center, Department of Medicine, Hamad Medical Corporation, Doha, Qatar*

Correspondence should be addressed to Bijan Najafi, bnajafi@surgery.arizona.edu

Academic Editor: Neil D. Reeves

Objective. Asymmetric plantar temperature differences secondary to inflammation is a hallmark for the diagnosis and treatment response of Charcot foot syndrome. However, little attention has been given to temperature response to activity. We examined dynamic changes in plantar temperature (PT) as a function of graduated walking activity to quantify thermal responses during the first 200 steps. *Methods.* Fifteen individuals with Acute Charcot neuroarthropathy (CN) and 17 non-CN participants with type 2 diabetes and peripheral neuropathy were recruited. All participants walked for two predefined paths of 50 and 150 steps. A thermal image was acquired at baseline after acclimatization and immediately after each walking trial. The PT response as a function of number of steps was examined using a validated wearable sensor technology. The hot spot temperature was identified by the 95th percentile of measured temperature at each anatomical region (hind/mid/forefoot). *Results.* During initial activity, the PT was reduced in all participants, but the temperature drop for the nonaffected foot was 1.9 times greater than the affected side in CN group ($P = 0.04$). Interestingly, the PT in CN was sharply increased after 50 steps for both feet, while no difference was observed in non-CN between 50 and 200 steps. *Conclusions.* The variability in thermal response to the graduated walking activity between Charcot and non-Charcot feet warrants future investigation to provide further insight into the correlation between thermal response and ulcer/Charcot development. This stress test may be helpful to differentiate CN and its response to treatment earlier in its course.

1. Background

Charcot neuroarthropathy (CN) is a devastating complication of diabetes. It has a similar mortality rate as lower extremity ulceration and a twofold higher rate of major amputation compared to those without CN [1]. It has been estimated that 63% of CN patients will develop a foot ulcer [2]. The combination of foot ulcer and CN increases the risk of amputation 12-fold [3]. The increased mortality risk associated with CN appears to be independent of foot ulcer and other comorbidities [2].

What further complicates CN is that there is no clear definition for it [4]. There are no pathologic markers or diagnostic criteria. Therefore, the diagnosis relies on pattern recognition and clinical intuition [5]. Not surprisingly, the diagnosis can be missed up to 95% of the time [6] and the average diagnostic delay has been estimated at almost 7 months [7].

A significant number of CN patients either present or subsequently develop bilateral Charcot foot. A weighted average of studies reporting bilateral involvement suggests 21% (range 9%–75%) of CN patients will present or subsequently develop Charcot foot [8–14]. Of those studies reporting subsequent development of CN, point estimates for bilateral involvement ranged from 2 to 3.3 years (range 1–6 years) after initial presentation. However, 21% of cases presented at baseline are with bilateral involvement [8, 10, 14]. This suggests a window of opportunity for the prevention of bilateral CN development. Certainly, a goal for identifying CN earlier is an important diagnostic pursuit, as well.

The role of thermometry in the detection of CN has been well described [8, 15, 16]. Armstrong and Lavery reported baseline infrared dermal thermometry results for 39 patients presenting with unilateral acute CN [15]. After 15 minutes' rest, they found an average 8.8 ± 2.3°F (~4.9 ± 1.3°C) difference in temperature compared to the contralateral joint of interest (JOI). In a separate study, the same team reported specific mean joint differences of 7.3°F (~4.1°C), 8.0°F (~4.4°C), and 8.8°F (~4.9°C) for the ankle Chopart and Lisfranc's joint, respectively [16]. Temperature differences correlate highly with radiographic changes [15] and with markers of bone turnover [17]. Offloading treatment should continue until temperature equilibration with the contralateral JOI [15] or within 2°C [18] is achieved. It is, however, unclear how temperature gradients changes are considered as a function of activity level. In this study, we examined temperature gradient changes of plantar temperature as a function of number of steps in patients with type 2 diabetes and peripheral neuropathy (DPN) including with and without acute CN.

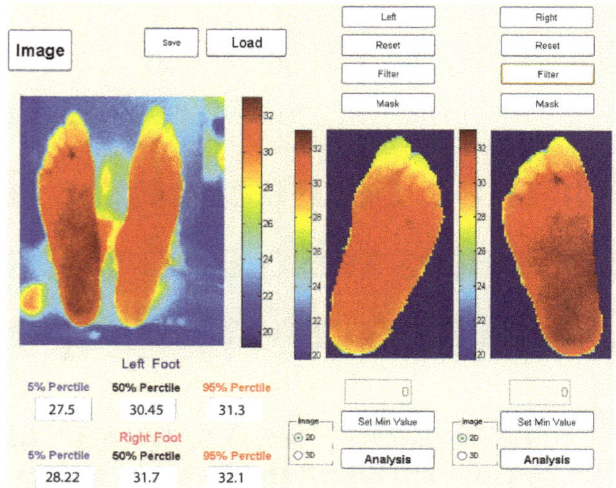

Figure 1: A purpose-designed image processing toolbox was developed using Matlab (version 7.4, The MathWorks, Inc., Natick, MA, USA), to isolate each foot from the thermal image and extract plantar temperature in three anatomical regions of foot including hind-, mid-, and forefoot.

2. Research Design and Methods

The study was conducted at a single academic medical center as part of a multinational collaborative study of lower extremity disease in diabetes. The study received ethical approval; participants were informed of the nature of the study and signed an informed consent form. Participants were included if they had type 2 diabetes diagnosed by their primary care physician and exhibited loss of protective sensation using 10-gram monofilament at 1–3 sites in the following locations: hallux, 1st, 3rd, and 5th metatarsal heads [19]. Patients with major foot amputation and inability to walk a distance of 100 m without assistance were excluded. The diagnosis of unilateral acute CN was made by a single clinician using previously described clinical criteria of swelling, redness, and local temperature gradient [20–22].

All participants walked for two predefined paths of 50 and 150 steps (total 200 steps). A validated wearable gait analysis technology (LEGSys, Biosensics LLC, MA, USA) [23–25] was used to assess gait and quantify the number of steps. All subjects were examined in prescribed footwear. In CN patients, this included nine with removable cast walkers, one with surgical sandal, and five with prescribed shoes. A thermal camera (Fluke Co., Model i25) was used to monitor plantar temperature at baseline after foot acclimatization and immediately after each walking trial. The subject was asked to sit in a podiatric examination chair with their legs parallel to the transverse plane and their shoes and socks removed for a 5-minute environment acclimatization period for baseline assessment. This was done to allow the subject's feet to equilibrate to room temperature. All subsequent thermal images (approximately at 50 steps and 200 steps) were taken with shoes and socks removed immediately after each walking trial. Due to the intermittent measurement at 50 steps, there was a slight delay (approximately 30 seconds) between continuation of the subsequent walking trial. We assumed that the change in plantar temperature is not rapid and thus this delay should have a negligible effect on assessing plantar temperature.

A custom image processing toolbox (Figure 1) was designed using MATLAB version 7.4 (R2007z) (The MathWorks, Inc., Natick, MA, USA), to automatically isolate each foot from the thermal image using an edge detection algorithm. The toolbox also afforded manual enhancement and noise removal prior to the analysis. This is critical to accurately identify inflammatory hot spots and measure dynamic changes in plantar temperature. Using an automated masking algorithm, plantar temperature changes were measured in three independent anatomical regions (hind/mid/fore-foot). We estimated the 5th, 50th, and 95th temperature percentiles at each region. For the purpose of this study, only the 95th percentile value representing a hot spot was reported.

Paired sample Student's t-test was used to examine intra-subject PT differences between feet. A two-sample Student's t-test assuming equal variance was used between groups. ANOVA test (N-way analysis of variance) with linear model was used to examine the dependency of PT change on footwear type, gender, age, and active diabetic foot ulcer (DFU). Statistical significance was set at 0.05.

3. Results

Thirty-two eligible subjects (age: 56.6 ± 8.6 years, BMI = 30.3 ± 4.9 Kg/m^2, 87% male) were recruited. Fifteen subjects were diagnosed with CN and 17 as non-CN. Eight CN and nine non-CN participants had DFU. Nine CN participants wore casts, one sandal, and five wore prescribed shoes. Eight non-CN participants wore their habitual shoes, six wore prescription shoes, and three wore surgical sandals. At baseline, CN demonstrated a significant 1.84 ± 1.3°C

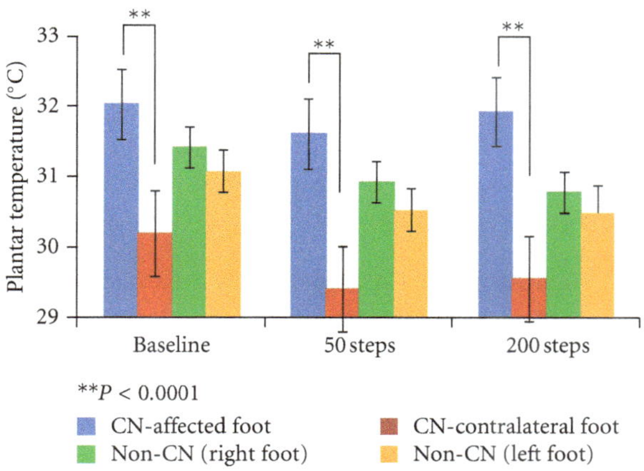

FIGURE 2: Plantar temperature in hot spot recognized in the midfoot region.

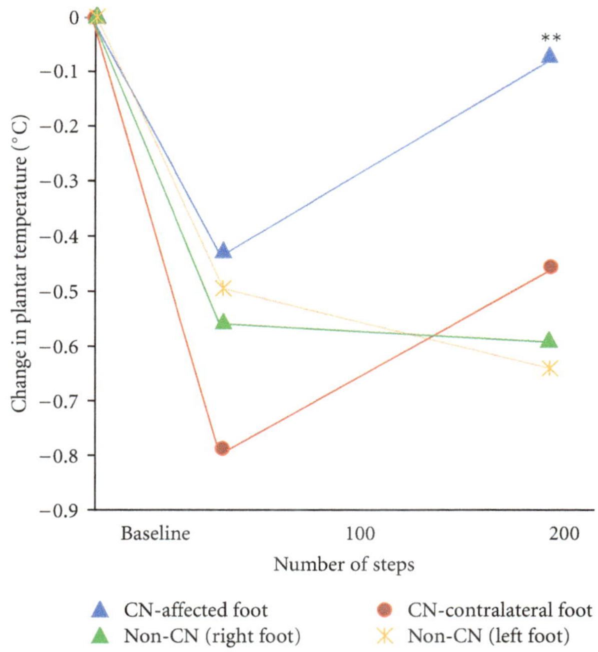

FIGURE 3: Change in plantar temperature as a function of walking steps for the hot spots recognized in the midfoot region.

difference ($P < 0.0001$) between the feet at JOI and for all plantar regions (Figure 2). No significant difference was observed in non-CN ($P > 0.3$). Upon activity initiation, plantar temperature was reduced in all participants, but the drop for nonaffected foot as well as non-CN was significantly lower by a factor of 1.9 than the affected side ($P = 0.04$). Interestingly, plantar temperature in CN was sharply increased by prolong walking beyond of 50 steps with slope of 0.25 deg/100 steps for both feet, while no difference was observed in non-CN between 50 and 200 steps ($P > 0.5$, Figure 3). At 200 steps, plantar temperature on the CN side was still higher than the contralateral foot and non-CN ($P < 0.0001$).

Multivariable analysis suggested PT asymmetry measured at baseline as well as after each walking trial is independent of DFU, gender, age, and type of footwear ($P > 0.1$) but significantly dependent on presence of CN ($P < 0.0001$). Using PT gradient criteria based on the JOI, the effect size between CN and non-CN group was increased by 61% at 50 steps compared to baseline ($d = 1.20$ and $r = 0.52$ at baseline versus $d = 1.94$ and $r = 0.70$ at 50 steps).

4. Discussion

The current study reports a simple objective method to characterize asymmetry in plantar temperature as a function of graduated walking activity. This technique characterizes the PT hot spot (95th percentile) at each plantar region instead of manual comparison of plantar temperature between two feet.

We found that all participants experienced initial temperature decrease in both feet after 50 steps. But the slope of PT cooling to baseline was significantly slower in the affected foot. Consequently, the temperature difference between CN affected and contralateral foot is magnified after walking 50 steps ($d = 1.20$ and $r = 0.52$ at baseline versus $d = 1.94$ and $r = 0.70$ at 50 steps).

The initial drop in plantar temperature in early-walking steps may be due to regulation of microvascular flow in response to cyclic loading and relaxation. Silver-Thorn [26] by applying a cyclic loading and unloading to human healthy tissue demonstrated that skin perfusion is initially increased in response to early loading and dropped with further increases in pressure or prolong loading till reaching to a steady-state level (first pulse response). Then, again it is increased followed by decreasing to the initial value in response to unloading (second pulse response or hyperemia response), whereas little to no tissue reperfusion was observed during prolong relaxation period without cyclic stress. Therefore, cyclic activities like walking may actually increase the cumulative plantar skin perfusion as a function of time (or time integral) compared to prolong relaxing (e.g., sitting, lying, and offloading) or prolong loading (e.g., standing) conditions. Thus, this skin perfusion regulation in response to cyclic stress may explain the initial drop in plantar temperature in early steps compared to baseline (relaxation) for healthy skin when other factors contributing to increase in skin temperature (e.g., friction, metabolic cost, etc.) are still negligible. Considering that the most of walking episodes are short (often less than 50 steps per episode) [27], this regulation mechanism is of key importance in regulating foot temperature during activity of daily living. A failure in the above-explained skin perfusion regulation in response to cyclic plantar stress may explain the lack of drop in temperature in the CN-affected foot.

In non-CN, the temperature remained the same after continued activity from 50 steps up to 200 steps, but temperature was lower relative to the temperature at baseline. In CN, there was, however, a significant increase in temperature at 200 steps compared to 50, significantly higher than temperature difference between 50 and 200 steps in non-CN. These interesting findings merit further study as a potential stress test for prediction of unilateral or bilateral CN and subsequent ulcer development.

The sharp increase in plantar temperature in CN group after continued activity beyond 50 steps could be explained by a complex interplay between local metabolic status [28, 29], propensity for an ill-defined inflammatory overreaction [5, 29], perfusion status [30], the physical state of plantar tissue, and limited joint mobility which may increase skin friction or metabolic cost. There could be an empiric support for these findings from Johnson, who reported a sharp increase in plantar temperature in Charcot patients and postulated that it could be explained by hyperemia in Charcot foot [31]. According to Boulton et al., "It has been theorized that the site of pathology was within the arteriovenous shunts, which normally are under control of the sympathetic system. Loss of this function will result in blood being routed rapidly to the venous side of the capillary bed, increasing the local pO2, thereby decreasing the distal perfusion to the cells" [32]. These results also support that modulating duration of continuous steps and/or prolong standing during daily activity could be helpful for reducing the trauma in patients with CN or DFU [27, 33–35].

The temperature differences in our study differ from others at baseline [15, 16]. This could be due to the duration of acclimatization, use of a thermal imager as opposed to an infrared dermal thermometer, and aggregation of temperature into regions of the foot as opposed to manual point testing. Additionally, we have eliminated any bias towards absolute temperature measurements by using the 95th percentile values.

This study has few limitations. First, we were not able to control the stage of Charcot foot development. It is likely that some patients were in a coalescence phase. The magnitude of the differences between groups merit further investigation in stages 0 and 1 patients. It is entirely plausible that these patients are likely to have a higher thermal gradient. Second, we did not standardize the offloading footwear and, while our population was easily robust enough to assess temperature gradient, it was not sufficiently powered to perform a stratified analysis by stage and offloading footwear type. Third, due to limitations in technology, a short delay was required for assessing plantar temperature after each walking path. However, since the change in plantar temperature is not rapid, we assumed that the effect of this delay (approximately 30 seconds) for assessing change in plantar temperature as a function of walking is negligible. Another study should be addressed to validate this hypothesis.

The observed differential thermal response to walking initiation between Charcot and non-Charcot feet warrants future investigation to provide further insight into the correlation between activity dosing and thermal response. It may also lend valuable insight into identifying an "inflammatory trigger" that may ultimately provide an early-warning sign [36] or increased sensitivity for subsequent unilateral or bilateral CN development or clinical expression of foot ulcer. The importance of improved sensitivity and earlier diagnoses of CN was recently described by Wukich and colleagues. In their retrospective review of 22 CN patients, they emphasized the importance of identifying and aggressively treating stage 0 patients [6]. This was defined as patients with diabetes-related sensory neuropathy presenting following foot and ankle insult with local swelling, redness, and warmth and radiographic signs absent for fracture and normal alignment [37, 38]. The group that was identified and treated for 4 weeks developed significantly less complications (14%) versus the group that was identified and treated after 8 weeks (67%) [6].

In conclusion, the variability in thermal response to the initiation of walking between Charcot and non-Charcot feet warrants future investigation to potentially provide further insight into the correlation between thermal response and ulcer/Charcot development.

Authors' Contribution

B. Najafi researched data, wrote the paper, reviewed/edited the paper, contributed to discussion; G. Grewal recruited the subjects and analyzed the data. R. Menzies and T. Talal screened and recruited patients and, assisted in data collection, and contributed to discussion. M. Zirie contributed in discussion, J. Wrobel reviewed/edited researched data, wrote the paper, reviewed/edited the paper; contributed to discussion and D. G. Armstrong researched data, reviewed/edited the paper, and contributed to discussion.

Conflict of Interests

The authors declared no conflict of interests.

Acknowledgments

This study was supported by a Grant from the Qatar National Research Foundation (Award No. NPRP08-499-3-109). The content is solely the responsibility of the authors and does not necessarily represent the official views of the Qatar National Research Foundation. The authors would like to thank Dr. Manish Bharara for reviewing, editing and contributing to the discussion and interpretation of results.

References

[1] A. Gazis, N. Pound, R. Macfarlane, K. Treece, F. Game, and W. Jeffcoate, "Mortality in patients with diabetic neuropathic osteoarthropathy (Charcot foot)," *Diabetic Medicine*, vol. 21, no. 11, pp. 1243–1246, 2004.

[2] M. W. Sohn, T. A. Lee, R. M. Stuck, R. G. Frykberg, and E. Budiman-Mak, "Mortality risk of charcot arthropathy compared with that of diabetic foot ulcer and diabetes alone," *Diabetes Care*, vol. 32, no. 5, pp. 816–821, 2009.

[3] M. W. Sohn, R. M. Stuck, M. Pinzur, T. A. Lee, and E. Budiman-Mak, "Lower-extremity amputation risk after charcot arthropathy and diabetic foot ulcer," *Diabetes Care*, vol. 33, no. 1, pp. 98–100, 2010.

[4] L. C. Rogers, R. G. Frykberg, D. G. Armstrong et al., "The charcot foot in diabetes," *Diabetes Care*, vol. 34, no. 9, pp. 2123–2129, 2011.

[5] W. Jeffcoate, "The causes of the charcot syndrome," *Clinics in Podiatric Medicine and Surgery*, vol. 25, no. 1, pp. 29–42, 2008.

[6] D. K. Wukich, W. Sung, S. A. M. Wipf, and D. G. Armstrong, "The consequences of complacency: managing the effects of unrecognized charcot feet," *Diabetic Medicine*, vol. 28, no. 2, pp. 195–198, 2011.

[7] T. K. Pakarinen, H. J. Laine, S. E. Honkonen, J. Peltonen, H. Oksala, and J. Lahtela, "Charcot arthropathy of the diabetic foot. Current concepts and review of 36 cases," *Scandinavian Journal of Surgery*, vol. 91, no. 2, pp. 195–201, 2002.

[8] D. G. Armstrong, W. F. Todd, L. A. Lavery, L. B. Harkless, and T. R. Bushman, "The natural history of acute Charcot's arthropathy in a diabetic foot specialty clinic," *Diabetic Medicine*, vol. 14, no. 5, pp. 357–363, 1997.

[9] D. R. Clohisy and R. C. Thompson Jr., "Fractures associated with neuropathic arthropathy in adults who have juvenile-onset diabetes," *Journal of Bone and Joint Surgery A*, vol. 70, no. 8, pp. 1192–1200, 1988.

[10] J. Fabrin, K. Larsen, and P. E. Holstein, "Long-term follow-up in diabetic charcot feet with spontaneous onset," *Diabetes Care*, vol. 23, no. 6, pp. 796–800, 2000.

[11] S. A. Herbst, K. B. Jones, and C. L. Saltzman, "Pattern of diabetic neuropathic arthropathy associated with the peripheral bone mineral density," *Journal of Bone and Joint Surgery B*, vol. 86, no. 3, pp. 378–383, 2004.

[12] M. S. Myerson, M. R. Henderson, T. Saxby, and K. W. Short, "Management of midfoot diabetic neuroarthropathy," *Foot and Ankle International*, vol. 15, no. 5, pp. 233–241, 1994.

[13] S. Sinha, C. S. Munichoodappa, and G. P. Kozak, "Neuro-arthropathy (Charcot joints) in diabetes mellitus (clinical study of 101 cases)," *Medicine*, vol. 51, no. 3, pp. 191–210, 1972.

[14] H. B. Leung, Y. C. Ho, and W. C. Wong, "Charcot foot in a Hong Kong Chinese diabetic population," *Hong Kong Medical Journal*, vol. 15, no. 3, pp. 191–195, 2009.

[15] D. G. Armstrong and L. A. Lavery, "Monitoring healing of acute Charcot's arthropathy with infrared dermal thermometry," *Journal of Rehabilitation Research and Development*, vol. 34, no. 3, pp. 317–321, 1997.

[16] D. G. Armstrong, L. A. Lavery, P. J. Liswood, W. F. Todd, and J. A. Tredwell, "Infrared dermal thermometry for the high-risk diabetic foot," *Physical Therapy*, vol. 77, no. 2, pp. 169–177, 1997.

[17] R. Bem, A. Jirkovská, M. Dubský et al., "Role of quantitative bone scanning in the assessment of bone turnover in patients with Charcot foot," *Diabetes Care*, vol. 33, no. 2, pp. 348–349, 2010.

[18] N. L. Petrova and M. E. Edmonds, "Charcot neuro-osteoarthropathy—current standards," *Diabetes/Metabolism Research and Reviews*, vol. 24, supplement 1, pp. S58–S61, 2008.

[19] A. J. Boulton, D. G. Armstrong, S. F. Albert et al., "Comprehensive foot examination and risk assessment: a report of the task force of the foot care interest group of the American Diabetes Association, with endorsement by the American Association of Clinical Endocrinologists," *Diabetes Care*, vol. 31, no. 8, pp. 1679–1685, 2008.

[20] D. K. Wukich and W. Sung, "Charcot arthropathy of the foot and ankle: modern concepts and management review," *Journal of Diabetes and Its Complications*, vol. 23, no. 6, pp. 409–426, 2009.

[21] D. K. Wukich, W. Sung, S. A. M. Wipf, and D. G. Armstrong, "The consequences of complacency: managing the effects of unrecognized Charcot feet," *Diabetic Medicine*, vol. 28, no. 2, pp. 195–198, 2011.

[22] D. G. Armstrong and E. J. Peters, "Charcot's arthropathy of the foot," *Journal of the American Podiatric Medical Association*, vol. 92, no. 7, pp. 390–394, 2002.

[23] B. Najafi, J. L. Helbostad, R. Moe-Nilssen, W. Zijlstra, and K. Aminian, "Does walking strategy in older people change as a function of walking distance?" *Gait and Posture*, vol. 29, no. 2, pp. 261–266, 2009.

[24] B. Najafi, T. Khan, and J. Wrobel, "Laboratory in a box: wearable sensors and its advantages for gait analysis," in *Proceedings of the IEEE Engineering in Medicine & Biology Society*, vol. 2011, pp. 6507–6510, August 2011.

[25] K. Aminian, B. Najafi, C. Büla, P. F. Leyvraz, and P. Robert, "Spatio-temporal parameters of gait measured by an ambulatory system using miniature gyroscopes," *Journal of Biomechanics*, vol. 35, no. 5, pp. 689–699, 2002.

[26] M. B. Silver-Thorn, "Investigation of lower-limb tissue perfusion during loading," *Journal of Rehabilitation Research and Development*, vol. 39, no. 5, pp. 597–608, 2002.

[27] B. Najafi, R. T. Crews, and J. S. Wrobel, "The importance of time spent standing for those at risk of diabetic foot ulceration," *Diabetes Care*, vol. 33, no. 11, pp. 2448–2450, 2010.

[28] R. G. Frykberg and R. Belczyk, "Epidemiology of the Charcot foot," *Clinics in Podiatric Medicine and Surgery*, vol. 25, no. 1, pp. 17–28, 2008.

[29] W. J. Jeffcoate, F. Game, and P. R. Cavanagh, "The role of proinflammatory cytokines in the cause of neuropathic osteoarthropathy (acute Charcot foot) in diabetes," *The Lancet*, vol. 366, no. 9502, pp. 2058–2061, 2005.

[30] S. A. Shapiro, K. B. Stansberry, M. A. Hill et al., "Normal blood flow response and vasomotion in the diabetic Charcot foot," *Journal of Diabetes and Its Complications*, vol. 12, no. 3, pp. 147–153, 1998.

[31] J. T. Johnson, "Neuropathic fractures and joint injuries. Pathogenesis and rationale of prevention and treatment," *Journal of Bone and Joint Surgery A*, vol. 49, no. 1, pp. 1–30, 1967.

[32] A. J. M. Boulton, J. H. B. Scarpello, and J. D. Ward, "Venous oxygenation in the diabetic neuropathic foot: evidence of arteriovenous shunting?" *Diabetologia*, vol. 22, no. 1, pp. 6–8, 1982.

[33] D. G. Armstrong and A. J. M. Boulton, "Activity monitors: should we begin dosing activity as we dose a drug?" *Journal of the American Podiatric Medical Association*, vol. 91, no. 3, pp. 152–153, 2001.

[34] B. Najafi, R. T. Crews, and J. S. Wrobel, "Incorporating standing time into physical activity assessment of patients at risk of diabetic foot ulceration," in *Proceedings of the 70th American Diabetes Association Scientific Sessions (ADA '10)*, Orlando, Fla, USA, June, 2010.

[35] J. S. Wrobel and B. Najafi, "Diabetic foot biomechanics and gait dysfunction," *Journal of Diabetes Science and Technology*, vol. 4, no. 4, pp. 833–845, 2010.

[36] D. K. Wukich, W. Sung, S. A. M. Wipf, and D. G. Armstrong, "The consequences of complacency: managing the effects of unrecognized Charcot feet," *Diabetic Medicine*, vol. 28, no. 2, pp. 195–198, 2011.

[37] G. V. Yu and J. R. Hudson, "Evaluation and treatment of stage 0 Charcot's neuroarthropathy of the foot and ankle," *Journal of the American Podiatric Medical Association*, vol. 92, no. 4, pp. 210–220, 2002.

[38] T. Shibata, K. Tada, and C. Hashizume, "The results of athrodesis of the ankle for leprotic neuroarthropathy," *Journal of Bone and Joint Surgery A*, vol. 72, no. 5, pp. 749–756, 1990.

2

Impact of Endothelial Microparticles on Coagulation, Inflammation, and Angiogenesis in Age-Related Vascular Diseases

Margaret Markiewicz,[1] Erin Richard,[2] Natalia Marks,[3] and Anna Ludwicka-Bradley[1]

[1] *Division of Rheumatology and Immunology, Medical University of South Carolina, 114 Doughty Street, STB, Charleston, SC 29425, USA*
[2] *Department of Biology, College of Charleston, Rita Liddy Hollings Science Center, Charleston, SC 29424, USA*
[3] *Department of Radiology, Maimonides Medical Center, Brooklyn, NY 11219, USA*

Correspondence should be addressed to Margaret Markiewicz; markiewi@musc.edu

Academic Editor: Barbara Shukitt-Hale

Endothelial microparticles (EMPs) are complex vesicular structures that originate from plasma membranes of activated or apoptotic endothelial cells. EMPs play a significant role in vascular function by altering the processes of inflammation, coagulation, and angiogenesis, and they are key players in the pathogenesis of several vascular diseases. Circulating EMPs are increased in many age-related vascular diseases such as coronary artery disease, peripheral vascular disease, cerebral ischemia, and congestive heart failure. Their elevation in plasma has been considered as both a biomarker and bioactive effector of vascular damage and a target for vascular diseases. This review focuses on the pleiotropic roles of EMPs and the mechanisms that trigger their formation, particularly the involvement of decreased estrogen levels, thrombin, and PAI-1 as major factors that induce EMPs in age-related vascular diseases.

1. Introduction

Vascular diseases are among the most common causes of morbidity and mortality, and both number and severity of morbid vascular conditions increase with age. Regulations of angiogenesis, coagulation, and inflammation are very important issues in vascular biology, both in normal physiology and pathology [1]. It is now well established that disruption of endothelial integrity represents a crucial event in the initiation and development of cardiovascular (CV) diseases. Numerous studies have reported that microparticles (MPs) play an important role in endothelial dysfunction. Endothelial dysfunction occurs when a perturbed homeostatic endothelium disrupts vascular competency resulting in reduced vasodilatation and increased proinflammatory and prothrombotic properties of the vascular network [2]. Recently, MPs originating from various cells have been found to be associated with several vascular related diseases. Moreover, exposed procoagulant phospholipids and specific receptors at the surface of MPs act as biomessengers linking inflammation, coagulation, and angiogenesis [3–5].

Although MPs were first described as "cellular debris" that are believed to have no biological significance, recent studies documented that MPs of endothelial and other origins are biological effectors in inflammation, vascular injury, angiogenesis, and thrombosis [6–8]. MPs isolated from granulation tissue are derived from endothelial cells, monocytes, platelets, erythrocytes [9–13], and myofibroblasts [8]. They exchange biological signals and information intercellularly and each kind of MP carries the antigens and receptors of the cells they originated. MPs may transfer part of their components and content to the selected target cells, thus mediating cell activation, phenotypic modification, and reprogramming of cell function [14]. Although 70% to 90% of all circulating MPs in the peripheral blood of healthy individuals are derived from platelets [15], marked elevations of all kinds of MPs have been observed in many vascular diseases. Specifically, endothelium-derived microparticles (EMPs) represent a relatively small (5–15%) but very important subset of all circulating microparticles [16–18]. This number may vary in different cardiovascular and inflammatory diseases [18, 19]. New insights into endothelial dysfunction and alterations in angiogenesis are emerging from studies of vascular microparticles, particularly endothelial microparticles in elderly populations.

Age-related CV diseases are considered a major concern for the elderly. Vascular aging with impairment of endothelial cell function leads to altered angiogenesis, a key factor in the etiology of various cardiovascular disorders. 73% of individuals aged 60–79 have a CV disease, including stroke, hypertension, or heart failure, and at >79 years of age prevalence of these diseases increased to 86% in females and 82% in males (2012 NHLBI Fact Book) [20]. Recently published data have shown that these diseases are the leading cause of death for individuals aged >65 [21] and morbidity increased from 32% for individuals aged 66 to 48% for individuals aged 85. An important factor which significantly decreases the incidence of coronary heart diseases in postmenopausal women is estrogen [22–24]. In women already having coronary artery disease or ischemic stroke, the therapeutic benefit of estrogen is not clear [25, 26] although it has been reported that estrogen induces rapid vasodilation, exerts anti-inflammatory activity, and regulates vascular cell growth, migration, and protection of cardiomyocytes from injury [27], all of which prevent atherosclerotic deterioration in vessels. This review focuses on the role of EMPs in angiogenesis, coagulation, and inflammation during age-related vascular diseases and the contribution of estrogen to these diseases.

2. Endothelial Microparticles and Factors That Stimulate Their Formation and Release

EMPs are small vesicles that are released from endothelial cells and can be found circulating in the blood. Defined by their small size (0.1 to 1.0 μm), they are a heterogeneous population of vesicles which are shed from plasma membranes in response to cell activation, injury, angiogenesis/neovascularization, and/or apoptosis. EMPs consist of a small amount of cytosol surrounded by a plasma membrane and display negatively charged phospholipids on their surface that can initiate and accelerate coagulation [28]. Circulating EMPs have been demonstrated as a marker of preeclampsia [29, 30], acute coronary syndromes [31], and severe hypertension [30, 32, 33] suggesting their association with pathological processes within the endothelium [34]. Furthermore, circulating EMP levels are also implicated in the progression of atherosclerotic lesions, heart failure, arrhythmias, inflammatory vascular disease, sickle anemia, and endotoxemia [35].

EMPs can display differing characteristics that are reflective of specific thrombotic and inflammatory conditions [36]. Jimenez et al. demonstrated that the surface antigens of EMPs are distinctive depending on the type of endothelial cell injury, as in apoptosis *versus* activation. High levels of the surface antigens E-selectin, intracellular adhesion molecule-1 (ICAM-1), and vascular cell adhesion molecule-1 (VCAM-1) are on EMPs derived from activated endothelial cells. In contrast, the low levels of these antigens are on EMPs derived from apoptotic endothelial cells. Platelet cell adhesion molecule (PECAM-1), endoglin, and vascular endothelial-cadherin (VE-cadherin) are at low levels on EMPs derived from activated ECs [37–40] (Figure 1). Additionally, EMPs generated from apoptotic endothelial cells have higher levels of phosphatidylserine on their surface and different phospholipid composition and oxidation status compared with EMPs generated from activated endothelial cells [41, 42]. These data suggest that there are distinct mechanisms for the formation of EMPs in apoptotic and activated cells [43] and several studies suggest that these types of EMPs have different functions in vascular diseases [40, 44].

Both inflammatory cytokines and coagulation factors participate in the generation of EMPs (Figure 2).

Recently, it has been shown that p38 mitogen-activated protein kinase (MAPK) is a critical molecule in the production of proinflammatory EMPs and increased ICAM-1 production by endothelial cells, providing a paracrine loop to enhance the endothelial response to inflammation [46]. *In vitro* studies have shown that the proinflammatory agent, TNFα, activates endothelial cells and induces release of EMPs [47] (Figure 2). Another potent stimulus for EMP formation both *in vivo* and *in vitro* is angiotensin II (Ang II) [3]. This effect is mediated by Ang II receptor type I that signals through NADPH oxidase and Rho kinase. Furthermore, in Ang II-infused apoliprotein E (ApoE −/−) hyperlipidemic mice, a model of significant endothelial dysfunction, Ang II has been shown to increase EMP formation by a redox-sensitive and blood-pressure-independent process [2].

Another important factor PAI-1 (plasminogen activator inhibitor type 1) plays an important role in the formation of EMPs. It has been shown by Brodsky et al. that PAI-1 promotes formation of EMPs with reduced transmembrane asymmetry of phospholipids in a dose dependent manner. This occurrence may be responsible for the observed increase in *in vitro* thrombin generation. These findings could possibly link elevated levels of PAI-1 with endothelial dysfunction and tendency toward thrombosis [48–50]. Increased levels of PAI-1 might serve as an initiator of EMP formation followed by increased procoagulant activity and thrombin generation [50]. In addition, it is also known that thrombin stimulates PAI-1 synthesis [51] suggesting constant production of these two factors. All these data indicate that formation of EMPs links together inflammation, coagulation, and angiogenesis and causes the impairment of the last two phenomena (Figure 3).

Among many signaling molecules, T-cadherin (T-cad) on the surface of ECs might be upregulated and may serve as a characteristic marker of EC activation and stress. Recently, Philippova et al. have demonstrated a mechanism of T-cad-dependent signaling in the vascular endothelium. The authors identified that T-cadherin levels in plasma are increased in early atherosclerosis and correlate with endothelial dysfunction, which may lead to increased release of EMPs from ECs [52].

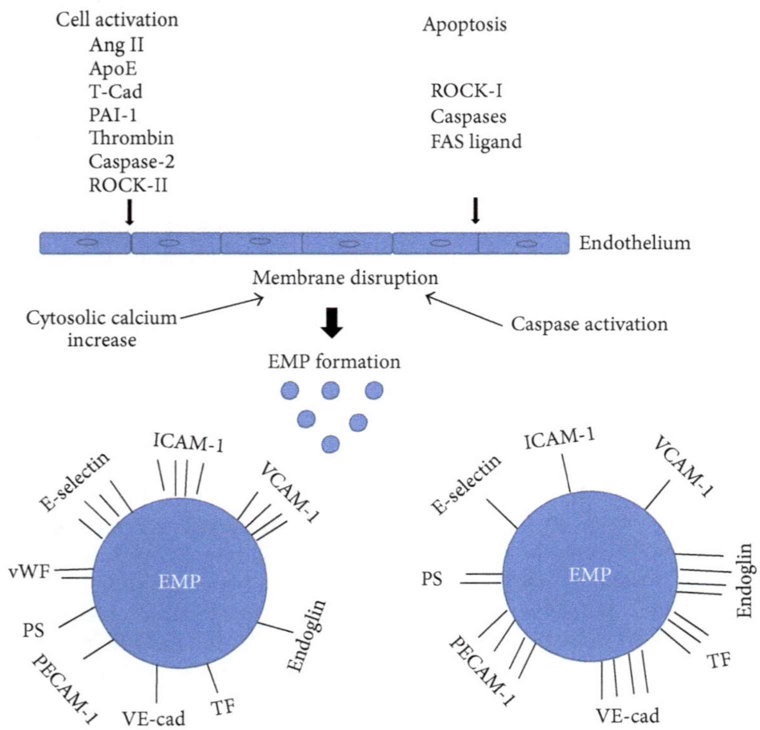

FIGURE 1: Differences in antigen expression of EMPs derived from activation versus apoptosis of endothelial cells. Endothelial cell activators, angiotensin II (Ang II), apoliprotein E (ApoE), T-cadherin (T-Cad), plasminogen activator inhibitor-1 (PAI-1), and thrombin, cause cytosolic calcium increase which leads to endothelial cell membrane disruption. Caspase-2 activates ROCK-II independently of cell death [45]. Apoptosis inducers including Rho activated kinase (ROCK-I), caspases, and FAS ligand activate caspases and cause membrane disruption in endothelial cells. Both activators of cell activation and apoptosis lead to vesiculation and EMP generation. Bars represent level of antigen on the surface of the EMP. 4 bars: high level of antigen; 1 bar: low level of antigen. EMP antigens: E-selectin, intracellular adhesion molecule-1 (ICAM-1), vascular cell adhesion molecule-1 (VCAM-1), platelet cell adhesion molecule-1 (PECAM-1), endoglin, vascular endothelial-cadherin (VE-cadherin), tissue factor (TF), phospholipid (PS), and von Willebrand factor (vWf). This figure was prepared based on [13, 37–40, 42, 45].

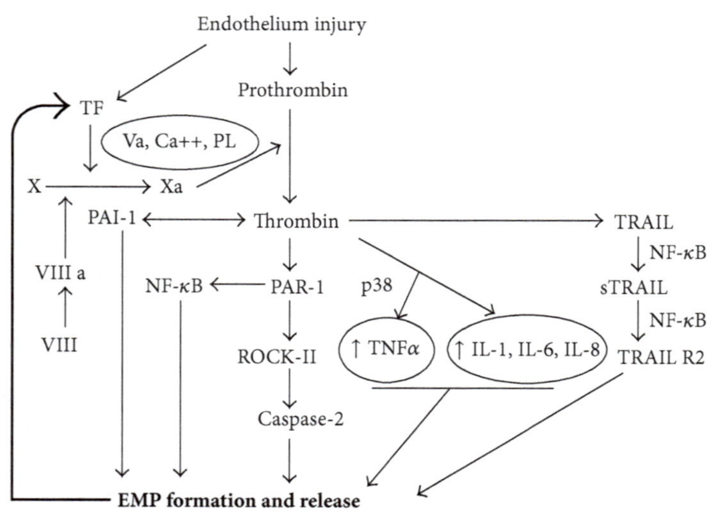

FIGURE 2: Signaling pathways involved in thrombin induced EMP formation. EMPs carry TF, the main initiator of the extrinsic pathway of the coagulation cascade. Cofactor VIIIa known as a von Willebrand factor activates factor X to Xa in the presence of factor Va, calcium, and phospholipids (PL), which results in the generation of thrombin. Thrombin induces tumor necrosis factor alpha (TNFα) via p38 (mitogen activated protein kinase) and interleukins 1, 6, and 8 (Il-1, IL-6, and IL-8), which both lead to formation of EMPs. Thrombin, via proteolytically activated receptor-1 (PAR-1), induces nuclear factor kappa B (NF-κB), which directly induces EMP formation. PAR-1 also induces Rho kinase (ROCK- II) which activates caspase-2 leading to EMPs formation. Thrombin via (tumor necrosis factor related apoptosis inducing ligand) TRAIL activates sTRAIL, which is synthesized to TRAIL R2. This process requires the activation of NF-κB.

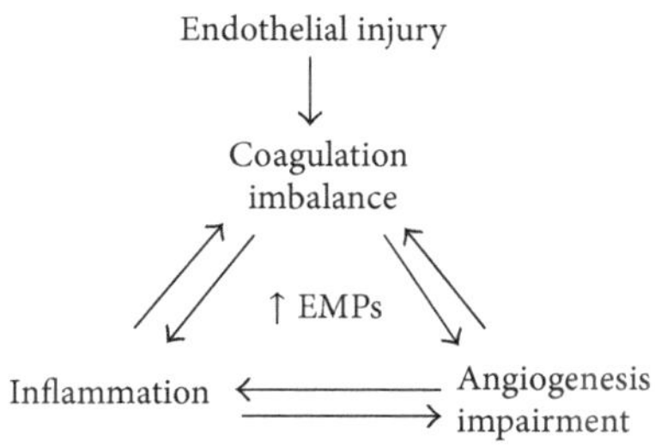

FIGURE 3: EMPs link inflammation, coagulation, and angiogenesis.

3. Endothelial Microparticles in Coagulation and Vascular Aging

Increasing evidence has also accumulated to implicate an impaired coagulation system in many vascular diseases. This coagulation imbalance is the net result of activation of coagulation, impaired activity of natural coagulation inhibitors, and suppressed fibrinolysis [53]. Activation of coagulation proteases, for example, thrombin, is one of the earliest events following tissue injury [54]. Thrombin modulates tissue repair responses by altering vascular permeability, stimulating endothelial cell, fibroblast, and neutrophil migration, and promoting their spreading and adhesion [55]. It activates various cell types and induces secretion of several proimmune, profibrotic, and proinflammatory factors [45, 56, 57]. Additionally, thrombin induces generation of EMPs. Recent studies by Sapet et al. have shown that release of EMPs by endothelial cells in response to thrombin involves a group of genes that regulate angiogenesis and are linked to the cytoskeleton reorganization family. Among these genes, Rho-kinase ROCK-II was transcribed at a high rate and was identified as a target of thrombin in EMP generation [58]. The involvement of caspase-2 in ROCK-II activation, independent of cell death, points out a novel signaling pathway that emphasizes the proteolytic activity of caspase in EMP generation in response to cell activation [58] (Figure 1). However, further studies are needed to determine the molecular mechanisms involved in EMP release. EMP release is initiated when thrombin binds to its receptor, proteolytically activated receptor-1 (PAR-1), which induces gene transcription that is mediated by thrombin via TRAIL/Apo2L, a cytokine belonging to the tumor necrosis factor alpha (TNFα) superfamily. This mechanism of EMP generation depends on the nuclear factor (NF) κB activation and involves the soluble form of TRAIL, which is secreted by the endothelial cells under thrombin or inflammatory stimulation [4, 59] (Figure 2).

Phospholipids expressed on EMPs bind coagulation factors leading to a prothrombotic state [60] and an increase in procoagulant activity of tissue factor (TF). These phospholipids are exposed on the outer membrane of MP and are considered to be the main initiators of the coagulation cascade [28]. Additionally, it has been demonstrated that sphingosine 1-phosphate (S1P) strongly potentiates thrombin-induced TF expression in ECs suggesting its role in blood coagulation [61]. S1P has also been shown to be involved in the process of angiogenesis and inflammation [62–64]. Another important role of MPs is their contribution to the development of platelet- and fibrin-rich thrombi at sites of vascular injury via the recruitment of cells and the accumulation of TF. Data suggest that EMP-mediated coagulation has clinical significance; for example, an association between the number of circulating MPs and the risk of thrombolytic complication has been reported [19]. Because EMPs interact with coagulation proteins and with inflammatory or vascular cells, their role in cardiovascular diseases has been intensively studied. It has also been observed by Jy et al. that EMPs carry von Willebrand factor (vWf) and factor VIII that promote platelet aggregates and increase their stability [65] (Figure 1). Moreover, the authors postulated that EMPs released during vascular injury may arrest bleeding by rapid interaction with platelets via membrane-associated vWf multimers and adhesions to stabilized platelet aggregates in the microenvironment. Sabatier demonstrated that EMPs also carry TF and bind to monocytes causing further TF expression and resulting in enhanced transmigration of monocytes through endothelial junction [66, 67].

One of the important key genes for aging-associated cardiovascular disorders is plasminogen activator inhibitor-1 (PAI-1), a main inhibitor of fibrinolysis. The expression of PAI-1 is not only elevated in the elderly but also significantly induced in a variety of pathologies associated with the process of aging [68]. Increased levels of PAI-1 and its procoagulant activity have been recognized as hallmarks of endothelial dysfunction in vascular aging (Figure 4). Furthermore, elevated levels of PAI-1 were found in Werner syndrome, a disease characterized by premature aging [68, 69] and atherosclerosis, which in advanced stages may lead to myocardial infarction and death. Recently, it has been shown that EMPs expressing both activators and inhibitors of coagulation have fibrinolytic properties that counteract their procoagulant activities, which may enable them to contribute to haemostatic balance [70]. It has been observed that endothelial and leukocyte microparticles generate fibrinolytic activity, whereas erythrocyte and platelet microparticles do not have this property. Additionally, different plasminogen activators were identified on leukocyte microparticles, urokinase-type plasminogen activator (uPA), and EMPs where tissue plasminogen activator (tPA) has been found. The authors provide evidence that microparticles with plasminogen activators are rare in healthy populations but are observed more frequently in pathological conditions [70] suggesting that plasmin generation on microparticles may be important in the modulation of hemostatic balance. Therefore, complex functions of EMPs have an ambivalent role both in physiological and pathological conditions, either promoting or inhibiting coagulation, inflammation, or angiogenesis. However, the precise mechanism has not yet been explored.

4. Endothelial Microparticles in Inflammation

There is increasing evidence that inflammation is a potent activator of coagulation pathways. Inflammatory mediators increase several procoagulant factors, inhibit endogenous anticoagulants, and attenuate the fibrinolytic response [71].

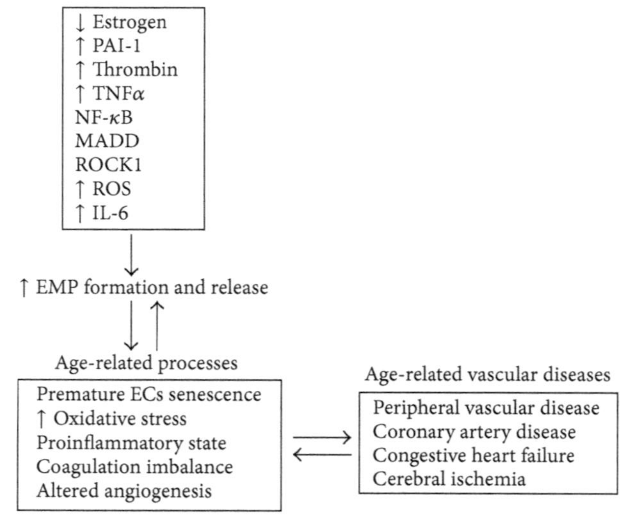

Figure 4: Factors contributing to EMP formation in age-related vascular diseases.

However, the interaction between these two systems is bidirectional, as coagulation is also capable of modulating inflammatory activity. Thrombin mediated inflammatory molecules such as IL-8 and IL-1Ra and IL-1 participate in EMP release [4, 59] (Figure 2) and are key factors involved in coagulation, inflammation, and angiogenesis. Inflammation and coagulation are linked processes in many diseases and EMPs may amplify the responses by activating the endothelium. It has been reported that in addition to activation of D-dimers and C-reactive proteins in coagulation, the inflammatory cytokine IL-6 is associated with mortality, declines in all measures of function, and leads to the frailty phenotype in the elderly [72]. Recently, it has been shown that increased levels of IL-6 are present in aged aortas and that aging induces a proinflammatory phenotype in vascular smooth muscle cells (VSMC) due in part to increased signaling of toll-like receptor 4 (TLR4) and its signaling adaptor MYD 88 [73]. These observations support the notion of a high prevalence of proinflammatory conditions in advanced age. All of these factors lead to increased generation of EMPs and impaired coagulation, inflammation, and angiogenesis in CV diseases (Figures 3 and 4).

5. Endothelial Microparticles and Their Effect on Vascular Function in the Elderly

The process of angiogenesis is complex and requires endothelial cells (ECs) to detach from pericytes and the extracellular matrix (ECM), proliferate, invade the surrounding tissues, migrate, and differentiate to form capillary tubes that connect to newly developed vascular networks leading to vascular stabilization [74–76]. Defective angiogenesis has been found in many vascular diseases and it has been established that EMPs play an important role in this process. MPs can act on angiogenesis directly through ligand/receptor interaction or indirectly by modulating production of soluble factors involved in endothelial cell differentiation, proliferation, migration, and adhesion [62]. Brodsky et al. have shown that in low concentration, EMPs did not affect the endothelium. However, increased levels of circulating EMPs are an important factor in the pathophysiology of CV diseases, directly affecting the endothelium and other circulating cells [77]. One of the mechanisms mediating these changes may be increased oxidative stress. Brodsky et al. have demonstrated that EMPs directly impair vasorelaxation via diminishing production and/or bioavailability of nitric oxide. This result was correlated with increased superoxide levels in aortic rings isolated from rats and cultured endothelial cells treated with microparticles [77]. Other studies have demonstrated that MPs of endothelial origin induce the expression of endothelial cyclooxygenase type 2, different adhesion molecules, release of cytokines, and impaired release of nitric oxide from vascular endothelial cells [78]. High EMP levels may be considered a biomarker of vascular damage [79]. A pathological concentration ($\geq 10^5$) of EMPs affects angiogenesis by diminishing the cell proliferation rate and decreasing the total capillary length of human umbilical vein endothelial cells (HUVEC) plated on a matrigel substrate [80]. Moreover, HUVECs or human microvascular endothelial cells (HMVECs) treated with EMPs demonstrated disorganized tube formation in the presence or absence of VEGF [80]. This data suggests that EMPs regulate EC function and disrupt growth factor signaling. Many aspects of endothelial cell function and angiogenic capacity are also altered with age. Impairments in the regulation of vascular tone, coagulation, and hemostasis contribute to damage of the vascular system and dysfunctional angiogenesis [81–83]. Recently, *in vitro* studies published by Burger et al. have proved that a long term culture of mouse aortic ECs leads to a senescent phenotype with increased ROCK activity and formation of MPs (Figure 4). Furthermore, it has been shown that MPs promote premature EC senescence through the stimulation of endothelial cell ROS production [84] (Figure 4). Brodsky et al. demonstrated a significant increase in the number of circulating EMPs in obesity-induced diabetes rats as well as premature endothelial cell senescence and vasculopathy. This disorder was characterized by impaired vasorelaxation, nitric oxide production, and defective angiogenesis. An increased number of circulating EMPs have been identified in patients with certain diseases, such as hypertension, coronary artery disease, acute coronary syndrome, and stroke [81]. In patients with established endothelial dysfunction, levels of circulating EMPs are inversely correlated with the amplitude of flow-mediated dilation, independent of blood pressure [11, 85–87]. Another study published by Thomasow et al. has shown elevated levels of $CD31^+$ (PECAM-1), which are suggestive of EC apoptosis, in severe and mild chronic obstructive pulmonary disease (COPD) and emphysema. $CD31^+$ EMPs were positively related to emphysema and were inversely associated with pulmonary microvascular blood flow. In contrast, $CD62E^+$ (E-selectin) EMPs indicative of endothelial activation were elevated in severe COPD and hyperinflation. These cellular markers may involve endothelial apoptosis in the pathogenesis of emphysema and COPD [88]. Previous studies have demonstrated an impairment of cell proliferation, migration, tube formation, and sprouting in older individuals (>65 years, male or female) when compared to their younger counterparts (<65 years, male or female) suggesting that these changes contribute to the decrease in effective blood vessel growth and repair mechanisms in the elderly [89]. A decrease of proangiogenic factors and loss of circulating endothelial progenitor cells (EPCs) have also been observed with increased aging (>50 years, male), which may lead to compromised angiogenesis [90]. Furthermore, age-related changes in EPC number and function may directly correlate with the degree of senescent endothelial impairment [91]. Furthermore, in older men (>60 years) with myocardial infarction, circulating microparticles selectively impair the nitric oxide transduction pathway in endothelial cells, which contributes to the general vasomotor dysfunction observed after myocardial infarction [33]. Additionally, an environmental alteration such as a decrease in ECM proteins particularly fibrillar collagen production and small leucine rich proteoglycans (SLRPs) [92] and changes in the expression of matrix metalloproteinases (MMPs) have also been observed with increased aging [93]. EMPs are clearly implicated in the impairment of angiogenesis in vascular diseases associated with aging however, the specific pathways through which EMPs augment this process are unknown. Moreover, EMPs may be one of the major factors leading to reduced effectiveness of therapies for treating impaired angiogenesis in humans and should be further explored.

6. Endothelial Microparticles and Estrogen in Age-Related Vascular Diseases

Aging and estrogen loss are strongly linked. Furthermore, estrogen levels have been connected to thrombin generation, a central molecule in the coagulation cascade in postmenopausal women [94]. Estrogen plays an extraordinary role in normal vascular development and vascular diseases. It has been shown that estrogen directly modulates angiogenesis via multiple pathways. In particular, estradiol increases migration, proliferation, and formation of capillary-like networks of HUVECs [95] by the classic estrogen receptor (ER) pathway [96–98]. Most reports have concentrated on the role of ERs in mediating big vessel relaxation and contraction. In a rat model of acute myocardial infarction it has been shown that estradiol promotes myocardial angiogenesis by increasing microvascular density through estrogen receptors [99]. Furthermore, in ovariectomized rats it has been demonstrated that an increased number of genes in the aged heart, including TNF and MAP kinase-activating death domain protein (MADD), play a role in the release of EMPs [100–102] (Figure 4). Another *in vivo* study has shown that ovariectomy in female rats is associated with reduced PAI-1 expression, while estrogen replacement counteracts this change promoting EMP formation [103]. *In vitro* studies have demonstrated that estrogen induced PAI-1 expression is implicated in HUVEC horizontal migration [103]. Other mechanisms have also been revealed to be involved in the proangiogenic effect of estrogen including increased expression of both VEGF and its receptors [104, 105] and bFGF [106], as well as expression of vascular adhesion molecules [107]. Moreover, estrogen is known to enhance nitric oxide production and release by endothelial cells [108]. Studies published by Reed and Edelberg have suggested that a physiological decrease in the concentration of steroid hormones (e.g., estrogen and testosterone) as a result of menopause and "chronological aging" may contribute both directly and indirectly to subsequent deficits in the synthesis and function of the angiogenic growth factor TGF-β [109].

In humans endogenous estrogen contributes to the anticoagulant, anti-inflammatory, and antithrombotic properties of the endothelium. The numbers of endothelium, platelet, and monocyte-derived microparticles have been found to be elevated in low-estrogen menopausal women. The authors implied that increased numbers of procoagulant microparticles provide a resource to study mechanisms for cardiovascular risk development in newly menopausal women [110]. On the other hand, studies demonstrated by Rank et al. [111] had shown that hormone replacement therapy in postmenopausal women increased the concentration of MPs derived from platelets. The EMP levels were unchanged excluding their primary role in the initiation of a thromboembolic event in these women [112]. Another study has shown that EMP concentration was diminished in older patients (>80 years, male or female) but MP procoagulant activity was preserved [113] in comparison to younger patients. The older patients had higher incidence of hypertension and stable coronary disease. The authors suggested that a decreased EMP level was associated with age and any effect of gender was ruled out by multivariate analysis. The study performed by Mateos-Caceres [78] had shown an increased level of circulating EMPs in elderly (>66 years) male and female patients with acute stroke and that TNF activated EMPs were the major player in stroke induction. Furthermore, Simak et al. demonstrated that circulating EMP phenotypes may be associated with the severity, lesion volume, and outcome of acute ischemic stroke (AIS) in male patients (>78 years) [113]. On the other hand, studies published by Williams et al. have shown that in elderly patients of both genders (>66 years), EMP levels were similar in AIS and stroke mimic patients [114]. Moreover, they demonstrated that EMPs were generated via activation and not by apoptosis/necrosis of endothelial cells. This suggested that EMPs may not be an appropriate marker for AIS, given the incapability to distinguish between AIS and stroke mimic. The tree-city cohort studies have shown that increased thrombin generation is an independent predictor of AIS in elderly women suggesting that hypercoagulability may play an important role in the pathogenesis of AIS [115]. Furthermore, the population-based cohort studies published by Hoekstra et al. indicated that elevated plasma PAI-1 levels are a strong risk factor for stroke at old age in people of both genders; however, the 4G/5G polymorphism variant of PAI-1 is associated with reduced incidence of stroke [116]. Furthermore, PAI-1 has been suggested as a gene predisposing peripheral hypertension. It has been shown that the single polymorphism PAI-1 4G/5G genotype is associated with higher central systolic, diastolic, and mean arterial blood pressure in women (>70 years), while no association was found in men [117] suggesting gender specific biology of PAI-1 in addition to an advanced age specific factor. Moreover, elevated levels of circulating MPs have been reported in patients (>58 years, male or female) with acute myocardial infarction and coronary artery disease [118]. Studies published by Sinning et al. [119] have shown that circulating EMPs, but not MPs of other cellular origin, are a strong predictor of cardiovascular mortality and major cardiovascular events in patients (>66 years, male or female) with coronary artery disease and pulmonary hypertension [120]. All these data may indicate that estrogen probably does not exert its protective effects on CV diseases through the EMP axis. However, more analyses are needed in order to confirm if a direct connection occurs between estrogen and EMPs in age-related vascular diseases (Figure 4).

7. Conclusions

Endothelial microparticles, as pleiotropic factors, play a role in both physiological and pathological conditions and thus may contribute to regulation of vascular homeostasis. EMPs not only reflect the stage of disease but also play a causative role in the development of various vascular diseases. They can modulate coagulation, and their elevated levels have been observed in many conditions associated with inflammation and angiogenesis. The prothrombotic properties and proinflammatory effects of microparticles on endothelial cells affect vascular aging and lead to structural changes in the heart and other organs. Thrombin and PAI-1 seem to be key factors involved in EMP generation in age-related vascular disease. Furthermore, in age-related vascular diseases, steroid hormones are among the factors that have been shown to have an influence on vascular homeostasis. Specifically, estrogen plays a regulatory function on vessel inflammation, injury, and repair. Lack of estrogen has been suggested to be directly involved in the endothelial cell injury with EMP release that is observed in ischemic diseases. However, the direct link between EMP generation, EMP release, and estrogen is understudied and the further investigation of cellular and molecular mechanisms of these correlations is imperative for understanding and providing a basis for new translational investigations. Furthermore, circulating EMPs show great promise not only as biomarkers in the diagnostics of vascular diseases but also as a target for the treatment of these disorders, especially in elderly patients.

Acknowledgments

The authors wish to thank Dr. R. M. Silver for critically reviewing this paper and for the editorial assistance. This work was conducted in a facility constructed with support from the National Institutes of Health (NIA), Grant no. K01AG031909 (MM) from Extramural Research Facilities Program of the National Center for Research.

References

[1] W. Liu, N. Reinmuth, O. Stoeltzing et al., "Antiangiogenic therapy targeting factors that enhance endothelial cell survival," *Seminars in Oncology*, vol. 29, no. 3, pp. 96–103, 2002.

[2] D. H. Endemann and E. L. Schiffrin, "Endothelial dysfunction," *Journal of the American Society of Nephrology*, vol. 15, no. 8, pp. 1983–1992, 2004.

[3] D. Burger, A. C. Montezano, N. Nishigaki, Y. He, A. Carter, and R. M. Touyz, "Endothelial microparticle formation by angiotensin II is mediated via ang II receptor type I/NADPH Oxidase/rho kinase pathways targeted to lipid rafts," *Arteriosclerosis, Thrombosis, and Vascular Biology*, vol. 31, no. 8, pp. 1898–1907, 2011.

[4] A. S. Leroyer, F. Anfosso, R. Lacroix et al., "Endothelial-derived microparticles: biological conveyors at the crossroad of inflammation, thrombosis and angiogenesis," *Thrombosis and Haemostasis*, vol. 104, no. 3, pp. 456–463, 2010.

[5] A. P. Owens and N. MacKman, "Microparticles in hemostasis and thrombosis," *Circulation Research*, vol. 108, no. 10, pp. 1284–1297, 2011.

[6] C. M. Boulanger, "Microparticles, vascular function and hypertension," *Current Opinion in Nephrology and Hypertension*, vol. 19, no. 2, pp. 177–180, 2010.

[7] C. M. Boulanger and F. Dignat-George, "Microparticles: an introduction," *Arteriosclerosis, Thrombosis, and Vascular Biology*, vol. 31, no. 1, pp. 2–3, 2011.

[8] V. J. Moulin, D. Mayrand, H. Messier, M. C. Martinez, C. A. Lopez-Vallé, and H. Genest, "Shedding of microparticles by myofibroblasts as mediator of cellular cross-talk during normal wound healing," *Journal of Cellular Physiology*, vol. 225, no. 3, pp. 734–740, 2010.

[9] P. Wolf, "The nature and significance of platelet products in human plasma," *The British Journal of Haematology*, vol. 13, no. 3, pp. 269–288, 1967.

[10] R. J. Berckmans, R. Nieuwland, A. N. Böing, F. P. H. T. M. Romijn, C. E. Hack, and A. Sturk, "Cell-derived microparticles circulate in healthy humans and support low grade thrombin generation," *Thrombosis and Haemostasis*, vol. 85, no. 4, pp. 639–646, 2001.

[11] A. S. Leroyer, H. Isobe, G. Lesèche et al., "Cellular origins and thrombogenic activity of microparticles isolated from human atherosclerotic plaques," *Journal of the American College of Cardiology*, vol. 49, no. 7, pp. 772–777, 2007.

[12] F. Meziani, A. Tesse, and R. Andriantsitohaina, "Microparticles are vectors of paradoxical information in vascular cells including the endothelium: role in health and diseases," *Pharmacological Reports*, vol. 60, no. 1, pp. 75–84, 2008.

[13] G. N. Chironi, C. M. Boulanger, A. Simon, F. Dignat-George, J. Freyssinet, and A. Tedgui, "Endothelial microparticles in diseases," *Cell and Tissue Research*, vol. 335, no. 1, pp. 143–151, 2009.

[14] S. F. Mause and C. Weber, "Microparticles: protagonists of a novel communication network for intercellular information exchange," *Circulation Research*, vol. 107, no. 9, pp. 1047–1057, 2010.

[15] L. L. Horstman and Y. S. Ahn, "Platelet microparticles: a wide-angle perspective," *Critical Reviews in Oncology/Hematology*, vol. 30, no. 2, pp. 111–142, 1999.

[16] M. N. A. Hussein, E. W. Meesters, N. Osmanovic, F. P. H. T. M. Romijn, R. Nieuwland, and A. Sturk, "Antigenic characterization of endothelial cell-derived microparticles and their detection ex vivo," *Journal of Thrombosis and Haemostasis*, vol. 1, no. 11, pp. 2434–2443, 2003.

[17] V. Combes, A. Simon, G. Grau et al., "In vitro generation of endothelial microparticles and possible prothrombotic activity

in patients with lupus anticoagulant," *Journal of Clinical Investigation*, vol. 104, no. 1, pp. 93–102, 1999.

[18] M. C. Martínez, A. Tesse, F. Zobairi, and R. Andriantsitohaina, "Shed membrane microparticles from circulating and vascular cells in regulating vascular function," *The American Journal of Physiology—Heart and Circulatory Physiology*, vol. 288, no. 3, pp. H1004–H1009, 2005.

[19] M. Diamant, M. E. Tushuizen, A. Sturk, and R. Nieuwland, "Cellular microparticles: new players in the field of vascular disease?" *European Journal of Clinical Investigation*, vol. 34, no. 6, pp. 392–401, 2004.

[20] 2012 NHLBI Fact Book, Chapter 4, Disease Statistics: Prevalence of Common Cardiovascular and Lung Diseases, US., 2007–2011.

[21] Morbidity & Mortality: 2012 Chart Book on Cardiovascular, Lung, and Blood Diseases.

[22] P. E. Belchetz, "Hormonal treatment of postmenopausal women," *The New England Journal of Medicine*, vol. 330, no. 15, pp. 1062–1071, 1994.

[23] F. Grodstein, M. J. Stampfer, J. E. Manson et al., "Postmenopausal estrogen and progestin use and the risk of cardiovascular disease," *The New England Journal of Medicine*, vol. 335, no. 7, pp. 453–461, 1996.

[24] S. E. Dick, D. E. DeWitt, and B. D. Anawalt, "Postmenopausal hormone replacement therapy and major clinical outcomes: a focus on cardiovascular disease, osteoporosis, dementia, and breast and endometrial neoplasia," *The American Journal of Managed Care*, vol. 8, no. 1, pp. 95–104, 2002.

[25] S. Hulley, D. Grady, T. Bush et al., "Randomized trial of estrogen plus progestin for secondary prevention of coronary heart disease in postmenopausal women," *The Journal of the American Medical Association*, vol. 280, no. 7, pp. 605–613, 1998.

[26] C. M. Viscoli, L. M. Brass, W. N. Kernan, P. M. Sarrel, S. Suissa, and R. I. Horwitz, "A clinical trial of estrogen-replacement therapy after ischemic stroke," *The New England Journal of Medicine*, vol. 345, no. 17, pp. 1243–1249, 2001.

[27] T. Simoncini, "Mechanisms of action of estrogen receptors in vascular cells: relevance for menopause and aging," *Climacteric*, vol. 12, no. 1, pp. 6–11, 2009.

[28] O. Morel, F. Toti, B. Hugel et al., "Procoagulant microparticles: disrupting the vascular homeostasis equation?" *Arteriosclerosis, Thrombosis, and Vascular Biology*, vol. 26, no. 12, pp. 2594–2604, 2006.

[29] F. Bretelle, F. Sabatier, D. Desprez et al., "Circulating microparticles: a marker of procoagulant state in normal pregnancy and pregnancy complicated by preeclampsia or intrauterine growth restriction," *Thrombosis and Haemostasis*, vol. 89, no. 3, pp. 486–492, 2003.

[30] M. J. VanWijk, K. Boer, R. J. Berckmans et al., "Enhanced coagulation activation in preeclampsia: the role of APC resistance, microparticles and other plasma constituents," *Thrombosis and Haemostasis*, vol. 88, no. 3, pp. 415–420, 2002.

[31] Z. Mallat, H. Benamer, B. Hugel et al., "Elevated levels of shed membrane microparticles with procoagulant potential in the peripheral circulating blood of patients with acute coronary syndromes," *Circulation*, vol. 101, no. 8, pp. 841–843, 2000.

[32] R. A. Preston, W. Jy, J. J. Jimenez et al., "Effects of severe hypertension on endothelial and platelet microparticles," *Hypertension*, vol. 41, no. 2, pp. 211–217, 2003.

[33] C. M. Boulanger, A. Scoazec, T. Ebrahimian et al., "Circulating microparticles from patients with myocardial infarction cause endothelial dysfunction," *Circulation*, vol. 104, no. 22, pp. 2649–2652, 2001.

[34] D. Burger and R. M. Touyz, "Cellular biomarkers of endothelial health: microparticles, endothelial progenitor cells, and circulating endothelial cells," *Journal of the American Society of Hypertension*, vol. 6, no. 2, pp. 85–99, 2012.

[35] A. S. Shet, O. Aras, K. Gupta et al., "Sickle blood contains tissue factor-positive microparticles derived from endothelial cells and monocytes," *Blood*, vol. 102, no. 7, pp. 2678–2683, 2003.

[36] L. L. Horstman, W. Jy, J. J. Jimenez, and Y. S. Ahn, "Endothelial microparticles as markers of endothelial dysfunction," *Frontiers in Bioscience*, vol. 9, pp. 1118–1135, 2004.

[37] J. J. Jimenez, W. Jy, L. M. Mauro, C. Soderland, L. L. Horstman, and Y. S. Ahn, "Endothelial cells release phenotypically and quantitatively distinct microparticles in activation and apoptosis," *Thrombosis Research*, vol. 109, no. 4, pp. 175–180, 2003.

[38] A. F. Tramontano, R. Lyubarova, J. Tsiakos, T. Palaia, J. R. Deleon, and L. Ragolia, "Circulating endothelial microparticles in diabetes mellitus," *Mediators of Inflammation*, vol. 2010, Article ID 250476, 8 pages, 2010.

[39] S. H. van Ierssel, E. M. van Craenenbroeck, V. M. Conraads et al., "Flow cytometric detection of endothelial microparticles (EMP): effects of centrifugation and storage alter with the phenotype studied," *Thrombosis Research*, vol. 125, no. 4, pp. 332–339, 2010.

[40] P. J. Yong, C. H. Koh, and W. Shim, "Endothelial microparticles: missing link in endothelial dysfunction?" *European Journal of Preventive Cardiology*, vol. 20, no. 3, pp. 496–512, 2013.

[41] J. Huber, A. Vales, G. Mitulovic et al., "Oxidized membrane vesicles and blebs from apoptotic cells contain biologically active oxidized phospholipids that induce monocyte-endothelial interactions," *Arteriosclerosis, Thrombosis, and Vascular Biology*, vol. 22, no. 1, pp. 101–107, 2002.

[42] M. J. VanWijk, E. VanBavel, A. Sturk, and R. Nieuwland, "Microparticles in cardiovascular diseases," *Cardiovascular Research*, vol. 59, no. 2, pp. 277–287, 2003.

[43] N. MacKman and G. E. Davis, "Blood coagulation and blood vessel development: is tissue factor the missing link?" *Arteriosclerosis, Thrombosis, and Vascular Biology*, vol. 31, no. 11, pp. 2364–2366, 2011.

[44] P. Rautou, A. S. Leroyer, B. Ramkhelawon et al., "Microparticles from human atherosclerotic plaques promote endothelial ICAM-1-dependent monocyte adhesion and transendothelial migration," *Circulation Research*, vol. 108, no. 3, pp. 335–343, 2011.

[45] A. Ludwicka-Bradley, E. Tourkina, S. Suzuki et al., "Thrombin upregulates interleukin-8 in lung fibroblasts via cleavage of proteolytically activated receptor-I and protein kinase C-γ activation," *The American Journal of Respiratory Cell and Molecular Biology*, vol. 22, no. 2, pp. 235–243, 2000.

[46] A. M. Curtis, P. F. Wilkinson, M. Gui, T. L. Gales, E. Hu, and J. M. Edelberg, "p38 mitogen-activated protein kinase targets the production of proinflammatory endothelial microparticles," *Journal of Thrombosis and Haemostasis*, vol. 7, no. 4, pp. 701–709, 2009.

[47] D. B. Peterson, T. Sander, S. Kaul et al., "Comparative proteomic analysis of PAI-1 and TNF-alpha-derived endothelial microparticles," *Proteomics*, vol. 8, no. 12, pp. 2430–2446, 2008.

[48] M. Franchini, "Hemostasis and aging," *Critical Reviews in Oncology/Hematology*, vol. 60, no. 2, pp. 144–151, 2006.

[49] G. A. Zimmerman, "Thinking small, but with big league consequences: procoagulant microparticles in the alveolar space," *The American Journal of Physiology—Lung Cellular and Molecular Physiology*, vol. 297, no. 6, pp. L1033–L1034, 2009.

[50] S. V. Brodsky, K. Malinowski, M. Golightly, J. Jesty, and M. S. Goligorsky, "Plasminogen activator inhibitor-1 promotes formation of endothelial microparticles with procoagulant potential," *Circulation*, vol. 106, no. 18, pp. 2372–2378, 2002.

[51] J. P. Rerolle, A. Hertig, G. Nguyen, J. D. Sraer, and E. P. Rondeau, "Plasminogen activator inhibitor type 1 is a potential target in renal fibrogenesis," *Kidney International*, vol. 58, no. 5, pp. 1841–1850, 2000.

[52] M. Philippova, Y. Suter, S. Toggweiler et al., "T-cadherin is present on endothelial microparticles and is elevated in plasma in early atherosclerosis," *European Heart Journal*, vol. 32, no. 6, pp. 760–771, 2011.

[53] M. A. Krupiczojc, C. J. Scotton, and R. C. Chambers, "Coagulation signalling following tissue injury: focus on the role of factor Xa," *International Journal of Biochemistry and Cell Biology*, vol. 40, no. 6-7, pp. 1228–1237, 2008.

[54] R. C. Chambers, "Procoagulant signalling mechanisms in lung inflammation and fibrosis: novel opportunities for pharmacological intervention?" *The British Journal of Pharmacology*, vol. 153, supplement 1, pp. S367–S378, 2008.

[55] A. Ludwicka-Bradley, G. Bogatkevich, and R. M. Silver, "Thrombin-mediated cellular events in pulmonary fibrosis associated with systemic sclerosis (scleroderma)," *Clinical and Experimental Rheumatology*, vol. 22, no. 3, supplement 33, pp. S38–S46, 2004.

[56] B. G. Bachhuber, I. J. Sarembock, L. W. Gimple, and G. K. Owens, "α-thrombin induces transforming growth factor-β1 mRNA and protein in cultured vascular smooth muscle cells via a proteolytically activated receptor," *Journal of Vascular Research*, vol. 34, no. 1, pp. 41–48, 1997.

[57] A. Ludwicka-Bradley, R. M. Silver, and G. S. Bogatkevich, "Coagulation and autoimmunity in scleroderma interstitial lung disease," *Seminars in Arthritis and Rheumatism*, vol. 41, no. 2, pp. 212–222, 2011.

[58] C. Sapet, S. Simoncini, B. Loriod et al., "Thrombin-induced endothelial microparticle generation: identification of a novel pathway involving ROCK-II activation by caspase-2," *Blood*, vol. 108, no. 6, pp. 1868–1876, 2006.

[59] S. Simoncini, M. Njock, S. Robert et al., "Trail/Apo2L mediates the release of procoagulant endothelial microparticles induced by thrombin in vitro: a potential mechanism linking inflammation and coagulation," *Circulation Research*, vol. 104, no. 8, pp. 943–951, 2009.

[60] T. Ueba, T. Haze, M. Sugiyama et al., "Level, distribution and correlates of platelet-derived microparticles in healthy individuals with special reference to the metabolic syndrome," *Thrombosis and Haemostasis*, vol. 100, no. 2, pp. 280–285, 2008.

[61] H. Takeya, E. C. Gabazza, S. Aoki, H. Ueno, and K. Suzuki, "Synergistic effect of sphingosine 1-phosphate on thrombin-induced tissue factor expression in endothelial cells," *Blood*, vol. 102, no. 5, pp. 1693–1700, 2003.

[62] M. C. Martinez and R. Andriantsitohaina, "Microparticles in angiogenesis: therapeutic potential," *Circulation Research*, vol. 109, no. 1, pp. 110–119, 2011.

[63] H. Obinata and T. Hla, "Sphingosine 1-phosphate in coagulation and inflammation," *Seminars in Immunopathology*, vol. 34, no. 1, pp. 73–91, 2012.

[64] M. Markiewicz, S. S. Nakerakanti, B. Kapanadze, A. Ghatnekar, and M. Trojanowska, "Connective tissue growth factor (CTGF/CCN2) mediates angiogenic effect of S1P in human dermal microvascular endothelial cells," *Microcirculation*, vol. 18, no. 1, pp. 1–11, 2011.

[65] W. Jy, J. J. Jimenez, L. M. Mauro et al., "Endothelial microparticles induce formation of platelet aggregates via a von Willebrand factor/ristocetin dependent pathway, rendering them resistant to dissociation," *Journal of Thrombosis and Haemostasis*, vol. 3, no. 6, pp. 1301–1308, 2005.

[66] F. Sabatier, V. Roux, F. Anfosso, L. Camoin, J. Sampol, and F. Dignat-George, "Interaction of endothelial microparticles with monocytic cells in vitro induces tissue factor-dependent procoagulant activity," *Blood*, vol. 99, no. 11, pp. 3962–3970, 2002.

[67] W. Jy, A. Minagar, J. J. Jimenez et al., "Endothelial microparticles (EMP) bind and activate monocytes: elevated EMP-monocyte conjugates in multiple sclerosis," *Frontiers in Bioscience*, vol. 9, pp. 3137–3144, 2004.

[68] M. Cesari, M. Pahor, and R. A. Incalzi, "Plasminogen activator inhibitor-1 (PAI-1): a key factor linking fibrinolysis and age-related subclinical and clinical conditions," *Cardiovascular Therapeutics*, vol. 28, no. 5, pp. e72–e91, 2010.

[69] C. J. Epstein, G. M. Martin, A. L. Schultz, and A. G. Motulsky, "Werner's syndrome a review of its symptomatology, natural history, pathologic features, genetics and relationship to the natural aging process," *Medicine*, vol. 45, no. 3, pp. 177–221, 1966.

[70] R. Lacroix and F. Dignat-George, "Microparticles as a circulating source of procoagulant and fibrinolytic activities in the circulation," *Thrombosis Research*, vol. 129, supplement 2, pp. S27–S29, 2012.

[71] S. Q. van Veen, J. C. M. Meijers, M. Levi, T. M. van Gulik, and M. A. Boermeester, "Effects of intra-abdominal administration of recombinant tissue plasminogen activator on coagulation, fibrinolysis and inflammatory responses in experimental polymicrobial peritonitis," *Shock*, vol. 27, no. 5, pp. 534–541, 2007.

[72] F. Tita-Nwa, A. Bos, A. Adjei, W. B. Ershler, D. L. Longo, and L. Ferrucci, "Correlates of D-dimer in older persons," *Aging—Clinical and Experimental Research*, vol. 22, no. 1, pp. 20–23, 2010.

[73] Y. Song, H. Shen, D. Schenten, P. Shan, P. J. Lee, and D. R. Goldstein, "Aging enhances the basal production of IL-6 and CCL2 in vascular smooth muscle cells," *Arteriosclerosis, Thrombosis, and Vascular Biology*, vol. 32, no. 1, pp. 103–109, 2012.

[74] J. Folkman and Y. Shing, "Angiogenesis," *The Journal of Biological Chemistry*, vol. 267, no. 16, pp. 10931–10934, 1992.

[75] V. Djonov, M. Schmid, S. A. Tschanz, and P. H. Burri, "Intussusceptive angiogenesis. Its role in embryonic vascular network formation," *Circulation Research*, vol. 86, no. 3, pp. 286–292, 2000.

[76] J. Li, Y. Zhang, and R. S. Kirsner, "Angiogenesis in wound repair: angiogenic growth factors and the extracellular matrix," *Microscopy Research and Technique*, vol. 60, no. 1, pp. 107–114, 2003.

[77] S. V. Brodsky, F. Zhang, A. Nasjletti, and M. S. Goligorsky, "Endothelium-derived microparticles impair endothelial function in vitro," *The American Journal of Physiology—Heart and Circulatory Physiology*, vol. 286, no. 5, pp. H1910–H1915, 2004.

[78] P. J. Mateos-Caceres, J. J. Zamorano-Leon, P. Rodriguez-Sierra, C. Macaya, and A. J. Lopez-Farre, "New and old mechanisms

associated with hypertension in the elderly," *International Journal of Hypertension*, vol. 2012, Article ID 150107, 10 pages, 2012.

[79] K. H. Jung, K. Chu, S. T. Lee et al., "Circulating endothelial microparticles as a marker of cerebrovascular disease," *Annals of Neurology*, vol. 66, no. 2, pp. 191–199, 2009.

[80] A. Mezentsev, R. M. H. Merks, E. O'Riordan et al., "Endothelial microparticles affect angiogenesis in vitro: role of oxidative stress," *The American Journal of Physiology—Heart and Circulatory Physiology*, vol. 289, no. 3, pp. H1106–H1114, 2005.

[81] P. Davizon and J. A. López, "Microparticles and thrombotic disease," *Current Opinion in Hematology*, vol. 16, no. 5, pp. 334–341, 2009.

[82] V. L. T. Ballard and J. M. Edelberg, "Targets for regulating angiogenesis in the ageing endothelium," *Expert Opinion on Therapeutic Targets*, vol. 11, no. 11, pp. 1385–1399, 2007.

[83] P. E. Gates, W. D. Strain, and A. C. Shore, "Human endothelial function and microvascular ageing," *Experimental Physiology*, vol. 94, no. 3, pp. 311–316, 2009.

[84] D. Burger, D. G. Kwart, A. C. Montezano et al., "Microparticles induce cell cycle arrest through redox-sensitive processes in endothelial cells: implications in vascular senescence," *Journal of the American Heart Association*, vol. 1, no. 3, Article ID e001842, 2012.

[85] N. Amabile, P. Rautou, A. Tedgui, and C. M. Boulanger, "Microparticles: key protagonists in cardiovascular disorders," *Seminars in Thrombosis and Hemostasis*, vol. 36, no. 8, pp. 907–916, 2010.

[86] Z. Mallat, B. Hugel, J. Ohan, G. Lesèche, J. Freyssinet, and A. Tedgui, "Shed membrane microparticles with procoagulant potential in human atherosclerotic plaques: a role for apoptosis in plaque thrombogenicity," *Circulation*, vol. 99, no. 3, pp. 348–353, 1999.

[87] R. Lacroix, F. Sabatier, A. Mialhe et al., "Activation of plasminogen into plasmin at the surface of endothelial microparticles: a mechanism that modulates angiogenic properties of endothelial progenitor cells in vitro," *Blood*, vol. 110, no. 7, pp. 2432–2439, 2007.

[88] M. A. Thomashow, D. Shimbo, M. A. Parikh et al., "Endothelial microparticles in mild chronic obstructive pulmonary disease and emphysema. The multiethnic study of atherosclerosis chronic obstructive pulmonary disease study," *The American Journal of Respiratory and Critical Care Medicine*, vol. 188, no. 1, pp. 60–68, 2013.

[89] J. M. Edelberg and M. J. Reed, "Aging and angiogenesis," *Frontiers in Bioscience*, vol. 8, pp. s1199–s1209, 2003.

[90] J. M. Hill, G. Zalos, J. P. J. Halcox et al., "Circulating endothelial progenitor cells, vascular function, and cardiovascular risk," *The New England Journal of Medicine*, vol. 348, no. 7, pp. 593–600, 2003.

[91] C. Heiss, S. Keymel, U. Niesler, J. Ziemann, M. Kelm, and C. Kalka, "Impaired progenitor cell activity in age-related endothelial dysfunction," *Journal of the American College of Cardiology*, vol. 45, no. 9, pp. 1441–1448, 2005.

[92] M. Markiewicz, Y. Asano, S. Znoyko, Y. Gong, D. K. Watson, and M. Trojanowska, "Distinct effects of gonadectomy in male and female mice on collagen fibrillogenesis in the skin," *Journal of Dermatological Science*, vol. 47, no. 3, pp. 217–226, 2007.

[93] T. Koike, R. B. Vernon, M. D. Gooden, E. Sadoun, and M. J. Reed, "Inhibited angiogenesis in aging: a role for TIMP-2," *Journals of Gerontology A*, vol. 58, no. 9, pp. 798–805, 2003.

[94] C. N. Bagot, M. S. Marsh, M. Whitehead et al., "The effect of estrone on thrombin generation may explain the different thrombotic risk between oral and transdermal hormone replacement therapy," *Journal of Thrombosis and Haemostasis*, vol. 8, no. 8, pp. 1736–1744, 2010.

[95] D. E. Morales, K. A. McGowan, D. S. Grant et al., "Estrogen promotes angiogenic activity in human umbilical vein endothelial cells in vitro and in a murine model," *Circulation*, vol. 91, no. 3, pp. 755–763, 1995.

[96] H. W. Schnaper, K. A. McGowan, S. Kim-Schulze, and M. C. Cid, "oestrogen and endothelial cell angiogenic activity," *Clinical and Experimental Pharmacology and Physiology*, vol. 23, no. 3, pp. 247–250, 1996.

[97] C. D. Venkov, A. B. Rankin, and D. E. Vaughan, "Identification of authentic estrogen receptor in cultured endothelial cells: a potential mechanism for steroid hormone regulation of endothelial function," *Circulation*, vol. 94, no. 4, pp. 727–733, 1996.

[98] S. Kim-Schulze, K. A. McGowan, S. C. Hubchak et al., "Expression of an estrogen receptor by human coronary artery and umbilical vein endothelial cells," *Circulation*, vol. 94, no. 6, pp. 1402–1407, 1996.

[99] X. Jin, Y. C. Chen, W. Q. Liu, H. Y. Wang, B. Wang, and Z. Zeng, "Estradiol promote myocardial anglogenesis in a rat model of acute myocardial infarction through estrogen receptors," *Sichuan Da Xue Xue Bao Yi Xue Ban*, vol. 39, no. 3, pp. 398–401, 2008.

[100] K. L. Hamilton, L. Lin, Y. Wang, and A. A. Knowlton, "Effect of ovariectomy on cardiac gene expression: inflammation and changes in SOCS gene expression," *Physiological Genomics*, vol. 32, no. 2, pp. 254–263, 2008.

[101] A. S. Pechenino, L. Lin, F. N. Mbai et al., "Impact of aging versus estrogen loss on cardiac gene expression: estrogen replacement and inflammation," *Physiological Genomics*, vol. 43, no. 18, pp. 1065–1073, 2011.

[102] A. A. Knowlton and A. R. Lee, "Estrogen and the cardiovascular system," *Pharmacology and Therapeutics*, vol. 135, no. 1, pp. 54–70, 2012.

[103] S. Gopal, S. Garibaldi, L. Goglia et al., "Estrogen regulates endothelial migration via plasminogen activator inhibitor (PAI-1)," *Molecular Human Reproduction*, vol. 18, no. 8, pp. 410–416, 2012.

[104] D. W. Losordo and J. M. Isner, "Estrogen and angiogenesis: a review," *Arteriosclerosis, Thrombosis, and Vascular Biology*, vol. 21, no. 1, pp. 6–12, 2001.

[105] R. R. Greb, O. Heikinheimo, R. F. Williams, G. D. Hodgen, and A. L. Goodman, "Vascular endothelial growth factor in primate endometrium is regulated by oestrogen-receptor and progesterone-receptor ligands in vivo," *Human Reproduction*, vol. 12, no. 6, pp. 1280–1292, 1997.

[106] M. Rusnati, G. Casarotti, S. Pecorelli, G. Ragnotti, and M. Presta, "Estro-progestinic replacement therapy modulates the levels of basic fibroblast growth factor (bFGF) in postmenopausal endometrium," *Gynecologic Oncology*, vol. 48, no. 1, pp. 88–93, 1993.

[107] M. C. Cid, H. K. Kleinman, D. S. Grant, H. W. Schnaper, A. S. Fauci, and G. S. Hoffman, "Estradiol enhances leukocyte binding to tumor necrosis factor (TNF)-stimulated endothelial cells via an increase in TNF-induced adhesion molecules E-selectin, intercellular adhesion molecule type 1, and vascular cell adhesion molecule type 1," *Journal of Clinical Investigation*, vol. 93, no. 1, pp. 17–25, 1994.

[108] M. C. Cid, H. W. Schnaper, and H. K. Kleinman, "Estrogens and the vascular endothelium," *Annals of the New York Academy of Sciences*, vol. 966, pp. 143–157, 2002.

[109] M. J. Reed and J. M. Edelberg, "Impaired angiogenesis in the aged," *Science of Aging Knowledge Environment*, vol. 2004, no. 7, p. pe7, 2004.

[110] M. Jayachandran, R. D. Litwiller, W. G. Owen, and V. M. Miller, "Circulating microparticles and endogenous estrogen in newly menopausal women," *Climacteric*, vol. 12, no. 2, pp. 177–184, 2009.

[111] A. Rank, R. Nieuwland, K. Nikolajek et al., "Hormone replacement therapy leads to increased plasma levels of platelet derived microparticles in postmenopausal women," *Archives of Gynecology and Obstetrics*, vol. 285, no. 4, pp. 1035–1041, 2012.

[112] A. Forest, E. Pautas, P. Ray et al., "Circulating microparticles and procoagulant activity in elderly patients," *Journals of Gerontology A*, vol. 65, no. 4, pp. 414–420, 2010.

[113] J. Simak, M. P. Gelderman, H. Yu, V. Wright, and A. E. Baird, "Circulating endothelial microparticles in acute ischemic stroke: a link to severity, lesion volume and outcome," *Journal of Thrombosis and Haemostasis*, vol. 4, no. 6, pp. 1296–1302, 2006.

[114] J. B. Williams, E. C. Jauch, C. J. Lindsell, and B. Campos, "Endothelial microparticle levels are similar in acute ischemic stroke and stroke mimics due to activation and not apoptosis/necrosis," *Academic Emergency Medicine*, vol. 14, no. 8, pp. 685–690, 2007.

[115] L. Carcaillon, M. Alhenc-Gelas, Y. Bejot et al., "Increased thrombin generation is associated with acute ischemic stroke but not with coronary heart disease in the elderly: the three-city cohort study," *Arteriosclerosis, Thrombosis, and Vascular Biology*, vol. 31, no. 6, pp. 1445–1451, 2011.

[116] T. Hoekstra, J. M. Geleijnse, C. Kluft, E. J. Giltay, F. J. Kok, and E. G. Schouten, "4G/4G genotype of PAI-1 gene is associated with reduced risk of stroke in elderly," *Stroke*, vol. 34, no. 12, pp. 2822–2828, 2003.

[117] H. M. Björck, P. Eriksson, U. Alehagen et al., "Gender-specific association of the plasminogen activator inhibitor-1 4G/5G polymorphism with central arterial blood pressure," *The American Journal of Hypertension*, vol. 24, no. 7, pp. 802–808, 2011.

[118] E. Steogonekpień, E. Stankiewicz, J. Zalewski, J. Godlewski, K. zmudka, and I. Wybrańska, "Number of microparticles generated during acute myocardial infarction and stable angina correlates with platelet activation," *Archives of Medical Research*, vol. 43, no. 1, pp. 31–35, 2012.

[119] J. Sinning, J. Losch, K. Walenta, M. Böhm, G. Nickenig, and N. Werner, "Circulating CD31+/Annexin V+ microparticles correlate with cardiovascular outcomes," *European Heart Journal*, vol. 32, no. 16, pp. 2034–2041, 2011.

[120] N. Amabile, C. Heiss, W. M. Real et al., "Circulating endothelial microparticle levels predict hemodynamic severity of pulmonary hypertension," *The American Journal of Respiratory and Critical Care Medicine*, vol. 177, no. 11, pp. 1268–1275, 2008.

3

Use of Physical and Intellectual Activities and Socialization in the Management of Cognitive Decline of Aging and in Dementia

Myuri Ruthirakuhan, Angela C. Luedke, Angela Tam, Ankita Goel, Ayaz Kurji, and Angeles Garcia

Department of Medicine (Geriatrics) and Centre for Neuroscience, Queen's University, Kingston, ON, Canada K7L 5A2

Correspondence should be addressed to Angeles Garcia, garciaa@providencecare.ca

Academic Editor: Richard F. Gillum

Lifestyle nonpharmacological interventions can have a deep effect on cognitive aging. We have reviewed the available literature on the effectiveness of physical activity, intellectual stimulation, and socialization on the incidence of dementia and on the course of dementia itself. Even though physical activity appears to be beneficial in both delaying dementia onset and in the course of the disease, more research is needed before intellectual stimulation and socialization can be considered as treatments and prevention of the disease. Through our paper, we found that all three nonpharmacological treatments provide benefits to cognition and overall well-being in patients with age-related cognitive impairments. These interventions may be beneficial in the management of dementia.

1. Introduction

Alzheimer's disease (AD) is a neurodegenerative disorder with devastating consequences [1]. Despite being the most common cause of dementia, affecting approximately 5.4 million Americans [2] and almost 50% of people over the age 85 [3], no cure has yet been discovered. Efforts are also focusing on the development of more effective strategies to slow the progression of AD to increase the quality of life of those affected. Even a two-year delay in disease onset would reduce the prevalence of AD among Americans by two million people within fifty years [4]. If an intervention that delayed the onset of AD by five years had been applied back in 1997, we would have seen a 50% reduction in AD incidence [4]. Research on strategies to slow the development and progression of AD is arguably more important now than ever before, since the number of people with AD is expected to nearly triple over the next forty years [4], and dementia is the most important contributor to disability in the elderly [5].

Among others, three nonpharmacological interventions are particularly relevant as they might positively influence cognition, general functioning, and overall quality of life. These three strategies are *physical exercise*, *intellectual stimulation*, and *social interaction*. While there are studies that evaluate the role of individual and multimodal interventions on AD, there is a lack of literature on the combination of all three. The purpose of this paper is to review key areas of the literature that focus on the effects of physical exercise, intellectual stimulation, and socialization strategies on AD evolution, as they collectively play an important role in the management of Alzheimer's disease. Physical exercise encapsulates both aerobic exercises (e.g., walking and cycling) and nonaerobic exercises (e.g., strength and resistance training; flexibility and balance exercises). For intellectual stimulation, we examine studies that have evaluated the prognostic effects of either cognitive hobbies (e.g., reading, word puzzles, and card games) or cognitive training (e.g., computer training games/paradigms that target specific cognitive domains such as memory and attention). Social interaction is defined as the participation of an AD patient in group-related activities, such as mealtime conversations, support groups, or other forms of social engagement.

Evidence-based nonpharmacological interventions are an essential part of any management plan, especially for geriatric populations in whom the harmful effects of polypharmacy are a major concern. Nonpharmacological strategies are sometimes even more effective than pharmacological interventions and are empowering to proactive individuals who seek to gain greater personal control over their mental and physical health. We suggest that comprehensive AD management plans should include evidence-based nonpharmacological strategies.

2. Methods

Electronic databases (PubMed, Web of Science, and MEDLINE) were searched for the period from 1980 to 2012 with the combination of key words: AD, dementia, incident AD, aging, cognition, cognitive aging, exercise, aerobic exercise, resistance training, cognitive reserve, intellectual stimulation, cognitive stimulation, hobbies, cognitive training, memory training, brain games, leisure activities, socialization, loneliness, social network, support groups, quality of life, activities of daily living, nonpharmacological, and treatment. We included studies that examined the preservation of cognition in AD populations and AD incidence.

3. Physical Activity

The health benefits attributed to physical activity are numerous and well known. Exercise has been associated with a lower incidence in many chronic diseases, such as coronary heart disease [6], type 2 diabetes [7], obesity [8], cancer [9], bone loss [10], and high blood pressure [11]. We have reviewed the effects of physical exercise on cognition.

Higher cardiorespiratory fitness has been related to higher scores on tests of cognitive function [12]. A meta-analysis of randomized controlled trials examining the relationship between exercise and cognition showed modest improvements in attention, processing speed, executive function, and memory among older adults in the treatment arms [13]. This is highly relevant for the elderly population, as it suggests that physical activity can serve as a preventative measure against age-related cognitive decline [14].

Several large longitudinal studies followed older adults without cognitive impairments at baseline and measured rate of incident dementia to clarify the relationship between physical activity and incident cognitive loss. A large prospective study by Podewils et al. identified an inverse relationship between physical activity and dementia risk [15]. Compared to no exercise, physical activity has been linked with reduced risks of developing cognitive impairment and dementia [16] with the risk for dementia being further reduced with increasing levels of physical activity. Larson and colleagues found that persons who exercised three or more times per week had a reduced risk of developing dementia compared to those who exercised less, and the reduction was more marked among those with the poorest physical function at baseline [17]. These results were corroborated by Buchman et al. who found that participants in the lowest percentiles of physical activity had more than twice the risk of developing dementia than those in the highest percentiles of physical activity [18]. Furthermore, Lautenschlager et al. demonstrated that these results might be transferable to adults with mild cognitive impairment (MCI), and, thus, at high risk for dementia; participants who underwent exercise training showed modest improvements in cognition after six months [19]. Physical exercise has, therefore, been recommended as a preventative measure of mild cognitive impairment and dementia [20, 21].

There is much less research focusing on the effect of physical activity in AD patients. This may be due to the challenges of implementing an exercise regime while managing the behavioral and emotional disturbances in AD patients, particularly in the later stages of the disease. However, the results in the available literature are promising. Early research involving AD patients in nonrandomized controlled trials showed significant cognitive improvements among participants who underwent cycling training and somatic and isotonic-relaxation exercises [22, 23].

Physical exercise may have beneficial effects in AD patients beyond cognition as well. A meta-analysis on 30 randomized controlled trials that employed exercise, behavioral and environmental manipulations in patients with cognitive impairment found exercise had positive effects on strength and cardiovascular fitness in addition to improvements in behavior and cognition [24–26]. Further evidence supporting multifaceted positive effects of exercise on AD can be traced to recent randomized controlled trials of physical exercise regimes on AD patients (Table 1).

Compared to controls, patients in the intervention programs showed better physical functioning (functional reach, walking, and mobility). After treatment, these patients also showed improved performance of activities of daily living (ADLs), and less cognitive decline and cognitive improvement in some cases. Physical exercise, therefore, appears to be beneficial for AD patients. While the majority of the studies did not find any differences in depression, one study by Steinberg found increased depression and decreased quality of life in patients who underwent the exercise intervention [31]. Further research into the effect of physical exercise on mood and quality of life in AD patients is, therefore, required.

When considering the role of exercise on AD, it is important to note that any positive results may be due to a placebo effect, even in randomized controlled trials. However, due to the varied nature of the outcome measures used in these studies, it is unlikely that every intervention group demonstrated significant gains over the controls due to a placebo effect alone. Furthermore, control group members never appeared to show any improvement and often showed higher rates of functional and cognitive decline.

The majority of the reviewed studies employed aerobic exercise as a component to their therapy. Yet, two studies demonstrated that nonaerobic activity, such as strength and flexibility training, might also be beneficial to AD patients

Table 1: Summary of randomized controlled trials of physical exercise regimes in AD patients.

Study	Length and frequency	Type of exercise	Sample	MMSE (baseline mean)	Outcome measures	Major findings
Kemoun et al. [27]	15 wks; 1 h sessions 3x/wk	Aerobic, balance, and endurance	$n_{ex} = 16$ $n_c = 15$	12.6	Walking speed, stride length, double limb support time, and ERFC	Higher ERFC and walking parameter scores in exercise group; positive correlation between walking parameters and ERFC scores
Miu et al. [28]	3 mos; ~1 h sessions 2x/wk	Aerobic, flexibility	$n_{ex} = 36$ $n_c = 49$	20 (median)	SF-12, 6 min walk, functional reach, BBS, MMSE, ADAS-Cog, and CSDD	Improvement in walking and functional reach in exercise group
Roach et al. [29]	16 wks; 15–30 min sessions 5x/wk	Strength, flexibility, endurance, and balance	$n_{ex} = 28$ $n_{soc} = 25$ $n_{walk} = 29$	10.7	ACIF, 6 min walk, and MMSE	Improved transfer in exercise group
Rolland et al. [30]	1 yr; 1 h session 2x/wk	Aerobic, strength, flexibility, and balance	$n_{ex} = 67$ $n_c = 67$	8.8	Katz Index of ADLs, walking speed, get-up-and-go, one-leg balance, MNA, NPI, and MADRS	Less decline in overall ADLs in exercise group
Steinberg et al. [31]	12 wks; ~3x/wk	Aerobic, strength, balance, and flexibility	$n_{ex} = 14$ $n_c = 13$	20.1	YPAS, 8-ft walk, JTT, sit-to-stand, MMSE, BNT, HVLT, ADQRL, NPI, CSDD, and SCB	Improved performance in JTT and sit-to-stand, increased depression, and decreased ADQRL in exercise group
Venturelli et al. [32]	24 wks; 30 min sessions 4x/wk	Mobility, aerobic	$n_{ex} = 12$ $n_c = 12$	13	6 min walk, Barthel Index of ADLs, and MMSE	Improvements in walking and ADLs, slower decline in MMSE in exercise group
Vreugdenhil et al. [33]	4 mos; >30 mins daily	Strength, balance, and aerobic	$n_{ex} = 20$ $n_c = 20$	22.9	ADAS-Cog, MMSE, functional reach, Timed Up and Go, sit-to-stand, Barthel Index of ADLs, GDS, CIBIC-plus, and Zarit Burden Interview	Improved scores on ADAS-Cog, MMSE, CIBIC-plus, functional reach, Timed Up and Go, sit-to-stand, and ADLs in exercise group
Yàgüez et al. [34]	6 wks; 1.5 h sessions 1x/wk	Flexibility, eye-hand coordination	$n_{ex} = 15$ $n_c = 12$	22.1	CANTAB-Expedio	Improvements in attention, visual memory recognition, and working memory in exercise group

$n_{ex}, n_c, n_{soc}, n_{walk}$: number of participants in exercise program, control group, social conversation group, and walking group, respectively. ACIF: Acute Care Index of Function, ADAS-Cog: Alzheimer's Disease Assessment Scale-Cognitive Subscale, ADL: activities of daily living, ADQRL: Alzheimer's Disease Quality Related Life Scale, BBS: Berg Balance Scale, BNT: Boston Naming Test, CANTAB-Expedio: The Cambridge Neuropsychological Test Automated Battery, CIBIC-plus: Clinician's Interview-Based Impression of Change Plus Caregiver Input, CSDD: Cornell Scale for Depression in Dementia, ERFC: Rapid Evaluation of Cognitive Function, GDS: Geriatric Depression dcale, HDS: Hamilton Depression Scale, HVLT: Hopkins Verbal Learning Test, JTT: Jebsen Total Time, MADRS: Montgomery-Asberg Depression Rating Scale, MMSE: Mini-Mental State Examination, MNA: Mini-Nutritional Assessment, NPI: Neuropsychiatric Inventory, SCB: Screen for Caregiver Burden, SF-12: SF-12 Quality of Life Questionnaire, SF-36: Short-Form Health Survey, SIP: Sickness Impact Profile, and YPAS: Yale Physical Activity Survey.

[29, 34]. Studies involving cognitively normal adults and nonaerobic exercises offer insight into the potential effects of nonaerobic activity and cognitive decline. Cassilhas et al. found that participants who underwent resistance training showed significant improvements in memory measures compared to controls [35]. Liu-Ambrose and colleagues, who used a combination of resistance and balance exercises as their intervention, saw significant improvements in response inhibition in their intervention group while the control group deteriorated [36]. Resistance training may, therefore, provide protective effects for cognition. The effect of stretch exercises, such as yoga, on cognition has been briefly examined; Oken and colleagues found no cognitive differences between their control and yoga groups after treatment [37]. However, more research into stretch exercises and cognition is required to draw more definitive conclusions.

Future studies may investigate which types of exercises, or combinations of exercises, yield the greatest benefit specifically to AD patients. It is important to mention that some of the aforementioned randomized controlled trials [27, 29, 30, 32] were conducted on participants recruited from long-term care facilities, and thus were likely to be in the more moderate-advanced stages of the disease. These studies demonstrate not only the feasibility of the exercise programs in AD patients but also that patients can benefit greatly from physical exercise even in moderate-to-severe stages of the disease.

Enhanced neuroplasticity might be underlying the improvements seen. Colcombe and colleagues demonstrated that older adults without dementia who performed aerobic exercises had greater grey and white matter volumes compared to adults who engaged in stretching and toning exercises [38]. Exercise has also been associated with functional connectivity between brain networks often affected by age, such as the default mode, frontal parietal, and frontal executive networks, in older adults without dementia [39]. While randomized controlled trials in AD patients examining the relationship between neuroplasticity and exercise are underway, correlational studies examining brain volumes and cardiorespiratory fitness have been done. In AD patients, cardiorespiratory fitness has been associated with brain volume. VO_2^{peak}, peak oxygen consumption, has been positively correlated with greater whole brain volume and white matter volume [40], notably in the inferior parietal lobule, hippocampal, and parahippocampal regions [41]. Future results of randomized controlled trials will improve our knowledge in this field of research.

Overall, physical activity offers promising outcomes for cognition and physical health in the elderly population and AD patients.

4. Intellectual Activity

Engagement in intellectually stimulating activities has been linked with reduced risk of developing AD and intellectual stimulation has been widely explored as a nonpharmacological treatment option for dementia [42].

Among cognitively normal older persons, randomized control trials employing intellectual training concluded that cognitive interventions produce protective and potentially long lasting positive effects in various cognitive domains as well as activities of daily living [43]. There is also evidence that frequent engagement in hobbies, including reading, puzzles, and games, for at least six hours per week reduces the risk of incident dementia [44]. The concept of intellectual stimulation as a preventative measure for dementia in healthy older adults can be parallel to the notion of building a "compensatory mechanism" or "cognitive reserve" [45–48].

Cognitive reserve refers to the hypothesis that individual differences shaped by inherent characteristics and external sources including intelligence, years of education, occupation, and intellectual activities, may provide neural protective support against dementia [45–47]. It has been argued that these collective life experiences may contribute to building cognitive reserve and, thus, provide skills to compensate for AD pathology [45–47]. In other words, a greater cognitive reserve might delay the appearance of dementia despite the presence of neuropathology, after which a rapid progression of cognitive decline may ensue once pathology is significant enough to result in AD diagnosis. Thus, AD patients with higher education and occupation accomplishments suffer more rapid decline in cognitive abilities when compared to AD patients with less education and occupational attainment following diagnosis [49]. Another study by Helzner and colleagues [50] investigated the relationship between premorbid leisure activity and rate of cognitive decline in AD patients. Leisure activities were classified into four categories: intellectual, social, physical, and other. Higher-frequency participation in intellectual leisure activities prior to AD diagnosis was associated with delayed AD onset followed by faster cognitive decline. The study by Helzner and colleagues [50] provides evidence for the benefits of intellectual stimulation on slowing down AD development.

Besides reducing the risk of dementia, cognitive interventions later in life may affect functional decline in AD. Treiber and colleagues [51] explored the association between engaging in cognitively stimulating activities in late life and the rate of cognitive decline in incident AD. This study included a wide range of intellectual activities that required varying levels of cognitive demand, for example, completing puzzles, reading, watching television, listening to music, and cooking. The results suggested that higher-frequency participation in stimulating activities in early stages of dementia resulted in slower cognitive decline. However, as time progressed there was an overall decrease in participation in activities, which might reflect the nature of AD in terms of functional abilities.

Intellectual stimulation can be divided into several categories including cognitive stimulation, cognitive training, and cognitive rehabilitation (Table 2) [48, 52–54]. Each type of stimulation targets various cognitive domains including memory and attention, or even more generally, activities of daily living [55]. The focus of this paper is to investigate the literature on the link between intellectual stimulation and rate of cognitive decline in patients with dementia.

4.1. Cognitive Stimulation and Reality Orientation in Dementia. Cognitive stimulation therapy (CS) encompasses a variety of mentally stimulating activities and is less formal than other forms of cognitive training [53]. In addition, cognitive stimulation can be passive, such as listening to music, or active, such as playing a game [53]. The goal of CS is to enhance a wide range of functioning, including social skills, often through group discussions [48, 56]. An earlier randomized control trial included a total of 167 participants (97 in the treatment group and 70 in the control group). This study examined the relationship between CS, cognitive functioning, and quality of life [57]. The CS group participated in activities including crafts, games, and singing compared to a control group who received no intervention. The sessions ran for seven weeks and consisted of a total of 14 sessions, one 45-minute session twice a

Table 2: Summary of trials involving cognitive interventions in AD patients.

Study	Length and frequency	Type of stimulation	Sample	MMSE (baseline mean)	Outcome measures	Major findings
Buschert et al. [59]	6 months; 2 hours 1x/wk	Multicomponent intervention with focus on CS	$n_{ex} = 8$ $n_c = 7$	Experimental: 24.5 Control: 25.3	(i) MMSE (ii) ADAS-Cog (iii) TMT (iv) RBANS story memory and recall (v) QoL-AD (vi) MADRS	(i) No significant benefit
Chapman et al. [58]	8 wks; 90-minute sessions 1x/wk	Cognitive stimulation	$n_{ex} = 28$ $n_c = 26$	20.87	(i) MMSE (ii) ADAS-Cog (iii) TFLS NPI-irritability and apathy (iv) QoL-AD (v) CBIC	(i) Modest positive effects on language, global and functional abilities, and emotional wellbeing in experimental group compared to control group just treated with donepezil
Spector et al. [57]	7 wks; 45-minute sessions 2x/wk	Cognitive stimulation	$n_{ex} = 97$ $n_c = 70$	Experimental: 14.2 Control: 14.8	(i) MMSE (ii) ADAS-Cog (iii) QoL-AD (iv) HCS (v) Cornell Scale for Depression in Dementia (vi) CAPE-BRS (vii) CDR	(i) Significant improvement on the MMSE, ADAS-COG, and QoL-AD
Onder et al. [60]	25 wks; 30-minute sessions 3x/wk	Reality orientation	$n_{ex} = 70$ $n_c = 67$	Experimental: 20.2 Control: 19.9	(i) MMSE (ii) ADAS-Cog (iii) Functional status: Barthel Index, (iv) IADL (v) NPI (vi) Family caregiver outcomes: HRSD, HRSA, Caregiver Burden Inventory, SF-36	(i) Small improvement in MMSE and ADAS-COG
Loewenstein et al. [64]	12–16 weeks; 45-minute sessions 2x/wk	Cognitive rehabilitation/cognitive training	$n_{ex} = 25$ $n_c = 19$	Experimental: 23.40 Control: 24.53	(i) The face-name association task: (ii) Orientation (iii) The continuous performance test (iv) Procedural object-memory evaluation (v) Modified Making-Change-For-A-Purchase Task (vi) Balancing-A-Checkbook Task (vii) RMBPC (viii) B-ADLS (ix) CES-D (x) IQCODE	(i) Training specific improvement in orientation, face-name recall, processing speed, and making change compared to control group receiving mental stimulation

Table 2: Continued.

Study	Length and frequency	Type of stimulation	Sample	MMSE (baseline mean)	Outcome measures	Major findings
Davis et al. [65]	5 weeks; 1-hour sessions 1x/wk; home practice 30 minutes per day 6x/wk	Cognitive training	$n_{ex} = 19$ $n_c = 18$	Experimental: 21.84 Control: 22.78	(i) MMSE (ii) WMS-R logical memory (iii) WMS-R visual reproduction (iv) WAIS-R digit span (v) VSAT (vi) Controlled oral word association test (vii) Category fluency (viii) Finger taping test (ix) GDS (x) Quality of life patient	(i) Improvement in attention, recall of personal information, and face-name recall compared to mock control group (ii) Results did not extend to other neuropsychological tests or quality of life
Koltai et al. [67]	Group program: 5 wks; 1-hour sessions 1x/wk Individual program: 6 wks; 1-hour sessions 1x/wk with caregiver involvement in last 10–15 minutes	Cognitive rehabilitation/cognitive training	$n_{ex} = 14$ $n_c = 8$	Experimental: 22.9 Control: 26.6	(i) GDS and relative GDS (ii) EMQ and relative EMQ (iii) CERAD (iv) MMSE	(i) No significant differences between the experimental group and the wait-list control group (ii) Participants with insight about self-deficits perceived greater gains in memory compared to participants with no insight
Quayhagen et al. [66]	8 weeks; 1-hour sessions 5x/wk	Cognitive training	$n_{AD} = 103$ $n_c = 103$ (i) Numbers in each group (cognitive training, dyadic counseling, dual supportive seminar, and early-stage day care) not specified	Not reported	(i) Immediate memory composite: WMS-R Logical Memory 1 and visual reproduction 1, DRS (memory) (ii) Delayed memory composite: WMS logical memory 2, visual reproduction 2 (iii) Verbal fluency composite: controlled oral word association, DRS (initiation) (iv) Problem solving composite: geriatric coping schedule, DRS (conceptualization) (v) Memory and Behavior Problems Checklist (part A)	(i) Improvement in memory and communication with caregiver (ii) Other types of interventions (dual support seminar, early-stage daycare) had positive effects on communication and interactions

Table 2: Continued.

Study	Length and frequency	Type of stimulation	Sample	MMSE (baseline mean)	Outcome measures	Major findings
Cahn-Weiner et al. [71]	6 wks; 45-minute sessions 2x/wk	Memory training	$n_{ex} = 17$ $n_c = 17$	Experimental: 24.3 Control: 25.1	(i) HVLT-R (ii) BVMT-R (iii) BNT (iv) COWA (v) JLO (vi) TMT (Parts A and B) (vii) ADL questionnaire (viii) EMQ	(i) No significant effects

n_{ex}, n_c, n_{AD}: number of participants in intellectual stimulation program, control group, and group diagnosed with AD. MMSE: Mini-Mental state examination, ADAS-Cog: Alzheimer's Disease Assessment Scale-Cognitive Subscale, TMT: Trail Making Test, RBANS: Repeatable Battery for the Assessment of Neuropsychological Status Versions A (before testing) and B (after testing), QoL-AD: quality of life-Alzheimer's disease, MADRS: Montgomery-Asberg Depression Rating Scale, TFLS: Texas Functional Living Scale, NPI: Neuropsychiatric Inventory, CIBIC: Clinician's Interview-Based Impression of Change, HCS: Holden Communication Scale, CAPE-BRS: The Clifton Assessment Procedures for the Elderly-Behaviour Rating Scale, CDR: The Clinical Dementia Rating Scale, IADL: instrumental activities of daily living, HRSD: Hamilton Rating Scales for Depression, HRSA: Hamilton Rating Scales for Anxiety, SF-36: The Medical Outcomes Study 36-Item Short-Form General Health Survey, RMBPC: The Revised Memory and Behavior Problems Checklist, B-ADLS: The Bayer Activities of Daily Living Scale, CES-D: The Center for Epidemiological Studies-Depression Scale, IQCODE: the informant questionnaire of the cognitive decline in the elderly scale, WMS-R: Wechsler Memory Scale-Revised, WAIS-R: Wechsler Adult Intelligence Scale-Revised, VSAT: The Verbal Series Attention Test, GDS: Geriatric Depression Scale, EMQ: Everyday Memory Questionnaire, CERAD: Consortium to Establish a Registry for Alzheimer's Disease Test Battery, DRS: The Mattis Dementia Rating Scale, HVLT-R: Hopkins Verbal Learning Test Revised, BVMT-R: Brief Visual Spatial Memory Test Revised, BNT: Boston Naming Test, COWA: Controlled Oral Word Association Test, and JLO: Judgment of Line Orientation.

week. Assessment measures included cognitive tests and measures of quality of life, communication, behavior, global functioning, depression, and anxiety. The results indicated positive effects of CS on cognitive functioning as well as ADLs. Other studies found CS to be beneficial on measures of language [58], emotional wellbeing [58], and cognitive tests [57]. Unfortunately, not all studies found significant benefits of CS on dementia patients [59].

Reality orientation (RO) is a component of CS and focuses on orienting the individual with AD to person, place and time [52, 56]. Studies on RO in dementia indicate slight advantages on cognitive tests [60, 61]. A recent Cochrane review of fifteen randomized control trials investigated the effectiveness of RO and some CS in AD [56]. The review included 718 participants, with 407 participants in the treatment group and 311 in the control group. Intervention length varied between four weeks and 24 months, with sessions ranging from 30 to 90 minutes. Overall cognitive functioning was improved in AD patients receiving RO and CS, with some studies indicating additional positive changes to social and communicative functioning and quality of life [56].

Based on the current literature on the efficacy of CS and RO on decline in AD, it appears that both forms of intervention may provide encouraging results for slowing decline and improving quality of life [52, 56].

4.2. Cognitive Training and Cognitive Rehabilitation in Dementia. Cognitive training (CT) targets individual or multiple cognitive domains through teaching specific skills. It aims to improve functioning in the targeted area as well as the possibility of extending the improvements to more general functioning and other cognitive domains [54, 62]. Similarly, cognitive rehabilitation (CR) aims at improving daily functioning by identifying individualized strengths and weaknesses [56, 63]. Due to the significant amount of overlap between CT and CR, both interventions are sometimes combined [62].

Several reviews on CT suggest mixed outcomes in terms of effectiveness as a treatment option for AD [52, 62]. While several studies show improvement in specific cognitive domains targeted by training [64–66], others fail to report any significant changes [67] or extend results to more general functioning [65]. A Cochrane review by Clare and Woods [62] concluded that CT and CR provided no positive or negative effects on cognitive performance in AD compared to control groups. Conversely, Small and colleagues [68] found CT to have a negative impact on mood in patients with dementia and in their caregivers. A meta-analysis showed that CT had modest positive effects on various aspects of cognition, including learning, memory, executive and general functioning, and depression [55]. A randomized control trial using CR alone found that goal performance and satisfaction was improved compared to the control groups receiving relaxation therapy [63].

Another review investigated the literature on CT in preventing incident AD, preventing MCI conversion to AD, and slowing AD progression [48, 69]. The results suggested that CT may be most beneficial to healthy elderly and at risk individuals with MCI as opposed to AD treatment [48].

There is a lack of a consensus in the literature as to whether CT can ameliorate symptoms of AD [52, 62]. Although some studies show promising results for CT [55], others reveal improvement only in specific areas of cognitive training, such as learning personal information and aspects of attention [65]. CR, on the other hand, might produce more general benefits to cognitive functioning [63].

4.3. Specific Cognitive Domain Training in Dementia. Targets of intellectual stimulation can also be divided into unidomain and multidomain. While most cognitive interventions target multidomain areas of cognition and functioning, some are specific to memory training. Although some studies suggest memory rehabilitation can improve specific memory function with sufficient time and caregiver involvement [70], a randomized control study focusing on mnemonic memorization strategies found no significant difference between the treatment and control groups [71].

4.4. Comparing Interventions. Ballard and colleagues recently reviewed CT, CS, CR, and memory aids and concluded that all forms of intervention may offer modest effects, with most benefit attributed to CS [52]. In comparing CT and CS, both resulted in improvement of activities of daily living; however, only CS resulted in improvement in behavior [53, 72]. There are several reasons to explain differences in effectiveness of treatment types. There can be a significant overlap between types of intellectual stimulation, making it difficult to identify which types of interventions are most effective. The fact that some studies implementing only memory training were included in reviews of cognitive training [55] might also contribute to mixed findings in reviews of CT and cloud the effectiveness of each type of treatment. Moreover, differences in the past history and disease stages of the patients might also explain different results. Diversity in methodologies, such as sample size, variations in inclusion criteria, inconsistent outcome measures and protocols, also renders between study comparisons problematic [55]. In addition, not all studies control for medications such as cholinesterase inhibitors, which might contribute to positive effects along with stimulating activities [53].

Nonetheless, intellectual stimulation is a promising tool for slowing the progression of AD. More randomized control trials that compare generalizability of training programs, long-term effects, and rate of cognitive decline across different intervention types are needed to assess the most effective form of intellectual stimulation.

5. Socialization

AD patients' feelings of incompetence, along with societal misconceptions, may accelerate the progression of AD [73]. So far, the relevance of the social environment surrounding an individual with AD has been mostly overlooked, but the results of increased social engagement on risk of dementia open the opportunity to incorporate socialization therapies in AD.

5.1. Influence of Increased Socialization on Incident Dementia. The cognitive reserve hypothesis, as previously described [45–47], includes social engagement as an important skill set for delaying the development of AD. An increase in social engagement with the surrounding environment can be correlated with angiogenesis, synaptogenesis, and neurogenesis [74]. Fratiglioni et al. also explained the relevance of stress reduction in cognition through the stress hypothesis [74] and increased social engagement is associated with improved self-esteem [73]. The importance of social engagement in reducing the risk of AD can be further supported by the vascular hypothesis. It is important to note that vascular risk factors, which could be reduced with increased social engagement, can contribute to the pathogenesis and progression of AD [74, 75].

Table 3 showcases the importance of social engagement on the prevention of AD, there is a lack of research on the effects of social engagement on AD prognosis. Collaborative research in the fields of sociology, psychology, neuroscience, and medicine will be important in this area.

5.2. Influence of Socialization on AD Population. Many AD patients sense that their cognitive impairment isolates them from other people leading to anxiety, depression, societal withdrawal, and decreased self-confidence. Manipulating the social environment around AD patients may help them regain a sense of self-worth and a better attitude towards life. This may improve eating and exercise habits and social interactions, which may result in improved AD prognosis [73].

Shaping how cognitively normal individuals relate to AD patients can play an important role in improving patients' social environment and interactions [73]. It is extremely important that surrounding healthy individuals (friends, family members, etc.) maintain a supportive atmosphere towards AD patients to ensure that, regardless of their cognitive abilities, they have a place in society and that their identity is valued. After multiple experiences, MacRae [73] reported that married AD patients whose spouses encouraged them to live life as normally as possible, and to remain socially engaged, preserved a "positive sense of self while living with dementia." This led to healthier eating habits and increased physical exercise and participation in cognitively and socially stimulating activities, thereby improving quality of life [73].

In further support of how a positive social atmosphere can benefit individuals with AD, Keller et al. [81] analyzed how shared mealtimes can enhance social engagement. With disease progression, alterations must be made to accommodate for changes in eating conduct (difficulties with using utensils or wandering), swallowing ability, and the ability to prepare food safely. Therefore, an event that was once a traditional social occasion may become an event filled with tension, frustration, and disappointment. As a result, the social experience associated with mealtimes may become limited and possibly nonexistent. However, reports show that AD patients benefit from shared mealtimes by getting motivated through another's physical presence to improve their attentional, planning, and decision making abilities [81].

Loneliness is widely reported by patients with dementia, arising from the feeling of not having anyone to relate to, dissatisfaction with one's way of living, and social isolation. Recent studies have attempted to reduce this sense of "loneliness" and assess its effects on cognition [76]. Pitkala et al. [75] examined the effects of enhancing social stimulation on cognitive outcomes in the elderly and patients with mild dementia. Volunteers were divided into three social intervention groups, according to their preference: (1) art, inspiring activities, and discussions, (2) exercise and discussions, and (3) therapeutic writing and discussions. Within each group, they were further divided into intervention or placebo. Participants in the intervention groups improved significantly over the course of 3 months on the Alzheimer's Disease Assessment Scale (ADAS-Cog) compared to control groups. Furthermore, a health-related quality of life (HRQol) questionnaire conducted at baseline and at 12 months revealed significant improvements in quality of life in the social intervention groups [75].

Support groups are another intervention aimed to assist with the psychosocial difficulties that patients diagnosed with early-stage dementia face [82]. A clinical trial compared quality of life (QOL), depression, and family communication outcomes between an early-stage memory loss (ESML) support group and a wait-list (WL) control group [83]. The ESML condition involved 90-minute weekly sessions for 9 weeks. The WL condition did not participate in the social support groups, but received educational material from their local Alzheimer's Association group and were encouraged to contact relevant support services should any questions or concerns arise. Results showed that in comparison to control participants, ESML participants expressed better QOL and less depressive symptoms after 9 weeks. Furthermore, the improved QOL among ESML participants was associated with an improvement of cognition and family communication [83].

Results have shown that although caregivers are willing to help their loved ones; at times at a personal cost, AD caregivers have a much higher chance of being clinically depressed than age-matched controls [84, 85]. Thus, many psychosocial therapies have been explored to primarily help caregivers, which frequently lead to better care of patients. Mittelman explains that individualized counseling and involvement in caregiver support groups result in long-lasting lower caregiver distress, even at followups at one and three years later [86]. Furthermore, lower distress and depressive symptoms were observed across caregivers for patients with varying dementia severity, living conditions, and after death of the patient [86].

It appears that enhanced social interactions may decrease the risk of AD and improve patients' QOL, self-confidence, and possibly prognosis. Although it appears that socialization is important in supporting cognitive abilities in the normal elderly, further research is needed to clarify how and to what extent socialization benefits patients with AD.

Table 3: Summary of studies on the effect of socialization on incident dementia.

Study	Length and frequency	Protocol	Sample	MMSE (baseline mean)	Outcome measures	Major findings
Wilson et al. [76]	4 years; annual check up	Longitudinal clinicopathological cohort study	$n = 823$		(i) Clinical diagnosis of AD (ii) Change in measures of global cognition and specific cognitive functions	(i) Loneliness associated with cognitive decline and development of AD
Wang et al. [77]	Data collection (9 years)	Longitudinal population-based study	$n = 776$	27.3	(i) Frequency of social and leisure activities engaged 6.4 years before diagnosis (ii) Baseline MMSE (iii) MMSE of incident dementia cases	(i) Socially and mentally stimulating activity may preserve mental functioning in the elderly, reducing risk of dementia
Friedland et al. [78]		Questionnaire data collection	$n_{AD} = 193$ $n_{HC} = 358$		(i) Monthly involvement in possible 26 nonoccupational activities at early adulthood and middle adulthood	(i) AD patients are less active in midlife than HC participants
Bennet et al. [79]	6-7 years	Longitudinal, epidemiological clinicopathological cohort study	$n = 89$	25.8 (not used in analysis)	(i) Annual clinical evaluation (ii) Brain autopsy at death (iii) Social network size (number of individuals seen at least once/month)	(i) Larger social network sizes observed in participants with higher level of cognition
Fratiglioni et al. [80]	3 years	Longitudinal community-based study	$n_{HC} = 1203$	>23	(i) Social network at baseline, clinical evaluation at baseline and 3 years	(i) Limited social network ties and interaction increased risk of developing dementia

n_{HC}, n_{AD}: number of participants in healthy control group and group diagnosed with AD. MMSE: Mini-Mental State Examination.

6. Multimodal Therapy

Given that physical exercise, intellectual stimulation, and socialization have individually shown to benefit AD patients, we summarize the results of multimodal interventions, combining at least two of the three activity types.

Coelho et al. [87] found that participants who engaged in an exercise program while simultaneously completing cognitive tasks had significantly higher scores ($P < 0.001$) than the control group on the Frontal Assessment Battery, which measures frontal lobe cognitive function. Furthermore, participants in the control group demonstrated decreased executive and visuospatial abilities through lower scores on a clock drawing test. The physical exercise program consisted of aerobic, flexibility and balance exercises, and resistance training. Cognitive tasks included generating words according to specific criteria (e.g., flowers, animals) or reacting to sensory stimuli such as verbal commands. These findings suggest that there is a place for physical exercise combined with intellectual stimulation in AD management.

Arkin [88] provides further support for the use of multimodal intervention through a study of 24 AD patients engaged in exercise (aerobic and weight training), cognitive tasks (taking place before, during, and after exercise), and social activities. Compared to controls, the 4-year intervention group experienced no decline in several cognitive measures: MMSE, Clinical Dementia Rating Scale, verbal fluency, Boston Naming, and WAIS-R Comprehension. Burgener et al. [89] conducted a trial in which 24 early-AD patients received a multimodal intervention (exercise, cognitive behavioral therapy, and support group) and were compared to 19 patient control group who received attention-control educational programs. In addition to physical and behavioral outcome benefits, there was a significant difference in MMSE scores between the intervention and control groups, not present at baseline. As such, both studies suggest that multimodal intervention programs can help delay the cognitive decline characteristic of AD.

It is important to note, however, that evidence supporting multimodal intervention is not yet conclusive. A pilot study of 14 AD patients by Maci et al. [90] found that participants engaged in a multimodal program of exercise (balance, gait, and coordination), cognitive stimulation, and socialization (talking/singing with other participants) led to reduced depression and improved anxiety and quality of life. However, there were no significant between-group differences in cognition as measured by the MMSE and Frontal Assessment Battery. It is possible that behavioral improvements may have been secondary to the very small sample size. Conflicting findings such as these indicate the need for further research in this area.

While the impact of multimodal interventions (and perhaps even each intervention independently) on reducing cognitive decline in AD remains unclear, it appears that patients may benefit in other ways from physical exercise, intellectual stimulation, and socialization. More research into the effects of multimodal therapies is required.

7. Conclusions

In summary, this paper highlights key research on the effectiveness of nonpharmacological treatment options, specifically exercise, intellectual stimulation, and socialization, on the progression of AD. Based on our findings in the literature, all three intervention strategies may provide positive effects on cognition and overall wellbeing. More specifically, physical exercise appears to benefit various aspects of cognition in AD patients including stabilization of MMSE scores, and improved attention, memory and recognition, and ability to perform ADLs. It has also been demonstrated that regular exercise is helpful in reducing the risk of AD development and progression. Future studies should include a broader range of exercises to determine the most effective exercise regime for AD patients. Increased social interaction has been shown to benefit Alzheimer's patients by minimizing one's sense of loneliness, isolation, stress, and vascular factors that contribute to cognitive decline. It can also improve patients' sense of self-worth. However, limited studies exist on the benefits of socialization on cognition in the AD population. Studies focusing on these areas would help verify if a social component would provide more than simply behavioral benefits. In addition, intellectual stimulation may benefit AD patients by improving their cognition, emotional and social wellbeing as well as performance of ADLs. However, inconsistent results on the effectiveness of intellectual stimulation in delaying cognitive decline in AD patients demonstrate the need for further research.

It is necessary for future research to identify and address limitations found in the current literature. Patient recruitment can be a significant challenge in those with moderate-to-advanced AD due to the necessary comprehension levels for study completion. In addition, as dementia progresses, patients may become increasingly tired and frustrated, leading to higher attrition rates. Some of the studies do not provide adequate characterization of the enrolled population, rendering comparisons difficult. The ability to make between-study comparisons is further limited by the broad range of physical, cognitive, and social activities used in nonpharmacological therapies. Determining which nonpharmacological therapy is the most beneficial to the AD population is difficult due to the widespread and overlapping positive effects of each activity. As the goal of this paper was to provide a general overview of nonpharmacological interventions in AD, we were limited in our ability to produce statistical analysis. Therefore, a meta-analysis is suggested in order to obtain quantitative results.

Based on the literature presented in this paper, patients experience less depression and improved quality of life, ability to perform ADLs, and social relationships. Most importantly, interventions that combine physical exercise and socialization with cognitive stimulation are often highly enjoyable for patients, leading to participants expressing their approval by saying: "This has been the only thing I have found that feels like I am doing something to help myself" [89]. Thus, the aforementioned nonpharmacological therapies are recommended in AD management.

Authors' Contribution

The first three authors contributed equally to this work.

References

[1] J. L. Cummings, "Alzheimer's disease," *New England Journal of Medicine*, vol. 351, no. 1, pp. 56–67, 2004.

[2] W. Thies and L. Bleiler, "Alzheimer's disease facts and figures," *Alzheimer's and Dementia*, vol. 7, no. 2, pp. 208–244, 2011.

[3] A. L. Fitzpatrick, L. H. Kuller, D. G. Ives et al., "Incidence and prevalence of dementia in the cardiovascular health study," *Journal of the American Geriatrics Society*, vol. 52, no. 2, pp. 195–204, 2004.

[4] R. Brookmeyer, S. Gray, and C. Kawas, "Projections of Alzheimer's disease in the United States and the public health impact of delaying disease onset," *American Journal of Public Health*, vol. 88, no. 9, pp. 1337–1342, 1998.

[5] R. M. Sousa, C. P. Ferri, D. Acosta et al., "Contribution of chronic diseases to disability in elderly people in countries with low and middle incomes: a 10/66 Dementia Research Group population-based survey," *The Lancet*, vol. 374, no. 9704, pp. 1821–1830, 2009.

[6] K. E. Powell, P. D. Thompson, C. J. Caspersen, and J. S. Kendrick, "Physical activity and the incidence of coronary heart disease," *Annual Review of Public Health*, vol. 8, pp. 253–287, 1987.

[7] A. M. Kriska, S. N. Blair, and M. A. Pereira, "The potential role of physical activity in the prevention of non-insulin-dependent diabetes mellitus: the epidemiological evidence," *Exercise and Sport Sciences Reviews*, vol. 22, pp. 121–143, 1994.

[8] S. N. Blair and S. Brodney, "Effects of physical inactivity and obesity on morbidity and mortality: Current evidence and research issues," *Medicine and Science in Sports and Exercise*, vol. 31, no. 11, pp. S646–S662, 1999.

[9] I. M. Lee, "Physical activity and cancer prevention—data from epidemiologic studies," *Medicine and Science in Sports and Exercise*, vol. 35, no. 11, pp. 1823–1827, 2003.

[10] D. Bonaiuti, B. Shea, R. Iovine et al., "Exercise for preventing and treating osteoporosis in postmenopausal women," *Cochrane Database of Systematic Reviews*, no. 3, Article ID CD000333, 2002.

[11] S. N. Blair, N. N. Goodyear, L. W. Gibbons, and K. H. Cooper, "Physical fitness and incidence of hypertension in healthy normotensive men and women," *Journal of the American Medical Association*, vol. 252, no. 4, pp. 487–490, 1984.

[12] A. D. Brown, C. A. McMorris, R. S. Longman et al., "Effects of cardiorespiratory fitness and cerebral blood flow on cognitive outcomes in older women," *Neurobiology of Aging*, vol. 31, no. 12, pp. 2047–2057, 2010.

[13] P. J. Smith, J. A. Blumenthal, B. M. Hoffman et al., "Aerobic exercise and neurocognitive performance: a meta-analytic review of randomized controlled trials," *Psychosomatic Medicine*, vol. 72, no. 3, pp. 239–252, 2010.

[14] K. I. Erickson and A. F. Kramer, "Aerobic exercise effects on cognitive and neural plasticity in older adults," *British Journal of Sports Medicine*, vol. 43, no. 1, pp. 22–24, 2009.

[15] L. J. Podewils, E. Guallar, L. H. Kuller et al., "Physical activity, APOE genotype, and dementia risk: findings from the Cardiovascular Health Cognition Study," *American Journal of Epidemiology*, vol. 161, no. 7, pp. 639–651, 2005.

[16] D. Laurin, R. Verreault, J. Lindsay, K. MacPherson, and K. Rockwood, "Physical activity and risk of cognitive impairment and dementia in elderly persons," *Archives of Neurology*, vol. 58, no. 3, pp. 498–504, 2001.

[17] E. B. Larson, L. Wang, J. D. Bowen et al., "Exercise is associated with reduced risk for incident dementia among persons 65 years of age and older," *Annals of Internal Medicine*, vol. 144, no. 2, pp. 73–81, 2006.

[18] A. S. Buchman, P. A. Boyle, L. Yu, R. C. Shah, R. S. Wilson, and D. A. Bennett, "Total daily physical activity and the risk of AD and cognitive decline in older adults," *Neurology*, vol. 78, no. 17, pp. 1323–1329, 2012.

[19] N. T. Lautenschlager, K. L. Cox, L. Flicker et al., "Effect of physical activity on cognitive function in older adults at risk for Alzheimer disease: a randomized trial," *Journal of the American Medical Association*, vol. 300, no. 9, pp. 1027–1037, 2008.

[20] J. E. Ahlskog, Y. E. Geda, N. R. Graff-Radford, and R. C. Petersen, "Physical exercise as a preventive or disease-modifying treatment of dementia and brain aging," *Mayo Clinic Proceedings*, vol. 86, no. 9, pp. 876–884, 2011.

[21] M. Weih, Ü. Degirmenci, S. Kreil, and J. Kornhuber, "Physical activity and alzheimer's disease: a meta-analysis of cohort studies," *The Journal of Gerontopsychology and Geriatric Psychiatry*, vol. 23, no. 1, pp. 17–20, 2010.

[22] L. Palleschi, F. Vetta, E. De Gennaro et al., "Effect of aerobic training on the cognitive performance of elderly patients with senile dementia of Alzheimer type," *Archives of Gerontology and Geriatrics*, vol. 22, no. 1, pp. 47–50, 1996.

[23] G. F. Lindenmuth and B. Moose, "Improving cognitive abilities of elderly Alzheimer's patients with intense exercise therapy," *American Journal of Alzheimer's Care and Related Disorders and Research*, vol. 5, no. 1, pp. 31–33, 1990.

[24] P. Heyn, B. C. Abreu, and K. J. Ottenbacher, "The effects of exercise training on elderly persons with cognitive impairment and dementia: a meta-analysis," *Archives of Physical Medicine and Rehabilitation*, vol. 85, no. 10, pp. 1694–1704, 2004.

[25] C. A. Alessi, E. Yoon, J. F. Schnelle, N. R. Al-Samanai, and P. A. Cruise, "A randomized trial of a combined physical activity and environmental intervention in nursing home residents: do sleep and agitation improve?" *Journal of the American Geriatrics Society*, vol. 47, no. 7, pp. 784–791, 1999.

[26] L. Teri, L. E. Gibbons, S. M. McCurry et al., "Exercise plus behavioral management in patients with Alzheimer disease: a randomized controlled trial," *Journal of the American Medical Association*, vol. 290, no. 15, pp. 2015–2022, 2003.

[27] G. Kemoun, M. Thibaud, N. Roumagne et al., "Effects of a physical training programme on cognitive function and walking efficiency in elderly persons with dementia," *Dementia and Geriatric Cognitive Disorders*, vol. 29, no. 2, pp. 109–114, 2010.

[28] D. K. Miu, S. L. Szeto, and Y. F. Mak, "A randomised controlled trial on the effect of exercise on physical, cognitive and affective function in dementia subjects," *Asian Journal of Gerontology and Geriatrics*, vol. 3, no. 1, pp. 8–16, 2008.

[29] K. E. Roach, R. M. Tappen, N. Kirk-Sanchez, C. L. Williams, and D. Loewenstein, "A randomized controlled trial of an activity specific exercise program for individuals with Alzheimer disease in long-term care settings," *Journal of Geriatric Physical Therapy*, vol. 34, no. 2, pp. 50–56, 2011.

[30] Y. Rolland, F. Pillard, A. Klapouszczak et al., "Exercise program for nursing home residents with Alzheimer's disease: a 1-year randomized, controlled trial," *Journal of the American Geriatrics Society*, vol. 55, no. 2, pp. 158–165, 2007.

[31] M. Steinberg, J. M. Sheppard Leoutsakos, L. J. Podewills, and C. G. Lyketsos, "Evaluation of a home-based exercise program in the treatment of Alzheimer's disease: the Maximizing Independence in Dementia (MIND) study," *International Journal of Geriatric Psychiatry*, vol. 24, no. 7, pp. 680–685, 2009.

[32] M. Venturelli, R. Scarsini, and F. Schena, "Six-month walking program changes cognitive and ADL performance in patients with Alzheimer," *American Journal of Alzheimer's Disease and other Dementias*, vol. 26, no. 5, pp. 381–388, 2011.

[33] A. Vreugdenhil, J. Cannell, A. Davies, and G. Razay, "A community-based exercise programme to improve functional ability in people with Alzheimer's disease: a randomized controlled trial," *Scandinavian Journal of Caring Sciences*, vol. 26, no. 1, pp. 12–19, 2012.

[34] L. Yágüez, K. N. Shaw, R. Morris, and D. Matthews, "The effects on cognitive functions of a movement-based intervention in patients with Alzheimer's type dementia: a pilot study," *International Journal of Geriatric Psychiatry*, vol. 26, no. 2, pp. 173–181, 2011.

[35] R. C. Cassilhas, V. A. R. Viana, V. Grassmann et al., "The impact of resistance exercise on the cognitive function of the elderly," *Medicine and Science in Sports and Exercise*, vol. 39, no. 8, pp. 1401–1407, 2007.

[36] T. Liu-Ambrose, M. G. Donaldson, Y. Ahamed et al., "Otago home-based strength and balance retraining improves executive functioning in older fallers: a randomized controlled trial," *Journal of the American Geriatrics Society*, vol. 56, no. 10, pp. 1821–1830, 2008.

[37] B. S. Oken, D. Zajdel, S. Kishiyama et al., "Randomized, controlled, six-month trial of yoga in healthy seniors: effects on cognition and quality of life," *Alternative Therapies in Health and Medicine*, vol. 12, no. 1, pp. 40–47, 2006.

[38] S. J. Colcombe, K. I. Erickson, P. E. Scalf et al., "Aerobic exercise training increases brain volume in aging humans," *Journals of Gerontology*, vol. 61, no. 11, pp. 1166–1170, 2006.

[39] M. W. Voss, R. S. Prakash, K. I. Erickson et al., "Plasticity of brain networks in a randomized intervention trial of exercise training in older adults," *Froniers in Aging Neuroscience*, vol. 2, p. 32, 2010.
[40] J. M. Burns, B. B. Cronk, H. S. Anderson et al., "Cardiorespiratory fitness and brain atrophy in early Alzheimer disease," *Neurology*, vol. 71, no. 3, pp. 210–216, 2008.
[41] R. A. Honea, G. P. Thomas, A. Harsha et al., "Cardiorespiratory fitness and preserved medial temporal lobe volume in alzheimer disease," *Alzheimer Disease and Associated Disorders*, vol. 23, no. 3, pp. 188–197, 2009.
[42] R. S. Wilson, D. A. Bennett, J. L. Bienias et al., "Cognitive activity and incident AD in a population-based sample of older persons," *Neurology*, vol. 59, no. 12, pp. 1910–1914, 2002.
[43] M. Valenzuela and P. Sachdev, "Can cognitive exercise prevent the onset of dementia? systematic review of randomized clinical trials with longitudinal follow-up," *American Journal of Geriatric Psychiatry*, vol. 17, no. 3, pp. 179–187, 2009.
[44] T. F. Hughes, C. C. H. Chang, J. Vander Bilt, and M. Ganguli, "Engagement in reading and hobbies and risk of incident dementia: the MoVIES project," *American Journal of Alzheimer's Disease and other Dementias*, vol. 25, no. 5, pp. 432–438, 2010.
[45] Y. Stern, "What is cognitive reserve? Theory and research application of the reserve concept," *Journal of the International Neuropsychological Society*, vol. 8, no. 3, pp. 448–460, 2002.
[46] N. Scarmeas and Y. Stern, "Cognitive reserve and lifestyle," *Journal of Clinical and Experimental Neuropsychology*, vol. 25, no. 5, pp. 625–633, 2003.
[47] N. Scarmeas and Y. Stern, "Cognitive reserve: implications for diagnosis and prevention of Alzheimer's disease," *Current Neurology and Neuroscience Reports*, vol. 4, no. 5, pp. 374–380, 2004.
[48] L. Mowszowski, J. Batchelor, and S. L. Naismith, "Early intervention for cognitive decline: can cognitive training be used as a selective prevention technique?" *International Psychogeriatrics*, vol. 22, no. 4, pp. 537–548, 2010.
[49] Y. Stern, S. Albert, M. X. Tang, and W. Y. Tsai, "Rate of memory decline in AD is related to education and occupation: cognitive reserve?" *Neurology*, vol. 53, no. 9, pp. 1942–1947, 1999.
[50] E. P. Helzner, N. Scarmeas, S. Cosentino, F. Portet, and Y. Stern, "Leisure activity and cognitive decline in incident Alzheimer disease," *Archives of Neurology*, vol. 64, no. 12, pp. 1749–1754, 2007.
[51] K. A. Treiber, M. C. Carlson, C. Corcoran et al., "Cognitive stimulation and cognitive and functional decline in Alzheimer's disease: the Cache County Dementia Progression Study," *The Journals of Gerontology, Series B*, vol. 66, no. 4, pp. 416–425, 2011.
[52] C. Ballard, Z. Khan, H. Clack, and A. Corbett, "Nonpharmacological treatment of Alzheimer disease," *Canadian Journal of Psychiatry*, vol. 56, no. 10, pp. 589–595, 2011.
[53] F. Yu F, K. M. Rose, S. C. Burgener et al., "Cognitive training for early-stage Alzheimer's disease and dementia," *Journal of Gerontological Nursing*, vol. 35, no. 3, pp. 23–29, 2009.
[54] A. F. Kurz, S. Leucht, and N. T. Lautenschlager, "The clinical significance of cognition-focused interventions for cognitively impaired older adults: a systematic review of randomized controlled trials," *International Psychogeriatrics*, vol. 23, no. 9, pp. 1364–1375, 2011.
[55] D. I. Sitzer, E. W. Twamley, and D. V. Jeste, "Cognitive training in Alzheimer's disease: a meta-analysis of the literature," *Acta Psychiatrica Scandinavica*, vol. 114, no. 2, pp. 75–90, 2006.
[56] B. Woods, E. Aguirre, A. E. Spector, and M. Orrell, "Cognitive stimulation to improve cognitive functioning in people with dementia," *Cochrane Database of Systematic Reviews*, no. 2, Article ID CD005562, 2012.
[57] A. Spector, L. Thorgrimsen, B. Woods et al., "Efficacy of an evidence-based cognitive stimulation therapy programme for people with dementia: randomised controlled trial," *British Journal of Psychiatry*, vol. 183, pp. 248–254, 2003.
[58] S. B. Chapman, M. F. Weiner, A. Rackley, L. S. Hynan, and J. Zientz, "Effects of cognitive-communication stimulation for Alzheimer's disease patients treated with donepezil," *Journal of Speech, Language, and Hearing Research*, vol. 47, no. 5, pp. 1149–1163, 2004.
[59] V. C. Buschert, U. Friese, S. J. Teipel et al., "Effects of a newly developed cognitive intervention in amnestic mild cognitive impairment and mild Alzheimer's disease: a pilot study," *Journal of Alzheimer's Disease*, vol. 25, no. 4, pp. 679–694, 2011.
[60] G. Onder, O. Zanetti, E. Giacobini et al., "Reality orientation therapy combined with cholinesterase inhibitors in Alzheimer's disease: randomised controlled trial," *British Journal of Psychiatry*, vol. 187, pp. 450–455, 2005.
[61] A. Spector, S. Davies, B. Woods, and M. Orrell, "Reality orientation for dementia: a systematic review of the evidence of effectiveness from randomized controlled trials," *Gerontologist*, vol. 40, no. 2, pp. 206–212, 2000.
[62] L. Clare and B. Woods, "Cognitive rehabilitation and cognitive training for early-stage Alzheimer's disease and vascular dementia," *Cochrane Database of Systematic Reviews*, no. 4, Article ID CD003260, 2008.
[63] L. Clare, D. E. J. Linden, R. T. Woods et al., "Goal-oriented cognitive rehabilitation for people with early-stage alzheimer disease: a single-blind randomized controlled trial of clinical efficacy," *American Journal of Geriatric Psychiatry*, vol. 18, no. 10, pp. 928–939, 2010.
[64] D. A. Loewenstein, A. Acevedo, S. J. Czaja, and R. Duara, "Cognitive rehabilitation of mildly impaired Alzheimer disease patients on cholinesterase inhibitors," *American Journal of Geriatric Psychiatry*, vol. 12, no. 4, pp. 395–402, 2004.
[65] R. N. Davis, P. J. Massman, and R. S. Doody, "Cognitive intervention in Alzheimer disease: a randomized placebo-controlled study," *Alzheimer Disease and Associated Disorders*, vol. 15, no. 1, pp. 1–9, 2001.
[66] M. P. Quayhagen, M. Quayhagen, R. R. Corbeil et al., "Coping with dementia: evaluation of four nonpharmacologic interventions," *International Psychogeriatrics*, vol. 12, no. 2, pp. 249–265, 2000.
[67] D. C. Koltai, K. A. Welsh-Bohmer, and D. E. Schmechel, "Influence of anosognosia on treatment outcome among dementia patients," *Neuropsychological Rehabilitation*, vol. 11, no. 3-4, pp. 455–475, 2001.
[68] G. W. Small, P. V. Rabins, P. P. Barry et al., "Diagnosis and treatment of Alzheimer disease and related disorders: consensus statement of the American Association for Geriatric Psychiatry, the Alzheimer's Association, and the American Geriatrics Society," *Journal of the American Medical Association*, vol. 278, no. 16, pp. 1363–1371, 1997.
[69] L. J. Thal, "Prevention of Alzheimer disease," *Alzheimer Disease and Associated Disorders*, vol. 20, no. 2, pp. S97–S99, 2006.
[70] L. P. De Vreese, M. Neri, M. Fioravanti, L. Belloi, and O. Zanetti, "Memory rehabilitation in Alzheimer's disease: a review of progress," *International Journal of Geriatric Psychiatry*, vol. 16, no. 8, pp. 794–809, 2001.

[71] D. A. Cahn-Weiner, P. F. Malloy, G. W. Rebok, and B. R. Ott, "Results of a randomized placebo-controlled study of memory training for mildly impaired Alzheimer's disease patients," *Applied Neuropsychology*, vol. 10, no. 4, pp. 215–223, 2003.

[72] E. Farina, F. Mantovani, R. Fioravanti et al., "Evaluating two group programmes of cognitive training in mild-to-moderate AD: is there any difference between a "global" stimulation and a "cognitive-specific" one?" *Aging and Mental Health*, vol. 10, no. 3, pp. 211–218, 2006.

[73] H. MacRae, "Self and other: the importance of social interaction and social relationships in shaping the experience of early-stage Alzheimer's disease," *Journal of Aging Studies*, vol. 25, pp. 445–456, 2011.

[74] L. Fratiglioni, S. Paillard-Borg, and B. Winblad, "An active and socially integrated lifestyle in late life might protect against dementia," *The Lancet Neurology*, vol. 3, no. 6, pp. 343–353, 2004.

[75] K. H. Pitkala, P. Routasalo, H. Kautiainen, H. Sintonen, and R. S. Tilvis, "Effects of socially stimulating group intervention on lonely, older people's cognition: a randomized, controlled trial," *American Journal of Geriatric Psychiatry*, vol. 19, no. 7, pp. 654–663, 2011.

[76] R. S. Wilson, K. R. Krueger, S. E. Arnold et al., "Loneliness and risk of Alzheimer disease," *Archives of General Psychiatry*, vol. 64, no. 2, pp. 234–240, 2007.

[77] H. X. Wang, A. Karp, B. Winblad, and L. Fratiglioni, "Late-life engagement in social and leisure activities is associated with a decreased risk of dementia: a longitudinal study from the Kungsholmen Project," *American Journal of Epidemiology*, vol. 155, no. 12, pp. 1081–1087, 2002.

[78] R. P. Friedland, T. Fritsch, K. A. Smyth et al., "Patients with Alzheimer's disease have reduced activities in midlife compared with healthy control-group members," *Proceedings of the National Academy of Sciences of the United States of America*, vol. 98, no. 6, pp. 3440–3445, 2001.

[79] D. A. Bennett, J. A. Schneider, Y. Tang, S. E. Arnold, and R. S. Wilson, "The effect of social networks on the relation between Alzheimer's disease pathology and level of cognitive function in old people: a longitudinal cohort study," *The Lancet Neurology*, vol. 5, no. 5, pp. 406–412, 2006.

[80] L. Fratiglioni, H. X. Wang, K. Ericsson, M. Maytan, and B. Winblad, "Influence of social network on occurrence of dementia: a community-based longitudinal study," *The Lancet*, vol. 355, no. 9212, pp. 1315–1319, 2000.

[81] H. H. Keller, L. S. Martin, S. Dupuis, R. Genoe, H. G. Edward, and C. Cassolato, "Mealtimes and being connected in the community-based dementia context," *Dementia*, vol. 9, no. 2, pp. 191–213, 2010.

[82] R. G. Logsdon, S. M. McCurry, and L. Teri, "Evidence-based interventions to improve quality of life for individuals with dementia," *Alzheimer's Care Today*, vol. 8, no. 4, pp. 309–318, 2007.

[83] R. G. Logsdon, K. C. Pike, S. M. McCurry et al., "Early-stage memory loss support groups: outcomes from a randomized controlled clinical trial," *Journals of Gerontology*, vol. 65, no. 6, pp. 691–697, 2010.

[84] M. S. Mittelman, S. H. Ferris, E. Shulman et al., "A comprehensive support program: effect on depression in spouse-caregivers of AD patients," *Gerontologist*, vol. 35, no. 6, pp. 792–802, 1995.

[85] M. S. Mittelman, C. Epstein, and A. Pierzchala, *Counselling the Alzheimer's Caregiver: A Resource for Health Care Professionals*, American Medical Association, Chicago, Ill, USA, 2001.

[86] M. S. Mittelman, D. L. Roth, D. W. Coon, and W. E. Haley, "Sustained benefit of supportive intervention for depressive symptoms in caregivers of patients with Alzheimer's disease," *American Journal of Psychiatry*, vol. 161, no. 5, pp. 850–856, 2004.

[87] F. G. M. Coelho, L. P. Andrade, R. V. Pedroso et al., "Multimodal exercise intervention improves frontal cognitive functions and gait in Alzheimer's disease: a controlled trial," *Geriatriatrics and Gerontolology International*. In press.

[88] S. Arkin, "Language-enriched exercise plus socialization slows cognitive decline in Alzheimer's disease," *American Journal of Alzheimer's Disease and other Dementias*, vol. 22, no. 1, pp. 62–77, 2007.

[89] S. C. Burgener, Y. Yang, R. Gilbert, and S. Marsh-Yant, "The effects of a multimodal intervention on outcomes of persons with early-stage dementia," *American Journal of Alzheimer's Disease and other Dementias*, vol. 23, no. 4, pp. 382–394, 2008.

[90] T. Maci, F. Le Pira, G. Quattrocch, S. Di Nuovo, V. Perciavalle, and M. Zappia, "Physical and cognitive stimulation in Alzheimer disease. The GAIA Project: a pilot study," *American Journal of Alzheimers Disease and other Dementias*, vol. 27, no. 2, pp. 107–113, 2012.

Elevated Serum Carboxymethyl-Lysine, an Advanced Glycation End Product, Predicts Severe Walking Disability in Older Women: The Women's Health and Aging Study I

Kai Sun,[1] Richard D. Semba,[1] Linda P. Fried,[2] Debra A. Schaumberg,[3] Luigi Ferrucci,[4] and Ravi Varadhan[5]

[1] *Department of Ophthalmology, Johns Hopkins University School of Medicine, Baltimore, MD 21287, USA*
[2] *Mailman School of Public Health, Columbia University, New York, NY 10032, USA*
[3] *Division of Preventive Medicine, Department of Medicine, Brigham and Women's Hospital, Harvard Medical School, Boston, MA 02215, USA*
[4] *Longitudinal Studies Section, Clinical Research Branch, National Institute on Aging, Baltimore, MD 21225, USA*
[5] *Department of Medicine, Johns Hopkins University School of Medicine, Baltimore, MD 21287, USA*

Correspondence should be addressed to Richard D. Semba, rdsemba@jhmi.edu

Academic Editor: Benedetta Bartali

Advanced glycation end products (AGEs) have been implicated in the pathogenesis of sarcopenia. Our aim was to characterize the relationship between serum carboxymethyl-lysine (CML), a major circulating AGE, and incident severe walking disability (inability to walk or walking speed <0.4 m/sec) over 30 months of followup in 394 moderately to severely disabled women, ≥ 65 years, living in the community in Baltimore, Maryland (the Women's Health and Aging Study I). During followup, 154 (26.4%) women developed severe walking disability, and 23 women died. Women in the highest quartile of serum CML had increased risk of developing of severe walking disability in a multivariate Cox proportional hazards model, adjusting for age and other potential confounders. Women with elevated serum CML are at an increased risk of developing severe walking disability. AGEs are a potentially modifiable risk factor. Further work is needed to establish a causal relationship between AGEs and walking disability.

1. Introduction

Mobility difficulties are common among older adults and are associated with poor quality of life [1], increased need for care, and are predictive of death [2–4]. Understanding the processes that lead to disability is important in order to develop strategies to prevent or delay disability in older adults. Lifestyle factors that may influence the pathway to disability include diet. Diet has been incompletely characterized in relation to the development of disability. Recent studies suggest that advanced glycation end products (AGEs), which are active biomolecules formed by the non-enzymatic covalent binding of sugars with proteins and other molecules, may be related to muscle strength and physical performance [5, 6]. The western diet is high in AGEs, which are formed in high concentrations in foods that are prepared at high temperatures. Thus, some foods are considered an important exogenous source of AGEs. AGEs are thought to be absorbed in the process of digestion, circulate in the blood, and can be deposited in different organs and tissues [7].

Sarcopenia, or loss of muscle strength and muscle mass, is an important factor underlying mobility difficulties such as slow walking speed in older adults [8]. Older adults have increased cross-linking of collagen and deposition of AGEs in skeletal muscle [9]. In aging animals, cross-linking of collagen is associated with increased muscle stiffness, reduced muscle function [10, 11], and accumulation of AGEs

[12]. AGEs may also play a role in sarcopenia through upregulation of inflammation and endothelial dysfunction in the microcirculation of skeletal muscle through the receptor for AGEs, or RAGE [13]. AGE-induced cross-linking of is collagen elevated in older adults [14] and has been shown to increase the stiffness of human articular cartilage [15].

The relationship between circulating AGEs and the development of disability has not been characterized in older adults. We hypothesized that women with elevated serum carboxymethyl-lysine (CML), an advanced glycation end product, had an increased risk of developing severe walking disability. To address this hypothesis, we examined the relationship between serum CML concentrations and severe walking disability among older women living in the community.

2. Subjects and Methods

2.1. Study Population. Subjects in this study were women who participated in the Women's Health and Aging Study I (WHAS I), a population-based study designed to evaluate the causes and course of physical disability in older disabled women living in the community. WHAS I participants were recruited from an age-stratified random sample of women aged 65 years and older selected from Medicare enrollees residing in 12 contiguous-zip-code areas in Baltimore [16]. Women were screened to identify self-reported physical disability that was categorized into four domains. The domains of disability were ascertained in a 20- to 30-minute home interview that included questions related to (1) mobility and exercise tolerance, that is, walking for a quarter of a mile, walking up 10 steps without resting, getting in and out of bed or chairs; (2) upper extremity function, that is, raising your arms up over your head, using your fingers to grasp or handle, lifting or carrying something as heavy as ten pounds; (3) higher functioning tasks (a subset of instrumental activities of daily living, not including heavy housework, that is, using the telephone, doing light housework, preparing your own meals, shopping for personal items); (4) basic self-care tasks (a subset of nonmobility dependent activities of daily living, i.e., bathing or showering, dressing, eating, using the toilet). WHAS I enrolled the one-third most disabled women ages 65 and older, those with disability in two or more domains. Of the 1409 women who met study eligibility criteria, 1002 agreed to participate in the study in 1992. There were no major differences in sociodemographic or reported health characteristics between eligible participants and those who declined to participate [16].

At the 12-month follow-up visit (as baseline for the present study), 879 women returned for followup, of which 580 received a blood draw. CML was measured in 531 women who had walking speed measurements available. 119 had severe walking disability, 412 did not have severe walking disability, and of whom 394 who had at least one follow-up visit thereafter were included in the present study. Laboratory measurements of serum CML were done at the 12-month follow-up visit rather than at enrollment because of a greater availability of serum aliquots from this visit.

2.2. Data Collection. Standardized questionnaires were administered in the participant's home by trained interviewers. Race was assessed in a questionnaire as black, white, or other, current smoking as yes or no, and education as 0–8, 9–11, 12, or more than 12 years as the highest level of formal education achieved. Two weeks later, a trained registered full-time study nurse practitioner examined each study participant in her home, using a standardized evaluation of physical performance and physical exam. Approximately 75% of women also consented to phlebotomy performed during a separate visit by a trained phlebotomist who followed a standardized protocol. The definitions for the chronic diseases reported in this study were adjudicated by WHAS coinvestigators based on standardized algorithms that combined information from the questionnaire, physical examination, and physician contact [16]. The Mini-Mental State Examination (MMSE) was administered at enrollment. Further details on the methods and sampling design of the WHAS studies are published elsewhere [16].

The participant was asked to walk over a 4-meter course for each follow-up visit. Participants were instructed to stand with both feet at the starting line and to start walking after a specific verbal command. Timing began when the command was given. In this test, the subject could use a cane, a walker, or other walking aid, but not the aid of another person. The times to complete the first meter and the entire path were recorded. The test was repeated three times, twice at the woman's usual pace, and once at her fastest possible pace. The speed of the faster of the two usual-pace walks was used in the analyses. The length of the walk expressed in meters divided by the time in seconds was used to calculate the average walking speed [16]. Women were categorized as having severe walking disability based upon being unable to walk or having a walking speed < 0.4 m/sec [17]. The 0.4 m/sec cut-off point was approximately at the top of the lowest quartile in the WHAS population at baseline [18] and has been shown to predict functional dependence [19]. Demographic characteristics, self-rated health, and information about appetite and eating were measured in the WHAS questionnaires. Chronic diseases were adjudicated by WHAS coinvestigators based on the questionnaire, physical examination, and physician contact [16]. Vital status was determined through matching with the National Death Index from the 12-month follow-up visit, 1993–96 through the end of 2000. The study protocol was adherent to the Declaration of Helsinki. The Johns Hopkins University Institutional Review Board approved the study protocol, and written informed consent was obtained from all participants.

2.3. Laboratory Studies. Nonfasting blood samples were obtained by venipuncture between 9 AM and 2 PM. Blood samples were delivered to Quest Diagnostics Laboratories (formerly Ciba-Corning Laboratories, Baltimore, MD) on the day of blood drawing for complete blood count and creatinine measurements. Serum creatinine was measured using the Jaffe method. Processing, aliquoting, and freezing were carried out at the Core Genetics Laboratory of the Johns

Hopkins University School of Medicine following a standardized protocol. Blood samples were stored continuously at −70°C until the time of analyses of serum carboxymethyl-lysine (CML). CML is well characterized, circulating AGE, and one of the dominant AGEs in tissue proteins [20]. CML was measured using a competitive ELISA (AGE-CML ELISA, Microcoat, Penzberg, Germany) [21]. This assay has been validated [22], is specific, and shows no cross-reactivity with other compounds [21]. Measurements were performed in duplicate according to the protocol of the manufacturers, and the results were averaged. The within-assay and between-assay coefficients of variation for serum CML were 3% and 4%, respectively.

2.4. Statistical Analysis. Continuous variables were compared using Wilcoxon rank-sum test. Categorical variables were compared using chi-square tests. Body mass index (BMI) was categorized as underweight (<18.5 kg/m^2), normal range (18.5–24.9 kg/m^2), overweight (≥25–29.9 kg/m^2) and obese (≥30 kg/m^2) [23]. An MMSE score of <24 was defined as cognitive impairment [24]. Renal insufficiency was defined as estimated glomerular filtration rate of <60 mL/min/1.73 m^2 using the Modification of Diet in Renal Disease equation of Levey and colleagues [25]. Plasma CML was divided into quartiles, and the cut-off between quartiles was 452.6, 558.8, and 689.1 ng/mL. Grouped-time Cox proportional hazards models [26] were used to examine the associations between serum AGEs and the risk of developing severe walking disability because severe walking disability was determined at six-month intervals. The length of followup in longitudinal analyses was 30 months. Women who died, or refused further participation, or were lost to followup after a follow-up visit were censored according to their severe walking disability status at their last visit in the study.

During the 30 months following the original 12-month follow-up visit (as the baseline for the present study), there were 23 patients who died, 9 of them died after developing severe walking disability whereas 14 of them died with no severe walking disability until the last follow-up visit. Cox proportional hazards models were used to examine the associations between CML and risk of developing severe walking disability. As a highly significant association between slow walking speed and death has been previously described [27], it is a reasonable assumption that some women developed severe walking disability prior to death. For those who died without developing severe walking disability, first, the multiple imputation technique was used to impute the data and then the complete data was analyzed; second, the severe walking disability status known data only was analyzed with weighting by inverse probability weighting (IPW) on the data [28]; finally, two sensitivity analyses were applied to validate those two methods dealing with the incomplete data: (1) treating all missing data because of death as severe walking disability-free; (2) treating the missing data as severe walking disability developed [29]. The statistical program used was SAS 9.1 (SAS Institute, Cary, NC). The level of significance used in this study was $P < 0.05$.

3. Results

There were 394 women who did not have severe walking disability at baseline had serum carboxymethyl-lysine (CML) measurements available, and had at least one followup involved in the present study. One hundred fifty-four (26.4%) of the women developed severe walking disability during followup with an overall rate of severe walking disability of 14.8 per 100 person-years. The characteristics of women who did and did not develop severe walking disability during followup are shown in Table 1. Women who developed severe walking disability were older and more likely to be affected by congestive heart failure, peripheral artery disease, and diabetes. There were no significant differences between women who developed and those who did not develop walking disability by race, education, current smoking, MMSE score, body mass index, hypertension, coronary artery disease, stroke, depression, osteoarthritis, chronic obstructive pulmonary disease, and renal insufficiency. Compared with the group of lower three quartiles of CML, the patients in the group of highest quartile of CML were more likely to develop severe walking disability.

Univariate Cox proportional hazards models were used to examine the relationship between demographic and health characteristics and the development of severe walking disability (Table 2). Highest quartile of CML, older age, congestive heart failure, peripheral artery disease, and diabetes mellitus were associated with an increased risk of developing severe walking disability. Multivariable Cox proportional hazards model that adjusted for age, congestive heart failure, peripheral artery disease, diabetes mellitus, and renal insufficiency are shown in four scenarios (Table 3).

4. Discussion

The present study shows that older community-dwelling women with elevated serum CML are at increased risk of developing severe walking disability. These findings are consistent with a previous, cross-sectional study which showed that elevated plasma CML was associated with slow walking speed in older community-dwelling men and women [6]. The present study extends these findings and shows that elevated CML is an independent predictor of the development of severe walking disability.

These observations are consistent with the hypothesis that AGEs play a role in sarcopenia [13]. Increased AGEs may contribute to increased stiffness in muscle tissue and reduced viscoelastic properties of muscle and thus impair muscle function [9]. Collagen is the main structural component of the interstitial space of skeletal muscle and provides elasticity when muscles contract [30]. Aging muscle is characterized by an increase in pyridinium cross-linking of collagen, which is enzymatically derived, and the non-enzymatic accumulation of cross-linking AGEs. In adults without diabetes, the concentration of pentosidine, a major AGE in tissues, was found in skeletal muscle at greater than two times concentration in older compared with younger adults [9].

TABLE 1: Characteristics of women who developed and did not develop severe walking disability in the women's health and aging study I ($N = 394$).

Characteristic	Incident severe walking disability ($n = 104$)	No incident severe walking disability ($n = 290$)	P
Age category (years) (%)			
≤69	17.3	26.2	
70–74.9	22.1	27.6	
75–79.9	14.4	22.1	0.0005
80–84.9	14.4	10.0	
85–89.9	23.1	12.1	
≥90	8.7	2.0	
Race (white) (%)	69.2	75.5	0.21
Education < 12 years (%)	62.1	60.3	0.75
Current smoking (%)	15.4	10.0	0.14
Body mass index (kg/m^2) (%)			
<18.5	3.2	2.8	
18.5–24.9	27.7	23.2	0.83
25.0–29.9	35.1	36.8	
≥30	34.0	37.2	
MMSE score < 24 (%)	15.4	9.7	0.11
Hypertension (%)	57.7	56.2	0.79
Coronary heart disease (%)	24.0	22.1	0.68
Congestive heart failure (%)	14.4	7.2	0.029
Peripheral artery disease (%)	26.0	15.5	0.018
Stroke (%)	1.0	2.8	0.29
Diabetes mellitus (%)	23.1	11.7	0.005
Depression (%)	15.4	11.4	0.29
Chronic obstructive pulmonary disease (%)	29.8	25.9	0.44
Renal insufficiency (%)	58.4	52.5	0.30
Osteoarthritis (%)	57.7	53.5	0.46
CML highest quartile (%)	33.7	22.4	0.02

Tendons transfer the forces generated by muscles to bone and have elastic properties that affect the muscle tendon complex. AGEs are deposited in tendons and can affect their structural properties. In a rabbit model, cross-linking of collagen by nonenzymatic glycation increased the structural stiffness of Achilles tendon [31]. In humans, there was a sevenfold difference in concentrations of pentosidine in the patellar tendon in older compared with younger men [14]. Elevated AGEs are also associated with increased bone rigidity [32] which is thought to occur through cross-linking of collagen [33].

AGEs may also affect skeletal muscle and tendons through upregulation of inflammation via binding with RAGE [34]. The carboxymethyl-lysine (CML) adduct of AGEs has been identified as a signal-transducing ligand for RAGE, both *in vitro* and *in vivo* [35]. Ligand binding with RAGE triggers the induction of increased reactive oxygen species, activation of NADPH oxidase, and upregulation of inflammation through NF-κB and other signaling pathways [36, 37]. Inflammatory mediators that are upregulated through AGE and the NF-κB pathway include TNF-α, IL-6, and C-reactive protein [38].

A limitation of this study is that the results cannot necessarily be extrapolated to men or to less disabled women in the community. There are many different AGEs, and in the present study, CML was the only AGE that was measured in serum. However, other studies have shown that circulating CML has a moderate correlation with other AGEs in the blood such as pentosidine and methylglyoxal derivatives [39]. Serum CML concentrations show a moderate correlation with dietary intake of AGEs in older adults [39]. Serum CML concentrations have been reported to vary with dietary intake of AGEs [40], but these findings have not been corroborated by others [41, 42].

5. Conclusions

Older women with elevated plasma CML, an advanced glycation end product, had greater risk of developing severe walking disability. Whether modification of dietary intake of

TABLE 2: Univariate Cox proportional hazard models for demographic and health characteristics and incidence of severe walking disability in the women's health and aging study I ($N = 394$).

Characteristic	Univariate H.R.	95% C.I.	P
Age (years)			
≤69	1.00	—	—
70–74.9	1.18	0.64, 2.18	0.60
75–79.9	0.93	0.46, 1.86	0.83
80–84.9	1.96	0.99, 3.89	0.05
85–89.9	2.35	1.28, 4.34	0.006
≥90	5.04	2.25, 11.26	<0.0001
Race (white)	0.76	0.50, 1.16	0.19
Education < 12 years	1.12	0.75, 1.67	0.58
Current smoking	1.59	0.93, 2.70	0.09
Body mass index (kg/m^2)[1]			
<18.5	0.98	0.30, 3.25	0.98
18.5–24.9	1.00	—	—
25.0–29.9	0.75	0.45, 1.26	0.28
≥30	0.75	0.45, 1.27	0.28
MMSE < 24	1.59	0.93, 2.70	0.09
Hypertension	1.04	0.71, 1.54	0.84
Coronary heart disease	1.09	0.70, 1.71	0.70
Congestive heart failure	1.87	1.08, 3.24	0.03
Peripheral artery disease	1.74	1.12, 2.72	0.01
Stroke	0.46	0.06, 3.31	0.44
Chronic obstructive pulmonary disease	1.21	0.80, 1.85	0.37
Diabetes mellitus	1.79	1.13, 2.85	0.01
Depression	1.21	0.70, 2.09	0.49
Renal insufficiency	1.18	0.79, 1.75	0.42
Osteoarthritis	1.22	0.83, 1.81	0.32
CML highest quartile	1.68	1.11, 2.52	0.01

[1] For body mass index, 18.5–24.9 kg/m^2 was used as the reference category.

TABLE 3: Multivariate cox proportional hazard models for serum CML and development of severe walking disability, ($N = 394$)[1].

Scenario	H.R.[2]	95% C.I.	P
(1) All women with missing data had multiple simulations to impute severe walking disability status prior to death.	1.63	1.06, 2.49	0.03
(2) Inverse probability weighting method (IPW)	1.56	1.04, 2.36	0.03
(3) All women with missing data treated as censored, that is, no severe walking disability prior to death.	1.46	0.95, 2.23	0.08
(4) All women with missing data treated as developing severe walking disability prior to death.	1.54	1.04, 2.29	0.03

[1] All models adjusted for age, congestive heart failure, peripheral artery disease, diabetes mellitus, and renal insufficiency.
[2] Highest quartile of serum CML versus lower three quartiles.

AGEs can influence the pathway to disability in older adults is not known.

References

[1] E. J. Groessl, R. M. Kaplan, W. J. Rejeski et al., "Health-related quality of life in older adults at risk for disability," *American Journal of Preventive Medicine*, vol. 33, no. 3, pp. 214–218, 2007.

[2] J. Woo, S. C. Ho, and A. L. Yu, "Walking speed and stride length predicts 36 months dependency, mortality, and institutionalization in chinese aged 70 and older," *Journal of the American Geriatrics Society*, vol. 47, no. 10, pp. 1257–1260, 1999.

[3] Y. Rolland, V. Lauwers-Cances, M. Cesari, B. Vellas, M. Pahor, and H. Grandjean, "Physical performance measures as predictors of mortality in a cohort of community-dwelling older French women," *European Journal of Epidemiology*, vol. 21, no. 2, pp. 113–122, 2006.

[4] A. B. Newman, E. M. Simonsick, B. L. Naydeck et al., "Association of long-distance corridor walk performance with mortality, cardiovascular disease, mobility limitation, and disability," *Journal of the American Medical Association*, vol. 295, no. 17, pp. 2018–2026, 2006.

[5] M. Dalal, L. Ferrucci, K. Sun, J. Beck, L. P. Fried, and R. D. Semba, "Elevated serum advanced glycation end products and poor grip strength in older community-dwelling women," *Journals of Gerontology A*, vol. 64, no. 1, pp. 132–137, 2009.

[6] R. D. Semba, S. Bandinelli, K. Sun, J. M. Guralnik, and L. Ferrucci, "Relationship of an advanced glycation end product, plasma carboxymethyl-lysine, with slow walking speed in older adults: the InCHIANTI study," *European Journal of Applied Physiology*, vol. 108, no. 1, pp. 191–195, 2010.

[7] R. D. Semba, E. J. Nicklett, and L. Ferrucci, "Does accumulation of advanced glycation end products contribute to the aging phenotype?" *Journals of Gerontology A*, vol. 65, no. 9, pp. 963–975, 2010.

[8] F. Lauretani, C. R. Russo, S. Bandinelli et al., "Age-associated changes in skeletal muscles and their effect on mobility: an operational diagnosis of sarcopenia," *Journal of Applied Physiology*, vol. 95, no. 5, pp. 1851–1860, 2003.

[9] J. M. Haus, J. A. Carrithers, S. W. Trappe, and T. A. Trappe, "Collagen, cross-linking, and advanced glycation end products in aging human skeletal muscle," *Journal of Applied Physiology*, vol. 103, no. 6, pp. 2068–2076, 2007.

[10] M. E. T. Willems, G. R. Miller, and W. T. Stauber, "Force deficits after stretches of activated rat muscle-tendon complex with reduced collagen cross-linking," *European Journal of Applied Physiology*, vol. 85, no. 5, pp. 405–411, 2001.

[11] C. Ducomps, P. Mauriège, B. Darche, S. Combes, F. Lebas, and J. P. Doutreloux, "Effects of jump training on passive mechanical stress and stiffness in rabbit skeletal muscle: role of collagen," *Acta Physiologica Scandinavica*, vol. 178, no. 3, pp. 215–224, 2003.

[12] L. M. Snow, N. A. Fugere, and L. V. Thompson, "Advanced glycation end-product accumulation and associated protein modification in type II skeletal muscle with aging," *Journals of Gerontology A*, vol. 62, no. 11, pp. 1204–1210, 2007.

[13] G. W. Payne, "Effect of inflammation on the aging microcirculation: impact on skeletal muscle blood flow control," *Microcirculation*, vol. 13, no. 4, pp. 343–352, 2006.

[14] C. Couppé, P. Hansen, M. Kongsgaard et al., "Mechanical properties and collagen cross-linking of the patellar tendon in old and young men," *Journal of Applied Physiology*, vol. 107, no. 3, pp. 880–886, 2009.

[15] N. Verzijl, J. deGroot, C. Ben Zaken et al., "Crosslinking by advanced glycation end products increases the stiffness of the collagen network in human articular cartilage: a possible mechanism through which age is a risk factor for osteoarthritis," *Arthritis and Rheumatology*, vol. 46, no. 1, pp. 114–123, 2002.

[16] J. M. Guralnik, L. P. Fried, E. M. Simonsick, J. D. Kasper, and M. E. Lafferty, *The Women's Health and Aging Study: Health and Social Characteristics of Older Women with Disability*, National Institute on Aging, Bethesda, Md, USA, 1995, NIH Publication No. 95-4009.

[17] L. Ferrucci, T. B. Harris, J. M. Guralnik et al., "Serum IL-6 level and the development of disability in older persons," *Journal of the American Geriatrics Society*, vol. 47, no. 6, pp. 639–646, 1999.

[18] T. Rantanen, J. M. Guralnik, L. Ferrucci et al., "Coimpairments as predictors of severe walking disability in older women," *Journal of the American Geriatrics Society*, vol. 49, no. 1, pp. 21–27, 2001.

[19] M. E. Tinetti, S. K. Inouye, T. M. Gill, and J. T. Doucette, "Shared risk factors for falls, incontinence, and functional dependence: unifying the approach to geriatric syndromes," *Journal of the American Medical Association*, vol. 273, no. 17, pp. 1348–1353, 1995.

[20] S. Reddy, J. Bichler, K. J. Wells-Knecht, S. R. Thorpe, and J. W. Baynes, "Nε-(carboxymethyl)lysine is a dominant advanced glycation end product (AGE) antigen in tissue proteins," *Biochemistry*, vol. 34, no. 34, pp. 10872–10878, 1995.

[21] B. O. Boehm, S. Schilling, S. Rosinger et al., "Elevated serum levels of NE-carboxymethyl-lysine, an advanced glycation end product, are associated with proliferative diabetic retinopathy and macular oedema," *Diabetologia*, vol. 47, no. 8, pp. 1376–1379, 2004.

[22] X. Zhang, M. Frischmann, R. Kientsch-Engel et al., "Two immunochemical assays to measure advanced glycation end-products in serum from dialysis patients," *Clinical Chemistry and Laboratory Medicine*, vol. 43, no. 5, pp. 503–511, 2005.

[23] M. F. Folstein, S. E. Folstein, and P. R. McHugh, "Mini-Mental State' a practical method for grading the cognitive state of patients for the clinician," *Journal of Psychiatric Research*, vol. 12, no. 3, pp. 189–198, 1975.

[24] World Health Organization, "Physical status: the use and interpretation of anthropometry," Report of a WHO Expert Committee, World Health Organization, Geneva, Switzerland, 1995, WHO Technical Report Series 854.

[25] A. S. Levey, J. P. Bosch, J. B. Lewis, T. Greene, N. Rogers, and D. Roth, "A more accurate method to estimate glomerular filtration rate from serum creatinine: a new prediction equation," *Annals of Internal Medicine*, vol. 130, no. 6, pp. 461–470, 1999.

[26] R. L. Prentice and L. A. Gloeckler, "Regression analysis of grouped survival data with application to breast cancer data," *Biometrics*, vol. 34, no. 1, pp. 57–67, 1978.

[27] A. B. Newman, E. M. Simonsick, B. L. Naydeck et al., "Association of long-distance corridor walk performance with mortality, cardiovascular disease, mobility limitation, and disability," *Journal of the American Medical Association*, vol. 295, no. 17, pp. 2018–2026, 2006.

[28] J. Carpenter and M. Kenward, "A comparison of multiple imputation and inverse probability weighting for analyses with missing data," *Statistical Methods in Medical Research*, vol. 16, no. 3, pp. 199–218, 2007.

[29] C. Dufouil, C. Brayne, and D. Clayton, "Analysis of longitudinal studies with death and drop-out: a case study," *Statistics in Medicine*, vol. 23, no. 14, pp. 2215–2226, 2004.

[30] L. E. Gosselin, C. Adams, T. A. Cotter, R. J. Mccormick, and D. P. Thomas, "Effect of exercise training on passive stiffness in locomotor skeletal muscle: role of extracellular matrix," *Journal of Applied Physiology*, vol. 85, no. 3, pp. 1011–1016, 1998.

[31] G. K. Reddy, "Cross-linking in collagen by nonenzymatic glycation increases the matrix stiffness in rabbit Achilles tendon," *Experimental Diabesity Research*, vol. 5, no. 2, pp. 143–153, 2004.

[32] D. Vashishth, G. J. Gibson, J. I. Khoury, M. B. Schaffler, J. Kimura, and D. P. Fyhrie, "Influence of nonenzymatic glycation on biomechanical properties of cortical bone," *Bone*, vol. 28, no. 2, pp. 195–201, 2001.

[33] C. J. Hernandez, S. Y. Tang, B. M. Baumbach et al., "Trabecular microfracture and the influence of pyridinium and non-enzymatic glycation-mediated collagen cross-links," *Bone*, vol. 37, no. 6, pp. 825–832, 2005.

[34] G. Basta, "Receptor for advanced glycation endproducts and atherosclerosis: from basic mechanisms to clinical implications," *Atherosclerosis*, vol. 196, no. 1, pp. 9–21, 2008.

[35] T. Kislinger, C. Fu, B. Huber et al., "N^{ε}-(carboxymethyl)lysine adducts of proteins are ligands for receptor for advanced glycation end products that activate cell signaling pathways and modulate gene expression," *The Journal of Biological Chemistry*, vol. 274, no. 44, pp. 31740–31749, 1999.

[36] A. Bierhaus, T. Illmer, M. Kasper et al., "Advanced glycation end product (AGE)-mediated induction of tissue factor in cultured endothelial cells is dependent on RAGE," *Circulation*, vol. 96, no. 7, pp. 2262–2271, 1997.

[37] J. Li and A. M. Schmidt, "Characterization and functional analysis of the promoter of RAGE, the receptor for advanced glycation end products," *The Journal of Biological Chemistry*, vol. 272, no. 26, pp. 16498–16506, 1997.

[38] A. Bierhaus, S. Schiekofer, M. Schwaninger et al., "Diabetes-associated sustained activation of the transcription factor nuclear factor-κB," *Diabetes*, vol. 50, no. 12, pp. 2792–2808, 2001.

[39] J. Uribarri, W. Cai, M. Peppa et al., "Circulating glycotoxins and dietary advanced glycation endproducts: two links to inflammatory response, oxidative stress, and aging," *Journals of Gerontology A*, vol. 72, no. 4, pp. 427–433, 2007.

[40] M. Negrean, A. Stirban, B. Stratmann et al., "Effects of low- and high-advanced glycation endproduct meals on macro- and microvascular endothelial function and oxidative stress in patients with type 2 diabetes mellitus," *American Journal of Clinical Nutrition*, vol. 85, no. 5, pp. 1236–1243, 2007.

[41] R. D. Semba, A. Ang, S. Talegawkar et al., "Dietary intake associated with serum versus urinary carboxymethyl-lysine, a major advanced glycation end product, in adults: the Energetics Study," *European Journal of Clinical Nutrition*, vol. 66, no. 1, pp. 3–9, 2012.

[42] K. Šebeková, M. Krajčovičová-Kudláčková, R. Schinzel, V. Faist, J. Klvanová, and A. Heidland, "Plasma levels of advanced glycation end products in healthy, long-term vegetarians and subjects on a western mixed diet," *European Journal of Nutrition*, vol. 40, no. 6, pp. 275–281, 2001.

5

Self-Assessment of Adherence to Medication: A Case Study in Campania Region Community-Dwelling Population

Enrica Menditto,[1] Francesca Guerriero,[1] Valentina Orlando,[1] Catherine Crola,[2,3] Carolina Di Somma,[4] Maddalena Illario,[2,3] Donald E. Morisky,[5] and Annamaria Colao[6]

[1] *Center of Pharmacoeconomics (CIRFF), Federico II University, 80131 Naples, Italy*
[2] *Research and Development Board, Federico II University Hospital, 80131 Naples, Italy*
[3] *Translational Medical Sciences (DISMET), Federico II University, 80131 Naples, Italy*
[4] *IRCCS SDN, 80131 Naples, Italy*
[5] *Department of Community Health Sciences, UCLA Fielding School of Public Health, Los Angeles, CA 90095-1772, USA*
[6] *Department of Clinical Medicine and Surgery, Federico II University, 80131 Naples, Italy*

Correspondence should be addressed to Enrica Menditto; enrica.menditto@unina.it

Academic Editor: F. R. Ferraro

Objectives. The aim of the study was to assess self-reported medication adherence measure in patients selected during a health education and health promotion focused event held in the Campania region. The study also assessed sociodemographic determinants of adherence. *Methods.* An interviewer assisted survey was conducted to assess adherence using the Italian version of the 8-item Morisky Medication Adherence Scale (MMAS-8). Participants older than 18 years were interviewed by pharmacists while waiting for free-medical checkup. *Results.* A total of 312 participants were interviewed during the Health Campus event. A total of 187 (59.9%) had low adherence to medications. Pearson's bivariate correlation showed positive association between the MMAS-8 score and gender, educational level and smoking ($P < 0.05$). A multivariable analysis showed that the level of education and smoking were independent predictors of adherence. Individuals with an average level of education (odds ratio (OR), 2.21, 95% confidence interval (CI), 1.08–4.52) and nonsmoker (odds ratio (OR) 1.87, 95% confidence interval (CI), 1.04–3.35) were found to be more adherent to medication than those with a lower level of education and smoking. *Conclusion.* The analysis showed very low prescription adherence levels in the interviewed population. The level of education was a relevant predictor associated with that result.

1. Introduction

Medication adherence is a growing concern to healthcare systems as nonadherence to pharmacotherapy has been associated with adverse outcomes and higher costs of care.

Medication nonadherence is likely to grow as the population ages and as patients need to take more medications to treat chronic conditions. Several studies highlighted that the levels of adherence to treatment in patients with chronic diseases are inadequate showing rates that do not exceed 50%. Adherence and persistence to drug treatment represent the key factors necessary to gain a significant reduction in morbidity and mortality and to optimize the use of financial resources, but these aspects are widely underestimated in clinical practice and by patients [1–5]. The World Health Organization (WHO) estimates that the cost of nonadherence to drug therapy amounts to 125 million euros per year in Europe [6].

The approaches used to assess medication adherence include direct or indirect methods. Indirect methods include patient interviews, pill counts, refill records, and measurement of health outcomes. However, the most practical approach to apply in clinical practice is patient self-report. The advantages of assessing medication adherence by self-report included simplicity, speed, and viability of use [7]. The Morisky Medication Adherence Scale (MMAS-8) is one of the most commonly used self-reporting methods [8, 9].

In addition, the MMAS-8 provides information on behaviors associated with low adherence that may be unintentional (e.g., forgetfulness) or intentional (e.g., stopped taking medication(s) without telling the doctor, because they felt worse when they took it). Identification of these behaviors can facilitate tailoring of interventions to specific patient issues and is strongly related to concordance [7, 10].

Currently there are many studies evaluating the degree of adherence to treatment in patients with specific diseases [7, 11–13], while there seems to be a lack in the literature related to adherence to treatment in the general population.

The purpose of the current analysis was to evaluate adherence to medication in the general population during a prevention-related event held in Campania region (Southern Italy). The interview was carried out by administering the Italian version MMAS-8 questionnaire.

2. Materials and Methods

2.1. Setting. The prevention-related event was organized by the Health Campus, a nonprofit organization. It was established to carry out a continuous activity of dissemination and promotion of prevention through specific clinical screening and educational initiatives. The study is part of a larger activity that started in 2010 to assess the health status of the general population of the Campania Region, by providing free consultation, visits, and diagnostics for people coming to the outdoor hospital held in different public squares of Campania region during popular events [14].

The Health Campus focuses its energy and resources primarily on two major objectives: first, to provide specialist visits for disease prevention and early detection of risks to the health of Campania citizens; second, to promote dissemination of a culture of prevention that encourages a change in lifestyle for healthy living.

The Health Campus events periodically set up a disease prevention "Field Clinic," where early diagnosis tests are offered to the general public free of charge. Thus the public is encouraged to undergo specialist examinations and is informed about health risks and good practice habits to adopt for early diagnosis and screening.

The Health Campus is typically set up during large, popular events or at the request of public and/or private organizations.

2.2. Study Design. A cross sectional assisted interview survey was conducted by pharmacists on a population group selected during the Health Campus event held in Naples in April 2013 during the America's Cup.

People who were attending the event and were interested to undergo clinical evaluation and/or to take the opportunity of the available screening services, upon arrival, were selected as eligible if they were 18 years or older and taking at least one medication for at least one chronic condition. While waiting to receive a medical checkup, they were invited to the assessment of medication adherence and were interviewed by pharmacists. All participants provided their written informed consent to the study that was conducted in line with the Helsinki declaration for human studies.

The information collected included demographic data (i.e., age and gender), level of education (referred to Italian education system), smoking habit, number of drugs taken, and type of chronic disease present such as hypertension, diabetes, heart failure, COPD, renal failure, and osteoporosis. Self-reported adherence was assessed using the Italian validated version of the Morisky Medication Adherence Scale (MMAS-8) [15]. Use of the MMAS is protected by US copyright laws. Permission for use is required. This scale has been validated and used in many languages [12, 15, 16]. It consists of eight items that address specific behavior regarding medication assumption and both intentional and unintentional adherence (questionnaire used for interview is reported as Supplementary Material).

Scores on the Morisky Medication Adherence Scale can range from 0 to 8, scores < 6 reflecting low adherence, scores $\geq 6 < 8$ reflecting medium adherence, and scores $= 8$ reflecting high adherence [17].

In this study, none of the interviewed participants reported high adherence on the Morisky scale, so the dependent variable of patient adherence was dichotomized into 2 groups: low adherence (scores < 6) versus medium adherence (scores ≥ 6) [18].

The MMAS provides information on behaviors associated with low adherence that may be unintentional (e.g., forgetfulness) or intentional (e.g., stopped taking medication(s) without telling the doctor, because they felt worse when they took it) [7]. The MMAS-8 is divided into 4 items that assess intentional nonadherence and 4 items that assess unintentional nonadherence. We divided participants with low adherence into two categories: intentional nonadherent when majority of answers provided indicate a behavior that is not related to forgetfulness and unintentional nonadherent when majority of answers provided indicate a behavior that is related to forgetfulness.

2.3. Statistical Analyses. Baseline characteristics of the study population were analyzed using descriptive statistics and their degree of adherence, chi square test, and Student's t-test were used where appropriate. Pearson's correlation was used to assess bivariate association between adherence score and participant characteristic.

Additionally, associations between adherence and covariates were evaluated after accounting for other variables and predictors using logistic regression. The initial model included gender, smoking, and educational level. Factors were then sequentially eliminated from the multivariate model until only factors significant at the level of $P < 0.05$ remained in the final model. All analyses were performed using SPSS software version 17.1 for Windows (SPSS Inc., Chicago, IL, USA).

3. Results

312 patients were interviewed during the Health Campus event. The mean age was 61.8 (SD ±11.1) years. 57.4% of participants were women.

The characteristics of the analyzed population and the results of univariate association between low adherence on the Morisky scale and patient-reported factors are reported in Table 1.

TABLE 1: Univariate association between low adherence on the Morisky scale and patient-reported factors.

	Low adherence N = 187 (59.9%)	Medium adherence N = 125 (40.1%)	Total N = 312 (100.0%)	P value
Age group				0.58
Mean (±SD)	62.0 (11.4)	61.7 (10.8)	61.8 (11.1)	
18–60	75 (58.1)	54 (41.9)	129 (100.0)	
≥60	112 (61.2)	71 (38.8)	183 (100.0)	
Gender				0.03
Male	89 (66.9)	44 (33.1)	133 (100.0)	
Female	98 (54.7)	81 (45.3)	179 (100.0)	
Educational level				0.01
Primary school graduation	34 (68.0)	16 (32.0)	50 (100.0)	
Secondary school graduation	65 (69.9)	28 (30.1)	93 (100.0)	
High school graduation	55 (50.0)	55 (50.0)	110 (100.0)	
Degree graduation	33 (55.9)	26 (44.1)	59 (100.0)	
Number of medications				0.62
Mean (±SD)	2.33 (1.6)	2.15 (1.5)	2.26 (1.58)	
1	77 (56.6)	59 (43.4)	136 (100.0)	
2-3	71 (60.7)	46 (39.3)	117 (100.0)	
4-5	21 (67.7)	10 (32.3)	31 (100.0)	
≥6	18 (64.3)	10 (35.7)	28 (100.0)	
Smoking				0.03
No	136 (56.7)	104 (43.3)	240 (100.0)	
Yes	51 (70.8)	21 (29.2)	72 (100.0)	
Number of diseases				0.08
Mean (±SD)	1.58 (0.87)	1.46 (0.64)	1.53 (0.78)	
1	111 (59.4)	76 (40.6)	187 (100.0)	
2	52 (55.9)	41 (44.1)	93 (100.0)	
≥3	24 (75)	8 (25)	32 (100.0)	
Heart failure				0.58
No	171 (60.4)	112 (39.6)	283 (100.0)	
Yes	16 (55.2)	13 (44.8)	29 (100.0)	
COPD				0.35
No	183 (59.6)	124 (40.4)	307 (100.0)	
Yes	4 (80.0)	1 (20.0)	5 (100.0)	
Gastritis				0.42
No	172 (59.3)	118 (40.7)	290 (100.0)	
Yes	15 (68.2)	7 (31.8)	22 (100.0)	
Renal failure				0.68
No	185 (60.1)	123 (39.9)	308 (100.0)	
Yes	2 (50.0)	2 (50.0)	4 (100.0)	
Osteoporosis				0.15
No	168 (58.7)	118 (41.3)	286 (100.0)	
Yes	19 (73.1)	7 (26.9)	26 (100.0)	
Diabetes mellitus				0.51
No	163 (59.3)	112 (40.7)	275 (100.0)	
Yes	24 (64.9)	13 (35.1)	37 (100.0)	
Hypertension				0.76
No	87 (60.8)	56 (39.2)	143 (100.0)	
Yes	100 (59.2)	69 (40.8)	169 (100.0)	

18.9% of patients have a degree graduation, 35.3% of patients had high school graduation whereas 29.8% of patients attended secondary school graduation, and 16.0% finished the primary schools.

A total of 40.1% of patients had 2 or more diseases. More specifically, patients with hypertension were 169 (54.2%); 37 (11.9%) had type II diabetes; 29 (9.3%) had heart failure; 26 (8.3%) had osteoporosis; 22 (7.1%) had gastritis; 5 (1.6%) had COPD; and 4 (1.3%) had renal failure. A total of 37.5% of patients took from 2 to 3 drugs and 59.9% of patients have at least one disease. A total of 76.9% of patients were nonsmoking.

In the overall population, 59.9% of participants demonstrated low adherence and 40.1% medium adherence. Nobody showed high adherence. The mean score for the medication adherence scale was 4.95 (±1.52). Table 1 shows the characteristics of the population and the significant results ($P < 0.05$) of the univariate analyses examining the associations between scores on the Morisky scale and patient-reported factors.

Considering the frequency distribution of the MMAS-8 items, 42.6% of patients answered that they forgot to take their medicines, 47.1% of patients had problems taking their medicines in the last two weeks, 21.8% of patients have stopped taking their medicines without telling their doctor, 55.4% of patients stated that when they travel they forgot to bring along their medication, 20.2% of patients stated that when they feel like their condition is under control, they stop taking their medication, and 18.3% of patients felt hassled about sticking to their treatment plan. In conclusion, 19.9% of patients have difficulty remembering to take all their medications.

A total of 60.9% of nonadherent participants were intentional, 13.4% of nonadherent subjects were unintentional, and 25.7% of nonadherent participants did not fall within either category.

The number of medications prescribed, age, and number of diseases are not significant.

However, educational level, smoking habit, and gender were statistically significant ($P = 0.01$; 0.03; 0.03, resp.) (Table 1).

Univariate analysis showed that males have a higher risk of being low adherent than women (odds ratio (OR) 1.67, 95% confidence interval (CI), 1.05–2.66); the risk of being nonadherent to treatment for smokers is about double compared to nonsmokers (odds ratio (OR) 0.54, 95% confidence interval (CI) 0.30–0.95).

Only 2 factors remained as significant independent predictors of high adherence after logistic regression adjustment: level of education ($P = 0.03$) and smoking habit ($P = 0.03$) (Table 2).

People with high school graduation (odds ratio (OR), 2.21, 95% confidence interval (CI), 1.08–4.52) and nonsmokers (odds ratio (OR) 1.87, 95% confidence interval (CI), 1.04–3.35) are more adherent to treatment than those with lower education and smokers (Table 2).

TABLE 2: Association between adherence score with educational level and other significant variables in the regression analysis.

Variables	Odds ratio	IC 95%	P value
Gender			
Female	Reference		
Male	0.65	0.39–1.06	0.08
Smoker	Reference		
Nonsmoker	1.87	1.04–3.35	0.03
Educational level			
Primary school graduation	Reference		
Secondary school graduation	1.01	0.47–2.17	0.98
High school graduation	2.21	1.08–4.52	0.03
Degree graduation	1.63	0.74–3.62	0.23

4. Discussion

To the best of our knowledge, this is the first survey about adherence to medication that was carried out during a prevention event, among a population selected at the community level.

Previous studies on adherence have mostly been restricted to specific clinical populations, a specific disease, and/or a single treatment and the relevance of the outcomes to prescription drug users in general has been unclear [19]. Patient compliance to drug therapy is one of the most relevant issues in clinical practice as the success of a therapeutic intervention depends on the actual patient adherence to therapy. The noncompliance to treatment has direct consequences such as the distortion of the effectiveness of the treatment [20]. Furthermore, several observational studies raised many concerns about undertreatment in current clinical practice, because it leads to an increase in the number of hospitalizations and consequently an increase of the cost for the health system [21].

In industrialized countries, adherence to treatment by patients with chronic diseases is about 50% [22]. Our results are in line, showing 59.9% of low adherence to medications.

The main causes of poor adherence are the lack of motivation of the patients as well as low average education level, limited awareness about health, and the lack of perception of risk arising from treatment discontinuation [11]. This is in line with our results that showed that low level of education is a predictor of low adherence.

Moreover different studies indicate that 30% of the interviewed participants claim forgetfulness as the reason for their nonadherence, thus making it a prominent reason for nonadherence [23].

Using the MMAS-8, we were able to identify intentional and unintentional behaviors that cause low adherence [7]. About 42.6% of respondents say they do not take their medication regularly due to forgetfulness and 21.8% stop their treatment without speaking to their doctor. Intentional nonadherence indicates a lack of understanding and misconceptions regarding the chronicity of a health condition. This behavior can be related to lack of concordance, intended as the fact that the "prescriber and patient should come to an agreement about the regimen that the patient will take" [10]. Taking medications continuously and according to the instructions of the physician is an important aspect of drug treatment. This aspect, however, does not seem to be considered by the patients: our analysis showed that no more than 40.1% of patients have a medium level of adherence.

The interview was carried out by pharmacists. Several studies showed that interventions by pharmacists, often as a part of the care team, jointly with clinicians, have been found to be effective in improving medication adherence [24, 25]. However in Italy pharmacists are not sufficiently involved in adherence-related activities, despite the fact that pharmacists are the last point of contact with the patient before beginning the use of the medications [26]. Strategies should be formulated to achieve greater involvement of pharmacists in promoting adherence [27]. For this reason we chose to involve the pharmacist in the administration of the questionnaire as a way to improve awareness about adherence-related issues among pharmacists as well.

The European Innovation Partnership A1 Action Group on Active and Healthy Ageing, in 2012, has implemented joint initiatives between various European countries to improve the quality of the prescription and adherence to treatment [28]. Many intervention strategies that are currently being discussed among partners are aimed to promote coordinated and multidisciplinary intervention by involving all major stakeholders (general practitioners and specialists, pharmacists, nurses, family, health authorities, and pharmaceutical industry). The present initiative is part of the strategy carried out by the EIP-AHA A1 Action Group and provides preliminary data that might be useful for the further focused interventions.

4.1. Limitations of the Study. This study has some obvious limitations. Participation in this study was voluntary and, as a result, there may have been a selection bias. Population has not been selected on the basis of specific diseases or according to the number of medications prescribed. Nevertheless we assume that to be a minor limitation as the study was not aimed to assess adherence in specific conditions. Our results give a first overview about level of adherence and predictive factors. A larger population could provide more robust results. The assessment of adherence in our study was based on self-reporting. Questionnaires are a self-reporting tool that is relatively simple and economical to use, but it could overestimate the rate of medication adherence [29, 30].

5. Conclusion

In conclusion, we provided information about adherence levels in a population selected among participants to a prevention-related event. The analysis showed that adherence levels were mostly low. We found that a factor that could be associated with low levels of adherence was level of education which in turn is related to inadequate health literacy. Initiatives to raise awareness of the issue are needed as well as dissemination of the fundamental principles underlying control strategies of nonadherence to therapy. Performing such initiatives requires a *collective*, joint effort that involves different categories of stakeholders, from patient to health care providers and policy makers, whose role may be different depending upon the kind of initiative and health system organization.

Conflict of Interests

None of the authors had any potential conflict of interests including any financial, personal, or other relationships with other people or organizations since three years of the beginning of the submitted work that could inappropriately influence, or be perceived to influence, their work.

Acknowledgments

Use of the ©MMAS is protected by US copyright laws. Permission for use is required. A license agreement is available from Donald E. Morisky, ScD, ScM, MSPH, Professor, Department of Community Health Sciences, UCLA School of Public Health, 650 Charles E. Young Drive South, Los Angeles, CA 90095-1772, dmorisky@ucla.edu. The authors would like to thank Salvatore Riegler for his support during the revision of the paper.

References

[1] T. Wilke, S. Müller, and D. E. Morisky, "Toward identifying the causes and combinations of causes increasing the risks of nonadherence to medical regimens: combined results of two German self-report surveys," *Value in Health*, vol. 14, no. 8, pp. 1092–1100, 2011.

[2] R. Busse, M. Blümel, D. Scheller-Kreinsen, and A. Zentner, *Tackling Chronic Disease in Europe. Strategies, Interventions and Challenges*, Observatory Studies Series no. 20, 2010.

[3] J. K. Lee, K. A. Grace, and A. J. Taylor, "Effect of a pharmacy care program on medication adherence and persistence, blood pressure, and low-density lipoprotein cholesterol: a randomized controlled trial," *The Journal of the American Medical Association*, vol. 296, no. 21, pp. 2563–2571, 2006.

[4] L. Osterberg and T. Blaschke, "Adherence to medication," *The New England Journal of Medicine*, vol. 353, no. 5, pp. 487–497, 2005.

[5] M. C. Sokol, K. A. McGuigan, R. R. Verbrugge, and R. S. Epstein, "Impact of medication adherence on hospitalization risk and healthcare cost," *Medical Care*, vol. 43, no. 6, pp. 521–530, 2005.

[6] E. Sabaté, Ed., *Adherence to Long-Term Therapies: Evidence for Action*, World Health Organization, Geneva, Switzerland, 2003.

[7] M. Krousel-Wood, T. Islam, L. S. Webber, R. N. Re, D. E. Morisky, and P. Muntner, "New medication adherence scale versus pharmacy fill rates in seniors with hypertension," *American Journal of Managed Care*, vol. 15, no. 1, pp. 59–66, 2009.

[8] T. Xi, P. Isha, and C. Jongwha, "Review of the four item Morisky Medication Adherence Scale (MMAS-4) and eight item Morisky Medication Adherence Scale (MMAS-8)," *Innovations in Pharmacy*, vol. 5, no. 3, article 165, 2014.

[9] A. D. Oliveira-Filho, J. A. Barreto-Filho, S. J. F. Neves, and D. P. de Lyra, "Association between the 8-item Morisky Medication adherence Scale (MMAS-8) and blood pressure control,"

Arquivos Brasileiros de Cardiologia, vol. 99, no. 1, pp. 649–658, 2012.

[10] J. K. Aronson, “Compliance, concordance, adherence,” *British Journal of Clinical Pharmacology*, vol. 63, no. 4, pp. 383–384, 2007.

[11] D. E. Morisky, A. Ang, M. Krousel-Wood, and H. J. Ward, “Predictive validity of a medication adherence measure in an outpatient setting,” *The Journal of Clinical Hypertension*, vol. 10, no. 5, pp. 348–354, 2008.

[12] J. Yan, L.-M. You, Q. Yang et al., “Translation and validation of a Chinese version of the 8-item Morisky medication adherence scale in myocardial infarction patients,” *Journal of Evaluation in Clinical Practice*, vol. 20, no. 4, pp. 311–317, 2014.

[13] K. Reynolds, H. N. Viswanathan, C. D. O’Malley et al., “Psychometric properties of the osteoporosis-specific morisky medication adherence scale in postmenopausal women with osteoporosis newly treated with bisphosphonates,” *Annals of Pharmacotherapy*, vol. 46, no. 5, pp. 659–670, 2012.

[14] http://www.campussalute.it/.

[15] G. Fabbrini, G. Abbruzzese, P. Barone et al., “Adherence to anti-Parkinson drug therapy in the ‘rEASON’ sample of Italian patients with Parkinson’s disease: the linguistic validation of the Italian version of the ‘morisky medical adherence scale-8 items’,” *Neurological Sciences*, vol. 34, no. 11, pp. 2015–2022, 2013.

[16] H. K. Al-Qazaz, M. A. Hassali, A. A. Shafie, S. A. Sulaiman, S. Sundram, and D. E. Morisky, “The eight-item Morisky Medication Adherence Scale MMAS: translation and validation of the Malaysian version,” *Diabetes Research and Clinical Practice*, vol. 90, no. 2, pp. 216–221, 2010.

[17] D. E. Morisky, A. Ang, M. Krousel-Wood, and H. J. Ward, “Predictive validity of a medication adherence measure in an outpatient setting,” *Journal of Clinical Hypertension*, vol. 10, no. 5, pp. 348–354, 2008.

[18] M. Krousel-Wood, T. Islam, P. Muntner et al., “Association of depression with antihypertensive medication adherence in older adults: cross-sectional and longitudinal findings from CoSMO,” *Annals of Behavioral Medicine*, vol. 40, no. 3, pp. 248–257, 2010.

[19] L. Thunander Sundbom and K. Bingefors, “Women and men report different behaviours in, and reasons for medication non-adherence: a nationwide Swedish survey,” *Pharmacy Practice*, vol. 10, no. 4, pp. 207–221, 2012.

[20] D. E. Morisky, C. K. Malotte, P. Choi et al., “A patient education program to improve adherence rate with antitubercolosisi drug regimen,” *Health Education Wuarterly*, vol. 17, pp. 253–268, 2011.

[21] B. Hovstadius and G. Petersson, “Non-adherence to drug therapy and drug acquisition costs in a national population—a patient-based register study,” *BMC Health Services Research*, vol. 11, article 326, 2011.

[22] J. Dunbar-Jacob, J. A. Erlen, E. A. Schlenk, C. M. Ryan, S. M. Sereika, and W. M. Doswell, “Adherence in chronic disease,” *Annual Review of Nursing Research*, vol. 18, pp. 48–90, 2000.

[23] E. J. Unni and K. B. Farris, “Unintentional non-adherence and belief in medicines in older adults,” *Patient Education and Counseling*, vol. 83, no. 2, pp. 265–268, 2011.

[24] P. C. Lim and K. Lim, “Evaluation of a pharmacist-managed diabetes medication therapy adherence clinic,” *Pharmacy Practice*, vol. 8, no. 4, pp. 250–254, 2010.

[25] E. C. Chumney and L. C. Robinson, “The effects of pharmacist interventions on patients with polypharmacy,” *Pharmacy Practice*, vol. 4, no. 3, pp. 103–109, 2006.

[26] N. Fikri-Benbrahim, V. García-Cárdenas, L. Sáez-Benito, M. A. Gastelurrutia, and M. J. Faus, “Adherence: a review of education, research, practice and policy in Spain,” *Pharmacy Practice*, vol. 7, no. 3, pp. 125–138, 2009.

[27] L. S. Haugbølle and H. Herborg, “Adherence to treatment: practice, education and research in Danish community pharmacy,” *Pharmacy Practice*, vol. 7, no. 4, pp. 185–194, 2009.

[28] http://ec.europa.eu/research/innovation-union/index_en.cfm?section=active-healthy-ageing.

[29] E. Vermeire, H. Hearnshaw, P. van Royen, and J. Denekens, “Patient adherence to treatment: three decades of research. A comprehensive review,” *Journal of Clinical Pharmacy and Therapeutics*, vol. 26, no. 5, pp. 331–342, 2001.

[30] D. E. Morisky and M. R. Dimatteo, “Improving the measurement of self-reported medication nonadherence: final response,” *Journal of Clinical Epidemiology*, vol. 64, no. 3, pp. 262–263, 2011.

6

Alzheimer's Disease Clinical and Research Update for Health Care Practitioners

Philip A. DeFina,[1] Rosemarie Scolaro Moser,[2] Megan Glenn,[2] Jonathan D. Lichtenstein,[2] and Jonathan Fellus[1]

[1] *International Brain Research Foundation Inc., 227 Route 206 North, Building 2, Suite 101, Flanders, NJ 07836, USA*
[2] *RSM Psychology Center, LLC 3131 Princeton Pike, Building 5, Suite 110, Lawrenceville, NJ 08648, USA*

Correspondence should be addressed to Rosemarie Scolaro Moser; moserrs@comcast.net

Academic Editor: Michelle M. Mielke

Of the approximately 6.8 million Americans who have been diagnosed with dementia, over 5 million have been diagnosed with Alzheimer's Disease (AD). Due to the rise in the aging population, these figures are expected to double by 2050. The following paper provides an up-to-date review of clinical issues and relevant research. Research related to the methods of the earliest possible detection of AD is ongoing. Health care professionals should play a critical role in differentially diagnosing AD patients, as well as supporting their families. Novel interventions, including medications, natural supplements, and behavioral techniques, are constantly appearing in the literature. It is necessary for the health practitioner to remain current, regarding AD, as such information will facilitate better care for patients and their families.

1. Introduction

Approximately 6.8 million individuals in the United States are affected by dementia [1], and approximately 5.3 million have been diagnosed with Alzheimer's Disease (AD) [2]. As the elderly population continues to grow, these numbers are only expected to increase. AD has emerged as a serious public health concern, placing an immense burden on the individual, family, community, and health care resources.

AD most frequently presents with episodic memory impairment as the earliest and most prominent feature, with additional deficits in language, semantic memory, executive functioning, visuospatial abilities, and functional impairment that emerge over the disease course [3]. A common misconception is that AD is a "normal" or expected occurrence of aging, and it is part of the typical trajectory of age-related cognitive decline. Rather, healthy aging has been found to be associated with relatively stable performance on measures of cognitive functioning when measured longitudinally. However, cross-sectional studies have indicated that some domains of cognitive functioning do in fact decline with age [4]. As individuals live to advanced ages (e.g., over the age of 80), it can become more challenging to differentiate between the subtle cognitive declines that accompany aging and those that signify early dementia [5].

The trajectory of AD is characterized along a continuum, ranging from healthy aging to preclinical AD, mild cognitive impairment (MCI), and dementia. Pathological changes that underlie AD begin to accumulate for years, or even decades, before emotional, physical, or cognitive symptoms emerge, eventually reaching a threshold at which the onset of a gradual and progressive decline in cognition occurs [5]. Preclinical AD constitutes the presymptomatic phase during which characteristic neuropathological changes begin to emerge [6].

The transitional period between normal cognitive functioning and dementia is referred to as Mild Cognitive Impairment (MCI) [7]; the most common form, the one most likely to progress to AD, is amnestic MCI (a-MCI). Patients with a-MCI present with memory deficits greater than would be expected based on age and education; however functional abilities remain relatively preserved and independence intact [8]. Estimates of the annual incidence of individuals with MCI progressing to dementia range from 5 to 15% [9]. Regardless of this variation, annual conversion rate of those with MCI is far greater than the baseline incidence rate [4].

AD is often referred to as a "family disease" because of the tremendous impact that befalls the patient's immediate social support system. By identifying AD in its early stages, recommendations for the most current or efficacious interventions can be made, with the goal of slowing disease progression. Early detection may provide patients and their families with an opportunity to begin the discussion of future caregiving, finances, and end-of-life issues before the patient's autonomous decision-making skills deteriorate. Also, implementing caregiver interventions, such as referral to support groups, psychoeducation, and counseling or psychotherapy [9], can also assist patients and their families.

2. Epidemiology and Pathogenesis

Over the past 20 years, researchers have made great strides in the areas of AD, with respect to etiology, prevention, diagnosis, and treatment. However, while the exact etiology still remains a mystery, definitive diagnosis can only be made postmortem, and current treatments can only slow disease progression temporarily. Late-onset AD, the most common form of the disease, occurs in individuals over the age of 65. While researchers have not found any causal determinants for this particular type, they have identified several associated risk factors, including age, female gender, low educational and occupational attainment, prior head injury, sleep disorders (e.g., sleep apnea), estrogen replacement therapy, and vascular risk factors, such as diabetes, hypercholesterolemia, and hypertension [5, 10]. Additionally, the apolipoprotein E (APOE) gene has been recognized as conferring an increased likelihood of developing late-onset AD. Depending on the combination of APOE alleles that an individual possesses, he or she may have a three to eight times higher risk. The much rarer, early-onset from of AD, occurring in fewer than five percent of individuals with the disease, typically affects individuals between the ages of approximately thirty and sixty. This form of the disease is caused by one of three identified genetic mutations that are passed down in an autosomal dominant fashion among families: the amyloid precursor protein (APP), presenilin-1, and presenilin-2 genes [4, 10].

AD is characterized by progressive degenerative neuronal changes, with associated global deterioration of cognitive and personality functioning. This pathological sequence preferentially begins in the medial temporal lobe structures responsible for memory (the entorhinal cortex and hippocampus) and then progresses to the frontal, temporal, and parietal areas, with relative sparing of the motor and sensory cortical regions and subcortical regions [11]. The most widely held theory accounting for the pathological changes underlying disease process is the amyloid cascade hypothesis, positing that the primary, triggering event is the excessive accumulation and clumping together of beta-amyloid (Aβ), leading to the formation and deposition of amyloid plaques throughout the medial temporal lobe and cerebral cortex [12]. A resultant "cascade of events" occurs, including neuronal damage (and eventually death), disrupted neuronal communication, inflammation, and the initiation of a second abnormal protein process—the accumulation of neurofibrillary tangles (NFTs) [4, 13].

NFTs are composed of an abnormal form of the intraneuronal protein tau, which normally plays a role in structural support and cellular communication. Abnormal processes cause the tau protein to "misfold" and aggregate into NFTs, ultimately leading to a breakdown in neuronal function and communication and eventually cell death [14]. The accumulation of NFTs occurs in a hierarchical pattern, beginning primarily in the medial temporal lobe (especially, the entorhinal cortex), gradually progressing into the limbic system (hippocampus and amygdala), and eventually spreading throughout the neocortex [4, 11, 15]. There is evidence that the presence of both amyloid plaques and NFTs is required for AD to develop [8].

Researchers continue to search for tools that can offer the same degree of diagnostic certainty during life that postmortem brain tissue examinations offer. There are currently five biomarkers which show the most promise as indicators of AD pathology organized into two categories: biomarkers of beta-amyloid accumulation and biomarkers of neuronal degeneration or injury [16]. The accumulation of beta-amyloid can be detected through the use of radioactive tracers in conjunction with positron emission tomography (PET) imaging [17], as well as through the analysis of beta-amyloid levels in the cerebrospinal fluid (CSF) [18]. Analysis of CSF levels of tau has also been found to indicate neuronal degeneration associated with NFT accumulation [8, 18]. Fluorodeoxyglucose- (FDG-) PET imaging can be employed to detect hypometabolism in the temporoparietal region, which has been shown to effectively differentiate AD from normal controls [19]. Finally, structural magnetic resonance imaging (MRI) can be used to detect the characteristic pattern of pronounced atrophy in the medial temporal lobes that often occurs in mild to moderate AD [20].

While biomarker research holds promise for early detection and diagnosis of AD, standardized guidelines are still being developed for determining cut-points for diagnosis [8]. Thus, the use of biomarker data is currently indicated primarily for research purposes. Newly approved amyloid imaging techniques (via PET scan) are beginning to be used in order to supplement the results of other diagnostic evaluations.

3. Clinical Manifestations

In 2009, the National Institute on Aging and the Alzheimer's Association (NIA-AA) joined forces to develop new up-to-date guidelines for diagnosing AD based on the most current state of the evidence regarding the clinical and pathological processes of the disease. The official criteria were published in 2011 and are summarized as follows: (1) a gradual, progressive decline in cognition that represents a deterioration from a previous higher level; (2) cognitive or behavioral impairment evident in at least two of the following domains: episodic memory, executive functioning, visuospatial abilities, language functions, personality and/or behavior; (3) significant functional impairment that affects the individual's ability to carry out daily living activities; (4) the symptoms are not better accounted for by delirium or another mental disorder, stroke, another dementing condition (i.e., vascular dementia, frontotemporal dementia) or other neurological condition, or the effects of a medication [16]. The Diagnostic and Statistical Manual of Mental Disorders is a tool which is widely employed in clinical settings for diagnosing AD. The recently released version, the DSM-5, contains updated criteria for diagnosing AD which parallel the NIA-AA diagnostic guidelines. It is imperative for clinicians to familiarize themselves with these revised criteria, listed within the Neurocognitive Disorders section, as the criteria contained in the prior DSM-IV-TR are not reflective of the current state of the AD literature [21].

The initial presentation of AD typically involves anterograde amnesia resulting from progressive declines in episodic memory. Specific memory tests may reveal deficits in the encoding and consolidating of new information into long term memory as evidenced by rapid forgetting after a time delay and lack of improvement even when recognition cues are provided. On episodic memory tasks, AD patients commonly commit more errors of intrusion and perseveration, have difficulty employing semantic encoding tactics, and demonstrate less of a primacy effect when compared to normal elderly individuals [3, 5, 23]. As memory impairment begets functional decline, some of the first overt signs of AD often noted by family members include repeating oneself in conversations, misplacing items, becoming lost while driving (familiar routes), burning meals while cooking, and difficulty managing finances [4, 24]. With regard to remote memory, a pattern emerges in the early stages of the disease in which older memories are relatively spared, while those from the more recent past are lost [5, 23].

Deficits in semantic memory and language may become evident early in the course of AD, as well. These difficulties are thought to result from the degenerative disease process causing a breakdown in the brain's interconnected network of general knowledge for concepts, facts, words, and their meaning. Impairment may be detected on tests of verbal fluency, with the tendency to perform relatively worse on tasks requiring generation of words from a given category versus generation of words that begin with a particular letter of the alphabet. Patients are unable to employ clustering strategies to boost their performances and are also unaided by category retrieval cues [3, 23]. Given that AD leads to a loss of semantic knowledge, the failure to demonstrate semantic knowledge for a particular item or concept has been shown to be consistent across test methods [3]. Poor performance is also typically seen on confrontation naming tests and semantic categorization (i.e., of pictures) [5, 23]. Language discourse becomes increasingly filled with circumlocutions and overlearned phrases, accompanied by diminished meaning and spontaneity [23]. Decline in executive functioning can be seen on tests of complex problem solving, working memory, mental flexibility, and sequencing; deficits in these areas may be detected relatively early on tests such as the Tower of London puzzle, Porteus Maze task, Trail-Making Test, and Wisconsin Card Sorting Task and are implicated in the decline of instrumental activities of daily living (IADLs). Tests of immediate attention span and focus, such as digit span and mental control, may remain intact until later in the disease progression [3, 5, 23].

Visuospatial functioning tends not to be a prominent early feature of AD, but instead it regresses over the course of the disease [5]. In particular, visuoconstructional deficits may be apparent on the Clock Drawing task and on complex copying tasks using drawing or blocks [23, 24]. A hallmark indicator of AD is the patients' tendency to perform their copy of a design extremely close to, touching, or on top of the stimulus item [23]. Additionally, visuoperceptual and visual orientation abilities may become disturbed over time [5].

While extrapyramidal motor signs are more prominent in the latter stages of AD, patients may show deficits in ideomotor (skilled movement to verbal command or imitation) and ideational (performing a planned series of motor tasks to achieve a goal) praxis, even in the early stages of the disease [24]. This has implications for their ability to independently perform daily living tasks [23].

4. Diagnostic Approach

Determining the primary cause of cognitive decline can be challenging, given the common comorbidity of cerebrovascular disease, Lewy body disease, and AD [6, 8]. Additionally, temporal conditions, such as delirium, depression, anxiety, metabolic disorders, vitamin deficiencies, normal pressure hydrocephalus (NPH), and adverse reactions to medication, may resemble AD particularly in individuals who are young, newly symptomatic or whose symptoms are mild [24]. Neuropsychological testing can contribute to differentiating a true dementia process from a pseudo-dementia, as well as distinguishing between different forms of dementia. However, there are times when patients meet the diagnostic criteria for AD, and have a comorbid condition that may be contributing to cognitive impairment, thus causing a mixed dementia. The NIA-AA criteria differentiate between probable and possible AD and designate patients with mixed dementias to the latter category [16].

Table 1 offers a schematic for diagnostic guidance when evaluating a patient for dementia. Generally, when a clinician suspects changes in mental status, a screening test is performed to assess global cognitive abilities. The Mini-Mental State Examination (MMSE) is among the most widely researched instruments for screening cognitive impairment. This global assessment tool measures orientation to time and place, word recall, language abilities, attention and calculation, and visuospatial skills. The MMSE yields a perfect score of 30, with cut-off points between 24 and 26 suggesting dementia [25]. Age and education adjustments should be utilized for MMSE scoring, as performance may be affected by demographic factors, particularly education [25]. Temporal orientation and factual understanding of current events may be problematic even in early AD, which may be revealed by the MMSE.

Table 1: Diagnostic assessment for dementia.

(i) Initial exam
(signs to look for)
Poor orientation
Increased forgetfulness
Confusion in ADLs and IADLs
Language perseverations and circumlocutions
Change in personality and emotional status
Avoidance of typical activities and hobbies
Social isolation
(ii) Mental status screening-use NIAA criteria
(example of evaluation tools that may be used)
Mini mental state
Clock drawing
Mattis dementia screening
Montreal cognitive assessment
Clinical dementia rating scale
Geriatric depression scale
(iii) Interview for instrumental activities of daily living
(observations by family or caregiver report)
Medication use
Cooking
Driving
Financial management
(iv) Interview for general activities of daily living
(observations by family or caregiver report)
Bathing
Dressing
Toileting
(v) Assessment of visual motor skills
(signs to look for)
Ideomotor apraxia (skilled movement to verbal command or initiation)
Ideational apraxia (performing a planned series of tasks to achieve a goal)
Extrapyramidal motor signs
Constructional apraxia
Spatial conceptualization errors
(vi) Neuroimaging
CT
SPECT
MRI
PET
(vii) Neuropsychological testing
(skill areas to assess)
Estimate of premorbid IQ
Attention
Processing speed
Executive functioning
Planning, organization, mental flexibility
Memory
Working memory
Immediate recall
Delayed recall
Long term memory

Table 1: Continued.

Language
Naming
Semantic fluency
Evidence of perseverations
Evidence of circumlocution

The Montreal Cognitive Assessment (MoCA) was more recently developed to specifically detect the more subtle deficits associated with MCI [26]. Similar to the MMSE, scores on the MoCA range from 0 to 30, with the suggested cut-off for impairment being less than 26. However, the MoCA includes more difficult tasks, making it more sensitive in differentiating normal cognition from mild cognitive impairment. Individuals with MCI often score in the normal range on the MMSE and in the impaired range on the MoCA, highlighting the utility of the MoCA in detecting the earliest symptoms of AD [26].

A thorough patient history should be taken, preferably involving a knowledgeable spouse or other family member, in order to determine whether the onset and course of cognitive decline are gradual and progressive, as in AD, or sudden and/or stepwise, which may occur in the case of vascular dementia. An appropriate set of medical tests (i.e., neuroimaging, laboratory tests) may be conducted to rule out another neurological condition, medical illness, or another process which may be present, and patients are often referred for a neuropsychological assessment [8, 16].

The neuropsychologist should utilize a battery of assessment measures that are sensitive to the cognitive deficits seen in AD and capable of distinguishing between age-related cognitive decline, MCI, AD, and other forms of dementia. An example of such an abbreviated battery, used by the Alzheimer's Disease Centers (ADC) program of the NIA, incorporates measures of global cognition (MMSE), attention (Digit Span Forward & Backward), processing speed (Digit Symbol; Trail Making Test—Part A), executive functions (Trail Making Test—Part B), episodic memory (Logical Memory Story A—Immediate and Delayed Recall), and language (Category Fluency; Boston Naming) [27]. Additional evidence of episodic memory impairment may be gathered from word list memory tasks, which can help identify deficits in encoding, storage, and retrieval. Combined visuoconstructional and visual memory tasks may be used which require the patient to copy shapes and then to recall those shapes after a delay, both from memory and with recognition cues. A diverse range of skills may be assessed by administering a Clock Drawing task, including planning, visual attention, spatial orientation, and graphomotor control [28]. Finally, since many patients with dementia have never undergone previous neuropsychological assessment, an estimate of premorbid IQ may be obtained by administering a word list reading task, such as the Wechsler Test of Adult Reading (WTAR).

In addition to evaluating the patient's cognitive, the neuropsychologist will address functional issues related to the patient's personal safety and ability to perform instrumental activities of daily living (IADLs), such as driving, medication management, and financial management. Ability to perform basic activities of daily living (BADLs) must also be examined (e.g., toileting, bathing, and dressing), through observation, informant report, or rehabilitation specialists such as occupational therapists. The "gold standard" of formal measures for assessing the level of functional impairment is the Clinical Dementia Rating Scale (CDR) [29], which is a semistructured interview combining information from the patient and a knowledgeable informant. A global rating of dementia severity is calculated, along with the CDR sum of boxes score (CDR-SB), which allows for a detailed, continuous measure of the subtle differences between levels of impairment and has been found to be able to discriminate MCI from early AD [30].

5. Therapeutic Interventions

In the management of AD, a multimodal approach is warranted. Table 2 provides an outline of eight intervention areas to address. These interventions include pharmaceutical, nutraceutical, medical foods, neurophysiological, physical health, cognitive, behavioral, and future planning.

At this time, there are no established therapeutic interventions that have been found which can stop the progression or reverse the neural deterioration caused by AD. However, there are four FDA approved pharmaceuticals currently prescribed which temporarily halt or slow cognitive, functional, and behavioral decline. Three of the medications are cholinesterase inhibitors, namely, Donepezil, Rivastigmine, and Galantamine, which work to increase the levels of acetylcholine, a neurotransmitter in the brain that is involved in learning and memory. The cholinesterase inhibitors are indicated for the treatment of individuals in the mild to moderate stages of AD [31, 32]. Memantine works by increasing the levels of glutamate, another neurotransmitter implicated in learning and memory. This drug is indicated for the treatment of moderate to severe AD. There is also evidence that Memantine may provide added benefits for individuals with AD who are already taking Donepezil [33]. Overall, the benefits of AD drugs are limited, as they are effective for approximately one year and in only about half of individuals to whom they are prescribed [31].

Currently, there are no other evidence-supported treatments for AD, however ongoing research aims to find disease-modifying treatments. Consensus statements have pointed to a multifaceted approach for conquering AD, using a combination of drugs to target a number of factors associated with the disease process, including Aβ deposits, NFTs, inflammation, immune dysregulation, and insulin resistance [34]. Recent breakthroughs include results from a phase II clinical trial of IVIG, an immunotherapy agent, which was found to stabilize cognition and functioning, in a small sample of AD patients, for three years [35]. Another promising finding came from a pilot clinical trial of an intranasal insulin therapy for AD and a-MCI in which participants who underwent treatment experienced memory improvement and/or maintained their current level of overall cognitive and functional performance [36].

Additionally, Alpha GPC, phosphatidylserine, Huperzine A, and choline show promise as nutraceutical agents for enhancing cognitive performance and slowing cognitive decline. Alpha GPC, also known as L-Alpha Glycerylphosphorylcholine, a naturally occurring form of choline, acts as a parasympathomimetic acetylcholine precursor and has shown promise in improving cognitive symptoms related to AD, vascular dementia, and multi-infarct dementia. Phosphatidylserine is a widely abundant anionic phospholipid in the human body and has been shown to improve age-related cognitive changes. Huperzine A (a natural cholinesterase inhibitor) has been linked to improved memory performance in elderly people with benign forgetfulness, as well as patients with AD and vascular dementia. Cholinesterase inhibitors have been shown to have neuroprotective properties in patients with mild [37] as well as moderate-to-advanced AD [38].

Recently, there is the development of medical foods that are thought to have some promise in improving mental status: Axona, CerefolinNAC, and Souvenaid [39]. Each works via a different mechanism of action, and all are prescriptive supplements. However, Souvenaid is not currently available for use in the USA.

The application of translational models, such as through animal and cell research, has helped identify certain processes and elements that may deter the neuropathogenetic progression of AD [40]. Research has begun to explore nonpharmaceutical interventions through translational models that may reduce toxins and prevent cell loss including apoptosis. In other words, once applications of interventions on animals or cells are deemed successful, they can be translated or applied to human participants. Laser light therapy is one such intervention, and animal studies using infrared light treatment have documented positive results in mice with traumatic brain injury [41]. Stimulation of human mitochondrial processes and cell proliferation due to laser irradiation have also been demonstrated [42]. More recently, researchers revealed a significant reduction of Amyloid-B aggregates in neuroblastoma cells that were irradiated with intense 670 nm laser light, leading the authors to suggest that their approach might inspire a practical therapy for AD [43].

Ultimately, the most successful model of treatment for AD will likely include early detection and control of physical factors (diabetes, hypertension, hyperlipidemia), followed by application of multifaceted, disease-modifying interventions to prevent the early and continued loss of neurons and to reduce the toxins that result in further cell deterioration [34].

Changes in personality and behavioral disturbances affect most patients with AD and can range from disinterest and apathy to agitation, affective disinhibition, and restlessness. Specific behaviors can be difficult to manage, such as aimless wandering, emotional outbursts, stubbornness, paranoia, hallucinations, and depression. Behavioral interventions can complement medication management and include creating a structured, safe, low stress environment, promoting regular sleep and eating habits, minimizing unexpected changes, and employing redirection and distraction [44].

Table 2: Management of dementia: eight intervention areas to be addressed.

(i) Pharmaceutical interventions
(medications that may provide symptom relief for cognitive, emotional, and behavioral issues)
Donepezil
Rivastigmine
Galantamine
Memantine
Psychotropic (antidepressants, antianxiety, mood stabilizer, antipsychotic)
(ii) Nutraceutical interventions
(dietary supplements still in research stages)
Omega 3
Curcumin
Vitamin D
Alpha GPC
Phosphatidylserine
Choline
(iii) Medical foods interventions
(prescriptive)
Axona
CerefolinNAC
Souvenaid (not currently available in the USA)
(iv) Neurophysiological interventions
(still in research stages)
Cranioelectric stimulation
Transcranial magnetic stimulation
Neurofeedback
Laser light therapy
(v) Physical health interventions
Aerobic exercise
Medical management of disease
Diabetes
Hypertension
Hyperlipidemia
(vi) Cognitive interventions
Mental exercises/hobbies
Compensatory memory strategies and aids
Cognitive training
(vii) Behavioral interventions
(strategies to manage factors such as wandering, sundowning, agitation, disorientation, affective disinhibition, stubbornness, paranoia, irritability, apathy, and restlessness)
Occupational therapy safety assessment of home
Low stress calming environment
Regular sleep and meal schedules
Redirection and distraction
Minimization of unexpected changes in environment
Patient counseling and support groups in early stages
Caregiver strategies and resources through support groups and internet
In-home aide/assistant

Table 2: Continued.

Outpatient day program with all inclusive care
assisted living facility
(viii) Future planning interventions
Caregiver counseling to aid in life planning and decision making
Legal services for guardianship and capacity
Financial advisor for estate planning

Since ADLs such as self-care, personal hygiene, and dressing tend to worsen with the progression of the disease, patients with advanced AD require a greater level of caretaker commitment. Caregivers should be alerted to the challenges they will face as the disease progresses and be provided with appropriate coping skills, training, and interventions, through support groups and individual therapy. When at-home care is no longer an option, families will face the decision of placing their loved one in an assisted-living facility. Caregivers should not make this choice in isolation; mental health practitioners can help provide information and allow for the processing of the emotional weight of the decision and any mixed emotions of guilt, hurt, anger, and loss.

Considering that IADLs also decrease in AD, issues such as management of medical decisions, financial affairs, and cessation of driving will also emerge. When the patient is no longer able to perform basic math calculations, securing a financial advisor to oversee assets is often recommended. When insight becomes limited and memory is significantly compromised, medical decision-making and medication management may also need to be shifted to the hands of a caregiver. Pursuit of guardianship and capacity evaluations are not uncommon, especially when estate and legal issues need to be addressed.

6. Preventative Interventions

AD is believed to emerge as the result of a complicated interplay of genetic, environmental, and lifestyle factors. Due to this complex process, it is difficult to pinpoint a definitive prevention strategy; however, there is mounting evidence that modifying certain lifestyle factors may lower the risk of developing AD [45]. There is data to suggest that aerobic exercise may improve cognition [5] and serve a protective role in healthy older adults by inducing neuroplasticity in areas of the brain associated with episodic memory [46]. Additionally, physical activity has been found to improve scores on cognitive and functional measures in individuals with MCI and dementia [47].

As cardiovascular risk factors, such as diabetes, hypercholesterolemia, and hypertension, have been found to be associated with AD, it is hypothesized that preventing or managing these conditions may decrease the likelihood of developing AD [45]. Research has shown that healthy eating, specifically adhering to a Mediterranean diet, correlated with both a lower risk of cardiovascular disease and AD [48]. While there is ongoing research investigating the effects of various vitamins and dietary supplements in preventing AD, as of yet, clinical trials have not been able to prove their effectiveness [45].

In addition to maintaining physical health, engagement in cognitively stimulating as well as social activities seems important for promoting healthy brain functioning. Investigators have found that older adults who frequently participate in mentally demanding activities (i.e., reading, crossword puzzles) have decreased odds of developing AD [49]. Formal interventions involving cognitive training and time spent engaging in physical, cognitive, and social activities have been associated with a lower risk of developing dementia in healthy older adults, especially for individuals who participated in two or three of these endeavors [50].

7. Summary

Alzheimer's Disease (AD) is an increasingly common condition with projected increased incidence rates in the population. Fortunately, research geared towards enhancing disease-modifying and preventative interventions is gaining momentum. Neuropsychological evaluation continues to play a critical role in early detection and differential diagnosis of normal aging versus MCI and the various types of dementia. Health care practitioners can offer strategies and support for patients, as well as their families and caregivers, related to the disruptions that AD has upon daily functioning. As researchers continue to make strides in our understanding of the disease, it is imperative for clinicians to remain abreast of the dementia literature in order to assist patients in obtaining the most effective care.

Disclosure

Dr. Jonathan Fellus has been a consultant on the speakers bureau of and holds stock in the company Avanir.

Acknowledgments

This article is dedicated to the memory of Nathan Plafsky and the Nathan and Bernice Plafsky Center for the Aging Brain of the International Brain Research Foundation. The authors have no conflict of interests related to this article.

References

[1] NINDS, "Dementia: hope through research," 2012, http://www.ninds.nih.gov/disorders/detail_dementia.html.

[2] CDC, "Alzheimer's disease," 2010, http://www.cdc.gov/Features/Alzheimers/index.html.

[3] S. Weintraub, A. H. Wicklund, and D. P. Salmon, "The neuropsychological profile of Alzheimer disease," *Cold Spring Harbor Perspectives in Medicine*, vol. 2, no. 4, Article ID a006171, 2012.

[4] J. M. Burns and J. C. Morris, *Mild Cognitive Impairment and Early Alzheimer's Disease: Detections and Diagnosis*, John Wiley & Sons, 2008.

[5] M. W. Bondi, D. P. Salmon, and A. W. Kaszniak, "The neuropsychology of dementia," in *Neuropsychological Assessment of Neuropsychiatric and Neuromedical Disorders*, I. Grant and K. Adams, Eds., pp. 159–198, Oxford University Press, New York, NY, USA, 2009.

[6] C. R. Jack Jr., M. S. Albert, D. S. Knopman et al., "Introduction to the recommendations from the National Institute on Aging-Alzheimer's Association workgroups on diagnostic guidelines for Alzheimer's disease," *Alzheimer's and Dementia*, vol. 7, no. 3, pp. 257–262, 2011.

[7] R. C. Petersen, "Conceptual overview," in *Mild Cognitive Impairment: Aging to Alzheimer's Disease*, R. C. Petersen, Ed., pp. 1–14, Oxford University Press, New York, NY, USA, 2003.

[8] M. S. Albert, S. T. DeKosky, D. Dickson et al., "The diagnosis of mild cognitive impairment due to Alzheimer's disease: recommendations from the National Institute on Aging-Alzheimer's Association workgroups on diagnostic guidelines for Alzheimer's disease," *Alzheimer's and Dementia*, vol. 7, no. 3, pp. 270–279, 2011.

[9] Association As, "Alzheimer's disease facts and figures," 2012, http://www.alz.org/downloads/facts_figures_2012.pdf.

[10] NIA, *2011-2012 Alzheimer's Disease Progress Report: Intensifying the Research Effort*, 2012.

[11] H. Braak and E. Braak, "Neuropathological stageing of Alzheimer-related changes," *Acta Neuropathologica*, vol. 82, no. 4, pp. 239–259, 1991.

[12] D. J. Selkoe, "The molecular pathology of Alzheimer's disease," *Neuron*, vol. 6, no. 4, pp. 487–498, 1991.

[13] J. Hardy and D. J. Selkoe, "The amyloid hypothesis of Alzheimer's disease: progress and problems on the road to therapeutics," *Science*, vol. 297, no. 5580, pp. 353–356, 2002.

[14] J. Hoffman, *The Alzheimer's Project: Momentum in Science*, PublicAffairs/Home Box Office, New York, NY, USA, 2009.

[15] Z. Nagy, D. M. Yilmazer-Hanke, H. Braak, E. Braak, C. Schultz, and J. Hanke, "Assessment of the pathological stages of Alzheimer's disease in thin paraffin sections: a comparative study," *Dementia and Geriatric Cognitive Disorders*, vol. 9, no. 3, pp. 140–144, 1998.

[16] G. M. McKhann, D. S. Knopman, H. Chertkow et al., "The diagnosis of dementia due to Alzheimer's disease: recommendations from the National Institute on Aging-Alzheimer's Association workgroups on diagnostic guidelines for Alzheimer's disease," *Alzheimer's and Dementia*, vol. 7, no. 3, pp. 263–269, 2011.

[17] W. E. Klunk, H. Engler, A. Nordberg et al., "Imaging brain amyloid in Alzheimer's disease with pittsburgh compound-B," *Annals of Neurology*, vol. 55, no. 3, pp. 306–319, 2004.

[18] J. Q. Trojanowski, H. Vandeerstichele, M. Korecka et al., "Update on the biomarker core of the Alzheimer's disease neuroimaging initiative subjects," *Alzheimer's and Dementia*, vol. 6, no. 3, pp. 230–238, 2010.

[19] W. Jagust, "Positron emission tomography and magnetic resonance imaging in the diagnosis and prediction of dementia," *Alzheimer's and Dementia*, vol. 2, no. 1, pp. 36–42, 2006.

[20] M. Atiya, B. T. Hyman, M. S. Albert, and R. Killiany, "Structural magnetic resonance imaging in established and prodromal Alzheimer disease: a review," *Alzheimer Disease and Associated Disorders*, vol. 17, no. 3, pp. 177–195, 2003.

[21] APA, *Diagnostic and Statistical Manual of Mental Disorders*, American Psychiatric Association, Washington, DC, USA, 4th edition, 2000.

[22] J. D. Warren, P. D. Fletcher, and H. L. Golden, "The paradox of syndromic diversity in Alzheimer disease," *Nature Reviews*, vol. 8, no. 8, pp. 451–464, 2012.

[23] M. D. Lezak, *Neuropsychological Assessment*, Oxford University Press, New York, NY, USA, 5th edition, 2012.

[24] B. L. Malamut and L. M. Ryan, "Dementia: behavioral and cognitive aspectseds," in *Clinical Neurology of the Older Adult*, J. I. Sirven and B. L. Malamut, Eds., pp. 318–338, Wolters Kluwer Health/Lippincott Williams & Wilkins, Philadelphia, Pa, USA, 2nd edition, 2008.

[25] M. Mitrushina, "Cognitive screening methods," in *Neuropsychological Assessment of Neuropsychiatric and Neuromedical Disorders*, I. Grant and K. Adams, Eds., pp. 101–126, Oxford University Press, New York, NY, USA, 2009.

[26] Z. S. Nasreddine, N. A. Phillips, V. Bédirian et al., "The Montreal Cognitive Assessment, MoCA: a brief screening tool for mild cognitive impairment," *Journal of the American Geriatrics Society*, vol. 53, no. 4, pp. 695–699, 2005.

[27] S. Weintraub, D. Salmon, N. Mercaldo et al., "The Alzheimer's disease denters' Uniform Data Set (UDS): the neuropsychologic test battery," *Alzheimer Disease and Associated Disorders*, vol. 23, no. 2, pp. 91–101, 2009.

[28] M. Freedman, *Clock Drawing: A Neuropsychological Analysis*, Oxford University Press, 1994.

[29] J. C. Morris, "Clinical dementia rating: a reliable and valid diagnostic and staging measure for dementia of the Alzheimer type," *International Psychogeriatrics*, vol. 9, supplement 1, pp. 173–176, 1997.

[30] S. E. O'Bryant, L. H. Lacritz, J. Hall et al., "Validation of the new interpretive guidelines for the clinical dementia rating scale sum of boxes score in the national Alzheimer's coordinating center database," *Archives of Neurology*, vol. 67, no. 6, pp. 746–749, 2010.

[31] Association As, *Current Alzheimer's Treatments*, 2013.

[32] N. Herrmann, S. A. Chau, I. Kircanski, and K. L. Lanctôt, "Current and emerging drug treatment options for Alzheimers disease: a systematic review," *Drugs*, vol. 71, no. 15, pp. 2031–2065, 2011.

[33] P. N. Tariot, M. R. Farlow, G. T. Grossberg, S. M. Graham, S. McDonald, and I. Gergel, "Memantine treatment in patients with moderate to severe Alzheimer disease already receiving donepezil: a randomized controlled trial," *Journal of the American Medical Association*, vol. 291, no. 3, pp. 317–324, 2004.

[34] R. Duara, W. Barker, D. Loewenstein, and L. Bain, "The basis for disease-modifying treatments for Alzheimer's disease: the sixth snnual mild cognitive impairment symposium," *Alzheimer's and Dementia*, vol. 5, no. 1, pp. 66–74, 2009.

[35] N. Relkin, L. Bettger, D. Tsakanikas, and L. Ravdin, "Three year follow-up on the IVIG for Alzheimer's phase II study," *Alzheimer's & Dementia*, vol. 8, no. 4, article 589, 2012.

[36] S. Craft, L. D. Baker, T. J. Montine et al., "Intranasal insulin therapy for Alzheimer disease and amnestic mild cognitive impairment: a pilot clinical trial," *Archives of Neurology*, vol. 69, no. 1, pp. 29–38, 2012.

[37] A. Venneri, W. J. McGeown, and M. F. Shanks, "Empirical evidence of neuroprotection by dual cholinesterase inhibition in Alzheimer's disease," *Neuroreport*, vol. 16, no. 2, pp. 107–110, 2005.

[38] R. Howard, R. McShane, J. Lindesay et al., "Donepezil and memantine for moderate-to-severe Alzheimer's disease," *The New England Journal of Medicine*, vol. 366, no. 10, pp. 893–903, 2012.

[39] P. Thaipisuttikul and J. E. Galvin, "Use of medical foods and nutritional approaches in the treatment of Alzheimer's disease," *Clinical Practice*, vol. 9, no. 2, pp. 199–209, 2012.

[40] L. Hong, "Translational research in neurology: dementia," *Archives of Neurology*, vol. 69, no. 8, pp. 969–977, 2012.

[41] Q. Wu, W. Xuan, T. Ando et al., "Low-level laser therapy for closed-head traumatic brain injury in mice: effect of different wavelengths," *Lasers in Surgery and Medicine*, vol. 44, no. 3, pp. 218–226, 2012.

[42] W.-P. Hu, J.-J. Wang, C.-L. Yu, C.-C. E. Lan, G.-S. Chen, and H.-S. Yu, "Helium-neon laser irradiation stimulates cell proliferation through photostimulatory effects in mitochondria," *Journal of Investigative Dermatology*, vol. 127, no. 8, pp. 2048–2057, 2007.

[43] A. P. Sommer, J. Bieschke, R. P. Friedrich et al., "670 nm laser light and EGCG complementarily reduce amyloid-β aggregates in human neuroblastoma cells: basis for treatment of alzheimer's disease?" *Photomedicine and Laser Surgery*, vol. 30, no. 1, pp. 54–60, 2012.

[44] C. H. Sadowsky and J. E. Galvin, "Guidelines for the management of cognitive and behavioral problems in dementia," *Journal of the American Board of Family Medicine*, vol. 25, no. 3, pp. 350–366, 2012.

[45] National Institute on Aging NIoH, Department of Health and Human Services, *Preventing Alzheimer's Disease: What Do We Know?*, 2012.

[46] M. W. Voss, K. I. Erickson, R. S. Prakash et al., "Neurobiological markers of exercise-related brain plasticity in older adults," *Brain, Behavior, and Immunity*, vol. 28, pp. 90–99, 2013.

[47] P. Heyn, B. C. Abreu, and K. J. Ottenbacher, "The effects of exercise training on elderly persons with cognitive impairment and dementia: a meta-analysis," *Archives of Physical Medicine and Rehabilitation*, vol. 85, no. 10, pp. 1694–1704, 2004.

[48] N. Scarmeas, Y. Stern, M.-X. Tang, R. Mayeux, and J. A. Luchsinger, "Mediterranean diet and risk for Alzheimer's disease," *Annals of Neurology*, vol. 59, no. 6, pp. 912–921, 2006.

[49] R. S. Wilson, D. A. Bennett, J. L. Bienias et al., "Cognitive activity and incident AD in a population-based sample of older persons," *Neurology*, vol. 59, no. 12, pp. 1910–1914, 2002.

[50] A. Karp, S. Paillard-Borg, H.-X. Wang, M. Silverstein, B. Winblad, and L. Fratiglioni, "Mental, physical and social components in leisure activities equally contribute to decrease dementia risk," *Dementia and Geriatric Cognitive Disorders*, vol. 21, no. 2, pp. 65–73, 2006.

7

The Association between Seasonal Variation in Vitamin D, Postural Sway, and Falls Risk

Marie-Louise Bird,[1] Keith D. Hill,[2] Iain Robertson,[1] Madeleine J. Ball,[1] Jane K. Pittaway,[1] and Andrew D. Williams[1]

[1] *School of Human Life Sciences, University of Tasmania, Launceston, TAS 7250, Australia*
[2] *School of Physiotherapy, Curtin University, Perth, WA 6845, Australia*

Correspondence should be addressed to Marie-Louise Bird; birdm@utas.edu.au

Academic Editor: Alice Nieuwboer

Introduction. Low serum vitamin D levels are associated with increased postural sway. Vitamin D varies seasonally. This study investigates whether postural sway varies seasonally and is associated with serum vitamin D and falls. *Methods*. In a longitudinal observational study, eighty-eight independently mobile community-dwelling older adults (69.7 ± 7.6 years) were evaluated on five occasions over one year, measuring postural sway (force platform), vitamin D levels, fall incidence, and causes and adverse outcomes. Mixed-methods Poisson regression was used to determine associations between measures. *Results*. Postural sway did not vary over the year. Vitamin D levels varied seasonally ($P < 0.001$), peaking in summer. Incidence of falls ($P = 0.01$) and injurious falls ($P = 0.02$) were lower in spring, with the highest fall rate at the end of autumn. Postural sway was not related to vitamin D ($P = 0.87$) or fall rates, but it was associated with fall injuries (IRR 1.59 (CI 1.14 to 2.24, $P = 0.007$). *Conclusions*. Postural sway remained stable across the year while vitamin D varied seasonally. Participants with high values for postural sway demonstrated higher rates of injurious falls. This study provides important evidence for clinicians and researchers providing interventions measuring balance outcomes across seasons.

1. Introduction

Balance impairment is an important fall-risk factor [1], and increases in range of postural sway in the mediolateral direction in older adults are associated with increased fall-risk and rates [2]. Postural sway has been shown in older adults to be strongly related to other measures of balance [3]. Multivariate analysis reveals serum vitamin D levels as an independent variable associated with postural sway [4]. In individuals with suboptimal levels of vitamin D, balance and strength improve after supplementation [5], in particular postural sway [6]. Epidemiological studies have shown that vitamin D levels show seasonal variation [7, 8]. Lowest levels of serum vitamin D are recorded towards the end of winter, approximately four weeks after the shortest day of the year [8]. Overall, vitamin D supplementation did not reduce rate of falls (RaR 1.00, 95% CI 0.90 to 1.11; seven trials; 9324 participants) or risk of falling (RR 0.96, 95% CI 0.89 to 1.03; 13 trials; 26, 747 participants) but may do so in people with lower vitamin D levels before treatment [9]. Older adults are at risk for lower levels of serum vitamin D because of age-related changes in UVB absorption and skin capacity to synthesize vitamin D, reduction in activation in the kidneys, and reduced expression of vitamin D receptors in tissues [5].

There are many factors affecting fall-risk for older individuals, and although these may be different for inside and outside falls [10], strength and balance remain two important physical fall-risk factors. A recently published overview of the literature supports an assertion that age-related changes in postural reactions may be related to vitamin D status-mediated through either central nervous system integration or antigravity muscles as the effectors in postural responses [11]. Despite changes in vitamin D across the seasons [8], muscle strength in the quadriceps muscles has been shown to remain stable [12]. The relationship of postural sway to any potential increased winter fall rate and decreased levels of vitamin D has not been investigated.

The winter season sees an increase in injuries from falls and in the number of accidental deaths from falls [13]. Fracture rates from falls in older adults also increase at the end of the winter season [8], following two to eight weeks after the nadir in serum vitamin D levels. Research into seasonal variation in fall rates, however, has produced disparate results. Some studies report an increased rate of falls, for both inside and outside falls [13, 14]; however, significant seasonal variation in fall rates was not found in a three-year study [8] while, in a second study, seasonal variation in fall rates was reported in women but not in men [15].

Coincident static balance changes with any potential increased fall rates in winter have not been previously reported. The data presented here forms part of a larger study, from which two other papers with the same clinical trial registration have been published [12, 16]. The aim of this study was to determine differences in static balance (postural sway), vitamin D, incidence of falls, and type of fall serially at the end of each season over a 12-month period, in older community-living adults. A secondary aim was to determine associations between seasonal variations in these variables. We hypothesised that postural sway, falls, and vitamin D would show a seasonal variation and that there would be an inverse relationship between vitamin D and the other variables.

2. Materials and Methods

2.1. Study Design. At the end of consecutive seasons, static balance, vitamin D status, and fall rate were measured within a longitudinal study design. No intervention was implemented by study researchers, so that the study could identify natural variations that occur over the seasons. Data was collected over a three-week period in each season from end of spring 2009 to the end of spring 2010, with collection of data timed to coincide with expected peaks and troughs in serum vitamin D levels [8] in Australia at latitude 41 degrees south (Tasmania). After each assessment, participants were given an appointment for the next collection block in three months' time.

2.2. Participants. Independently living community-dwelling adults aged between sixty and eighty-five years were recruited through local print media and community clubs. All participants were able to ambulate independently. Exclusion criteria included recent or current acute medical conditions or an uncontrolled chronic condition. Daily intake of oral supplementation of vitamin D of greater than 800 international Units was also an exclusion criterion. Participants were also excluded if they had a history of neurological disease and were withdrawn if they suffered a medical condition while participating in the study that would impact on their ability to perform the physical tests. Liver and kidney disease both impact vitamin D metabolism, and any potential participants with either of these conditions were excluded.

A priori sample size calculation was based on a previous study reporting mediolateral sway range in a sample of community-dwelling older adults [17], and this indicated a minimum requirement of 81 completed participants (minimum effect size 2.5 mm sway; standard deviation (SD) 8 mm; power 0.8, alpha 0.05). Ninety-eight participants were recruited with the anticipation of a 15% drop-out rate. This repeated measures cohort study was designed to be able to detect differences in postural sway. This project received ethical approval from the Human Research Ethics Committee (Tasmania) Network (H0010561).

2.3. Outcome Measures. Postural sway range in the mediolateral sway direction was measured using a force platform (AMTI Accugait PJB 101, Massachusetts, USA) for thirty seconds under conditions of eyes open and closed, as well as with the additional challenge of using a 6.5 cm foam cushion (eyes open and eyes closed) (Airex Elite Balance Pad AG, Switzerland). Participants were asked to remain stationary with their arms by their sides and look straight ahead while standing on the force platform. No practice trials were given. Foot position (bare feet) was standardised with heels 4 cm apart using marked placement for the feet to ensure repeatability between testing occasions. Maximum excursion range during the 30 seconds was recorded.

Venous blood samples were collected and clotted, then centrifuged (1610 relative centrifugal force) for 15 minutes. The separated sera were aliquoted and stored until analysis at −80°C. Samples for each participant were analysed in the same batch to reduce interassay variation. Serum concentration of 25-hydroxy vitamin D was measured by direct, competitive chemiluminescent immunoassay in a commercial accredited laboratory, using LIAISON method (DiaSorin Inc., Stillwater, MN, USA).

Participants received an individually coded calendar for 12 months of the study on which to report any falls and associated details by date, including information regarding the location and cause of the fall. Information about the type of fall, any injuries that resulted, and if medical attention was sought was recorded. Diaries were returned each month via a free return paid envelope. This study utilised the WHO definition of a fall as "an event which results in a person coming to rest inadvertently on the ground or other lower level" [18].

2.4. Statistical Analysis. Annual cyclic trends were investigated by fitting a sine wave formula to data for postural sway and vitamin D, with the amplitude of the seasonal variation (in percentage change) and the annual mean values were estimated using repeated measures nonlinear regression, adjusted for age and gender. For secondary analysis the three monthly data were interpolated linearly to estimate intermediate values to correspond with the observed fall incident data. Mixed-methods Poisson regression was used to determine associations between falls, fall injuries, and postural balance and vitamin D. The association between postural balance and vitamin D and season was estimated using mixed-methods linear regression, adjusted for age, gender, and strength. For comparison, seasonal data for falls was grouped into autumn and winter and compared to spring and summer [14].

Table 1: Variations in serum vitamin D and dynamic and postural balance over 5 seasons.

Variable	End of spring	End of summer	End of autumn	End of winter	End of spring
ML sway EO (cm) mean (SD)	1.9 (0.7)	1.2 (0.6)	1.3 (0.5)	1.1 (0.5)	1.1 (0.5)
Range	0.7–5.0	0.4–3.8	0.6–2.8	0.4–3.6	0.5–2.5
Change from season 1 mean (95% CI)		−0.6 (−0.7 to −0.5)*	−0.6 (−0.7 to −0.4)*	−0.8 (−0.9 to −0.6)*	−0.7 (−0.8 to −0.4)*
ML sway EC (cm) mean (SD)	2.1 (0.9)	1.4 (0.7)	1.4 (0.7)	1.3 (0.8)	1.4 (0.8)
Range	0.8–4.7	0.4–3.8	0.6–4.2	0.6–5.2	0.5–4.9
Change from season 1 mean (95% CI)		−0.7 (−0.8 to −0.6)*	−0.7 (−0.8 to −0.6)*	−0.8 (−0.9 to −0.6)*	−0.7 (−0.9 to −0.6)*
Foam ML (cm) sway EO mean (SD)	3.8 (1.2)	2.8 (1.1)	3.0 (1.2)	2.4 (0.8)	2.6 (0.8)
Range	1.0–8.4	1.1–7.0	1.2–11.41	1.2–6.0	1.1–5.8
Change from season 1 mean (95% CI)		−1.0 (−1.2 to −0.7)*	−0.8 (−1.0 to −0.5)*	−1.2 (−1.5 to −1.0)*	−1.2 (−1.4 to −0.9)*
Foam ML (cm) sway EC mean (SD)	6.8 (2.7)	5.0 (1.7)	4.7 (2.1)	4.6 (1.9)	4.8 (1.9)
Range	2.0–28.7	1.7–10.5	2.0–14.0	2.0–11.9	1.9–16.2
Change from season 1 mean (95% CI)		−1.7 (−2.3 to −1.2)*	−2.1 (−2.6 to −1.5)*	−2.1 (−2.8 to −1.5)*	−2.1 (−2.8 to −1.3)*
Serum vitamin D (nmol/L) mean (SD)	60 (19)	68 (21)*	58 (21)	52 (21)*	59 (20)
Range	20–115	10–126	13–115	16–107	20–114
Change from season 1 mean (95% CI)		8 (6 to 11)	−2 (−5 to 1)	−8 (−11 to −5)	−2 (−5 to 1)

Data presented as mean (SD), changes from season one presented as mean change (95% CI) (adjusted for age, gender strength, and physical activity), *($P < 0.05$), ML: mediolateral, EO: eyes open, EC: eyes closed, cm: centimeter.

Physical activity using the CHAMPS questionnaire and muscle strength using the physiological profile assessment tools were recorded, and this information has been published elsewhere [12] but forms an integral part of the meta-analysis of this paper.

3. Results

3.1. Participants. Data from eighty-eight participants (70% females) are included in the final analysis. Five people did not attend appointments, and five people could not complete testing because of medical events. The participants had a mean (SD) age of 69.2 (6.5) years and body mass index 27.4 (3.9) $kg \cdot m^{-2}$. All participants were living in their own homes independently, with only 10% being sole occupants. Common chronic controlled health conditions included cardiovascular disease (39%) and arthritis (14%). Twenty-six percent of the participants reported the use of more than 4 medications.

3.2. Outcomes. Postural sway data for the five time points are provided in Table 1. All four balance measures had the highest sway scores (poorest balance) at the first end of spring measurement. All other seasonal measures were significantly different from this first time point (all $P < 0.05$), but no subsequent significant difference was seen after any other seasonal measures, indicating a lack of seasonal variation in this outcome ($P > 0.05$). No associations between postural sway and vitamin D were observed (all $P > 0.05$). Increased postural sway was associated with fall injuries (IRR 1.59 (CI 1.14 to 2.24) ($P = 0.007$) but not fall rates (IRR 1.36 (CI 0.95 to 1.97, $P = 0.09$).

Vitamin D levels for each of the seasons are reported in Table 1. There was 15% variation in this variable over the year, with a peak at the end of summer and the lowest values at the end of winter.

Seventy-five percent of fall diaries were posted on schedule while the remaining diaries were returned at the subsequent assessment appointment, resulting in a compliance of 100%. Thirty-three percent of the cohort (29 people) fell at least once, with 10% of the whole group falling multiple times (8 people). Over the duration of the study, 48 falls were recorded: 14 of these occurred inside the house, and 34 occurred outside. Six falls were due to fainting or dizziness and forty due to trip-related events, with one categorised as being pushed over (by a horse) and one not able to be categorised. Twenty-eight falls resulted in injury, with only four requiring medical treatment (including one fracture). Further details on season variation in location and type of fall

Table 2: Fall incidence, injury, location, and cause reported as grouped by season.

Season	Single falls	Multiple falls	Total number of falls	Inside	Outside	Injuries	Trips/slips	Faint
Spring	6	0	6	0	6	3	5	1
Summer	12	0	12	1	11	7	10	2
Autumn	15	2 × 2	19	9	10	12	18	1
Winter	11	0	11	4	7	6	9	2

are provided in Table 2. There were significantly fewer falls during spring than any other season ($P = 0.01$), with no other differences between the seasons recorded. Most falls occurred in May. When falls data were combined from autumn and winter seasons and compared to the combined spring and summer seasons, there were more falls reported in the combined autumn and winter seasons (30 compared to 18). Less injuries from falls were recorded in spring than any other season ($P = 0.02$), with no other seasonal differences recorded.

4. Discussion

This is the first cohort study to determine that no seasonal variation of postural sway occurs across 12 months in our population. Significant seasonal variation in serum vitamin D levels, with higher serum levels in summer, was recorded. There was a significant relationship between postural sway and the number of injurious falls observed, with lower values for sway range (i.e., better stability) associated with less fall injuries. The overall fall rates were higher in autumn/winter than spring/summer.

A significant learning effect was seen with all measures of mediolateral postural sway with time point one having larger ranges than all of the other time points (all $P > 0.05$). Further to this, there was no seasonal variation in postural sway under any of the four static balance test conditions measured (eyes open and closed on a firm surface or foam surface). Postural sway range has been used to identify those people with balance impairment [19], and it may be useful in describing the fall-risk status of a particular individual. Our data indicates that postural sway does not appear to be subject to changes across the year within a participant. It has been suggested that this measure is important in describing sensorimotor deficits or disability rather than functional abilities [20] and hence may not be subject to changes that may occur due to altered patterns of activity or sunlight exposure seen seasonally. The stability of this measure in a cohort across a year provides important information for researchers planning interventions designed to impact postural sway and clinicians who are measuring the effectiveness of their interventions. Familiarisation with postural sway measures is recommended.

Mediolateral sway range has been shown to be an independent fall-risk factor for indoor falls [10]. In our study, a lower proportion of falls occurred indoors (29%) compared to outdoors (71%), and although this is similar to other studies where more healthy samples have been reported as having a greater proportion of falls being outdoor falls (74%; [21]), it may be a reason why no association between sway range and fall incidence was seen. A trend for this association was evident and a larger sample size may have found a significant relationship between these two variables, as this study was powered to determine mediolateral sway changes not fall rates. An association between increased sway range and rate of injurious falls was recorded in our study, reinforcing the importance of this measure for those most at risk of injury.

Overall there was no significant relationship found between postural sway and vitamin D. As increased postural sway is linked to low levels of vitamin D [22], it may be that the levels of vitamin D were sufficient for this parameter even at their lowest levels in participants in this study and did not influence postural sway. If this threshold situation is true, it may be that seasonal variation in postural sway may be present in a population with much lower levels of vitamin D, but this is outside the scope of the current study.

Annual rates of falling for adults over 65 have been reported up to 40% [1], and although our cohort includes some adults between the ages of sixty and sixty-five, with a mean age of 69 years and a fall rate of thirty-three percent, our population appears to be representative of older community-dwelling adults in terms of fall rate. Fall rates in older-old adults (over 75 years) have been shown to vary seasonally [14], but consistent data for the general population of healthy older community-dwelling adults has not been previously reported. One previous study grouped the peak seasons of winter and autumn together and found differences in fall rates [14]. Manipulation of our data in a similar way reveals that there were more falls during the autumn/winter half year compared to spring/summer (Table 2). These seasonal differences may be related to intrinsic factors that may be subject to seasonal variation (e.g., vitamin D, physical activity, and muscle strength) [10] as well as seasonally related environmental factors (e.g., weather, temperature). Further research needs to investigate interventions to address potentially modifiable factors to reduce the increased falls risk in the autumn/winter period.

Our data indicates a higher rate of falls in summer than has previously been reported [14], perhaps due to activity characteristics of our cohort. Summer and winter falls differ between the genders, with more men falling due to slips in winter and more women falling due to trips in summer [23]. The high proportion of women in our study (79%) may be a factor in the high rate of summer falls observed. Gender differences may also need to be explored in future research in this area [15].

Another factor to consider is the relationship between fall status and vitamin D. Although 60 nmol/L has been determined to be the cutoff for fall-risk function [24], 16/48 falls (33%) occurred in participants in this study whose vitamin D was above that cutoff level. This may be explained by the higher proportion of summer time falls observed in our study. During summer months, with longer hours of daylight at this latitude, a large proportion of the falls occurred in the outside (13 of the 14 falls –93%) (Table 2). By contrast, in winter out-of-doors fall rate was reduced to 64%, indicating a higher winter time proportion of inside falls. For our generally healthy study population, it is likely that our participants were engaged in outdoor activities with higher associated risk of falls during the warmer weather; for example, several summer falls occurred while bushwalking.

Fall injuries, especially fractures, have been found to increase in winter; this includes both inside (hip) and out-of-doors falls (wrist) [25]. Studies in the area of seasonal variation in fracture rates provide good evidence for increased fracture rates from falls in winter, but these appear in populations with older participants than ours (mean age over 75 years) [8, 13]. Our study recorded few injuries that required medical attention, hence making it difficult to compare serious fall injury data.

5. Limitations

Although this study aimed to recruit independently living community-dwelling older adults, bias in the sample may be present, as volunteers to this type of research project may be more robust than the community members at large. The lack of more frail subgroups, including those with cognitive impairment, depression, or using walking aids, limits the generalisability of this study. This study provides some evidence that measurements of postural sway may be affected by some effect of test-retest learning, and this needs to be considered in future research.

6. Conclusion

This is the first study to investigate the effects of season and postural sway and found that postural sway remained stable over the 12 months. Higher mediolateral sway range was associated with higher rates of injurious falls. No relationship between vitamin D levels was found with postural sway and fall incidence. This study provides important evidence for clinicians and researchers that postural sway remains stable over an annual cycle but may be influenced by a learning effect.

Abbreviations

CI: Confidence intervals
EO: Eyes open
EC: Eyes closed
IRR: Incident rate ratio
ML: Mediolateral
RaR: Relative risk
RR: Relative rate
SD: Standard deviation.

Conflict of Interests

The authors declare that they have no conflict of interests.

Acknowledgments

Funding for this study was received from the Clifford Craig Medical Research Trust and the Physiotherapy Research Foundation (Australia).

References

[1] L. Rubenstein, "Falls in older people: epidemiology, risk factors and strategies for prevention," *Age and Ageing*, vol. 35, pp. 37–41, 2006.

[2] A. Bergland, G.-B. Jarnlo, and K. Laake, "Predictors of falls in the elderly by location," *Aging*, vol. 15, no. 1, pp. 43–50, 2003.

[3] Y. Lajoie and S. P. Gallagher, "Predicting falls within the elderly community: comparison of postural sway, reaction time, the Berg balance scale and the Activities-specific Balance Confidence (ABC) scale for comparing fallers and non-fallers," *Archives of Gerontology and Geriatrics*, vol. 38, no. 1, pp. 11–26, 2004.

[4] J. K. Dhesi, L. M. Bearne, C. Moniz et al., "Neuromuscular and psychomotor function in elderly subjects who fall and the relationship with vitamin D status," *Journal of Bone and Mineral Research*, vol. 17, no. 5, pp. 891–897, 2002.

[5] S. W. Muir and M. Montero-Odasso, "Effect of vitamin D supplementation on muscle strength, gait and balance in older adults: a systematic review and meta-analysis," *Journal of the American Geriatrics Society*, vol. 59, no. 12, pp. 2291–2300, 2011.

[6] J. K. Dhesi, S. H. D. Jackson, L. M. Bearne et al., "Vitamin D supplementation improves neuromuscular function in older people who fall," *Age and Ageing*, vol. 33, no. 6, pp. 589–595, 2004.

[7] I. A. F. van der Mei, A.-L. Ponsonby, O. Engelsen et al., "The high prevalence of vitamin D insufficiency across Australian populations is only partly explained by season and latitude," *Environmental Health Perspectives*, vol. 115, no. 8, pp. 1132–1139, 2007.

[8] J. A. Pasco, M. J. Henry, M. A. Kotowicz et al., "Seasonal periodicity of serum vitamin D and parathyroid hormone, bone resorption, and fractures: the Geelong Osteoporosis Study," *Journal of Bone and Mineral Research*, vol. 19, no. 5, pp. 752–758, 2004.

[9] L. D. Gillespie, M. C. Robertson, W. J. Gillespie et al., "Interventions for preventing falls in older people living in the community," *Cochrane Database of Systematic Reviews*, no. 2, Article ID CD007146, 2008.

[10] S. Pajala, P. Era, M. Koskenvuo, J. Kaprio, T. Törmäkangas, and T. Rantanen, "Force platform balance measures as predictors of indoor and outdoor falls in community-dwelling women aged 63–76 years," *Journals of Gerontology A*, vol. 63, no. 2, pp. 171–178, 2008.

[11] C. Annweiler, M. Montero-Odasso, A. M. Schott, G. Berrut, B. Fantino, and O. Beauchet, "Fall prevention and vitamin D in the elderly: an overview of the key role of the non-bone effects," *Journal of Neuro-engineering and Rehabilitation*, vol. 7, no. 1, article 50, 2010.

[12] M. L. Bird, K. D. Hill, I. K. Robertson et al., "Serum [25(OH)D] status, ankle strength and activity show seasonal variation in older adults: relevance for winter falls in higher latitudes," *Age and Ageing*, vol. 42, no. 2, pp. 181–185, 2013.

[13] S. Mirchandani, G. B. Aharonoff, R. Hiebert, E. L. Capla, J. D. Zuckerman, and K. J. Koval, "The effects of weather

and seasonality on hip fracture incidence in older adults," *Orthopedics*, vol. 28, no. 2, pp. 149–155, 2005.

[14] P.-Y. Yeung, P.-H. Chau, J. Woo, V. W.-T. Yim, and T. H. Rainer, "Higher incidence of falls in winter among older people in Hong Kong," *Journal of Clinical Gerontology and Geriatrics*, vol. 2, no. 1, pp. 13–16, 2011.

[15] A. J. Campbell, G. F. S. Spears, M. J. Borrie, and J. L. Fitzgerald, "Falls, elderly women and the cold," *Gerontology*, vol. 34, no. 4, pp. 205–208, 1988.

[16] J. K. Pittaway, K. D. K. Ahuja, J. M. Beckett et al., "Make vitamin D while the sun shines, take supplements when t doesn't: a longitudinal, observational study of older adults in Tasmania, Australia," *PLoS ONE*, vol. 8, no. 3, Article ID e59063, 2013.

[17] M.-L. Bird, K. Hill, M. Ball, and A. D. Williams, "Effects of resistance- and flexibility-exercise interventions on balance and related measures in older adults," *Journal of Aging and Physical Activity*, vol. 17, no. 4, pp. 444–454, 2009.

[18] http://www.who.int/mediacentre/factsheets/fs344/en.

[19] B. E. Maki, P. J. Holliday, and A. K. Topper, "A prospective study of postural balance and risk of falling in an ambulatory and independent elderly population," *Journals of Gerontology*, vol. 49, no. 2, pp. M72–M84, 1994.

[20] M. A. Hughes, P. W. Duncan, D. K. Rose, J. M. Chandler, and S. A. Studenski, "The relationship of postural sway to sensorimotor function, functional performance, and disability in the elderly," *Archives of Physical Medicine and Rehabilitation*, vol. 77, no. 6, pp. 567–572, 1996.

[21] K. Hill, J. Schwarz, L. Flicker, and S. Carroll, "Falls among healthy, community-dwelling, older women: a prospective study of frequency, circumstances, consequences and prediction accuracy," *Australian and New Zealand Journal of Public Health*, vol. 23, no. 1, pp. 41–48, 1999.

[22] M. Pfeifer, B. Begerow, H. W. Minne, C. Abrams, D. Nachtigall, and C. Hansen, "Effects of a short-term vitamin D and calcium supplementation on body sway and secondary hyperparathyroidism in elderly women," *Journal of Bone and Mineral Research*, vol. 15, no. 6, pp. 1113–1118, 2000.

[23] W. P. Berg, H. M. Alessio, E. M. Mills, and C. Tong, "Circumstances and consequences of falls in independent community-dwelling older adults," *Age and Ageing*, vol. 26, no. 4, pp. 261–268, 1997.

[24] H. A. Bischoff-Ferrari, B. Dawson-Hughes, H. B. Staehelin et al., "Fall prevention with supplemental and active forms of vitamin D: a meta-analysis of randomised controlled trials," *British Medical Journal*, vol. 339, Article ID b3692, 2009.

[25] H. A. Bischoff-Ferrari, J. E. Orav, J. A. Barrett, and J. A. Baron, "Effect of seasonality and weather on fracture risk in individuals 65 years and older," *Osteoporosis International*, vol. 18, no. 9, pp. 1225–1233, 2007.

8

Ready-to-Eat Cereal Consumption Patterns: The Relationship to Nutrient Intake, Whole Grain Intake, and Body Mass Index in an Older American Population

Ann M. Albertson,[1] A. Christine Wold,[2] and Nandan Joshi[3]

[1] *General Mills: Bell Institute of Health and Nutrition, James Ford Bell Technical Center, 9000 Plymouth Avenue North, Minneapolis, MN 55427, USA*
[2] *General Mills: Quality & Regulatory Operations, 1 General Mills Boulevand, BT 10-D-1, Minneapolis, MN 55426, USA*
[3] *General Mills India Pvt. Ltd., 601-Prudential, Hiranandani Business Park, Powai, Mumbai 400076, India*

Correspondence should be addressed to Ann M. Albertson, ann.albertson@genmills.com

Academic Editor: Nadine Sahyoun

Objective. To investigate the relationship between ready-to-eat (RTE) breakfast cereal consumption patterns and body mass index (BMI), nutrient intake, and whole grain intake in an older American population. *Design*. A cross-sectional survey of US households, collected by the NPD Group via the National Eating Trends (NET) survey. Main outcome measures include BMI, nutrient intake, and whole grain intake. *Subjects/Setting*. The sample included 1759 participants age 55 and older, which was divided into approximate quartiles based on intake of RTE breakfast cereal for the 2-week period (0 servings, 1–3 servings, 4–7 servings, and ≥8 servings). *Results*. In the multivariate linear regression analysis adjusted for energy and age; intake of dietary fiber, whole grains, and the majority of micronutrients examined were found to be positively associated with frequent RTE cereal consumption. The proportion of participants consuming less than the Estimated Average Requirement (EAR) was lower for the highest quartile of RTE cereal consumers compared to nonconsumers, for the majority of vitamins and minerals examined. Significant differences in BMI between RTE breakfast cereal intake groups were found for men. *Conclusion*. Results suggest that ready-to-eat breakfast cereals may contribute to the nutritional quality of the diets of older Americans. Prospective studies and experimental trials are needed to better evaluate the role of RTE cereal consumption in energy balance.

1. Introduction

According to US Department of Health and Human Services, Administration on Aging population estimates, the number of older Americans is expected to grow dramatically. By 2030, the number of adults aged 60+ is expected to increase to approximately 25% of the population, while the number of the oldest old (age 85+) is expected to double [1]. Adequate nutrition is an important factor in continued health and independence for older adults [2, 3].

Homebound elderly people who skip breakfast are more likely to have inadequate nutrient intakes [2]. Caloric needs typically drop with advancing age, while needs for certain micronutrients such as calcium, vitamin D, and vitamin B_{12} increase [4]. Thus the importance of choosing nutrient dense foods increases for this population. Several cross-sectional studies have found positive associations between breakfast consumption and RTE breakfast cereal consumption, and increased nutrient intake for adult and elderly adult populations [5–8]. RTE cereal provides a convenient and easy to prepare breakfast option, which can provide whole grains and dietary fiber, along with many vitamins and minerals. RTE breakfast cereal is also an important contributor of whole grain in the US diet, providing approximately 30% of daily whole grain intake [9]. Recently, whole grain intake was found to be inversely associated with BMI and abdominal body fat in an older American population [10].

Similar to other age groups, the prevalence of overweight and obesity in the elderly population is increasing [11]. An estimated 76.5% of men and 73.5% of women ≥60 years old are currently overweight or obese (BMI ≥ 25) while 36.6% of men and 42.3% of women ≥60 years old are estimated to be obese (BMI ≥ 30) [12]. Based on recent NHANES data, McKeown estimates 62.5% of men and 74.9% of women ages 60 to 69 years old are abdominally obese [10]. It has been suggested that abdominal obesity may be a better measure of obesity than BMI in an older population, since after the age of 60 this population tends to lose lean body mass, while increasing visceral body fat [13].

A number of cross-sectional studies have examined the association of ready-to-eat (RTE) cereal intake with nutrient intake and body weight status. RTE cereal consumption has been found to be positively associated with intake of a range of vitamins and minerals and inversely associated with body mass index (BMI) in child and adolescent populations [14, 15]. In addition, eating breakfast along with a pattern of frequent ready-to-eat cereal consumption is associated with lower BMI, higher nutrient intakes, and weight maintenance in adults [7, 16–19]. Research in older adults is lacking. Thus, we examined the association of RTE cereal consumption patterns with nutrient intake in a sample of older adults who participated in a cross-sectional survey. The association of RTE cereal consumption with BMI and percent overweight or obese (BMI ≥ 25) was also examined in this study.

2. Methods

Data collected as part of the National Eating Trends (NET) survey were analyzed. The NET survey is conducted by the NPD Group, a marketing information company that has been monitoring the intake of US households since 1980 through this survey [20]. As described previously, the General Mills Bell Institute of Health and Nutrition (BIHN) has developed a proprietary method for combining data from the NET survey's 14-day food diary data, with portion size estimates from the National Health and Nutrition Examination Survey (NHANES) 1999–2004, and nutrient and food group data from the University of Minnesota's Nutrient Data System for Research (NDSR) Version 34, 2008 (Nutrition Coordinating Center, Minneapolis, MN) [14]. This combined dataset allows for population based, food pattern comparisons of usual intake, based on categories of foods consumed.

2.1. Food Consumption Data. Annually, the NET survey samples 2,000 households representing approximately 10,000 individuals, and data from the March 2006 through February 2008 survey were used for this study. To be included in this study, the subjects must have completed at least 7 days of food reporting and have provided height and weight data for calculation of BMI. The NET survey included 1905 participants age 55 and older, of these 1759 completed at least 7 days of food diaries and provided height and weight data (92%). Of these 1759 participants, 46% were male, 54% were female, and 22% were ≥75 years old.

For the NET survey, each year the NPD Group collaborates with a third party to establish a mail access panel that is a cross-sectional group of US households (noninstitutionalized people in the contiguous 48 states). Survey targets are set for the following demographic factors (family versus nonfamily, age, household income, household size, age of head of household, employment status, race, and census region) based on US Census Bureau statistics. NPD uses historical response data to over-sample households with lower expected response rates and adjusts the target levels quarterly to obtain a demographically and geographically balanced sample. Panelists are recruited using mailing lists and mall interventions, and NET survey panelists are then randomly selected from active mail panelists (those who have returned at least 1 other survey). Participant incentives include selection from a range of gifts ($25 to $30 value). Approximately 72% of households provide completed surveys for at least 10 of the 14 days of the annual survey.

Recruitment and data collection were conducted across all 52 weeks of the year. Each household member was required to document food and beverage intake by maintaining a daily eating diary. The "person most responsible for meal preparation" was responsible for documenting the name and brand of all food consumed for all household members, including any additions with cooking or food preparation. Description of the meal occasion (breakfast, lunch, snack, etc.) and location (at home, away from home) was included in the diary along with food names, flavor descriptors, brand names, package types, product form, special nutritional attributes, and other details. Food diary records were mailed back on a daily basis for the 14 day period.

2.2. Food Diary Data Entry. The University of Minnesota's Nutrition Database System for Research (NDS-R) provided the nutrient and food group data for this study. The NDS-R system provides a comprehensive database of complete nutrient data for 156 nutrients or components, for over 18,000 foods. The database is updated on an ongoing basis and contains over 7,000 brand name products. NDS-R has over 100 food groups in the database and each food is assigned a food group. Completed food diaries were entered into NDS-R for calculation of nutrient intake and food groups. Foods reported by NET survey panelists were matched, based on food diary descriptions to foods included in the NDS-R database. The recipe module of the NDS software was used to assign nutrient values to foods with special attributes (low fat, calcium fortified, reduced sodium, etc.) which were not found in the database and each recipe was assigned an appropriate food group.

2.3. Portion-Size Data. NET panelists record the foods and beverages consumed by household members but not the quantities. This procedure is standard for panel surveys to minimize recorder burden and thus increase reliability. Portion-sizes were estimated by combining data from the NHANES 1999–2004. Serving weights for individual food codes were aggregated and then collapsed for like-foods to strengthen cell sizes, and smoothed to eliminate outliers. Age and gender-specific mean serving weights were thereby determined for over 800 food types; these portions were subsequently assigned to each food recorded and coded in the NET diary.

2.4. Data Tabulation. Of the 1905 older American adults who were included in the NET survey, 146 participants were excluded for not meeting the inclusion criteria. 94% of those in the analytic sample provided complete (14 days) food diaries. For the 6% of participants with 7 to 13 days of dietary information the estimated servings of RTE cereal were normalized to 14 to allow for placement in the study quartiles. The pattern established over the 7- to 13-day period was assumed to be constant for the full 14 days. For example if no RTE cereal was consumed in the days collected, no servings would be included for the full 14 days, or if 2 servings were consumed in 7 days, 4 servings would be assumed for the full 14-day period. Self-reported values for height and weight were provided by each individual in the study. BMI was calculated by using the formula: BMI = weight (lb)/height (in)^2 × 703.

Servings of whole grains consumed by study participants were estimated based on food group assignments in the NDS-R database. All grain-based foods in the NDSR database are categorized as being either "whole grain," "some whole grain" or "refined grain". To be assigned to the "whole grain" category the first grain ingredient in the product must be a whole grain. Foods assigned to the "some whole grain" category are products that contain whole grain ingredients, but the first grain ingredient is not a whole grain. "Refined grain" products are those that contain no whole grain ingredients. In this paper servings of whole grains were calculated by summing serving of foods classified as "whole grain" in the database.

2.5. Statistical Analysis. To examine whether RTE cereal consumption was associated with BMI, body weight status, whole grain, and nutrient intake a series of analysis of variance (ANOVA) models were conducted by approximate quartiles of RTE cereal intake. Slightly greater than one quarter of the participants were nonconsumers, which made breaks in intake levels approximate rather than exact quartiles of RTE cereal intake (Table 1).

Logistic regression modeling was conducted to examine the association between RTE cereal consumption pattern and odds of falling below Estimated Average Requirement (EAR) for micronutrients with an established intake level. Covariates included within the ANOVA and logistic regression models were energy and age. Values were adjusted for energy to see if RTE cereal consumption was associated with a more nutrient dense diet. Age was included as a covariate, because it is associated with both RTE cereal consumption and nutrient intake. The contrasts were examined between the possible pairs of cereal consumption categories using the Wald chi-square test.

Logistic regression was used to compare odds of being overweight or obese by level of RTE cereal consumption. The contrasts were examined between the possible pairs of cereal consumption categories using the Wald chi-square test. For both the ANOVA and logistic regression models examining the association of RTE cereal consumption with body weight age and age^2 were included as covariates. Age^2 was included because the relationship between BMI and age is not linear, around 60 years of age this relationship can change [13]. All analyses were stratified by sex, because it was hypothesized that the association of RTE cereal consumption with the measured outcomes may vary by sex.

An alpha level of 0.01 was used to determine the significance for the analysis of variance comparisons, except where otherwise noted. All analyses were performed using SAS version 9.2 (SAS Institute, Cary, NC).

3. Results

The sample size and RTE cereal consumption distribution are displayed in Table 1. With respect to findings related to food and nutrient intake, the objective of this study was to determine the relationship between RTE cereal quartile of consumption to nutrient intake. For both men and women in the sample, significant differences in nutrient intakes between the fourth quartile (Q4) compared to the lowest two quartiles (Q1 and Q2) of RTE cereal consumption were seen for most nutrients examined (Table 2). For males, Q4 intake of energy was higher compared to Q1 and Q2. After adjusting for energy and age there was a significantly lower ($P < 0.01$) intake of total fat, total saturated fat, total trans fat, and cholesterol among those in Q4 compared to Q1 and Q2. In addition among men, intakes of total carbohydrate, dietary fiber, total sugar, vitamin A, vitamin C, vitamin D, thiamin, riboflavin, niacin, vitamin B6, folate, vitamin B12, potassium, calcium, iron, magnesium, and zinc were significantly higher ($P < 0.01$) among those in Q4 compared to those in Q1 and Q2. There were no significant differences between intake of total protein, added sugar, or vitamin E across consumption patterns of RTE cereal. Sodium intake was not significantly different between the highest and lowest quartiles of intake. Similar relationships were found for women age 55+ (Table 3), with the exception of total sugar intake which was not significantly different across quartiles of RTE cereal intake.

In addition to significant differences in nutrient intake, this study found whole grain intake to be positively associated with RTE cereal consumption. For both men and women, average whole grain intake among those in Q4 of RTE cereal consumption was nearly double the whole grain intake of those in the Q1 (the nonconsumers) (Tables 2 and 3).

The percentage of participants in each quartile that fell below Estimated Average Requirement (EAR) for nutrients with established EAR amounts was examined (Table 4). A significant inverse linear relationship was found between the frequency of RTE cereal consumption and the percentage of participants failing to consume the EAR for a number of nutrients. In women, this relationship was found for all nutrients examined except vitamin D and E and for men, all but niacin and iron.

In examining the relationship of RTE cereal consumption patterns and BMI there were some significant differences found in mean BMI for all men and all women (Table 5). With respect to men, the adjusted mean BMI was significantly lower among those in Q4 compared to Q1 and Q2 ($P = 0.0332$). For women, there were significant differences between Q3 and Q4, but no significant differences between the highest and lowest quartiles of RTE cereal intake.

Table 1: Sample size and RTE cereal consumption distribution for adults 55+ from the 2007-2008 NET survey.

Gender/age	Sample size	Quartile of cereal consumption			
		Q1 0 Servings/14 d *n* (%)	Q2 1–3 Servings/14 d *n* (%)	Q3 4–7 Servings/14 d *n* (%)	Q4 8+ Servings/14 d *n* (%)
All adults ages 55+	1759	490 (27.9)	484 (27.5)	380 (21.6)	405 (23.0)
Males ages 55+	803	231 (28.8)	207 (25.8)	165 (20.6)	200 (24.9)
Females ages 55+	956	259 (27.1)	277 (29.0)	215 (22.5)	205 (21.4)

Table 2: Adjusted* mean daily nutrient intake for adult men, ages 55+, by quartile of cereal consumption.

Nutrient	Quartile of RTE cereal consumption				*P*
	Q1 0 Servings Mean ± SE	Q2 1–3 Servings Mean ± SE	Q3 4–7 Servings Mean ± SE	Q4 8+ Servings Mean ± SE	
Energy (kcal)	1826 ± 38[a]	1932 ± 39[ab]	2033 ± 45[bc]	2142 ± 43[c]	<0.0001
Total fat (g)	81 ± 1.6[a]	80 ± 1.8[a]	76 ± 2.0[b]	73 ± 1.9[c]	<0.0001
Total saturated fat (SFA) (g)	27 ± 0.6[a]	27 ± 0.7[a]	25 ± 0.8[b]	25 ± 0.7[b]	<0.0001
Total trans Fat (TRANS) (g)	5.2 ± 0.1[a]	5.3 ± 0.1[a]	5.0 ± 0.2[a]	4.4 ± 0.2[b]	<0.0001
Cholesterol (mg)	307 ± 8[a]	309 ± 8[a]	272 ± 8[b]	244 ± 6[c]	<0.0001
Total carbohydrate (g)	228 ± 5[a]	233 ± 5[a]	246 ± 7[b]	253 ± 6[b]	<0.0001
Dietary fiber (g)	16 ± 0.4[a]	16 ± 0.4[a]	18 ± 0.5[b]	19 ± 0.5[b]	<0.0001
Total sugar (g)	104 ± 4[a]	104 ± 3[a]	113 ± 4[b]	117 ± 4[b]	<0.0001
Added sugar (g)	69 ± 2[a]	67 ± 2[a]	68 ± 2[a]	67 ± 2[a]	0.7652
Total protein (g)	78 ± 1[a]	78 ± 1[a]	77 ± 2[a]	80 ± 1[a]	0.2402
Vitamin A (mcg rae)	735 ± 33[a]	724 ± 30[a]	805 ± 36[ab]	867 ± 29[b]	0.0020
Vitamin C (mg)	81 ± 3[a]	85 ± 4[a]	94 ± 4[ab]	99 ± 4[b]	0.0011
Vitamin D (mcg)	4.2 ± 0.2[a]	4.7 ± 0.2[ab]	5.3 ± 0.2[b]	6.5 ± 0.2[c]	<0.0001
Vitamin E (mg alpha-tocopherol)	6.5 ± 0.2[a]	6.6 ± 0.2[a]	7.3 ± 0.3[a]	7.3 ± 0.3[a]	0.0245
Thiamin (mg)	1.6 ± 0.03[a]	1.7 ± 0.03[b]	1.8 ± 0.04[c]	1.9 ± 0.04[d]	<0.0001
Riboflavin (mg)	2.1 ± 0.04[a]	2.2 ± 0.04[a]	2.4 ± 0.05[b]	2.6 ± 0.05[c]	<0.0001
Niacin (mg)	21.9 ± 0.4[a]	22.5 ± 0.4[a]	23.5 ± 0.5[b]	25.8 ± 0.5[c]	<0.0001
Vitamin B6 (mg)	1.6 ± 0.03[a]	1.7 ± 0.03[a]	1.9 ± 0.04[b]	2.3 ± 0.06[c]	<0.0001
Folate (mcg)	437 ± 8[a]	491 ± 9[b]	588 ± 12[c]	743 ± 20[d]	<0.0001
Vitamin B12 (mg)	5.1 ± 0.2[a]	5.3 ± 0.2[a]	5.6 ± 0.2[a]	7.0 ± 0.2[b]	<0.0001
Sodium (mg)	3509 ± 59[ab]	3584 ± 67[a]	3450 ± 75[ab]	3428 ± 69[b]	0.0146
Potassium (mg)	2544 ± 52[a]	2599 ± 51[a]	2775 ± 65[b]	2875 ± 61[b]	<0.0001
Calcium (mg)	759 ± 21[a]	781 ± 20[a]	895 ± 28[b]	987 ± 30[c]	<0.0001
Iron (mg)	13 ± 0.3[a]	14 ± 0.3[b]	16 ± 0.3[c]	19 ± 0.4[d]	<0.0001
Magnesium (mg)	248 ± 5[a]	252 ± 5[a]	274 ± 6[b]	294 ± 6[c]	<0.0001
Zinc (mg)	10.2 ± 0.2[a]	10.2 ± 0.2[ab]	10.8 ± 0.3[b]	12.3 ± 0.3[c]	<0.0001
Whole grains (servings/14 d)	5.4 ± 6 [a]	6.8 ± 5 [a]	8.8 ± 6[b]	13.0 ± 8[c]	<0.0001

[a,b,c,d]Means within the same row with the same letter are not significantly different ($P < 0.01$). *Adjusted for energy and age.

When comparing the rates of overweight and obesity across RTE cereal consumption levels in analysis adjusted for age and age^2, significant differences in mean % overweight or obese were found for males but not for females (Table 5). Among men, the rate of overweight and obesity (BMI $\geq$ 25) was lower among those in Q4 compared to Q1 and Q2 ($P = 0.0433$). Among men, the rate of obesity (BMI $\geq$ 30) was lower among Q4 compared to Q2. However, no significant differences were observed in other groups. For women, there were no significant differences between quartiles. Results were similar in analysis adjusted for age only (data not shown).

TABLE 3: Adjusted* mean daily nutrient intake for adult women, ages 55+, by quartile of RTE cereal consumption pattern.

Nutrient	Quartile of RTE cereal consumption Q1 0 Servings Mean ± SD	Q2 1–3 Servings Mean ± SD	Q3 4–7 Servings Mean ± SD	Q4 8+ Servings Mean ± SD	P
Energy (kcal)	1363 ± 24^{a}	1510 ± 28^{b}	1570 ± 32^{b}	1622 ± 33^{b}	<0.0001
Total fat (g)	60 ± 1.1^{a}	60 ± 1.2^{a}	58 ± 1.4^{b}	55 ± 1.4^{c}	<0.0001
Total saturated fat (SFA) (g)	20.0 ± 0.4^{a}	20.0 ± 0.5^{a}	19.3 ± 0.5^{ab}	18.7 ± 0.5^{b}	<0.0001
Total trans fat (TRANS) (g)	4.0 ± 0.1^{a}	4.0 ± 0.1^{a}	3.7 ± 0.1^{b}	3.3 ± 0.1^{c}	<0.0001
Cholesterol (mg)	216 ± 6^{a}	227 ± 5^{a}	212 ± 6^{a}	188 ± 5^{b}	<0.0001
Total carbohydrate (g)	183 ± 3^{a}	185 ± 4^{ab}	190 ± 4^{bc}	197 ± 5^{c}	<0.0001
Dietary fiber (g)	13 ± 0.3^{a}	13 ± 0.3^{a}	13 ± 0.3^{a}	15 ± 0.4^{b}	<0.0001
Total sugar (g)	88 ± 2^{a}	87 ± 3^{a}	91 ± 3^{a}	92 ± 3^{a}	0.0654
Added sugar (g)	58 ± 1^{a}	56 ± 1^{a}	56 ± 2^{a}	53 ± 2^{a}	0.1569
Total protein (g)	58 ± 1^{a}	59 ± 1^{a}	60 ± 1^{a}	61 ± 1^{a}	0.0648
Vitamin A (mcg rae)	588 ± 21^{a}	578 ± 18^{a}	631 ± 22^{ab}	679 ± 21^{b}	0.0005
Vitamin C (mg)	71 ± 3^{a}	68 ± 3^{a}	76 ± 3^{ab}	84 ± 3^{b}	0.0001
Vitamin D (mcg)	3.2 ± 0.1^{a}	3.8 ± 0.1^{b}	4.2 ± 0.1^{b}	4.9 ± 0.1^{c}	<0.0001
Vitamin E (mg alpha-tocopherol)	5.5 ± 0.2^{a}	5.2 ± 0.2^{a}	5.8 ± 0.2^{a}	5.9 ± 0.2^{a}	0.0336
Thiamin (mg)	1.20 ± 0.02^{a}	1.26 ± 0.02^{b}	1.34 ± 0.03^{c}	1.49 ± 0.03^{d}	<0.0001
Riboflavin (mg)	1.5 ± 0.03^{a}	1.7 ± 0.03^{b}	1.8 ± 0.04^{c}	2.0 ± 0.04^{d}	<0.0001
Niacin (mg)	16 ± 0.3^{a}	17 ± 0.3^{a}	18 ± 0.3^{b}	20 ± 0.4^{c}	<0.0001
Vitamin B6 (mg)	1.2 ± 0.02^{a}	1.3 ± 0.02^{a}	1.5 ± 0.03^{b}	1.8 ± 0.05^{c}	<0.0001
Folate (mcg)	344 ± 6^{a}	384 ± 7^{b}	471 ± 10^{c}	600 ± 16^{d}	<0.0001
Vitamin B12 (mg)	3.7 ± 0.1^{a}	4.0 ± 0.1^{ab}	4.4 ± 0.1^{b}	5.7 ± 0.2^{c}	<0.0001
Sodium (mg)	2640 ± 43^{a}	2697 ± 45^{a}	2622 ± 50^{a}	2585 ± 51^{a}	0.0263
Potassium (mg)	1988 ± 34^{a}	2036 ± 39^{a}	2095 ± 44^{a}	2246 ± 44^{b}	<0.0001
Calcium (mg)	597 ± 15^{a}	637 ± 15^{ab}	690 ± 17^{b}	765 ± 19^{c}	<0.0001
Iron (mg)	10 ± 0.2^{a}	11 ± 0.2^{a}	13 ± 0.2^{b}	15 ± 0.3^{c}	<0.0001
Magnesium (mg)	198 ± 4^{a}	202 ± 4^{a}	207 ± 5^{a}	230 ± 5^{b}	<0.0001
Zinc (mg)	7.6 ± 0.2^{a}	7.6 ± 0.1^{a}	8.1 ± 0.2^{a}	9.3 ± 0.2^{b}	<0.0001
Whole grain (servings/14 d)	6.1 ± 6^{a}	7.3 ± 6^{a}	8.8 ± 6^{b}	12.3 ± 7^{c}	<0.0001

[a,b,c,d] Means within the same row with the same letter are not significantly different ($P < 0.01$). *Adjusted for energy and age.

4. Discussion

Study results suggest that frequent RTE cereal consumption may be associated with better nutrient intake profiles and higher whole grain intake in older Americans. Among older men RTE cereal consumption may be associated with lower BMI. Key nutrients that are typically underconsumed in older American populations include protein, fiber, vitamins B12, D, and E, calcium, magnesium, and zinc. Nutrients for which overconsumption is a concern include fat, cholesterol, vitamin A, iron, and zinc. Frequent consumption of RTE cereal was found to be associated with higher intake of all key underconsumed nutrients expect protein, which was not significantly different between the groups. In addition, consumption of whole grains for Q4 was more than double than the Q1 (nonconsuming group). RTE cereal consumption was also associated with lower energy adjusted fat and cholesterol intakes.

It was not surprising to find the positive association between higher RTE cereal consumption with higher intakes of vitamins and minerals, as many RTE cereals are fortified with vitamins and minerals and other studies have found similar associations for both children and adults [7, 14, 15, 17, 21]. In addition, RTE cereal consumption is associated with greater intake of milk and calcium, as milk and RTE cereal are usually consumed together [19].

Breakfast intake and frequent RTE cereal consumption have been associated with lower BMI based on a number of cross-sectional studies [14–17]. However, BMI is not an ideal measure of body fatness or mortality risk for older individuals and several studies suggest abdominal circumference may be a better measure of overweight and obesity in an elderly population [13, 22]. This study has data only on BMI as no measure of waist circumference was gathered. In this study, significant associations between RTE cereal consumption and body weight were found only for men. This finding differs from Song's data for adults' ≥19 years of age, which found an inverse association between RTE cereal consumption and BMI for women but not men [17].

There are a number of strengths of this study. First, while many studies have data from only 2 to 4 days of food records;

Table 4: Percentage of adults 55+ falling below the Estimated Average Requirement (EAR) by RTE cereal consumption pattern.

Nutrient	Men					Women				
	Percent falling below EAR									
	Q1	Q2	Q3	Q4	*P*	Q1	Q2	Q3	Q4	*P*
Vitamin A	58.4^{a}	52.7^{a}	35.8^{b}	20.5^{c}	<0.0001	55.2^{w}	44.8^{x}	34.9^{y}	17.6^{z}	<0.0001
Vitamin C	58.0^{a}	53.1^{a}	38.2^{b}	40.0^{b}	<0.0001	55.2^{w}	50.2^{wx}	44.2^{xy}	35.6^{y}	0.0002
Vitamin E	95.2^{a}	96.1^{a}	91.5^{ab}	87.5^{b}	0.0042	97.3^{w}	97.8^{w}	94.4^{w}	95.6^{w}	0.1833
Thiamin	14.7^{a}	6.3^{b}	1.8^{bc}	0.5^{c}	<0.0001	29.3^{w}	15.2^{x}	9.3^{xy}	5.4^{y}	<0.0001
Riboflavin	3.9^{a}	1.0^{b}	0.0^{b}	0.0^{b}	0.0018	13.1^{w}	2.5^{x}	0.5^{x}	0.0^{x}	<0.0001
Niacin	3.9^{a}	3.9^{a}	2.4^{ab}	0.0^{b}	0.1547	14.3^{w}	8.7^{x}	4.7^{xy}	2.0^{z}	<0.0001
Vitamin B6	40.7^{a}	30.4^{b}	11.5^{c}	3.5^{d}	<0.0001	68.0^{w}	54.5^{x}	32.6^{y}	13.2^{z}	<0.0001
Folate	26.4^{a}	9.2^{b}	1.8^{c}	1.0^{c}	<0.0001	54.1^{w}	28.9^{x}	11.6^{y}	3.9^{z}	<0.0001
Vitamin B12	6.9^{a}	1.5^{b}	0.6^{b}	0.0^{b}	<0.0001	19.7^{w}	7.2^{x}	3.7^{xy}	1.0^{y}	<0.0001
Iron	1.7^{a}	1.5^{a}	0.0^{a}	0.0^{a}	0.1161	3.1^{w}	0.7^{x}	0.0^{x}	0.0^{x}	0.0025
Magnesium	90.9^{a}	89.9^{a}	82.4^{b}	69.5^{c}	<0.0001	91.5^{w}	82.0^{x}	79.5^{x}	67.8^{y}	<0.0001
Zinc	52.8^{a}	45.9^{a}	32.1^{b}	15.5^{c}	<0.0001	50.6^{w}	38.3^{x}	25.1^{y}	13.7^{z}	<0.0001
Calcium	74.0^{a}	67.2^{a}	49.7^{b}	34.0^{c}	<0.0001	95.8^{w}	89.5^{x}	88.4^{x}	77.1^{y}	<0.0001
Vitamin D	95.7^{a}	95.7^{a}	95.2^{ab}	87.0^{b}	0.0010	99.2	98.9	98.6	99.0	0.9305

[abcd]Proportions within the same row with same letters are not significantly different ($P < 0.01$) (men).
[wxyz]Proportions within the same row with same letters are not significantly different ($P < 0.01$) (women).

Table 5: Adjusted* mean body mass index for adults 55+ years and percent overweight or obese by quartile of cereal consumption (BMI ≥ 25) by RTE cereal consumption pattern (energy excluded).

		Quartile of RTE cereal consumption				
		Q1 0 Servings	Q2 1–3 Servings	Q3 4–7 Servings	Q4 8+ Servings	
Gender/age	Sample size	Mean BMI				Overall *P*
Male ages 55+	803	28.19^{a}	27.96^{a}	27.36^{ab}	26.93^{b}	0.0332
Female ages 55+	956	27.48^{ba}	28.22^{ba}	28.53^{a}	27.09^{b}	0.0607
		Percent overweight/obese				*P*
Male ages 55+	803	74.43^{a}	70.69^{a}	63.05^{b}	64.35^{b}	0.0433
Female ages 55+	956	61.11^{a}	63.40^{a}	62.57^{a}	58.81^{a}	0.7575
		Percent obese				
Male ages 55+	803	28.70^{ab}	30.61^{a}	24.42^{ab}	21.02^{b}	0.1111
Female ages 55+	956	28.63^{a}	33.19^{a}	32.46^{a}	28.84^{a}	0.5622

[a, b]Values within the same row with the same letter are not significantly different ($P < 0.05$).
*Mean values adjusted for age, age^2.

this study is based on 14 days of data. Measurement error due to within person coefficient of variation in food and nutrient intake is reduced in this study due to the collection of 14 days of dietary intake information. This study included a representative sample of an older US population. The sample size allowed for examining the association of RTE cereal consumption with nutrient intake and weight status in older adults, with analysis conducted separately for males and females. In addition, the nutrient and food group database NDSR is one of the most comprehensive databases available for diet research, including nutrients of interest such as vitamin D and few missing nutrient values.

One limitation of this study is that a number of factors that could potentially confound the association of RTE cereal with BMI were not assessed and therefore could not be adjusted for in the analysis. For example, it did not include any measure of physical activity or ability to perform daily activities. Therefore, we do not know if this consumption pattern was associated with other lifestyle patterns, such as higher levels of physical activity. Another limitation is that BMI is based on self-reported measures of height and weight, and this is not the most reliable measure since people tend to overestimate their height and underestimate weight. Another limitation is the lack of reported portion size data. Reporting of portion size is one of the most error prone areas of dietary assessment. Portion size values were imputed from NHANES data where respondents are trained and use a variety of estimation tools however; reporting error is a potential issue. Finally, data on intake of dietary nutrient supplements was not gathered. Consequently, the association of RTE cereal consumption with nutrient intake could not be examined in the context of vitamin and mineral intake for all sources. It is unknown if supplementation may help bridge the gap between usual nutrient intakes and dietary recommendations. RTE cereals are generally fortified and can contribute a significant proportion of nutrients to those who consume them.

Overconsumption of certain vitamins and minerals such as vitamin A, iron, and zinc can be a risk for older Americans who eat fortified products and use vitamin and mineral supplements [23]. A recent study found 37% of men and 47% of women age ≥51 years consume at least one vitamin or mineral supplement each day [23]. Data from the 1999-2000 NHANES found 63% of individuals ≥60 years in age consume some type of daily dietary supplements [24]. Many older Americans may be unaware of the risk of overconsumption of vitamins and minerals and more education about this concern is needed. In addition, food manufacturers need to consider this concern for the elderly population when deciding on how to fortify RTE cereal products.

The food grouping estimates in the NDSR database are not ideal of determining whole grain intake. Food items that were grouped as "some whole grain" were not included in this study due to the uncertainty of the amount of whole grain in the food. Foods grouped as "whole grain" were counted as all whole grain, when the food may have other ingredients and also may include some refined grains. The finding of higher levels of whole grain in the highest quartile of RTE cereal consumption makes sense considering the higher intake of fiber for this group and since RTE cereal is an important contributor of whole grain in the US diet.

5. Conclusion

Results suggest that ready-to-eat breakfast cereals may contribute to the nutritional quality of the diets of older Americans. Prospective studies and experimental trials are needed to better evaluate the role of RTE cereal consumption in energy balance.

Authors' Contribution

A. M. Albertson and N. Joshi contributed to research design. A. C. Wold wrote the introduction and discussion for the paper. A. M. Albertson wrote the methods and results for the paper. N. Joshi did the data analysis. All authors read and approved the final paper.

Acknowledgment

The authors acknowledge Arohi Bapna for helping in editing the paper.

References

[1] US Department of Health and Human Services, Administration on Aging, Aging Statistics Census Data & Population Estimates, http://www.aoa.gov/AoARoot/Aging_Statistics/future_growth/future_growth.aspx.

[2] J. R. Sharkey, L. G. Branch, N. Zohoori, C. Giuliani, J. Busby-Whitehead, and P. S. Haines, "Inadequate nutrient intakes among homebound elderly and their correlation with individual characteristics and health-related factors," *American Journal of Clinical Nutrition*, vol. 76, no. 6, pp. 1435–1445, 2002.

[3] B. E. Millen, J. C. Ohls, M. Ponza, and A. C. McCool, "The Elderly Nutrition Program: an effective national framework for preventive nutrition interventions," *Journal of the American Dietetic Association*, vol. 102, no. 2, pp. 234–240, 2002.

[4] S. Park, M. A. Johnson, and J. G. Fischer, "Vitamin and mineral supplements: barriers and challenges for older adults," *Journal of Nutrition for the Elderly*, vol. 27, no. 3-4, pp. 297–317, 2008.

[5] J. M. Kerver, E. J. Yang, S. Obayashi, L. Bianchi, and W. O. Song, "Meal and snack patterns are associated with dietary intake of energy and nutrients in US adults," *Journal of the American Dietetic Association*, vol. 106, no. 1, pp. 46–53, 2006.

[6] E. A. Gollub and D. O. Weddle, "Improvements in nutritional intake and quality of life among frail homebound older adults receiving home-delivered breakfast and lunch," *Journal of the American Dietetic Association*, vol. 104, no. 8, pp. 1227–1235, 2004.

[7] M. A. Galvin, M. Kiely, and A. Flynn, "Impact of ready-to-eat breakfast cereal (RTEBC) consumption on adequacy of micronutrient intakes and compliance with dietary recommendations in Irish adults," *Public Health Nutrition*, vol. 6, no. 4, pp. 351–363, 2003.

[8] K. J. Morgan and M. E. Zabik, "The influence of ready-to-eat cereal consumption at breakfast on nutrient intakes of individuals 62 years and older," *Journal of the American College of Nutrition*, vol. 3, no. 1, pp. 27–44, 1984.

[9] J. L. Bachman, J. Reedy, A. F. Subar, and S. M. Krebs-Smith, "Sources of food group intakes among the US population, 2001-2002," *Journal of the American Dietetic Association*, vol. 108, no. 5, pp. 804–814, 2008.

[10] N. M. McKeown, M. Yoshida, M. K. Shea et al., "Whole-grain intake and cereal fiber are associated with lower abdominal adiposity in older adults," *Journal of Nutrition*, vol. 139, no. 10, pp. 1950–1955, 2009.

[11] D. K. Houston, B. J. Nicklas, and C. A. Zizza, "Weighty concerns: the growing prevalence of obesity among older adults," *Journal of the American Dietetic Association*, vol. 109, no. 11, pp. 1886–1895, 2009.

[12] K. M. Flegal, D. Carroll, B. K. Kit, and C. L. Ogden, "Prevalence of obesity and trends in the distribution of body mass index among US adults, 1999–2010," *Journal of the American Medical Association*, vol. 307, no. 5, pp. 491–497, 2012.

[13] J. C. Seidell and T. L. S. Visscher, "Body weight and weight change and their health implications for the elderly," *European Journal of Clinical Nutrition*, vol. 54, supplement 3, pp. S33–S39, 2000.

[14] A. M. Albertson, G. H. Anderson, S. J. Crockett, and M. T. Goebel, "Ready-to-eat cereal consumption: its relationship with BMI and nutrient intake of children aged 4 to 12 years," *Journal of the American Dietetic Association*, vol. 103, no. 12, pp. 1613–1619, 2003.

[15] A. M. Albertson, S. G. Affenito, R. Bauserman, N. M. Holschuh, A. L. Eldridge, and B. A. Barton, "The relationship of ready-to-eat cereal consumption to nutrient intake, blood lipids, and body mass index of children as they age through adolescence," *Journal of the American Dietetic Association*, vol. 109, no. 9, pp. 1557–1565, 2009.

[16] S. Cho, M. Dietrich, C. J. P. Brown, C. A. Clark, and G. Block, "The effect of breakfast type on total daily energy intake and body mass index: results from the Third National Health and Nutrition Examination Survey (NHANES III)," *Journal of the American College of Nutrition*, vol. 22, no. 4, pp. 296–302, 2003.
[17] W. O. Song, O. K. Chun, S. Obayashi, S. Cho, and C. E. Chung, "Is consumption of breakfast associated with body mass index in US adults?" *Journal of the American Dietetic Association*, vol. 105, no. 9, pp. 1373–1382, 2005.
[18] L. R. Purslow, M. S. Sandhu, N. Forouhi et al., "Energy intake at breakfast and weight change: prospective study of 6,764 middle-aged men and women," *American Journal of Epidemiology*, vol. 167, no. 2, pp. 188–192, 2008.
[19] W. O. Song, O. K. Chun, J. Kerver, S. Cho, C. E. Chung, and S. J. Chung, "Ready-to-eat breakfast cereal consumption enhances milk and calcium intake in the US population," *Journal of the American Dietetic Association*, vol. 106, no. 11, pp. 1783–1789, 2006.
[20] The NPD Group, *National Eating Trends*, 2007-2008.
[21] B. A. Barton, A. L. Eldridge, D. Thompson et al., "The relationship of breakfast and cereal consumption to nutrient intake and body mass index: the National Heart, Lung, and Blood Institute Growth and Health Study," *Journal of the American Dietetic Association*, vol. 105, no. 9, pp. 1383–1389, 2005.
[22] T. L. S. Visscher, J. C. Seidell, A. Molarius, D. Van Der Kuip, A. Hofman, and J. C. M. Witteman, "A comparison of body mass index, waist-hip ratio and waist circumference as predictors of all-cause mortality among the elderly: the Rotterdam study," *International Journal of Obesity*, vol. 25, no. 11, pp. 1730–1735, 2001.
[23] R. S. Sebastian, L. E. Cleveland, J. D. Goldman, and A. J. Moshfegh, "Older adults who use vitamin/mineral supplements differ from nonusers in nutrient intake adequacy and dietary attitudes," *Journal of the American Dietetic Association*, vol. 107, no. 8, pp. 1322–1332, 2007.
[24] K. Radimer, B. Bindewald, J. Hughes, B. Ervin, C. Swanson, and M. F. Picciano, "Dietary supplement use by US adults: data from the National Health and Nutrition Examination Survey, 1999-2000," *American Journal of Epidemiology*, vol. 160, no. 4, pp. 339–349, 2004.

9

Sarcopenia, a Neurogenic Syndrome?

Ping Kwan

ST013a, Department of Rehabilitation Sciences, Hong Kong Polytechnic University, Hong Kong

Correspondence should be addressed to Ping Kwan; pkwan@polyu.edu.hk

Academic Editor: Louis Bherer

Sarcopenia is an aging-associated condition, which is currently characterized by the loss of muscle mass and muscle strength. However, there is no consensus regarding its characterization hitherto. As the world older adult population is on the rise, the impact of sarcopenia becomes greater. Due to the lack of effective treatments, sarcopenia is still a persisting problem among the global older adults and should not be overlooked. As a result, it is vital to investigate deeper into the mechanism underlying the pathogenesis of sarcopenia in order to develop more effective therapeutic interventions and to inscribe a more uniform characterization. The etiology of sarcopenia is currently found to be multifactorial, and most of the pharmacological researches are focused on the muscular factors in aging. Although the complete mechanism underlying the development of sarcopenia is still waiting to be elucidated, we propose in this article that the primary trigger of sarcopenia may be neurogenic in origin based on the intimate relationship between the nervous and muscular system, namely, the motor neuron and its underlying muscle fibers. Both of them are affected by the cellular environment and their physiological activity.

1. Introduction

Sarcopenia (Greek: *sarx* means "flesh," *penia* means "loss") is an age-related geriatric syndrome first described on a meeting in 1988 by Dr. Rosenberg as a phenomenon whereby the age-related decline in lean body mass affects ambulation, mobility, energy intake, overall nutrient intake and status, independence, and breathing [1]. More recently, sarcopenia is characterized by the gradual loss of muscle mass, muscle strength, and muscle function/quality in aging [2, 3]. However, there are studies indicating that sarcopenia should be referred only as the age-related loss in muscle mass whilst the age-related loss in muscle strength should be isolated as a new condition called "dynapenia" based on the evidences indicating that the loss of muscle mass and strength are two distinct processes with different pathophysiology [4].

Hitherto, there is no consistent data among a variety of prevalence studies probably due to the difference in study sample, definition of sarcopenia, and the assessment tool used [3]. For example, for the population of over 80 years old, American study of New Mexico Elder Health Survey has found that there were >40% of women and 50% of men who were sarcopenic whilst the NHANES III database study reveals that 11% of women and 7% of men were sarcopenic. Also, the Italian study of InCHIANTI cohort reveals that 15% of women and 70% of men were sarcopenic [3]. In summary, the prevalence of this syndrome depends on age, sex, race [3, 5–7], morbidity [7, 8], nutrition [9], and physical activity [10, 11].

Some studies indicate that sarcopenia leads to functional limitations, impaired mobility, disability, falls, and fractures, which in turn lead to the loss of independence, frailty, and increased risk of mortality [11–13]. In contrast, some studies indicate that the parameter of muscle mass may not relate to the functional status and mortality [4]. No matter whether sarcopenia may affect both the quality and quantity of life of individuals or not, there are no effective treatment for sarcopenia and its related outcomes yet. Pharmacological interventions currently present are not effective and possess a considerable level of side effects. These include hormonal (e.g., growth hormones, testosterones, estrogens, tibolone) and nonhormonal (e.g., losartan, telmisartan) interventions [14]. Hitherto, only exercise training except endurance training, especially by power training [11, 14], and with adequate nutrition [9] seems to be the relatively effective intervention with the least side effects. Together with the inconformity of sarcopenia characterization among different studies, it is imperative to explore deeper into the mechanism or etiology of sarcopenia which in turn will provide further insight into the development of more effective therapy as well as a better understanding of the rationale that leads to a better characterization of sarcopenia.

In this article, we aimed to provide another perspective on sarcopenia and propose that sarcopenia may be neurogenic in nature despite its muscle-related features. In the following sections, we will discuss first the definition of sarcopenia, followed by commonly accepted etiology of sarcopenia, and then the impact and overview of the physiological factors that link up the nervous and muscular system.

2. Definition of Sarcopenia

Despite the characterization of sarcopenia varied among different studies [2–4, 15, 16], the major impact of sarcopenia is the age-related progressive decline in muscle mass. Under normal circumstances, when a healthy individual is trying to perform a particular physical activity, the relevant muscles on the corresponding part of the body will start to generate strength or force by neural action potential-induced contraction. The part of the body moves only when the overall strength produced overcomes the weight exert by the corresponding body part and the resistance forces induced by the activity. It is commonly assumed that if every muscle fiber of a single type has the same rate of force generation and produces the same force, then the muscle strength shall be positively correlated with the number of muscle fibers present in the muscle. Thus, the loss of muscle mass shall at least partly contribute to the loss of muscle strength which in turn contribute to the decline in muscle function due to the impaired ability to overcome resistance forces involved in the physical activity. In fact, the association between muscle mass and strength was supported by early cross-sectional studies until recent longitudinal studies demonstrated that there may be a disassociation between age-related changes in muscle mass (sarcopenia) and strength (dynapenia), and there are distinct mechanisms accounting for each component [15, 16]. These recent evidences not only bring a new terminology "dynapenia" into the field but also a reconsideration of the mechanism and etiology that underlies the problems as well as examining the problem from other perspectives. However, according to the original definition of sarcopenia [1],

> *no decline with age is as dramatic or potentially more significant than the decline in lean body mass. In fact, there may be no single feature of age-related decline more striking than the decline in lean body mass in affecting ambulation, mobility, energy intake, overall nutrient intake and status, independence and breathing. Irwin H. Rosenberg, 1988*

Notwithstanding, the focus is on the decline of lean body mass, and if scrutinized carefully, the statement is actually referred to a phenomenon that relates to both the body mass and function but not the strength. Thus, "sarcopenia" in 1988 is defined as the change of body functions and behavior due to the loss of lean body mass. However, as strength is an independent predictor of body functions including falls and mortality [4, 16], it eventually replaces the body function and becomes part of the definition of sarcopenia in some studies [2, 3]. Since the definition of sarcopenia plays a central role in its research affecting the significance of its related research findings thereafter, we should have a consensus regarding this definition. Recently, some studies have pointed out the dissociation between the muscle mass and muscle strength [4, 15, 16] and have introduced the concept of "dynapenia" into the field; the strength parameter should be isolated from the definition of sarcopenia once again. However, when reading the original Albuquerque statement, it should be noted that Dr. Rosenberg has actually used the term "lean body mass" which includes the mass of muscles, blood, bones, and other nonfat tissues. All these tissues could experience aging and contribute to the decline in body function at a certain degree. Even the prefix "sarco" is commonly used to depict the muscles, and the Greek translation for "sarx" is only flesh whilst the one for muscle is "myx". As a result, the term "myopenia" may be more appropriate for the current pathological condition of the age-related decline in muscle mass.

Virtually all diseases and pathological conditions involve a change in body physiology in which a phenotype is determined by a myriad of molecular factors that weave different molecular cascades in an interlacing fashion. Interestingly, one physiological factor may link up to several diseases (e.g., inflammation involved in both Alzheimer's disease and Parkinson's disease) and one sort of disease may also have several underlying physiological factors (e.g., amyotrophic lateral sclerosis has several subtypes and each of which is associated with a different gene or protein). In the case of sarcopenia, although muscle wasting and muscle atrophy are main features of its pathology, it is not unique at least Cachexia has a similar characteristics and consequence as sarcopenia [8, 17, 18]. The certain degree of pathological overlapping suggests that at least some underlying molecular mechanisms are common to/shared between these pathologies. For instance, inflammation where proinflammatory cytokines and ubiquitin-proteasome degradation pathway are upregulated [17]. Despite the similarity and overlapping characteristics with cachexia, sarcopenia is a separate clinical condition with a certain degree of discrepancies. Sarcopenia is a chronic muscle wasting condition associated with a low grade systemic inflammation which is not necessary to be the pathological trigger whilst cachexia is an acute muscle wasting condition that only develops under an overlying inflammation [8, 17]. In summary, it may be more appropriate to account the loss of muscle mass in subtypes or in a way similar to the definition of amyotrophic lateral sclerosis. For example, the subtype with a muscle-in-origin etiology shall call "type I sarcopenia" whilst the subtype with a neuron-in-origin etiology shall call "type II sarcopenia". Or from the other perspective, the term "sarcopenia" shall be a pronoun for all types of chronic muscle mass decline and each of its subtypes is defined by one sort of etiological mechanism. For instance, the one shared with cachexia shall be called "cachexic sarcopenia" whilst the one shared with amyotrophic lateral sclerosis shall be called "Hawking's sarcopenia."

3. Commonly Accepted Etiology of Sarcopenia

Currently, the body physiology or the etiology of sarcopenia is believed to be affected by but not restricted to five main features: (1) aging, (2) genetics, (3) morbidity, (4) nutrition, and (5) activity. Nevertheless, it is certain that muscle mass, strength, function, and quality are determined by at least three cardinal physiological systems: (1) neurological system [15], (2) muscular system [15], and (3) circulatory system. Thus, it is not surprising that any diseases or conditions that affect or alter these physiological systems may contribute to the development of dynapenia and sarcopenia, for example, genetic factors, neurodegenerative diseases, hormonal dysregulatory diseases, autoimmune diseases, inflammation, malnutrition, physical injuries, and inactivity [5, 8, 12]. As the muscle function relies on the status of motor units (each of which consisted of a motor neuron, motor neurites (axons), neuromuscular junctions (NMJ), and muscle fibers) in addition to the circulation factors, the pathology of sarcopenia may be neurogenic, musculogenic (term created to differ from "myogenic"), synaptogenic (from NMJ), and/or vasculogenic (from blood vessels) (Figure 1).

3.1. Muscular Factors. Aging is a symplcetic ("sym": together; "plektos": braid) natural process of matters and contributes significantly to sarcopenia. For skeletal muscle, aging leads to a decline in muscle function. At the systemic level, both the upper and lower limbs of men and women have an age-associated sequential loss in muscle power, muscle strength, and muscle mass, starting from the age of 40 years, 30 years, and 24 years, respectively [19]. The age-related loss of muscle power is more rapid than the parallel loss of muscle strength which in turn is more rapid than the loss of muscle mass [12, 19]. The loss in muscle power and muscle strength is at least partly attributable to the reduction in muscle mass. At the molecular level, the loss of muscle power and muscle strength is further associated with a reduction in the amount of Ca^{2+} available for the mechanical response in muscles [20] and with a reduction in Ca^{2+} release in response to the mechanical action of muscles due to the age-associated reduction in dihydropyridine receptors at the t-tubule and sarcoplasmic reticulum membrane which in turn results in uncoupling of Ca^{2+} release channels or ryanodine receptors in type II muscle fibers [15, 19, 20]. On the myocellular level, skeletal muscle fibers are basically two types. Type I fibers are slow and oxidative which mainly operate in the weight bearing/antigravity functions, whilst type II fibers are fast and glycolytic which are mainly involved in the explosive actions (e.g., sprinting). Patients with sarcopenia manifested a reduction in the number of both type I/slow-twitch and type II/fast-twitch muscle fibers and an atrophy specific to the type II fibers (being more prominent in IIB fibers than IIA fibers) [12, 19]. This may be resulted from a hypotrophic or hypercatabolic state of muscle fibers which may be a cause or an effect of the denervation of motor units and/or the loss of motor neurons [21]. These are the common features of aging and are being more prominent in type II than type I fibers. However, the hypercatabolic state of muscle fibers may also attribute to the reduction in the number of satellite cells [22]. In other words, the loss of muscle mass is also partly attribute to the diminished ability of muscle self-repair due to the decreased number and impaired function of satellite cells [2, 22]. At the cellular level, aging is associated with a reduction in cell density of the satellite cell population in type II fibers as well as a diminished satellite cell proliferation capacity or a replicative senescence, which may relate to the shortening of telomeres [2, 22, 23].

3.2. Neurological Factors. On the neurological side, the loss of muscle power and muscle strength is associated with the age-related changes in motor units and in the degree of coactivation of antagonist muscles, respectively [19]. At the cellular level, aging is associated with a reduction in motor axon conduction velocity and the number of myelinated axons. Further, it is associated with a reduction in motor unit reinnervation after denervation, and with a reduction in the number of motor units and motor neurons specific to the type II muscle fibers [19, 21]. As the fast-twitch motor units are the determinant of the degree of power exerted by muscles, their loss in aging contributes to the loss in muscle power [19]. In fact, under normal aging process, a preferential denervation of type II muscle fibers occurs and these denervated fibers are then reinnervated by the axonal sprouting from slow motor neurons in a process called motor unit remodeling. However, if denervation outpaces reinnervation, then a population of denervated fibers will undergo atrophy and degeneration [24] due to the loss of trophic factors [25]. This process contributes to the loss of muscle mass at least partly by apoptosis [26]. At the molecular level, rat studies have shown that progressive denervation during aging have disrupted the precise overlapping between the presynaptic nerve terminal and the postsynaptic acetylcholine receptor (AChR) clusters at the NMJ [27]. Also, denervated muscles have elevated the expression of proapoptotic/atrophic factors including bax, caspase 3, 7, 8, and 10 [26] along with a reduction in the trophic factor signals including TrkB signaling via BDNF and NT-4/5 [27]. These in turn increase the apoptotic potential of myocytes. Thus, denervation seems to be the trigger for muscle loss.

3.3. Circulation Factors. Blood circulation is vital to the whole body and thus may also contribute to the pathology. Aging is associated with the changes in microcirculation and ultrastructure of the vascular endothelium [28], a decline in vascular endothelial functions [29], and a decline in exercise-induced blood flow which may be partly resulted from an age-related reduction in vasodilatory capacity and capillarization [28]. The reduced blood flow leads to a reduction in the exchange of oxygen, energy sources, metabolites, and heat between blood and the body cells. This results in a less trophic environment for the cells in the corresponding region [28].

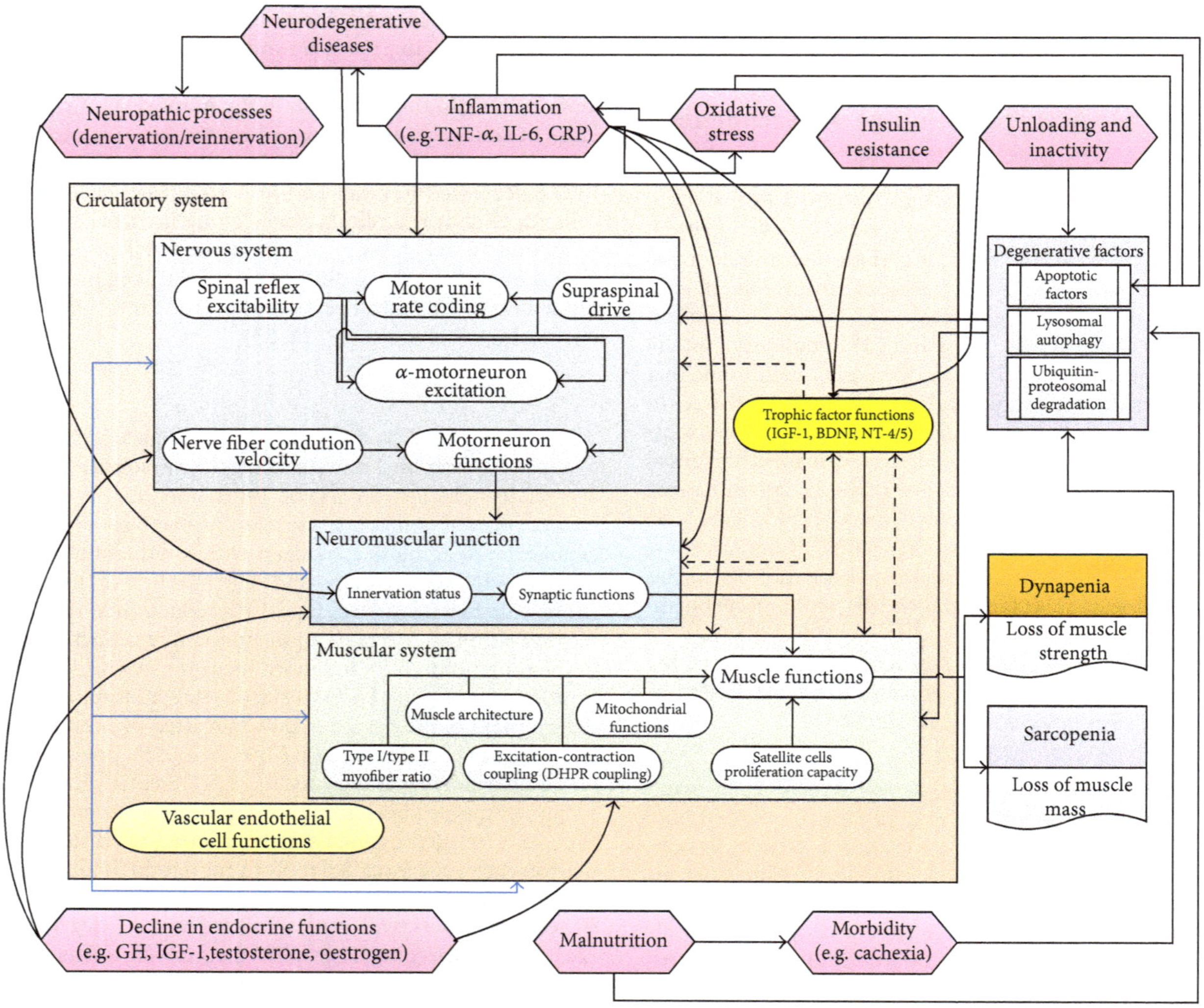

Figure 1: Summary of the neuromuscular mechanism and its relationship with the commonly accepted etiological factors of sarcopenia. The relationships between each of these factors are interlaced in a complex fashion. Black solid lines = positive regulators/reinforcements; black dash lines = positive regulators from the muscular system; red solid lines = negative regulators; blue solid lines = regulation by the circulation.

4. Common Pathophysiology Shared between the Aging Nervous System and the Aging Muscular System

According to most of the studies, contributors to the loss of muscle mass in sarcopenia are explained mainly by, but not limited to: (1) mitochondrial dysfunction, (2) elevation of oxidative stress, (3) inflamm-aging, (4) altered rate of protein turnover, (5) decreased hormones, growth factors, and proteins that maintain proper cellular functions, (6) declines in intake of essential nutrients, and (7) declines in physical activity [5, 12, 19, 21]. Interestingly, most of these contributors are not unique to the muscular system. They may also applicable to the nervous system.

4.1. Mitochondrial Dysfunction. Mitochondrial dysfunction may arise from the age-related decline in mitochondriogenesis [14, 30] and mitochondrial function. Both of which may be associated with an increase in the mitochondrial DNA damage by oxidative stress, changes in the mitochondrial respiratory chain enzymes, and changes in the mitochondrial proapoptotic proteins. Mitochondrial dysfunction results in an impaired mitochondrial oxidative function and energy production. These in turn affect cell viability through necrosis and/or apoptosis of both myocytes and neurons [21, 31].

4.2. Elevation of Oxidative Stress. Elevation of oxidative stress is commonly seen in aged animal cells with an increase in the oxidative species (e.g., H_2O_2 species, MDA/4-HAE, nitrotyrosine, catalase [32], iNOS [17]) and a decrease in the antioxidative species (e.g., MnSOD [32], G6PDH [33]). Also, accumulation of the oxidative stress-induced advanced age glycation end-product (AGE) and lipoxidation end-products (ALE) on the extracellular and intracellular proteins during aging impairs the activities of these proteins [21]. The consequence of an elevated oxidative stress in muscles is the iNOS-mediated downregulation of a set of myogenic proteins including CKM and MyoD [17], and the concomitant inhibition of general protein translation by both the phosphorylation of eIF2α and the inhibition of mTOR [17]. Additionally, aging upregulates the iNOS which correlates with an increase in caspase 2 and JNK signaling activity, this suggests the involvement of JNK-mediated apoptotic signaling [33]. In the perspective of the nervous system, oxidative stress may lead to an alteration in the balance between mitochondrial fission and fusion as well as an activation of the apoptotic pathway in neurons [34].

4.3. Inflamm-Aging (Aging-Associated Chronic Inflammation). Inflammation is intimately linked to the oxidative stress. Inflamm-aging is an age-related elevation of the baseline level of proinflammatory markers and cytokines (e.g., TNF-α, IL-6, CRP) [10]. The most representative cytokines are TNF-α and IL-6. TNF-α induce apoptosis directly through its iteraction with the death domain receptors which in turn leads to the activation of procaspase 8 [21, 26]; and indirectly through the activation of its downstream effectors, NF-κB, which activity is also elevated by aging [17]. Activated NF-κB upregulates MSTN/GDF8 [35], iNOS, and MuRF1 [17], these factors play a negative role in the trophic state of myocytes. Additionally, IL-6 plays a similar role by downregulating IGF-1 [2]. As a result, the anabolic potential of myocytes including the satellite cells is impaired due to (1) reduced expression of proteins involved in myogenesis and other relevant muscle growth processes (e.g., MRF, myogenin, MyoD, and CKM) [17, 26]; (2) elevated expression of MSTN which exerts its effect on muscle growth by regulating the Activin receptor-mediated pathway, MAPK pathway, and Akt/TORC1/p70S6K pathway [5]. Additionally, MSTN induces reactive oxygen species (ROS) production via NADPH oxidase and TNF-α. The elevated TNF-α in turn induces further MSTN production and the higher levels of MSTN promotes proteasome-mediated catabolism of intracellular proteins [35]. In addition to the muscular system, both oxidative stress and inflammation have great impacts on the nervous system as they are commonly disclosed in the neurodegenerative diseases [34, 36].

4.4. Altered Rate of Protein Turnover. Altered protein balance is one of the major features in aging cells. In myocytes, there is an age-associated change in expression of dystrophic factors (e.g., Id1, Id2 and Id3, etc.) [26] and trophic factors (e.g., MGF, etc.) [19]. Similarly, the expression profile of dystrophic/proapoptotic factors (e.g., bax and procaspase 3, etc.) [37] and trophic factors (e.g., CNTF, etc.) [19] in neurons are also altered by aging. The fate of a cell is determined by the balance between the rate of positive metabolism and the rate of negative metabolism which are positively correlated to the level of trophic signal (e.g., growth factor-mediated pathways) and atrophic/dystrophic signal (e.g., proapoptotic factor-mediated pathways), respectively. Thus, when the rate of negative metabolism exceeds the rate of positive metabolism, the cell will undergo atrophy and finally death by apoptosis. In the case of aging myocytes, despite the mechanism is not clear, the loss of multinucleated myocyte nuclei is suggested to be caused by apoptosis regulated by AIF-mediated caspase-independent DNA fragmentation. Unlike single-nucleated neurons, apoptosis of one single nucleus of the myocyte may not result in cell death [21]. Instead it will undergo an atrophy due to the decrease of the nuclear domain [19]. Together with the "use it or lose it" perspective (discuss in later section), this may explain the more remarkable reduction in the size of type II muscle fibers than that of the type I muscle fibers in sarcopenia. Additionally, this also suggested that myocytes may have a greater potential to resist death than neurons. At the transcription level, miRNAs may also contribute to the age-related alteration in protein turnover as they are capable of regulating protein expression. Many miRNA candidates altered their expression level during aging in both myocytes and neurons [38–40].

4.5. Decreased Hormones, Growth Factors, and Functional Proteins. Hormones, growth factors, and proteins that maintain proper cellular functions are associated with the trophic state of myocytes. Aging is associated with a decline in sex hormones in both male and female, for example, androgen and estrogen [2]. On the neurological side, the alteration in sex hormone levels may also affect brain functions as circulating sex hormones can penetrate the blood-brain barrier [41]. Additionally, aging is associated with a decline in growth factors and their relevant regulators affecting both myocytes and neurons, for example, (1) GH, which regulates the synthesis of IGF-1 [19] and the survival of neurons [42]; (2) IGFs, which stimulate amino acid and glucose transport and are important trophic factors to both myocytes [5, 12] and neurons [43–45]. IGF-1 regulates growth, differentiation, and regeneration of myocytes [12] by inducing hypertrophy pathways (e.g., PI3K and MAPK pathways) [5] whilst IGF-2 is associated with the proliferative action in adult muscles [12]; (3) CNTFs, which are important hypertrophic factors for both myocytes and neurons [12] and may play a role in the re-innervation of muscle fibers by motor neurons after muscle and nerve injury [5]. Apart from the growth factors, aging is also associated with a reduction in stress-induced expression of HSP70, which normally functioned as chaperones and expressed by both myocytes and neurons [21, 23]. HSP70 reduces the apoptotic potential of a cell by inhibiting the formation of apoptosome and functioning as an antagonist of AIF [21]. Thus, the age-associated decline in these candidates may have a serious consequence on both the muscular and nervous systems.

4.6. Malnutrition. Aging is commonly associated with a decline in the ability to utilize exogenous amino acids. This may be due but not limited to: (1) reductions in transmembrane amino acid transport for protein synthesis; (2) alterations in the whole body amino acid turnover which results in a reduced availability of substrate for protein synthesis; (3) alterations in the endogenous hormonal response; and/or (4) alterations in the response of muscle to the hormonal stimuli after meal intake [47]. The current recommended daily nutrition intake for the prevention of sarcopenia and frailty is 24–36 kcal and 0.8–1.2 g high quality protein per kg body weight [9]. Essential amino acids, in particular the branched-chain amino acids (BCAA) especially Leucine, are potent anabolic signals for protein accretion [47, 48], which requires ~0.7 kcal/g of muscle protein synthesized [47]. Therefore, lacking such nutrients may alter the protein turnover and thus contribute to the development of sarcopenia [8].

4.7. Disuse Atrophy. Physical inactivity, induced by either sedentary lifestyle or immobility due to illness/injury, is a trigger of muscle disuse atrophy [18]. At the molecular level, physical inactivity is associated with an inhibition of the IGF-1 hypertrophic signaling and a concomitant upregulation of proteasomal (ubiquitin) and lysosomal (autophagy) degradation signaling via FOXO proteins [18, 49]. This contributes to a reduced trophic state in myocytes. In contrast, increased physical activity level by resistance training enhances the muscle mass, muscle strength, and balance which in turn reduces the risk of physical limitation and/or the onset of frailty [11, 21]. The effect of exercise training is dose dependent. The higher the intensity involved in the training, the better the yield of the effect. Training at 60%–85% of the individual maximum voluntary strength can increase the muscle mass whilst more than 85% can also increase the rate of force development. The addition of a sensorimotor component to the exercise training program may also help improving the postural control in older persons [50]. In addition to the muscles, the influence of exercise training to the nervous system is also well described [51]. Interestingly, although having a positive impact on both muscle mass and strength, exercise trainings do not prevent the age-related impairment in muscle features. Recent studies reported that both the muscle size and functions are impaired in aged sprint-trained athletes. Similar to sarcopenia, type II muscle fibers were suffered from a more remarkable impairment than type I muscle fibers [52].

5. Use It or Loss It

On the neurological perspective, physical inactivity reflects a reduced activity of the corresponding motor units. Unused or seldom used neurons will undergo disuse degeneration which in turn results in a further disuse degeneration of its synaptically connected cells [53]. Thus, it is possible that the age-associated progressive denervation and the age-associated loss of muscle fibers are due to the disuse atrophy and degeneration of the NMJ and/or the motor neurons. This "use it or loss it" doctrine at least partly explains why there are more prominent type II motor unit atrophy and degeneration in sarcopenia and why sedentary individuals are more susceptible to sarcopenia. As sedentary individuals have less explosive actions, the frequency of usage and/or length of activation of the fast motor unit (type II fibers) is lesser than that of the slow motor unit (type I fibers) which is frequently engaged in the antigravity functions. Thus, the potential of disuse atrophy and degeneration for type II fibers is higher. In fact, age-related denervation, loss of motor units, and motor neurons are all being more prominent in the type II fibers in comparison to the type I fibers [19, 54]. Further, space flight studies reported that the loss of muscle mass, strength, and power are more prominent in the type I fibers than those of the type II fibers under microgravity [55]. These may be explained by the "use it or loss it" doctrine again. As gravity is reduced, the usage of slow motor unit is lesser than that of the fast motor unit. Hence the potential of disuse atrophy and degeneration for the type I fibers is higher. It is interesting to note that after the space flight, the type II fibers were also lesser. This may due to the reduction in gravity which leads to the reduction in resistance force for activity, and the type II motor units were then using lesser strength, energy, or power for the same work. As a result, they were susceptible to the disuse issue but to a lesser degree.

6. The Origin of Sarcopenia

Contributors to the development of sarcopenia discussed so far are common to both myocytes and neurons. Thus, the aforementioned contributors may be the systemic/general factors which may not necessary be the primary trigger in the etiology of sarcopenia but rather they may play a role in exacerbating the development process of sarcopenia upon triggering. Apparently, sarcopenia is linked to the interplay of assorted molecular cascades which involve a complex relationship between a variety of nucleic acids and proteins. Therefore, it is also possible that the pathology is originated from these multiple independent or synergistic triggers. Additionally, morbidity factors including neurodegenerative diseases and other pathological conditions may also have a direct or indirect role in the development of sarcopenia, that is, sarcopenia as a complication of other diseases.

By putting these pictures together, the development of sarcopenia may originate either from the following: (1) muscle fiber atrophy and degeneration which in turn leads to the denervation and loss of motor neuron (musculogenic); (2) synapse atrophy and degeneration of the NMJ which in turn leads to the atrophy and degeneration of muscle fibers (synaptogenic); (3) motor neuron atrophy and degeneration which in turn leads to the atrophy and degeneration of muscle fibers (neurogenic); (4) all of these. On the other hand, the exercise-induced hypertrophy of muscles may be explained either by (1) hypertrophy of the muscle fiber which in turn reinforces and stabilizes the synapses (muscle-induced); (2) hypertrophy of the synapses at the NMJ by synaptic facilitation through reinforcing signals and this in turn potentiates the trophic status of the muscle fibers (nerve induced); (3) both. Interestingly, the nervous system-based ideas seem more feasible due to (Figure 2) the following: (1) the trophic state of the muscle is determined by the net protein balance and some myogenic factors, e.g. myogenin, are strongly regulated by the electrical activity [25]; (2) some trophic factors, e.g. NT-4/5 and TrkB, are innervation dependent [56]; (3) some neurotrophic factors, CNTF, nourishes both the muscular and nervous system [57]; (4) the loss of muscle mass and strength albeit having different onset time, both of them are well maintained or decline slowly until the

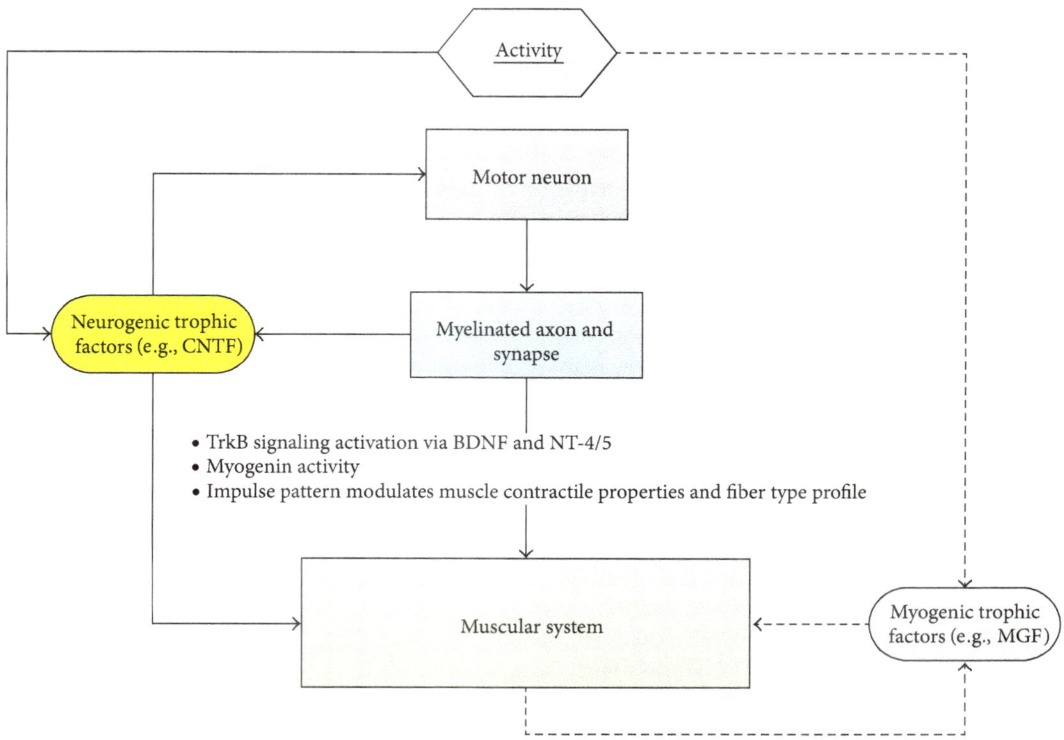

FIGURE 2: Relationship between the nervous system and the muscular system. (1) CNTF is released from the peripheral nerves and is one of the vital trophic factors for both the motor neuron and the myocytes. This growth factor is abundantly synthesized by Schwann cells. (2) MGF is locally released from the muscles and mainly activates satellite cells proliferation. (3) Some trophic factors (TrkB and myogenin) are innervation dependent. (4) Electrical impulse pattern modulates the muscle contractile properties and fiber-type profile.

age of 60 when a more rapid rate of decline commences. Coincidentally, the onset of age-associated denervation is also around the age of 60 [19]; (5) physiological change in the presynaptic terminal is greater than the postsynaptic terminal in aged animals [27]; (6) the nerve activity determines the muscle phenotype and this is mediated mainly by the Ras-MAPK pathway [25]; (7) the neurotrypsin-dependent NMJ degeneration results in a full sarcopenia phenotype in young adult mice [58].

7. One Picture Has Two Sides

Nature is amazing and sometimes surprising, this makes science even challenging and fascinating especially when analyzing a particular phenomenon with a different or even antagonistic logic. For example, although hypertrophic state is commonly considered to be important for the survival of cells, chronic hyperactivity of growth-promoting pathways may not possess any positive impacts. Animal studies reported that hyperactivation of the mTOR pathway, which originally promotes accretion and regulates initiation of translation, does not reverse the atrophy observed in obese muscles [59]. In contrast, when treated with the AMPK-agonists which inhibit the mTOR pathway, the translation capacity and the mass of obese muscle increased [59]. Thus, hyperactivity of mTOR may lead to a secondary resistance to the growth stimuli probably due to the negative feedback of a homeostatic effect [17]. Interestingly, some human studies reported that the muscle mass is higher in obese old persons than those with lesser obesity [60, 61]. This may be due to the decreased levels of SHBG which in turn results in an increased level of circulating androgens [61].

When we considered food intake as an important factor for the prevention of sarcopenia, caloric restriction without being malnutrition may have a positive impact on cells [59]. Animal studies shown that caloric restriction attenuates the progressive functional decline of organs [21]. At the cellular level, caloric restriction is associated with a decreased damage of peripheral nerve during aging by increasing the expression of chaperones and autophagic machineries [24]. It also ameliorates the loss of muscle mass, decreases abnormalities in the electron transport chain and diminished apoptotic potential in muscles [21]. Further, it is associated with neuronal protection against degeneration in animal CNS [62]. However, more ongoing investigations in humans are required to determine its efficacy in reality.

Every picture has two sides, like the above examples, although the nervous system may have an important vital role for the muscular system, the muscular system is also playing an important vital role for the nervous system as the muscle fibers are supplying the NGF-like factors to the motor neuron for its survival [63]. Thus, when considering the motor unit holistically, the common musculogenic model of sarcopenia is also valid.

8. Conclusion

Sarcopenia is an age-associated condition which links to multiple etiological factors ranging from external factors (physical activities, nutrients, and diseases) to internal factors (interplay between different cells, epigenetic profile of the cells, and congenital genetic configuration of an individual). In this article, we propose that sarcopenia may be neurogenic in origin due to the intimate relationship between the nervous system and the muscle cells. By summarizing the aforementioned evidences, it seems that the pathological importance at the presynaptic side (nerve side) precedes the postsynaptic side (muscle side). This presumption is in agreement with the age-associated degeneration of motor neurons [21]. Further, the age-associated denervation is more likely to be triggered by the disuse atrophy of synapse or even motor neurons. This is consistent with the fact that individuals with a sedentary life style or physical inactivity are usually more susceptible to sarcopenia compared to the physical active ones. However, more investigation is required in order to validate this belief. For example, to perform an in vitro experiment on the primary muscle cells which cultured with the necessary nervous-system-derived factors and observe whether the change in these factors would significantly affect the potential for sarcopenia development. But before that, a consensus for the definition of sarcopenia must be committed.

Conflict of Interests

The authors declare that they have no conflict of interests.

Acknowledgment

The authors of this paper certify that they comply with the guidelines for authorship and publishing in this Journal.

References

[1] I. H. Rosenberg, "Sarcopenia: origins and clinical relevance," *Journal of Nutrition*, vol. 127, no. 5, pp. 990–991, 1997.

[2] C. E. Lee, A. McArdle, and R. D. Griffiths, "The role of hormones, cytokines and heat shock proteins during age-related muscle loss," *Clinical Nutrition*, vol. 26, no. 5, pp. 524–534, 2007.

[3] G. A. Van Kan, "Epidemiology and consequences of sarcopenia," *Journal of Nutrition, Health and Aging*, vol. 13, no. 8, pp. 708–712, 2009.

[4] M. Visser and L. A. Schaap, "Consequences of sarcopenia," *Clinics in Geriatric Medicine*, vol. 27, no. 3, pp. 387–399, 2011.

[5] L. J. Tan, S. L. Liu, S. F. Lei, C. J. Papasian, and H. W. Deng, "Molecular genetic studies of gene identification for sarcopenia," *Human Genetics*, vol. 131, no. 1, pp. 1–31, 2011.

[6] E. M. Lau, H. S. Lynn, J. W. Woo, T. C. Kwok, and L. J. Melton III, "Prevalence of and risk factors for sarcopenia in elderly Chinese men and women," *The Journals of Gerontology A*, vol. 60, no. 2, pp. 213–216, 2005.

[7] J. S. W. Lee, T. W. Auyeung, T. Kwok, E. M. C. Lau, P. C. Leung, and J. Woo, "Associated factors and health impact of sarcopenia in older Chinese men and women: a cross-sectional study," *Gerontology*, vol. 53, no. 6, pp. 404–410, 2008.

[8] M. Muscaritoli, S. D. Anker, J. Argilés et al., "Consensus definition of sarcopenia, cachexia and pre-cachexia: joint document elaborated by Special Interest Groups (SIG) "cachexia-anorexia in chronic wasting diseases" and "nutrition in geriatrics"," *Clinical Nutrition*, vol. 29, no. 2, pp. 154–159, 2010.

[9] D. Volkert, "The role of nutrition in the prevention of sarcopenia," *Wiener Medizinische Wochenschrift*, vol. 161, no. 17-18, pp. 409–415, 2011.

[10] R. Roubenoff, "Physical activity, inflammation, and muscle loss," *Nutrition Reviews*, vol. 65, no. 12, Part 2, pp. S208–S212, 2007.

[11] E. Freiberger, C. Sieber, and K. Pfeifer, "Physical activity, exercise, and sarcopenia—future challenges," *Wiener Medizinische Wochenschrift*, vol. 161, no. 17-18, pp. 416–425, 2011.

[12] N. Garatachea and A. Lucía, "Genes and the ageing muscle: a review on geneticassociation studies," *Age*. In press.

[13] D. Bunout, M. P. de la Maza, G. Barrera, L. Leiva, and S. Hirsch, "Association between sarcopenia and mortality in healthy older people," *Australasian Journal on Ageing*, vol. 30, no. 2, pp. 89–92, 2011.

[14] F. Sanchis-Gomar, M. C. Gómez-Cabrera, and J. Viña, "The loss of muscle mass and sarcopenia: non hormonal intervention," *Experimental Gerontology*, vol. 46, no. 12, pp. 967–969, 2011.

[15] B. C. Clark and T. M. Manini, "Sarcopenia ≠ dynapenia," *Journals of Gerontology A*, vol. 63, no. 8, pp. 829–834, 2008.

[16] I. Janssen, "Evolution of sarcopenia research," *Applied Physiology, Nutrition, and Metabolism*, vol. 35, no. 5, pp. 707–712, 2010.

[17] D. T. Hall, J. F. Ma, S. D. Marco, and I. E. Gallouzi, "Inducible nitric oxide synthase (iNOS) in muscle wasting syndrome, sarcopenia, and cachexia," *Aging*, vol. 3, no. 8, pp. 702–715, 2011.

[18] A. Saini, S. Faulkner, N. Al-Shanti, and C. Stewart, "Powerful signals for weak muscles," *Ageing Research Reviews*, vol. 8, no. 4, pp. 251–267, 2009.

[19] M. R. Deschenes, "Effects of aging on muscle fibre type and size," *Sports Medicine*, vol. 34, no. 12, pp. 809–824, 2004.

[20] O. Delbono, K. S. O'Rourke, and W. H. Ettinger, "Excitation-calcium release uncoupling in aged single human skeletal muscle fibers," *Journal of Membrane Biology*, vol. 148, no. 3, pp. 211–222, 1995.

[21] A. J. Dirks and C. Leeuwenburgh, "The role of apoptosis in age-related skeletal muscle atrophy," *Sports Medicine*, vol. 35, no. 6, pp. 473–483, 2005.

[22] L. B. Verdijk, R. Koopman, G. Schaart, K. Meijer, H. H. C. M. Savelberg, and L. J. C. Van Loon, "Satellite cell content is specifically reduced in type II skeletal muscle fibers in the elderly," *American Journal of Physiology*, vol. 292, no. 1, pp. E151–E157, 2007.

[23] V. Renault, L. E. Thornell, G. Butler-Browne, and V. Mouly, "Human skeletal muscle satellite cells: aging, oxidative stress and the mitotic clock," *Experimental Gerontology*, vol. 37, no. 10-11, pp. 1229–1236, 2002.

[24] Y. C. Jang and H. Van Remmen, "Age-associated alterations of the neuromuscular junction," *Experimental Gerontology*, vol. 46, no. 2-3, pp. 193–198, 2011.

[25] S. Schiaffino, M. Murgia, A. L. Serrano, E. Calabria, and G. Pallafacchina, "How is muscle phenotype controlled by nerve activity?" *Italian Journal of Neurological Sciences*, vol. 20, no. 6, pp. 409–412, 1999.

[26] S. E. Alway, H. Degens, G. Krishnamurthy, and A. Chaudhrai, "Denervation stimulates apoptosis but not Id2 expression in hindlimb muscles of aged rats," *Journals of Gerontology A*, vol. 58, no. 8, pp. 687–697, 2003.

[27] S. A. Kulakowski, S. D. Parker, and K. E. Personius, "Reduced TrkB expression results in precocious age-like changes in neuromuscular structureneurotransmission, and muscle function," *Journal of Applied Physiology*, vol. 111, no. 3, pp. 844–852, 2011.

[28] H. Degens, "Age-related changes in the microcirculation of skeletal muscle," *Advances in Experimental Medicine and Biology*, vol. 454, pp. 343–348, 1998.

[29] L. A. Burton, M. E. McMurdo, and A. D. Struthers, "Mineralocorticoid antagonism: a novel way to treat sarcopenia and physical impairment in older people?" *Clinical Endocrinology*, vol. 75, no. 6, pp. 725–729, 2011.

[30] F. Derbré, M. C. Gomez-Cabrera, A. L. Nascimento et al., "Age associated low mitochondrial biogenesis may be explained by lack of response of PGC-1α to exercise training," *Age*, vol. 34, no. 3, pp. 669–679, 2012.

[31] L. J. Martin, "Mitochondrial pathobiology in ALS," *Journal of Bioenergetics and Biomembranes*, vol. 43, no. 6, pp. 569–579, 2011.

[32] P. M. Siu, E. E. Pistilli, and S. E. Alway, "Age-dependent increase in oxidative stress in gastrocnemius muscle with unloading," *Journal of Applied Physiology*, vol. 105, no. 6, pp. 1695–1705, 2008.

[33] M. Braga, A. P. S. Hikim, S. Datta et al., "Involvement of oxidative stress and caspase 2-mediated intrinsic pathway signaling in age-related increase in muscle cell apoptosis in mice," *Apoptosis*, vol. 13, no. 6, pp. 822–832, 2008.

[34] D. Nguyen, M. V. Alavi, K. Y. Kim et al., "A new vicious cycle involving glutamate excitotoxicity, oxidative stress and mitochondrial dynamics," *Cell Death & Disease*, vol. 2, article e240, 2011.

[35] S. Sriram, S. Subramanian, D. Sathiakumar et al., "Modulation of reactive oxygen species in skeletal muscle by myostatin is mediated through NF-κB," *Aging Cell*, vol. 10, no. 6, pp. 931–948, 2011.

[36] A. Machado, A. J. Herrera, J. L. Venero et al., "Peripheral inflammation increases the damage in animal models of nigrostriatal dopaminergic neurodegeneration: possible implication in Parkinson's disease incidence," *Parkinson's Disease*, vol. 2011, Article ID 393769, 10 pages, 2011.

[37] A. M. Robinson, D. B. Conley, M. J. Shinners, and R. C. Kern, "Apoptosis in the aging olfactory epithelium," *Laryngoscope*, vol. 112, no. 8, Part 1, pp. 1431–1435, 2002.

[38] X. Li, A. Khanna, N. Li, and E. Wang, "Circulatory miR34a as an RNAbased, noninvasive biomarker for brain aging," *Aging*, vol. 3, no. 10, pp. 985–1002, 2011.

[39] N. N. Hooten, K. Abdelmohsen, M. Gorospe, N. Ejiogu, A. B. Zonderman, and M. K. Evans, "microRNA expression patterns reveal differential expression of target genes with age," *PloS One*, vol. 5, no. 5, article e10724, 2010.

[40] M. W. Hamrick, S. Herberg, P. Arounleut et al., "The adipokine leptin increases skeletal muscle mass and significantly alters skeletal muscle miRNA expression profile in aged mice," *Biochemical and Biophysical Research Communications*, vol. 400, no. 3, pp. 379–383, 2010.

[41] Y. Ooishi, S. Kawato, Y. Hojo et al., "Modulation of synaptic plasticity in the hippocampus by hippocampus-derived estrogen and androgen," *Journal of Steroid Biochemistry and Molecular Biology*, vol. 131, no. 1-2, pp. 37–51, 2012.

[42] E. J. Sanders, W. Y. Lin, E. Parker, and S. Harvey, "Growth hormone promotes the survival of retinal cells in vivo," *General and Comparative Endocrinology*, vol. 172, no. 1, pp. 140–150, 2011.

[43] D. Ozdemir, B. Baykara, I. Aksu et al., "Relationship between circulating IGF-1 levels and traumatic brain injury-induced hippocampal damage and cognitive dysfunction in immature rats," *Neuroscience Letters*, vol. 507, no. 1, pp. 84–89, 2012.

[44] R. S. Akundi, L. Zhi, and H. Büeler, "PINK1 enhances insulin-like growth factor-1-dependent Akt signaling and protection against apoptosis," *Neurobiology of Disease*, vol. 45, no. 1, pp. 469–478, 2012.

[45] L. K. Tsai, Y. C. Chen, W. C. Cheng et al., "IGF-1 delivery to CNS attenuates motor neuron cell death but does not improve motor function in type III SMA mice," *Neurobiology of Disease*, vol. 45, no. 1, pp. 272–279, 2012.

[46] M. Amadio, G. Scapagnini, U. Laforenza et al., "Post-transcriptional regulation of HSP70 expression following oxidative stress in SH-SY5Y cells: the potential involvement of the RNA-binding protein HuR," *Current Pharmaceutical Design*, vol. 14, no. 26, pp. 2651–2658, 2008.

[47] S. Fujita and E. Volpi, "Amino acids and muscle loss with aging," *Journal of Nutrition*, vol. 136, no. 1, pp. 277S–280S, 2006.

[48] R. Koopman and L. J. C. Van Loon, "Aging, exercise, and muscle protein metabolism," *Journal of Applied Physiology*, vol. 106, no. 6, pp. 2040–2048, 2009.

[49] P. Zhang, X. Chen, and M. Fan, "Signaling mechanisms involved in disuse muscle atrophy," *Medical Hypotheses*, vol. 69, no. 2, pp. 310–321, 2007.

[50] F. Mayer, F. Scharhag-Rosenberger, A. Carlsohn, M. Cassel, S. Müller, and J. Scharhag, "The intensity and effects of strength training in the elderly," *Deutsches Ärzteblatt International*, vol. 108, no. 21, pp. 359–364, 2011.

[51] D. G. Sale, "Neural adaptation to resistance training," *Medicine and Science in Sports and Exercise*, vol. 20, 5 Supplement, pp. 135–145, 1988.

[52] M. T. Korhonen, A. Cristea, M. Alén et al., "Aging, muscle fiber type, and contractile function in sprint-trained athletes," *Journal of Applied Physiology*, vol. 101, no. 3, pp. 906–917, 2006.

[53] J. C. . McEachern and C. A. Shaw, "The plasticity-pathology continuum: defining a role for the LTP phenomenon," *Journal of Neuroscience Research*, vol. 58, no. 1, pp. 42–61, 1999.

[54] F. C. Wang, V. de Pasqua, and P. J. Delwaide, "Age-related changes in fastest and slowest conducting axons of thenar motor units," *Muscle & Nerve*, vol. 22, no. 8, pp. 1022–1029, 1999.

[55] R. H. Fitts, S. W. Trappe, D. L. Costill et al., "Prolonged space flight-induced alterations in the structure and function of human skeletal muscle fibres," *The Journal of Physiology*, vol. 588, Part 18, pp. 3567–3592, 2010.

[56] S. A. Kulakowski, S. D. Parker, and K. E. Personius, "Reduced TrkB expression results in precocious age-like changes in neuromuscular structureneurotransmission, and muscle function," *Journal of Applied Physiology*, vol. 111, no. 3, pp. 844–852, 2011.

[57] C. Guillet, P. Auguste, W. Mayo, P. Kreher, and H. Gascan, "Ciliary neurotrophic factor is a regulator of muscular strength in aging," *Journal of Neuroscience*, vol. 19, no. 4, pp. 1257–1262, 1999.

[58] L. Bütikofer, A. Zurlinden, M. F. Bolliger, B. Kunz, and P. Sonderegger, "Destabilization of the neuromuscular junction by proteolytic cleavage of agrin results in precocious sarcopenia," *FASEB Journal*, vol. 25, no. 12, pp. 4378–4393, 2011.

[59] D. L. Williamson, "Normalizing a hyperactive mTOR initiates muscle growth during obesity," *Aging*, vol. 3, no. 2, pp. 83–84, 2011.

[60] S. W. Park, B. H. Goodpaster, E. S. Strotmeyer et al., "Decreased muscle strength and quality in older adults with type 2 diabetes: the health, aging, and body composition study," *Diabetes*, vol. 55, no. 6, pp. 1813–1818, 2006.

[61] T. You, A. S. Ryan, and B. J. Nicklas, "The metabolic syndrome in obese postmenopausal women: relationship to body composition, visceral fat, and inflammation," *Journal of Clinical Endocrinology and Metabolism*, vol. 89, no. 11, pp. 5517–5522, 2004.

[62] S. Manzanero, M. Gelderblom, T. Magnus, and T. V. Arumugam, "Calorie restriction and stroke," :*.Experimental & Translational Stroke*, vol. 3, article 8, 2011.

[63] B. MacIntosh, P. Gardiner, and A. McComas, *Skeletal Muscle: Form and Function*, Human Kinetics, 2nd edition, 2006.

10

Older Primary Care Patients' Attitudes and Willingness to Screen for Dementia

Nicole R. Fowler,[1,2,3] Anthony J. Perkins,[1,2] Hilary A. Turchan,[1,2] Amie Frame,[1,2] Patrick Monahan,[3,4] Sujuan Gao,[3,4] and Malaz A. Boustani[1,2,3]

[1] *Indiana University Center for Aging Research, Indianapolis, IN 46202, USA*
[2] *Regenstrief Institute, Inc., Indianapolis, IN 46202, USA*
[3] *Indiana University School of Medicine, Indianapolis, IN 46202, USA*
[4] *Indiana University Department of Biostatistics, Indianapolis, IN 46202, USA*

Correspondence should be addressed to Nicole R. Fowler; fowlern@iupui.edu

Academic Editor: Elke Bromberg

Objective. To understand older primary care patients' perceptions of the risks and benefits of dementia screening and to measure the association between attitudes and screening behaviors. *Methods*. Eligible patients completed the Perceptions Regarding Investigational Screening for Memory in Primary Care (PRISM-PC) questionnaire and then were asked to undergo dementia screening by a telephone screening instrument. *Results*. Higher scores on the PRISM-PC questionnaire items that measure attitudes about benefits of screening were associated with decreased odds of refusing screening. Participants who refused screening had significantly lower PRISM-PC questionnaire scores on the items that measure perceived benefits compared to those who agreed to screening. Participants who refused screening were less likely to agree on screening for other conditions, such as depression and cancer. Participants who know someone with Alzheimer's disease (AD) were less likely to refuse screening. *Discussion*. Patients' attitudes about the benefits of dementia screening are associated with their acceptance of dementia screening.

1. Introduction

It is estimated that by 2050 there will be 11 to 19 million people in the United States of America (USA) living with dementia [1]. The incidence of dementia is also growing globally with a new patient being diagnosed approximately every 7 seconds [2]. Although there is currently no cure or proven prevention strategies for dementia, pharmacological and nonpharmacological interventions are available that may impact the symptoms of dementia [3, 4].

Despite rising incidence rates, many patients with dementia go unrecognized and never receive a cognitive evaluation or diagnosis. Estimates of undiagnosed dementia among older adults in the USA range from 45% to 80% [3, 5–7]. In 2013 the United States Preventive Services Task Force (USPSTF) concluded that the evidence to routinely screen for dementia in primary care is insufficient due to a lack of studies evaluating the risks, benefits, and patient perspectives of the value of dementia screening [8]. Understanding patients' attitudes about the risks and benefits of early identification of dementia is vital to assess the value of population-based dementia screening. In addition, this information allows for a better understanding of potential barriers and facilitators in the implementation of dementia screening programs in primary care settings [9].

The Perceptions Regarding Investigational Screening for Memory in Primary Care (PRISM-PC) questionnaire was developed by researchers at the Indiana University Center for Aging Research to identify the attitudes of older adults regarding screening for dementia in primary care. The purpose of this study is to understand primary care patients' perceptions of the risks and benefits of screening and early identification of dementia and to measure the association between patients' attitudes and behaviors of screening [10]. Based on our previous work, we hypothesized that many patients would report perceived benefits of early identification of dementia and that patient's acceptance of screening would be associated with the belief that early identification improves the patient-centered outcomes of the disease. Conversely, we hypothesized that refusal to be screened would be associated with the fear that early detection would result in being stigmatized or the loss of independence.

2. Methods

2.1. Study Population. Eligible patients were 65 years and older, had no diagnosis of dementia, had seen their primary care physician within the previous 12 months, and received their primary care at either St. Vincent Health or Community Health Network, both of which are located in Indianapolis, IN. Patients were excluded if they did not speak English, had hearing loss that precluded them from communicating via telephone, and had severe mental illness indicated in their medical record. This study was approved by the Institutional Review Boards of St. Vincent Hospital and the Community Health Network.

The research team obtained a list of eligible patients from the St. Vincent Health and Community Heath primary care office staff and appointment scheduling records. Eligible patients at the two sites were approached by telephone and offered the opportunity to participate in the study by research assistants from the Indiana University Center for Aging Research. All recruitment procedures complied with the Health Insurance Portability and Accountability Act and Institutional Review Board regulations. Informed consent was obtained from all patients who agreed to participate in the study.

2.2. Study Procedures and Instruments. The study uses The Perceptions Regarding Investigational Screening for Memory in Primary Care (PRISM-PC) questionnaire to measure patient's attitudes and perceived harms and benefits of screening for dementia. The PRISM-PC questionnaire includes 50 items with 12 items of capturing self-reported sociodemographic data and information regarding a participant's experience with or exposure to Alzheimer's disease and 38 items measuring the participant's perceptions of the acceptability, harms, and benefits of dementia screening. The PRISM-PC questionnaire uses the term Alzheimer's disease as a substitute for dementia since previous studies have shown that patients are more familiar with the term "Alzheimer's disease" than "dementia." Each item of the questionnaire is scored on a 1- to 5-point Likert scale with possible responses of strongly agree, agree, do not know, disagree, and strongly disagree for the following domains: benefits of dementia screening (8 items), stigma of dementia screening (10 items), negative effect of dementia screening on independence (6 items), suffering related to dementia screening (4 items), perceived acceptance of different types of dementia screening (6 items), perceived acceptance of screening for other conditions—colon cancer and depression (2 items), and the belief that a treatment for Alzheimer's disease is not currently available (2 items) [10].

IU-PBRN research assistants approached eligible individuals via telephone and explained the study. After obtaining consent, research assistant administered the PRISM-PC questionnaire and asked participants to undergo dementia screening. If participants agreed to screening, it was conducted during the same phone interview using the Telephone Instrument for Cognitive Screening (TICS). Participants who scored ≤ 30 screened positive for dementia and were referred to a specialist at either St. Vincent Health or Community Health Network for an evaluation and diagnostic assessment.

2.3. Statistical Analyses. Prior to conducting the analyses, responses on the PRISM-PC questionnaire were reverse-coded so that a higher score indicated stronger agreement on the items. To facilitate interpretation of the domain scores, we used a similar approach that is used to analyze scale scores on the SF-36 [11]. We converted all domains to the same metric by taking the sum of the reverse-coded responses and then transforming the sum to a 0 to 100 scale by subtracting the minimum possible score and dividing by the possible range. For a given domain, this meant that 0 represented strongly disagree on all items, 100 represented strongly agree on all items, and 50 represented neutral scores on all items.

For comparisons of groups of participants, we used t tests if the variables were continuous and Fisher's exact tests if the variables were categorical. To model the association of the PRISM-PC questionnaire domains with the dependent variable (acceptance versus refusal of telephone screening with the TICS), we used logistic regression and adjusted for covariates found to be significant or marginally significant ($P < 0.10$) in bivariate analyses. We reported the results in terms of odds ratios (ORs) and confidence intervals (CIs).

To determine if the scales derived from the phone administration of the PRISM-PC questionnaire showed the same internal consistency from prior studies when the PRISM-PC questionnaire was administered in person, we calculated Cronbach's alpha for each scale and compared it to previously published PRSIM-PC questionnaire findings [12]. For all statistical analyses, we used SAS statistical software version 9.3 (SAS Institute Inc., Cary, North Carolina).

3. Results

Sociodemographic characteristics and participants' experience with Alzheimer's disease are presented by study site in Table 1. There were no significant differences between the two study sites regarding prior experience with Alzheimer's disease. There were several significant differences between sites in sociodemographic characteristics. Participants from St. Vincent Health were significantly more likely to be married ($P < 0.05$), have higher levels of education ($P < 0.01$), and more likely to be African American ($P < 0.001$). Community Health Network participants tended to be older ($P = 0.05$) and more likely to live alone ($P = 0.06$).

Cronbach's alphas for the PRISM-PC questionnaire domain scales at the St. Vincent Health site were 0.85 for benefits of dementia screening, 0.74 for stigma, 0.72 for loss of independence, and 0.61 for suffering. Cronbach's alphas for

TABLE 1: Sociodemographic characteristics and experience with Alzheimer's disease of study participants from St. Vincent Health and Community Health Network.

	St. Vincent Health (n = 278) %	Community Health Network (n = 122) %	P value
Age, years			0.051
65–69	32.3	20.5	
70–74	20.6	22.1	
75–79	20.6	19.7	
≥80	26.5	37.7	
Gender			0.172
Female	66.9	73.8	
Race			<0.001
White	78.1	96.7	
African American	20.9	2.5	
Other	1.1	0.8	
Education, years			0.003
0–11	4.3	12.3	
≥12	95.7	87.7	
Housing status			0.063
Living alone	33.7	43.4	
Living with someone	66.3	56.6	
Marital status			0.030
Married	55.8	45.1	
Widowed	28.3	43.4	
Divorced	11.6	8.2	
Never married	4.3	3.3	
Income			0.124
<$10,000	4.1	5.1	
$10,000–$19,999	17.3	20.4	
$20,000–$39,999	28.4	38.8	
≥$40,000	50.2	35.7	
Do you have a relative or friend with Alzheimer's disease?			0.189
Yes	44.8	37.7	
Do you believe that you are at higher risk of Alzheimer's disease than others of your same age?			0.243
Yes	13.2	9.1	
Do you think you have more memory problems than others of your same age?			0.348
Yes	7.6	5.0	
Has a doctor told you that you have memory problems?			0.911
Yes	1.8	1.6	
Are you taking medication to help with memory?			0.733
Yes	2.2	1.6	

TABLE 2: Bivariate comparison of the sociodemographic characteristics and experience with Alzheimer's disease of study participants who accepted and refused screening for dementia[a] at St. Vincent Health and Community Health Network.

	St. Vincent Health (n = 278)			Community Health Network (n = 122)		
	Number (%) accepted	Number (%) refused	P value	Number (%) accepted	Number (%) refused	P value
Overall	173 (62.2)	105 (37.8)		78 (63.9)	44 (36.1)	
Age, years			0.780			0.071
65–69	55 (61.8)	34 (38.2)		19 (76.0)	6 (24.0)	
70–74	39 (68.4)	18 (31.6)		18 (66.7)	9 (33.3)	
75–79	34 (59.6)	23 (40.4)		16 (66.7)	8 (33.3)	
≥80	45 (61.6)	28 (38.4)		25 (54.4)	21 (45.6)	
Gender			0.844			0.292
Female	115 (61.8)	71 (38.2)		60 (66.7)	30 (33.3)	
Male	58 (63.0)	34 (37.0)		18 (56.2)	14 (43.8)	
Race			0.541			0.748
White	137 (63.1)	80 (36.9)		75 (63.6)	43 (36.4)	
African American	35 (60.3)	23 (39.7)		2 (66.3)	1 (33.3)	
Other	1 (33.3)	2 (66.7)		1 (100.0)	0 (0.0)	
Education, years			0.007			0.814
0–11	3 (25.0)	9 (75.0)		10 (66.7)	5 (33.3)	
≥12	170 (63.9)	96 (36.1)		68 (63.6)	39 (36.4)	
Housing status			0.733			0.063
Living alone	57 (61.3)	36 (38.7)		29 (54.7)	24 (45.3)	
Living with someone	116 (63.4)	67 (36.6)		49 (71.0)	20 (29.0)	
Marital status			0.550			0.865
Married	98 (63.6)	56 (36.4)		37 (67.3)	18 (32.7)	
Widowed	48 (61.5)	30 (38.5)		33 (62.3)	20 (37.7)	
Divorced	17 (53.1)	15 (46.9)		6 (60.0)	4 (40.0)	
Never married	9 (75.0)	3 (25.0)		2 (50.0)	2 (50.0)	
Income (N = 465)			0.122			0.205
<$10,000	5 (62.5)	3 (37.5)		4 (80.0)	1 (20.0)	
$10,000–$19,999	18 (52.9)	16 (47.1)		15 (75.0)	5 (25.0)	
$20,000–$39,999	41 (73.2)	15 (26.8)		20 (52.6)	18 (47.4)	
≥$40,000	73 (73.7)	26 (26.3)		25 (71.4)	10 (28.6)	
Do you have a relative or friend with Alzheimer's disease?			0.003			0.074
No	83 (54.2)	70 (45.8)		44 (57.9)	32 (42.1)	
Yes	89 (71.8)	35 (28.2)		34 (73.9)	12 (26.1)	
Do you believe that you are at higher risk of Alzheimer's disease than others of your same age?			0.106			0.511
No	144 (61.0)	92 (39.0)		69 (62.7)	41 (37.3)	
Yes	27 (75.0)	9 (25.0)		8 (72.7)	3 (27.3)	
Do you think you have more memory problems than others of your same age?			0.653			0.896
No	158 (61.7)	98 (38.3)		73 (64.0)	41 (36.0)	
Yes	14 (66.7)	7 (33.3)		4 (66.7)	2 (33.3)	
Has a doctor told you that you have memory problems?			0.917			0.679
No	170 (62.3)	103 (37.7)		77 (64.2)	43 (35.8)	
Yes	3 (60.0)	2 (40.0)		1 (50.0)	1 (50.0)	

TABLE 2: Continued.

	St. Vincent Health (*n* = 278)			Community Health Network (*n* = 122)		
	Number (%) accepted	Number (%) refused	*P* value	Number (%) accepted	Number (%) refused	*P* value
Are you taking medication to help with memory?			0.821			0.679
No	169 (62.1)	103 (37.9)		77 (64.2)	43 (35.8)	
Yes	4 (66.7)	2 (33.3)		1 (50.0)	1 (50.0)	

[a]Because our early work indicated that patients more readily understood the term "Alzheimer's disease" than the term "dementia," in this study we used Alzheimer's disease as a proxy for dementia.

TABLE 3: Bivariate comparison of the mean PRISM-PC questionnaire scores of study participants who accepted and refused screening for dementia at St. Vincent (St. V.) Health and Community Health Network (Community).

Domains and individual items[a]	St. V. Health Mean score (SD)			Community Mean score (SD)		
	Accepted screening (*n* = 173)	Refused screening (*n* = 105)	*P* Value	Accepted screening (*n* = 78)	Refused screening (*n* = 44)	*P* Value
Domain: benefits of dementia screening	73.8 (10.1)	67.7 (13.3)	<0.001	72.1 (9.5)	65.6 (12.8)	0.002
Domain: stigma of dementia screening	32.0 (11.4)	33.3 (9.2)	0.323	33.7 (11.5)	34.9 (9.3)	0.545
Domain: negative impact of dementia screening on independence	50.6 (12.6)	53.3 (13.8)	0.086	50.8 (11.1)	49.1 (11.8)	0.444
Domain: suffering related to dementia screening	59.0 (13.5)	58.6 (14.9)	0.828	59.1 (11.9)	53.0 (12.2)	0.009
Item in no domain: agreement with screening for colon cancer	3.3 (1.0)	3.2 (1.0)	0.242	3.2 (1.1)	2.8 (1.0)	0.083
Item in no domain: agreement with screening for depression	3.2 (1.0)	2.8 (1.0)	0.007	3.3 (1.0)	2.8 (1.0)	0.006
Item in no domain: belief that a treatment for Alzheimer's disease is not currently available	2.6 (0.9)	2.7 (0.8)	0.281	2.5 (0.9)	2.7 (0.7)	0.217

PRISM-PC: Perceptions Regarding Investigational Screening for Memory in Primary Care.
[a]For each domain, the table includes the individual item that was most relevant to our study objectives. The table also includes the 3 individual items that are not covered under any domain.

the Community Health Network sample were 0.81 for benefits, 0.78 for stigma, 0.78 for loss of independence, and 0.47 for suffering. These Cronbach alphas are comparable to or greater than the Cronbach alphas calculated from similar samples and in previously published PRISM-PC questionnaire studies when patients completed the PRISM-PC questionnaire in person and were asked to undergo dementia screening in person [10, 12].

The associations of demographic characteristics and prior AD experience with screening refusal are presented by site in Table 2. Overall there were no significant differences between dementia screening refusal at the two sites, 37.7% at St. Vincent and 36.1% at Community ($P = 0.746$). The only demographic variable significantly associated with screening refusal at the St. Vincent Health site was education. At St. Vincent Health only, participants with less than a high school education were more likely to refuse screening than the participants with at least a high school education. At both sites, participants without a relative or friend with AD were significantly more likely to refuse the screening (St. Vincent Health 45.8% versus 28.2%; $P = 0.003$ and Community Health Network 42.1% versus 26.1%; $P = 0.074$).

The association between screening refusal and the four domains on the PRISM-PC questionnaire and on individual questionnaire items are presented in Table 3. For both sites, participants who refused screening had significantly lower scores on the benefits domain than participants who agreed to screening. In addition, participants who refused screening at both sites were less likely to agree to question on the PRISM-PC questionnaire regarding annual screening for depression. At the Community Health Network site, participants who refused screening had significantly lower scores on the suffering domain, meaning they were more likely to agree on the items related to suffering as a result of screening for dementia.

TABLE 4: Logistic regression analysis of the odds of refusing to undergo screening for dementia at St. Vincent Health and Community Health Network.

Variable	St. Vincent Health Odds ratio (95% confidence interval)	St. Vincent Health *P* value	Community Health Network Odds ratio[a] (95% confidence interval)	Community Health Network *P* value
PRISM-PC questionnaire items				
High domain score: perception that dementia screening is beneficial	0.80 (0.70, 0.91)	0.001	0.79 (0.63, 0.98)	0.029
High domain score: suffering related to dementia screening	1.07 (0.97, 1.18)	0.200	0.89 (0.73, 1.08)	0.248
Perception that depression screening is beneficial	0.80 (0.62, 1.04)	0.100	0.63 (0.40, 0.99)	0.049
Have a relative or friend with AD	0.51 (0.30, 0.87)	0.014	0.43 (0.16, 1.12)	0.082
Lives alone	1.14 (0.64, 2.02)	0.662	2.18 (0.87, 5.44)	0.096
Education				
(>high school+ versus 0–11 years)	0.19 (0.05, 0.82)	0.025	1.38 (0.36, 5.25)	0.640
Age, years		0.648		0.573
65–69 (reference group)	1.00 [reference]		1.00 [reference]	
70–74	0.69 (0.32, 1.49)		1.71 (0.42, 6.93)	
75–79	1.17 (0.56, 2.45)		1.02 (0.24, 4.74)	
≥80	0.90 (0.44, 1.82)		2.01 (0.56, 7.25)	

PRISM-PC, Perceptions Regarding Investigational Screening for Memory in Primary Care.
[a]Odds ratios report a 5-point difference in the scale score.

Results from the logistic regressions are presented in Table 4. After adjusting for age and education, higher scores on the items in the benefits domain were significantly associated with decreased odds of refusing dementia screening at both sites. Additionally, at both sites, respondents who endorsed having a friend or relative with AD were less likely to refuse screening (St. Vincent Health AOR = 0.49; $P = 0.009$ and Community Health Network AOR = 0.39; $P = 0.052$).

4. Discussion

In our study of primary care patients at two different Indianapolis health care centers, we found that, despite different sociodemographic characteristics, predictors of who accepts and who declines dementia screening are similar. In this study, where participants completed the PRISM-PC questionnaire and dementia screening by phone, perceptions about the benefits of early identification remained a significant predictor of screening acceptance as did having a friend or relative with dementia. These results are consistent with previous studies that have administered the PRISM-PC questionnaire in person and administered dementia screening in person.

Findings form this study corroborate previous results that have shown that people's perceptions about the benefits of dementia screening are associated with their willingness to be screened. For example, the participants who had stronger agreement on the statements regarding the benefits of knowing about dementia earlier (e.g., ability to plan for the future) were more likely to accept screening. Of the various items of sociodemographic data that were gathered for our study, only level of education at the St. Vincent's Health System site was highly predictive of agreeing to be screened. The participants from the St. Vincent's Health System with less than a high school education were more likely to refuse screening than those with more than a high school education.

This study is the first to measure attitudes about dementia screening with the PRISM-PC questionnaire and offer screening by phone. The internal consistency reliability of the domain scales as measured by Cohen's Kappa was similar to those obtained from face-to-face administration of the PRISM-PC questionnaire and to those obtained in prior studies. In our sample, more than half (63.7%) of older primary care patients agreed to be screened for dementia by phone following completion of the PRISM-PC questionnaire. Despite the majority of participants agreeing, this rate is significantly less than our previous work that has found rates of people willing to be screened as high as 89.7% when we approached in person and screened in person [10].

A limitation of this study is that we do not know if participants had been screened for dementia as part of routine care, prior to being recruited for this study. However, none had a dementia diagnosis and less than 2% reported being told by their physician that they had memory problems.

In summary, the PRISM-PC questionnaire instrument is a valid tool to assess older primary care patients' perceptions about dementia screening, even when administered by phone. Across our work, in this study and others, belief in the benefits of recognizing dementia early is an important predictor of patient behaviors regarding screening and could be used in interventions designed to increase the uptake of dementia screening.

Conflict of Interests

The authors declare that there is no conflict of interests regarding the publication of this paper.

Acknowledgment

The authors would like to thank Laura Holtz for her assistance in preparation for this paper.

References

[1] P. D. Sloane, S. Zimmerman, C. Suchindran et al., "The public health impact of Alzheimer's disease, 2000–2050: potential implication of treatment advances," *Annual Review of Public Health*, vol. 23, pp. 213–231, 2002.

[2] C. P. Ferri, M. Prince, C. Brayne et al., "Global prevalence of dementia: a Delphi consensus study," *The Lancet*, vol. 366, no. 9503, pp. 2112–2117, 2005.

[3] M. Boustani, B. Peterson, L. Hanson, R. Harris, and K. N. Lohr, "Screening for dementia in primary care: a summary of the evidence for the U.S. Preventive Services Task Force," *Annals of Internal Medicine*, vol. 138, no. 11, pp. 927–I60, 2003.

[4] M. K. Jedrziewski, V. M.-Y. Lee, and J. Q. Trojanowski, "Lowering the risk of Alzheimer's disease: evidence-based practices emerge from new research," *Alzheimer's & Dementia*, vol. 1, no. 2, pp. 152–160, 2005.

[5] V. Kotagal, K. Langa, B. Plassman et al., "Factors associated with cognitive evaluations in the United States," *Neurology*, vol. 84, no. 1, pp. 64–71, 2015.

[6] M. Boustani, C. M. Callahan, F. W. Unverzagt et al., "Implementing a screening and diagnosis program for dementia in primary care," *Journal of General Internal Medicine*, vol. 20, no. 7, pp. 572–577, 2005.

[7] M. Boustani, L. Watson, B. Fultz, A. J. Perkins, and R. Druckenbrod, "Acceptance of dementia screening in continuous care retirement communities: a mailed survey," *International Journal of Geriatric Psychiatry*, vol. 18, no. 9, pp. 780–786, 2003.

[8] J. S. Lin, E. O'Connor, R. C. Rossom, L. A. Perdue, and E. Eckstrom, "Screening for cognitive impairment in older adults: a systematic review for the U.S. preventive services task force," *Annals of Internal Medicine*, vol. 159, no. 9, pp. 601–612, 2013.

[9] C. B. Cordell, S. Borson, M. Boustani et al., "Alzheimer's Association recommendations for operationalizing the detection of cognitive impairment during the Medicare Annual Wellness Visit in a primary care setting," *Alzheimer's & Dementia*, vol. 9, no. 2, pp. 141–150, 2013.

[10] N. R. Fowler, M. A. Boustani, A. Frame et al., "Effect of patient perceptions on dementia screening in primary care," *Journal of the American Geriatrics Society*, vol. 60, no. 6, pp. 1037–1043, 2012.

[11] J. E. Ware Jr. and C. D. Sherbourne, "The MOS 36-item short-form health survey (SF-36): I. Conceptual framework and item selection," *Medical Care*, vol. 30, no. 6, pp. 473–483, 1992.

[12] M. Boustani, A. J. Perkins, P. Monahan et al., "Measuring primary care patients' attitudes about dementia screening," *International Journal of Geriatric Psychiatry*, vol. 23, no. 8, pp. 812–820, 2008.

11

White Matter Lesion Assessment in Patients with Cognitive Impairment and Healthy Controls: Reliability Comparisons between Visual Rating, a Manual, and an Automatic Volumetrical MRI Method—The Gothenburg MCI Study

Erik Olsson,[1] Niklas Klasson,[1] Josef Berge,[1] Carl Eckerström,[1] Åke Edman,[1] Helge Malmgren,[1,2] and Anders Wallin[1]

[1] *Department of Neuroscience and Physiology, Institute of Psychiatry and Neurochemistry, The Sahlgrenska Academy, University of Gothenburg, 40530 Gothenburg, Sweden*
[2] *Department of Philosophy, Linguistics and Theory of Science, University of Gothenburg, 40530 Gothenburg, Sweden*

Correspondence should be addressed to Erik Olsson, erik.olsson@neuro.gu.se

Academic Editor: F. Richard Ferraro

Age-related white matter lesions (WML) are a risk factor for stroke, cognitive decline, and dementia. Different requirements are imposed on methods for the assessment of WML in clinical settings and for research purposes, but reliability analysis is of major importance. In this study, WML assessment with three different methods was evaluated. In the Gothenburg mild cognitive impairment study, MRI scans from 152 participants were used to assess WML with the Fazekas visual rating scale on T2 images, a manual volumetric method on FLAIR images, and FreeSurfer volumetry on T1 images. Reliability was acceptable for all three methods. For low WML volumes (2/3 of the patients), reliability was overall lower and nonsignificant for the manual volumetric method. Unreliability in the assessment of patients with low WML with manual volumetry may mainly be due to intensity variation in the FLAIR sequence used; hence, intensity standardization and normalization methods must be used for more accurate assessments. The FreeSurfer segmentations resulted in smaller WML volumes than the volumes acquired with the manual method and showed deviations from visible hypointensities in the T1 images, which quite likely reduces validity.

1. Introduction

Age-related white matter lesions (WML) mainly affect information processing speed and executive function [1] and entail an increased risk for cognitive decline and disability [2]. In a meta-analytic study, high hazard ratios were also reported for incident stroke (3.3) and dementia (1.9) [3], but results from studies on WML association to dementia subtypes are inconclusive [4–6]. The prevalence of WML increases with age, and in a population study, 51% of randomly selected healthy subjects aged 44–48 had WML [7]. For the age range 60–64, all had WML, and 49% of these had at least one large (>12 mm) WML region [8].

In magnetic resonance (MR) imaging, white matter hypointensities in T1 weighted images, and white matter hyperintensities in T2 weighted and FLAIR images are regarded as visualizations of WML. The conditions for demarcation of WML are enhanced in FLAIR images due to suppression of the signal from free fluid. In contrast to T2 and T1 weighted images, this suppression causes fluid filled cavities in FLAIR images to be hypointensive and excluded from WML by the intensity definition. However, the intensity suppression in the FLAIR sequence entails incident imaging artifacts in the border region between WML and free fluid, for example, in the periventricular region [9]. WML visible in MR imaging reflect demyelinization, axonal loss, gliosis, or edema. However, WML MR imaging comprises no lucid separation between these pathological substrates.

It is customary to use CT or MR imaging of WML among the diagnostic criteria for subcortical vascular dementia, for example, in Erkinjuntti et al. [10]. However, standardization of WML estimation is needed in order to establish uniform diagnostic criteria in clinical practice. Visual rating is simple and fast and therefore an important candidate method for standardized clinical use. There are several visual rating methods for WML research purposes [11, 12]. Among these, the Fazekas visual rating [13, 14] is frequently used in research, and it has been shown to have good reliability compared to two other rating scales [12], but the results on its correlation to volumetrical assessment diverge. For example, the Fazekas visual rating has shown the highest [11] and lowest [15] correlation to volumetrical assessment compared to other visual rating scales. Manual volumetrical assessments have shown higher reliability than visual rating scales [11, 15] and would be valuable in clinical settings if made less labour intensive. In Gouw et al. [16], visual rating of WML and WML volumetry had similar correlations to neuropsychological performance, but in Garrett et al. [17], a correlation to neuropsychological performance was only found using WML volumetry and not in visual WML rating. Several segmentation and thresholding techniques have been used to manually assess WML volume in the literature, but one of the few techniques with a methodological description is reported in Gurol et al. [18].

Several automatic volumetry methods have been developed for WML classification [19–21]. FreeSurfer is one of these methods, and it contains automatic assessment of neuroanatomical subregions as well as WML hypointensity volumes. FreeSurfer has been frequently used for neuroanatomical subregional volumetry and has been shown to be comparable in accuracy to manual labeling for many tasks [22, 23] and to perform well compared to other automated segmentation tools [24]. However, few publications have reported FreeSurfer WML volumes at all, and only one study reports intermethod reliability figures [25]. The latter study also reported that regional WML predicted executive dysfunction. One study found that total WML was significant for AD versus controls [26], and another found that total WML predicted functional decline almost as well as the best predicting regional WML regions [5].

Reliability analysis is the first step in assessing the accuracy of a WML method, and the often reported excellent or near excellent reliability may be a reason why methodological issues about reliability have not always been given enough attention. The aim of the present study was to compare three types of assessment methods of total WML in a clinical sample in order to examine different aspects of their reliability and to determine features in need of further methodological development. The Fazekas rating was included in this study because of its simplicity. The manual MRIcron WML volumetry method was included on the basis of a presumed superiority in accuracy. FreeSurfer WML volumetry was included because of the automatic assessment of WML as well as the need for further validation because of the common use of the method.

2. Method

In the Gothenburg mild cognitive impairment (MCI) study, subjects between 40 and 86 years of age (mean 65.6, SD 7.7 years) with subjective or objective cognitive impairment were recruited from the Memory Clinic at the Sahlgrenska University Hospital. The selection process has been described in more detail by Eckerström et al. [27]. Exclusion criteria were acute somatic disease, severe psychiatric disorder, pseudodementia, and substance abuse or confusion caused by drugs. Controls were recruited from other medical studies and senior citizen organizations, and baseline exclusion criteria were subjective or objective signs of cognitive disorder. The study was approved by the Ethics Committee of the University of Gothenburg, and the subjects gave their informed consent to participate in the study.

The study subjects were biannually assessed and classified according to the Global Deterioration Scale (GDS) [28]. Subjects with a GDS 2 or GDS 3 score received an MCI classification. MCI subjects remaining in the GDS 2 to GDS 3 range at followup were classified as "MCI stable," while MCI subjects receiving a GDS 4 (mild dementia) or higher classification at followup were classified as "MCI converting." Twenty eight controls, 69 MCI stable, 9 MCI converting, and 46 dementia subjects were included in the present study. WML was measured on the first 1.5T MR imaging acquisitions in the study, between the years 2005 and 2007.

Imaging was performed on a Siemens Symphony 1.5T scanner. Axial T2 weighted images were used for the Fazekas rating, coronal FLAIR images were manually segmented in the MRIcron software, and coronal T1 weighted images were analyzed with the FreeSurfer package (stable release version 4.0.5). In Table 1, the scan parameters used in the study are presented. All raters and operators were blinded for header data like identity and cognitive status of the subject. This study report was outlined to be in accordance with the guidelines for reliability studies in Kottner et al. [29].

2.1. Visual Rating. WML severity was rated using modifications of the Fazekas scale [13]. Periventricular WML and deep WML were not rated separately, in accordance with the recommendations by Fazekas et al. [30], but only three grades were used as in Inzitari et al. [14] in contrast to the original four-graded Fazekas scale, and in the present study, grade 1 also included possible absence of WML. For each subject, the slice with the largest WML occurrence visible was used to determine the WML load as belonging to one of three grades. The assessments were performed independently by two raters (J. Berge and J. Eldblom) who compared the images with the template images in axial orientation of the different grades of WML given by [14]. Metrical measurements were not used. Only cerebral WML were included in the ratings. The raters J. Berge and J. Eldblom had substantial knowledge of neuroanatomy and went through limited training in visual rating before entering the study assessment.

2.2. MRIcron. Cerebral WML segmentation and intensity thresholding were performed on 1.5T coronal 5 mm FLAIR images using the MRIcron software with a modification (see later) of the method used in Gurol et al. [18]. The segmentation method involves an initial rough manual demarcation of WML, separating them from noncerebral

Table 1: Scan parameters 1.5T Siemens Symphony (Syngo MR 200-4A 4VA25A).

		2D FLAIR Coronal	T2 2D TSE Axial	T1 3D MPR Coronal
Repetition time	ms	8780	5410	1610
Echo time	ms	112	104	2.38
Number of averages		1	2	1
Flip angle	°	150	150	15
Slice thickness	mm	5	5	1
Spacing between slices	mm	5.5	6	1
Acquisition pixel size	mm	1.3 * 0.9	0.9 * 0.4	1.0 * 1.0
Reconstruction pixel size	mm	0.45 * 0.45	0.45 * 0.45	0.49 * 0.49
Matrix size		512 * 416	512 * 416	512 * 416
Field of view	mm	230 * 187	230 * 187	250 * 203

regions and septum pellucidum, as in Holland et al. [31], within the same intensity span, followed by an intensity threshold set to separate WML from adjacent tissue types. In the Gothenburg MCI cohort, artifactual image intensity differences between slices and between series (using the same FLAIR sequence) were common. No automatic intensity normalization between patients was done, but in order to consistently analyze each patient's series in similar intensity settings, the MRIcron grayscale mapping was used on a window setting containing all brain tissue in a certain slice (containing the quadrigeminal plate). Due to intensity inhomogeneities, the manual volumetry method adapted from Gurol et al. [18] required a modification towards a more WML-specific manual segmentation, where the contour of the WML was demarcated quite closely. One rater (E. Olsson) demarcated 152 subjects, while a second rater (J. Berge) independently demarcated 27 randomly selected subjects for the determination of interrater reliability. The rater E. Olsson has longstanding experience in MRI segmentation, and the rater J. Berge went through substantial training in the manual WML volumetrical method before entering the study assessment.

2.3. FreeSurfer. Hypointensity volumetrics determined as WML were estimated by an operator (N. Klasson) running the FreeSurfer analysis (stable release version 4.0.5). FreeSurfer is a highly automatic image analysis suite and is available for download online (http://surfer.nmr.mgh.harvard.edu/). FreeSurfer uses a probabilistic atlas generated from manually segmented MR scans to execute the segmentation. The probabilistic information has been mapped into Talairach space so that each location therein contains specific probabilities for each tissue type. Given a specific location and tissue type, the probabilities are given as (1) a Gaussian intensity distribution, (2) probability of occurrence, and (3) probability of neighboring tissue types. During segmentation, a number of processes take place including motion correction and intensity normalization, removal of nonbrain tissue, Talairach registration, and labeling of voxels into tissue types. An initial labeling takes place where each voxel is assigned its most probable tissue type. An iterative algorithm then uses the found tissue probabilities to calculate new probabilities for the voxel labels. This process continues until no changes of tissue types take place. Manual edits were done by the operator (N. Klasson) to reduce inaccuracies in white and grey matter classification. The segmentation process has been described in detail elsewhere [22, 23].

2.4. Statistical Methods. The distribution of WML volumes in the Gothenburg MCI study was right skewed, and normality could not be assumed, not even after log transformation. The statistical analyses were done in SPSS 19. The reliability analyses comprised Spearman correlation, intraclass correlation (ICC) (with two-way mixed, absolute agreement and single measurements model), and Kendall's tau. Tertile selection was performed on the manual MRIcron volumetry distribution. Differences in reliability between the highest WML tertile and the lower tertiles were tested with Fischer's r to z transformation. For differences between raters and methods, Wilcoxon matched pairs test and Bland-Altman plots were used.

3. Results

3.1. Study Characteristics. The study characteristics for the controls, MCI stable, and dementia groups are presented in Table 2. Dementia patients had significantly lower MMSE scores than all other groups, had significantly lower education than stable MCI, and were significantly older than stable MCI. All three WML assessment methods detected significant associations between WML estimate and age (Fazekas 0.385, manual MRIcron 0.334, automatic FreeSurfer 0.524).

3.2. Reliability. Regarding interrater reliability, the Spearman rho coefficient was 0.89 with regard to the modified Fazekas visual rating scale and 0.60 regarding the manual MRIcron WML volumetry. The rho value was 0.65 for the intermethod correlation between FreeSurfer automatic WML volumetry and manual WML volumetry (Table 3). No significant systematic differences between raters were found for Fazekas visual rating or for MRIcron manual volumetry in the Wilcoxon matched pairs test (details not shown), but the FreeSurfer automatic volumetry differed significantly from the manual MRIcron volumetry. Almost all FreeSurfer volumes were lower than the corresponding manual MRIcron volume (Figure 1).

In order to evaluate reliabilities in the dense and the sparse parts of the data distribution (Figure 2), respectively, the WML volumes were separated into tertiles (Table 3). For the aggregated lower two tertiles, the Fazekas interrater reliability (Spearman's rho) measured 0.65, and for the upper WML tertile 0.92, this difference was significant. The manual MRIcron interrater reliability was nonsignificant for the lower two tertiles (which make up about 10 percent of the whole volume range) but significant for the upper WML tertile with an interrater reliability of 0.94. For the anterior part of the brain taken separately, there was still no significant

TABLE 2: Study characteristics. P-values were assessed by the two-tailed t-test except gender where chi square was used. Gr 4 is group 4 Dementia. Gr 2 and MCI-s are stable MCI. MCI-c is converting MCI. Gr 2 and Gr 4 had significantly lower scores than the group specified in the cell for the pertaining variable; for example, Gr 2 (stable MCI) had significantly lower age than group 4 (dementia group). There was no significant difference in gender.

	1 Controls		2 MCI-s		3 MCI-c		4 Dementia		Gr 2	Gr 4
	Mean	SD	Mean	SD	Mean	SD	Mean	SD	$P < 0.05$	$P < 0.05$
Age	66.5	8.2	63.9	7.2	65.6	7.2	67.6	8.0	4	
Education years	11.7	2.3	11.8	3.4	12.6	4.5	10.4	3.7		2
MMSE	29.3	0.4	28.3	1.9	28.4	1.7	25.3	2.9		1, 2, 3
	Count		Count		Count		Count			
Gender M/F	9/19		31/38		6/3		21/25		ns	

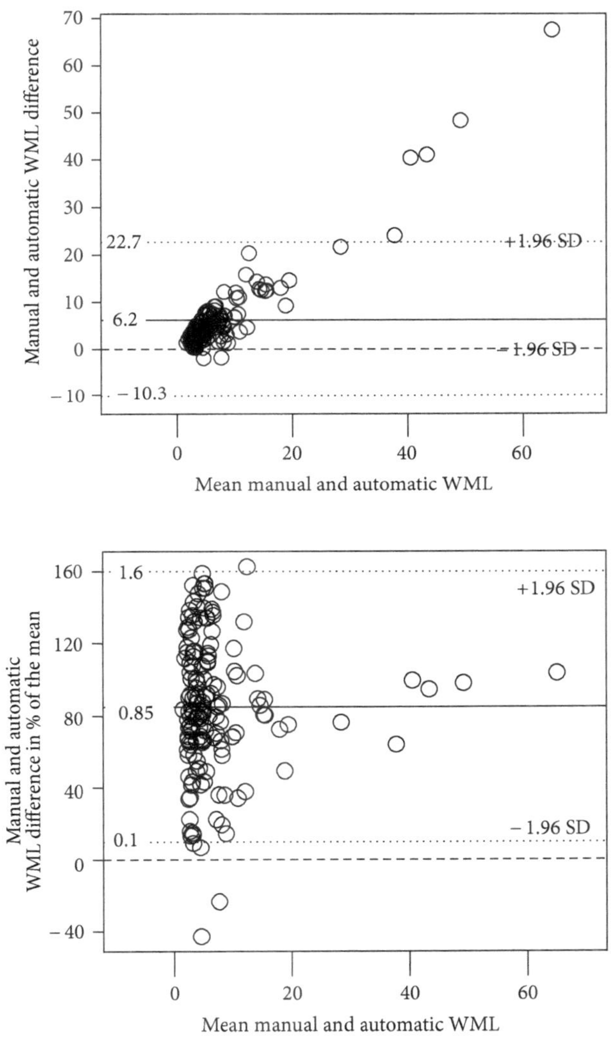

FIGURE 1: Bland-Altman plots of the intermethod differences (manual MRIcron minus automatic FreeSurfer WML volumes in cm^3). The x-axes contain mean WML volumes; the y-axis contains absolute differences in (a) and fractional differences of mean volume in (b). The dashed line designates the no differences level.

reliability for the lower aggregated WML tertiles, but it was significant for the posterior part with a rho value of 0.56. For the intermethod reliability between the manual MRIcron volumetry and the automatic FreeSurfer volumetry, the rho value was also lower, 0.38 in the lower aggregated tertiles, than in the upper tertiles, 0.74.

For ICC values, see Table 3. The reason why we do not report them in the text is stated in Section 4.

Table 3: Inter-rater and inter-method reliability. *Correlation was significant at the 0.05 level (2-tailed). **Correlation was significant at the 0.01 level (2-tailed). ManWML is manual MRIcron volumetry; $n = 27$. Anterior is the manual MRIcron assessed volume anterior of the quadrigeminal plate. Posterior is the manual MRIcron assessed volume posterior of the quadrigeminal plate. ManWML versus AutoWML is the manual MRIcron volumetry correlation to the automatic FreeSurfer volumetry. Rho below T3 is the Spearman correlation, and ICC below T3 is the intraclass correlation in the lower two tertiles. Rho in T3 is the Spearman correlation and ICC in T3 the intraclass correlation in the highest tertile. The reliability was significantly higher in the highest tertile for all methods.

	Kendall's tau-b	ICC	ICC below T3	ICC in T3	Rho	Rho below T3	Rho in T3
			Inter-rater reliability				
Fazekas	0.88**	0.87**	0.65**	0.86**	0.89**	0.65**	0.92**
ManWML	0.45*	0.97**	0.19	0.95**	0.60**	−0.03	0.94**
Anterior					0.63**	0.23	0.94**
Posterior					0.82**	0.56*	1.00**
			Inter-method reliability				
ManWML versus AutoWML	0.48**	0.51**	0.14**	0.44**	0.65**	0.38**	0.74**

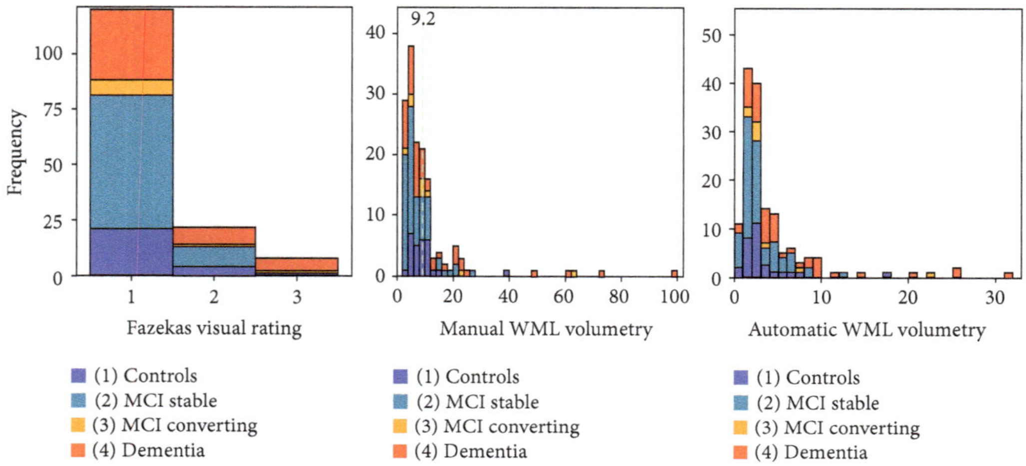

Figure 2: Histograms of WML distribution in the three methods compared. (a) Fazekas visual rating (grade). (b) Manual MRIcron volumetry (cm^3). Dashed green line shows tertile 2 cut off. (c) Automatic FreeSurfer volumetry (cm^3).

Figure 3(a) shows the Bland-Altman (BA) plots of absolute volume interrater differences in the manual MRIcron method, demonstrating increasing differences with higher volumes. However, the variation in rater differences was larger in the assessments of the lowest range of the WML volumes embracing about 80% of the subjects. When comparing the difference as a percentage of the mean measures of each subject (Figure 3(b)), the variation was even more pronounced with regard to the lowest part of the WML volumes, while there was no clear indication of an increase in rater differences with larger volumes.

The intermethod BA plots (Figure 1) for the manual MRIcron volumetry and automatic FreeSurfer volumetry showed a similar pattern as the interrater BA plots, with a pronounced variation for low WML volumes in Figure 1(b).

4. Discussion

4.1. Reliability. Conventional interrater reliabilities were acceptable for the Fazekas rating and the manual MRIcron volumetry. The intermethod reliability for the manual MRIcron and automatic FreeSurfer methods was also acceptable. It is common to evaluate reliability in WML research with intraclass correlation (ICC) with excellent results, for example, in Gao et al. and Smith et al. [11, 25]. However, it is misleading to use such an analysis in a data structure where the distribution is skewed, with very sparse data points in the upper third of the volume range. While showing an excellent reliability for the whole sample, like previous studies, the ICC in the lower aggregated tertiles for the manual method was nonsignificant (Table 3). The density of low-burden WML (Figure 2) probably represents a very common clinical distribution, and reliability analysis must under these conditions be performed and interpreted with caution.

The finding in the present study of lower reliability in the Fazekas rating with lower WML burden is congruent with the finding by Wardlaw et al. [32] where cohorts with lower WML burden showed lower reliability. The higher reliability for high WML burden has been considered as a ceiling effect, but there might as well be floor effects in visual rating [33]. Presumed ceiling and floor effects do not disqualify visual rating as a candidate for clinical use, but such effects would

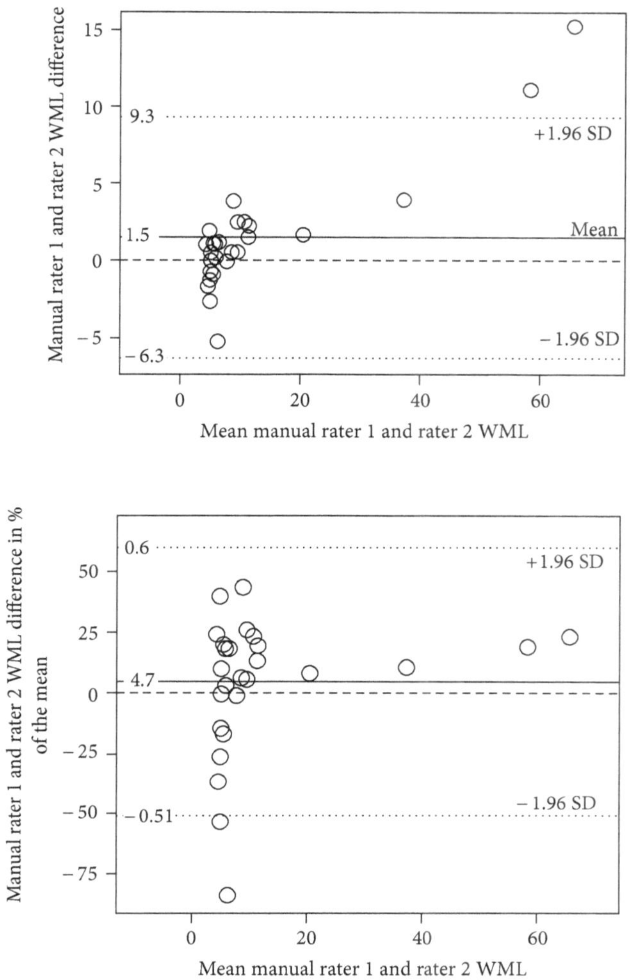

FIGURE 3: (a) and (b) Bland-Altman plots of the interrater differences for the manual MRIcron WML method in cm^3. The x-axes contain mean WML volumes; the y-axis contains absolute differences in (a) image and fractional difference of mean volume in (b). The dashed line designates the no differences level.

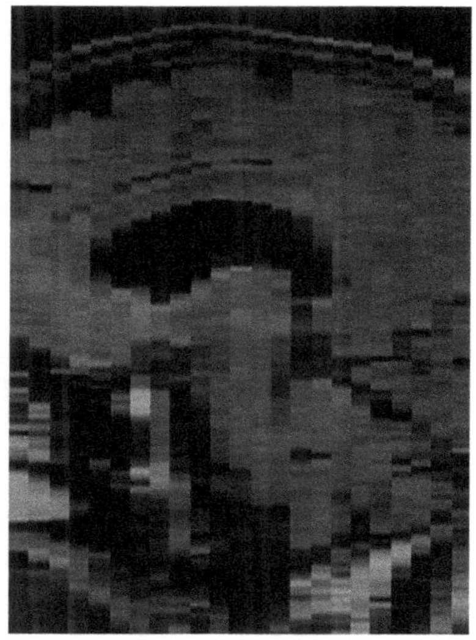

FIGURE 4: Sagittally reformatted slice from an example subject showing the common anterior intensity shift between the fourth and fifth slices in the coronal 2D FLAIR sequence.

in general lower the usefulness for WML research, for example, the possibility to find valid correlations with psychometrics.

The nonsignificant Spearman correlation in the aggregated lower tertiles between manual MRIcron volumetry raters could possibly be due to the high density of data affecting the rank order of the ratings. It is unclear if the high Spearman correlation for high-burden WML implies an overestimation of the reliability due to the sparse data density (leading to less error with ranked data) or if there really was a higher reliability as the BA plot of fractional differences seems to imply (Figure 3(b)). In our opinion, the low reliability in low-burden WML is most probably not due to the combination of high density of data and the nature of the Spearman correlation. Rather, it may be a real rater- and intermethod variation as is visible in the BA plots which seem to indicate an increased variation in the lowest quarter of the volume range. The higher rater variation in low WML may in turn be due to difficulties in the handling of intensity distortion affecting the thresholding step in the manual volumetry.

Intensity inhomogeneities in MR images and variation in grayscale level between scan series result in inconsistent classifications of hyperintensities that in turn introduce measurement errors in the manual WML assessment. In order to assess WML volumes as accurately as possible under conditions with varying intensity levels through the image slices of a subject, a methodology was chosen where the thresholding was adjusted as a compromise to best fit the visible WML volume through all image slices of a subject's brain. Since the localization and extent of WML vary, the accuracy of the thresholding can be expected to be decreased by these intensity distortions. A particular shift in grayscale level was observed in the anterior part of all FLAIR image series (Figure 4), which may be due to gradient eddy currents or cross talk between 2D FLAIR slices [34, 35]. The unreliability for low WML seems to emanate mainly from the anterior half of the image data, and the intensity shift in the anterior part may well be a reason for more complex considerations in the thresholding of low WML burden cases. For higher WML volumes, the thresholding step in general only affects the amount of WML selected, but for lower volumes, the thresholding more often affected the presence or absence of WML in a slice, which means a more straightforward thresholding with higher volumes. In short, increased complexity in the thresholding may be the main cause of an increased rater variation for low WML volumes.

The FreeSurfer suite includes intensity normalization steps which to some extent will limit intensity distortion, but that also may extinguish some of the hypointensities. Further, the T1 MR sequence used for the FreeSurfer volumetry does in general have lower WML definition and somewhat smaller areas of WML hypointensities compared to the

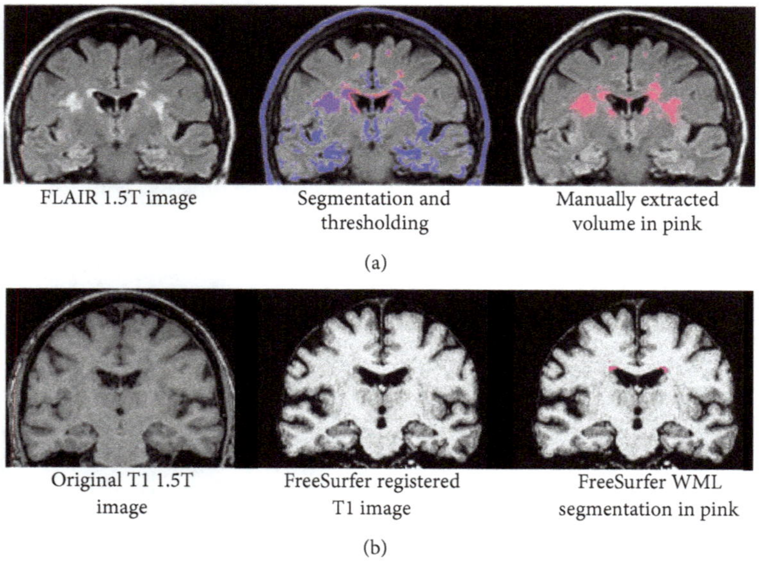

FIGURE 5: 1.5T MR images from a patient with severe-burden WML showing the differences in scan sequence and WML detection between manual MRIcron volumetry (a) and automatic FreeSurfer volumetry (b).

hyperintensities in the FLAIR sequence. A visual inspection of the T1 weighted images and the FreeSurfer segmentations confirmed that the substantial deviations between the volumetrical methods in the detection of WML in various locations may mainly be due to the lower definition in the T1 weighted images. The FreeSurfer segmentation often omitted large amounts of deep WML seen in the FLAIR images (Figure 5). On few occasions, FreeSurfer classified sulcal cortical voxels as WML. Occasionally, FreeSurfer detected more WML in the periventricular region than visible in the T1 weighted images. Compared to WML seen in FLAIR images, the amount of WML found by FreeSurfer still was lower even in the periventricular regions. The T1 MRI images in Figures 5 and 6 are examples showing that the noise level makes the detection of punctate WML a difficult task, nevertheless FreeSurfer detects several punctate WML patches in this region. The single punctate WML patch in the FLAIR slice in Figure 6 is hardly visible in the T1 slice, and it is conceivable that no punctuate WML patch in this location is detected in FreeSurfer. In some cases, FreeSurfer detected small punctate WML not detected in the manual volumetry (Figure 6(b)), but occasionally, it detected less punctate WML than the manual volumetry (Figure 6(c)). Hence, FreeSurfer seems to detect punctate WML in a largely random way. However, a more accurate punctate WML detection may be a disadvantage in dementia research since punctate WML often originate from perivascular spaces and have been found to have low progression [36]. In short, the FreeSurfer volumetry generally detects less WML, which is likely due to a combination of the method, the characteristics of WML, and the visibility of WML in T1 weighted images and leads to larger differences between the methods when measuring larger WML volumes (Figure 1).

WML progression generally begins in the periventricular region and subsequently expands radially to more peripheral locations [37]. The skewness of the distribution of WML, with a low fraction of high-burden WML subjects also in the dementia part of the sample, can be expected to exist also for clinical samples in general. The statistical atlas used in FreeSurfer was generated from a small sample (http://surfer.nmr.mgh.harvard.edu/fswiki/Buckner40Testing), where high-burden WML cases might be rare or lacking. An atlas generated with a low frequency of high-burden exposure may contribute to the FreeSurfer inability to find deep WML.

4.2. Limitations. The Fazekas rating was performed by comparing the largest WML aggregation to the templates, and no metrical measurements were used which possibly affected the classification of the subjects close to the Fazekas definitions of the metrical borders. The visual rating in three grades differs from the design in other studies, which limits the comparability of results. It is not feasible to use a zero grade WML in T2 images with any accuracy, and in a later control of the FLAIR images, it was ascertained that no subjects with complete absence of WML were present in the study. In visual rating, the FLAIR sequence can be expected to be advantageous compared to the T2 sequence due to the signal suppression of free fluid in FLAIR images. However, the FLAIR sequence in this study had coronal orientation and 5 mm slice thickness, which made it unsuitable to use with the axial template images. Therefore, the axial T2 scan sequence was used.

In the manual method, the basal ganglia nuclei in FLAIR images often had no clear intensity separation from white matter, which may have contributed to an inaccurate volume assessment in this region. The hyperintensities along the ventricular lining in the basal ganglia region were included in the manually assessed WML, which may be unsuitable and possibly confound the differentiation, primarily in patients

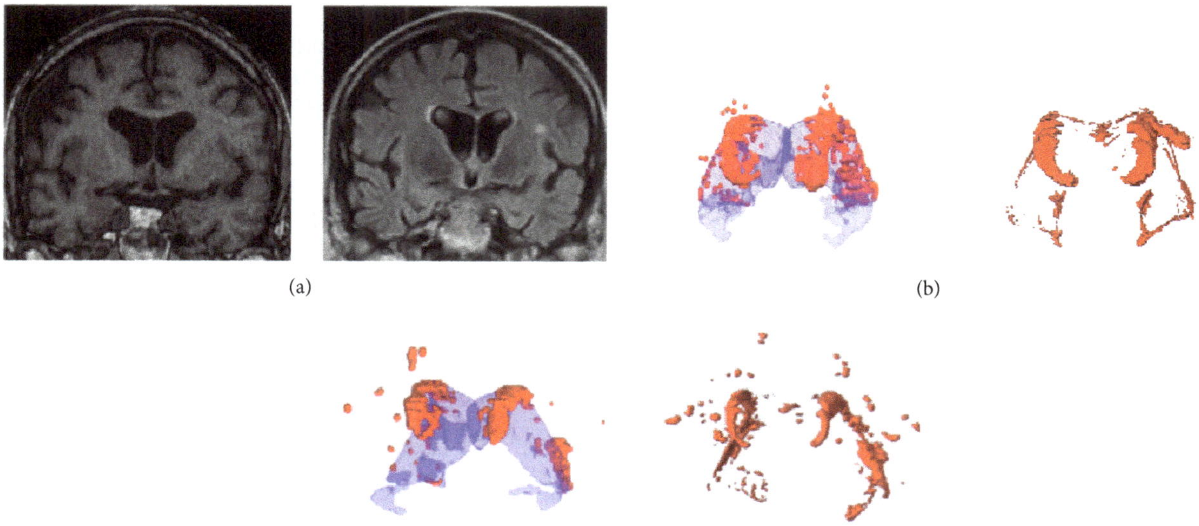

(c)

FIGURE 6: 3D visualizations and MRI images of WML assessed by FreeSurfer and in manual volumetry. (a) MRI images of a dementia patient. The left image shows a T1 original image used in the FreeSurfer assessment where there are FreeSurfer findings of punctate WML. The FLAIR image to the right in the corresponding position contains a large punctate WML patch close to the superior cortical part of the left insula which is hardly visible in the T1 image. (b) The same dementia patient with WML burden (in red) at approximately the same manually extracted high-burden WML volume as the control subject. FreeSurfer assessment is shown to the left with the lateral ventricles visualized in transparent blue, and manual volumetry is shown to the right. (c) Control subject with WML burden (in red) at approximately the same manually extracted high-burden WML volume as the dementia patient. FreeSurfer assessment is shown to the left with the lateral ventricles visualized in transparent blue. Manual volumetry is shown to the right.

with low WML volumes. The different scan sequences used in the different methods confound the methodological comparison; for example, only the FLAIR sequence does to some extent show separate intensity ranges for fluid filled cavities and WML. By contrast, in T1 and T2 sequences, fluid-filled cavities have intensities in the same range as WML.

The moderate interrater correlation for the manual volumetry could possibly be a consequence of intensity distortions in the FLAIR images. Although steps were taken in the thresholding methodology to minimize the impact of intensity distortions, sample tests of WML volume using different thresholdings unveiled considerable variation in measurements. The FLAIR sequence had obvious intensity inhomogeneities, and no automatic intensity normalization was performed which may limit the possibilities to interpret the present findings further.

5. Conclusions

Reliability analysis showed acceptable overall results but with lower reliability for all methods in the lower aggregated tertiles. Despite excellent overall reliability for manual volumetry, no significant reliability was found in the lower aggregated tertiles. Hence, the results of intraclass correlation in WML samples, that is, commonly skewed, might be misleading, and reliability analysis of WML methods should be considered with caution. Image intensity distortion seems to be the major cause of the reliability deficits. Optimized MR imaging, postscan intensity standardization and normalization are quite likely among the most important factors to consider for more accurate measurements of WML. FreeSurfer comprised lower volumes than the manual method, probably due to the T1 sequence it uses, and was not able to detect punctuate WML in a consistent manner.

5.1. Future Directions. A medically oriented follow-up paper focusing on the predictive power of the different WML measurements is being prepared. In another study, we intend to refine the visual comparison between the methods, using a larger sample of subjects and coregistration of images from different scan series. Finally, our long-term goal is an improved manual method that excludes thresholding but includes an adequate intensity normalization.

Conflict of Interests

The authors have no actual or potential conflict of interests with the work in the present study, either financial or otherwise.

Acknowledgments

This study was supported by Sahlgrenska University Hospital, Swedish Research Council, Swedish Brain Power, and Wilhelm och Martina Lundgrens Vetenskapsfond. The authors thank Erik Joas and Anne Ingeborg Berg for statistical advice, Johannes Eldblom for visual rating, and Mattias Göthlin and Ewa Styrud for data base assistance.

References

[1] J. D. Schmahmann, E. E. Smith, F. S. Eichler, and C. M. Filley, "Cerebral white matter: neuroanatomy, clinical neurology, and neurobehavioral correlates," *Annals of the New York Academy of Sciences*, vol. 1142, pp. 266–309, 2008.

[2] D. Inzitari, G. Pracucci, A. Poggesi et al., "Changes in white matter as determinant of global functional decline in older independent outpatients: three year follow-up of LADIS (leukoaraiosis and disability) study cohort," *BMJ*, vol. 339, article b2477, 2009.

[3] S. Debette and H. S. Markus, "The clinical importance of white matter hyperintensities on brain magnetic resonance imaging: systematic review and meta-analysis," *BMJ*, vol. 341, article c3666, 2010.

[4] S. Bombois, S. Debette, A. Bruandet et al., "Vascular subcortical hyperintensities predict conversion to vascular and mixed dementia in MCI patients," *Stroke*, vol. 39, no. 7, pp. 2046–2051, 2008.

[5] D. B. Wakefield, N. Moscufo, C. R. Guttmann et al., "White matter hyperintensities predict functional decline in voiding, mobility, and cognition in older adults," *Journal of the American Geriatrics Society*, vol. 58, no. 2, pp. 275–281, 2010.

[6] Y. Zhang, N. Schuff, C. Ching et al., "Joint assessment of structural, perfusion, and diffusion MRI in Alzheimer's disease and frontotemporal dementia," *International Journal of Alzheimer's Disease*, vol. 2011, Article ID 546871, 11 pages, 2011.

[7] W. Wen, P. S. Sachdev, J. J. Li, X. Chen, and K. J. Anstey, "White matter hyperintensities in the forties: their prevalence and topography in an epidemiological sample aged 44-48," *Human Brain Mapping*, vol. 30, no. 4, pp. 1155–1167, 2009.

[8] W. Wen and P. Sachdev, "The topography of white matter hyperintensities on brain MRI in healthy 60- to 64-year-old individuals," *NeuroImage*, vol. 22, no. 1, pp. 144–154, 2004.

[9] W. M. Bailey, "Fast Fluid Attenuated Inversion Recovery (FLAIR) imaging and associated artefacts in Magnetic Resonance Imaging (MRI)," *Radiography*, vol. 13, no. 4, pp. 283–290, 2007.

[10] T. Erkinjuntti, D. Inzitari, L. Pantoni et al., "Research criteria for subcortical vascular dementia in clinical trials," *Journal of Neural Transmission, Supplement*, no. 59, pp. 23–30, 2000.

[11] F. Q. Gao, R. H. Swartz, and P. Scheltens, "Complexity of MRI white matter hyperintensity assessments in relation to cognition in aging and dementia from the Sunnybrook Dementia Study," *Journal of Alzheimer's Disease*, vol. 26, supplement 3, pp. 379–388, 2011.

[12] P. Kapeller, R. Barber, R. J. Vermeulen et al., "Visual rating of age-related white matter changes on magnetic resonance imaging: scale comparison, interrater agreement, and correlations with quantitative measurements," *Stroke*, vol. 34, no. 2, pp. 441–445, 2003.

[13] F. Fazekas, J. B. Chawluk, and A. Alavi, "MR signal abnormalities at 1.5 T in Alzheimer's dementia and normal aging," *American Journal of Roentgenology*, vol. 149, no. 2, pp. 351–356, 1987.

[14] D. Inzitari, M. Simoni, G. Pracucci et al., "Risk of rapid global functional decline in elderly patients with severe cerebral age-related white matter changes: the LADIS study," *Archives of Internal Medicine*, vol. 167, no. 1, pp. 81–88, 2007.

[15] E. C. W. Van Straaten, F. Fazekas, E. Rostrup et al., "Impact of white matter hyperintensities scoring method on correlations with clinical data: the LADIS study," *Stroke*, vol. 37, no. 3, pp. 836–840, 2006.

[16] A. A. Gouw, W. M. Van Der Flier, E. C. W. Van Straaten et al., "Simple versus complex assessment of white matter hyperintensities in relation to physical performance and cognition: the LADIS study," *Journal of Neurology*, vol. 253, no. 9, pp. 1189–1196, 2006.

[17] K. D. Garrett, R. A. Cohen, R. H. Paul et al., "Computer-mediated measurement and subjective ratings of white matter hyperintensities in vascular dementia: relationships to neuropsychological performance," *Clinical Neuropsychologist*, vol. 18, no. 1, pp. 50–62, 2004.

[18] M. E. Gurol, M. C. Irizarry, E. E. Smith et al., "Plasma β-amyloid and white matter lesions in AD, MCI, and cerebral amyloid angiopathy," *Neurology*, vol. 66, no. 1, pp. 23–29, 2006.

[19] S. Klöppel, A. Abdulkadir, S. Hadjidemetriou et al., "A comparison of different automated methods for the detection of white matter lesions in MRI data," *NeuroImage*, vol. 57, no. 2, pp. 416–422, 2011.

[20] D. Mortazavi, A. Z. Kouzani, and H. Soltanian-Zadeh, "Segmentation of multiple sclerosis lesions in MR images: a review," *Neuroradiology*, vol. 54, no. 4, pp. 299–299-320, 2011.

[21] S. D. Smart, M. J. Firbank, and J. T. O'Brien, "Validation of automated white matter hyperintensity segmentation," *Journal of Aging Research*, vol. 2011, Article ID 391783, 5 pages, 2011.

[22] B. Fischl, D. H. Salat, E. Busa et al., "Whole brain segmentation: automated labeling of neuroanatomical structures in the human brain," *Neuron*, vol. 33, no. 3, pp. 341–355, 2002.

[23] B. Fischl, D. H. Salat, A. J. W. Van Der Kouwe et al., "Sequence-independent segmentation of magnetic resonance images," *NeuroImage*, vol. 23, supplement 1, pp. S69–S84, 2004.

[24] F. Klauschen, A. Goldman, V. Barra, A. Meyer-Lindenberg, and A. Lundervold, "Evaluation of automated brain MR image segmentation and volumetry methods," *Human Brain Mapping*, vol. 30, no. 4, pp. 1310–1327, 2009.

[25] E. E. Smith, D. H. Salat, J. Jeng et al., "Correlations between MRI white matter lesion location and executive function and episodic memory," *Neurology*, vol. 76, no. 17, pp. 1492–1499, 2011.

[26] C. Fennema-Notestine, D. J. Hagler Jr., L. K. McEvoy et al., "Structural MRI biomarkers for preclinical and mild Alzheimer's disease," *Human Brain Mapping*, vol. 30, no. 10, pp. 3238–3253, 2009.

[27] C. Eckerström, E. Olsson, M. Borga et al., "Small baseline volume of left hippocampus is associated with subsequent conversion of MCI into dementia: the Göteborg MCI study," *Journal of the Neurological Sciences*, vol. 272, no. 1-2, pp. 48–59, 2008.

[28] B. Reisberg, S. H. Ferris, M. J. De Leon, and T. Crook, "Global Deterioration Scale (GDS)," *Psychopharmacology Bulletin*, vol. 24, no. 4, pp. 661–623, 1988.

[29] J. Kottner, L. Audigé, S. Brorson et al., "Guidelines for reporting reliability and agreement studies (GRRAS) were proposed," *Journal of Clinical Epidemiology*, vol. 64, no. 1, pp. 96–106, 2011.

[30] F. Fazekas, R. Kleinert, H. Olfenbacher et al., "Pathologic correlates of incidental MRI white matter signal hyperintensities," *Neurology*, vol. 43, no. 9, pp. 1683–1689, 1993.

[31] C. M. Holland, E. E. Smith, I. Csapo et al., "Spatial distribution of white-matter hyperintensities in Alzheimer disease, cerebral amyloid angiopathy, and healthy aging," *Stroke*, vol. 39, no. 4, pp. 1127–1133, 2008.

[32] J. M. Wardlaw, K. J. Ferguson, and C. Graham, "White matter hyperintensities and rating scales—observer reliability varies

with lesion load," *Journal of Neurology*, vol. 251, no. 5, pp. 584–590, 2004.

[33] R. Mäntylä, T. Erkinjuntti, O. Salonen et al., "Variable agreement between visual rating scales for white matter hyperintensities on MRI," *Stroke*, vol. 28, no. 8, pp. 1614–1623, 1997.

[34] A. Simmons, P. S. Tofts, G. J. Barker, and S. R. Arridge, "Sources of intensity nonuniformity in spin echo images at 1.5 T," *Magnetic Resonance in Medicine*, vol. 32, no. 1, pp. 121–128, 1994.

[35] D. A. G. Wicks, G. J. Barker, and P. S. Tofts, "Correction of intensity nonuniformity in MR images of any orientation," *Magnetic Resonance Imaging*, vol. 11, no. 2, pp. 183–196, 1993.

[36] R. Schmidt, H. Schmidt, J. Haybaeck et al., "Heterogeneity in age-related white matter changes," *Acta Neuropathologica*, vol. 122, no. 2, pp. 171–185, 2011.

[37] C. DeCarli, E. Fletcher, V. Ramey, D. Harvey, and W. J. Jagust, "Anatomical mapping of white matter hyperintensities (WMH): exploring the relationships between periventricular WMH, deep WMH, and total WMH burden," *Stroke*, vol. 36, no. 1, pp. 50–55, 2005.

12

Redundant Vasodilator Pathways Underlying Radial Artery Flow-Mediated Dilation are Preserved in Healthy Aging

Kevin D. Ballard,[1] Michael E. Tschakovsky,[2] Amanda L. Zaleski,[1] Donna M. Polk,[1] Paul D. Thompson,[1] Francis J. Kiernan,[1] and Beth A. Parker[1,3]

[1] *Division of Cardiology, Hartford Hospital, 80 Seymour Street, Hartford, CT 06102, USA*
[2] *School of Kinesiology and Health Studies, Queen's University, 28 Division Street, Kingston, ON, Canada K7L 3N6*
[3] *Department of Health Sciences, University of Hartford, 200 Bloomfield Avenue, West Hartford, CT 06117, USA*

Correspondence should be addressed to Beth A. Parker; beth.parker@hhchealth.org

Academic Editor: Jack Cannon

Background. Blocking nitric oxide (NO) and vasodilator prostanoids (PN) does not consistently reduce flow-mediated dilation (FMD) in young adults. The impact of aging on the contribution of NO and PG to FMD is unknown. *Methods.* FMD was measured in older adults (n = 10, 65 ± 3 y) after arterial infusion of saline, N(G)-monomethyl-L-arginine (L-NMMA), and ketorolac + L-NMMA. Data were compared to published data in young adults. *Results.* L-NMMA reduced FMD in older adults (8.9 ± 3.6 to 5.9 ± 3.7%) although this was not statistically significant (P = 0.08) and did not differ (P = 0.74) from the reduction observed in young adults (10.0 ± 3.8 to 7.6 ± 4.7%; P = 0.03). Blocking PN did not affect FMD in young or older adults. In older adults, L-NMMA reduced (n = 6; range = 36–123% decrease), augmented (n = 3; 10–122% increase), or did not change FMD (n = 1; 0.4% increase). After PN blockade, FMD responses were reduced (n = 2), augmented (n = 6), or unaffected (n = 1). *Conclusions.* NO or PN blockade did not consistently reduce FMD in healthy older adults, suggesting the existence of redundant vasodilator phenotypes as observed previously in young adults.

1. Introduction

Conduit artery flow-mediated dilation (FMD) is a widely used noninvasive method to assess endothelial function. Diminished FMD is widely assumed to reflect impaired dilator function of nitric oxide (NO) [1], based on several studies reporting the absence or substantial attenuation of FMD following infusion of the NO synthase (NOS) inhibitor N(G)-monomethyl-L-arginine (L-NMMA) [2–6]. In support, a recent meta-analysis of 13 crossover studies utilizing L-NMMA infusion and temporary distal ischemia found a substantial contribution of NO (72%) to the conduit artery FMD response in healthy adults [7]. However, other studies failing to significantly alter FMD with L-NMMA [8–10] indicate potential involvement of additional vasodilators (such as vasodilator prostanoids (PN) [11] and endothelium-derived hyperpolarizing factor (EDHF) [12, 13]). Evidence of a concurrent or compensatory role of alternative dilators in health and disease [12, 14] suggests that these alternative vasodilators may be important for cardiovascular health. In support of this hypothesis, FMD following proximal cuff occlusion, which is only partially reduced by NO blockade [2], predicts future cardiovascular events as effectively as FMD following distal occlusion [15]. Consequently, interpreting conduit FMD as primarily mediated by NO release and endothelial dysfunction as a loss of the NO dilator system overlooks the relevance of redundant vasodilator systems for cardiovascular function and their potential as targets for therapies aimed at ameliorating cardiovascular risk with age and disease.

We recently investigated the mechanisms underlying radial artery (RA) FMD in young men and women, finding that blocking NO and PN reduced the vasodilator response to ischemia in some subjects but not in others [8]. For example, individual variability in the FMD response following L-NMMA and/or PN blockade by ketorolac was observed, and only half of the young subjects exhibited an observable (and fairly modest) effect of L-NMMA on RA FMD. As discussed above, these data suggest that variable and redundant dilator pathways contribute to conduit artery FMD in healthy young men and women. Whether these redundant vasodilator pathways are impacted by aging is unknown, as previous work investigating the contribution of NO and PN to rest and exercise limb hyperemia in aged humans has not been extended to FMD or has focused exclusively on the NO system [16–19]. Therefore, the present investigation extends our previous findings [8] by examining differences due to healthy aging on the vasodilator pathways underlying RA FMD, a model utilized in previous infusion studies [3, 4, 6, 9]. Specifically, we sought to determine whether aging impairs the FMD response that persists following single and combined NO and PN blockade [8]. We hypothesized that blocking NO and PN synthesis would more substantially reduce RA FMD in older adults, indicating impaired redundant vasodilator mechanisms with age that could deleteriously impact cardiovascular health.

2. Methods

2.1. Subjects. We enrolled healthy, nonsmoking older adults ($n = 10$, 5 men and 5 women, ages 60–79). Data from young adults ($n = 16$, 8 men and 8 women, ages 20–35) have been reported previously [8] and were used for comparison purposes in the present study. Both young and older individuals were excluded if they met the criteria described previously [8]. All participants provided written, informed consent as approved by the Institutional Review Board at Hartford Hospital.

2.2. Testing Procedures. Detailed methods have been described previously [8] and are identical in the present investigation. Interested subjects reported to the laboratory following a 12 h fast in which data for inclusion/exclusion criteria [8] were assessed. Next, a venous blood draw was performed for the analysis of whole blood viscosity, blood lipid levels, and hemoglobin (Clinical Laboratory Partners, Hartford, CT, USA) and resting blood pressure, heart rate, and anthropometrics were measured. On a separate day, enrolled participants reported to the laboratory for an invasive catheterization visit following a ≥8 h fast and abstinence from exercise, pain medications, and herbal supplements for ≥24 h.

2.3. Catheterization Visit. Detailed methods for the local infusion of study drugs have been described previously [8]. Briefly, to locally infuse saline and study drugs, a 20-gauge Teflon catheter was inserted into the left brachial artery at the level of the antecubital fossa following anesthetization of the overlying skin. A three-port connector in series with a catheter-transducer system was used to administer saline and study drugs via the arterial catheter. One port was used to measure arterial pressure while the two remaining ports allowed for drug infusions and continuous saline administration for flushing.

Following a 30 min supine rest period, saline was infused at 2 mL/min for 10 min to establish a control condition for any effects of infusate administration on FMD. Radial artery FMD was then performed. In brief, the RA was imaged ~10 cm distal to the antecubital fossa using a 5–12 MHz multifrequency linear-array transducer attached to a high-resolution ultrasound machine (Terason t3000; TeraTech Corp., Burlington, MA, USA). Using the same ultrasound machine Doppler velocity was also continuously measured using a 60° angle of insonation which remained constant throughout the study. Resting RA diameter and velocity were recorded for 1 min before the inflation (300 mmHg for 5 min) of a pneumatic occlusion cuff placed around the participant's wrist. Diameter and velocity were recorded continuously beginning 30 s before cuff deflation until 3 min after deflation. After a 10 min rest period and infusion of L-NMMA (Clinalfa, Laeufelfingen, Switzerland) for 10 min at 5 mg/mL, 2 mL/min, RA FMD was repeated to determine the impact of NO blockade. Following another 10 min rest period, ketorolac (Toradol; Abbott Labs, Abbott Park, IL, USA) was infused for 5 min at 600 μg/mL, 2 mL/min, immediately followed by a maintenance dose of L-NMMA for 5 min (5 mg/mL, 2 mL/min). RA FMD was then repeated a third time. Drug doses equaled or exceeded those used in previous studies successfully blocking NO and PN in the forearm [4, 6, 18, 20–22].

2.4. Diameter and Velocity Data Analysis. Radial artery FMD data were analyzed as reported previously [8]. Briefly, offline analysis of diameters and velocities was performed using Brachial Analyzer software (Medical Imaging Applications LLC, Coralville, IA, USA). Analyses were performed by a technician blinded to any subject information. Only end diastolic diameters, triggered by the corresponding Doppler waveform, were captured for diameter analyses. Radial artery FMD was expressed as percent change in dilation relative to baseline for each trial.

Mean velocity matched to the corresponding diameter was used to calculate shear stress in dyn/cm^2 [$4\mu\cdot V/D$; μ = blood viscosity (mPA·sec at 60 rpm); D = arterial diameter (cm); V = velocity (cm/sec)]. The postocclusion shear stress area under the curve (AUC SS) was calculated from cuff release until the time of peak diameter [23, 24] and used to normalize FMD [FMD/AUC SS]. Radial artery blood flow [RBF (mL/min) = blood velocity (cm/s) $*\ \pi\ *$ (radial diameter (cm)/2)^2 $*$ 60] and mean intra-arterial blood pressure (MAP (mmHg)) measured at the baseline of each trial were used to calculate radial vascular conductance [RVC = RBF/MAP $*$ 100].

2.5. Statistical Methods. Statistical analyses were performed with SPSS 19.0. A one-way ANOVA was performed to compare baseline differences between age groups. Two-way ANOVA was used to analyze RA FMD responses with trial (drug infusion) as the within-subject (repeated measures)

TABLE 1: Participant characteristics[a,b].

	Young (n = 16)[c]	Older (n = 10)
Age (years)*	28 ± 4	65 ± 3
BMI (kg/m^2)	25.1 ± 2.7	24.2 ± 3.7
SBP (mmHg)*	106 ± 10	119 ± 10
DBP (mmHg)*	65 ± 7	71 ± 6
HR (bpm)	58 ± 9	60 ± 8
LDL cholesterol (mmol/L)	2.4 ± 0.8	2.6 ± 0.5
HDL cholesterol (mmol/L)	1.6 ± 0.4	1.8 ± 0.4
Whole blood viscosity (mPA·s)	5.0 ± 0.7	4.9 ± 0.3
Hemoglobin (mg/dL)	14.2 ± 1.8	14.1 ± 0.8

[a]Data are means ± SD.
[b]BMI: body mass index; DBP: diastolic blood pressure; HDL: high-density lipoprotein; HR: heart rate; LDL: low-density lipoprotein; SBP: systolic blood pressure.
[c]Data from young participants have been published previously [8].
*Significant difference between age groups ($P < 0.05$).

factor, group as the between-subject factor, and a group-by-trial interaction. Significance was determined at $P \leq 0.05$ and a Tukey post hoc adjustment was applied to significant main effect and interaction comparisons. A chi square test was used to compare the number of young versus older adults who exhibited decreased RA FMD from saline to L-NMMA and then from L-NMMA to ketorolac + L-NMMA. Linear regression was performed to predict if the change in RA FMD from saline to L-NMMA was explained by select independent variables.

3. Results

3.1. Participant Characteristics. Characteristics for the young adults have been reported [8] and are summarized in Table 1 in comparison to older adults.

3.2. Baseline Hemodynamic Parameters across Infusion Trials. Means for resting RA diameter, RBF, MAP, and RVC between age groups measured immediately following infusions of saline, L-NMMA, and ketorolac + L-NMMA are shown in Table 2. In older adults, ketorolac + L-NMMA infusion increased ($P < 0.01$) MAP compared with saline. The lack of a significant trial ∗ group interaction ($P = 0.68$) indicates that the MAP response to combined infusion did not differ from the increase ($P < 0.01$) observed in young adults.

3.3. RA FMD Responses across Infusion Trials. One female participant in the older group was not included in the analysis between the L-NMMA and ketorolac + L-NMMA trials due to corruption of the video file during data acquisition. In older adults (n = 10) L-NMMA infusion decreased RA FMD by 26.5 ± 67.3% compared with saline (8.9 ± 3.6% to 5.9 ± 3.7%), although this was not statistically significant ($P = 0.08$) (Figure 1(a)). Furthermore, the lack of a significant trial ∗ group interaction ($P = 0.74$) indicates that the RA FMD response to L-NMMA infusion did not differ from the decrease (23.7 ± 37.0%) observed previously in young adults (10.0 ± 3.8% to 7.6 ± 4.7%; $P = 0.03$) (Figure 1(a)). Postocclusion AUC SS did not differ between trials or age groups (Figure 1(b)). Normalization to the shear stress stimulus abolished the effect of L-NMMA in both groups (trial ∗ group: $P = 0.75$) (Figure 1(c)). Individual RA FMD responses to L-NMMA in young adults have been reported previously [8] (Figure 2(a)). Compared with saline, RA FMD in older adults was decreased (n = 6, range = 36–123% decrease), augmented (n = 3, range = 10–122% increase), or unaffected (n = 1, 0.4% increase) following L-NMMA infusion (Figure 2(b)).

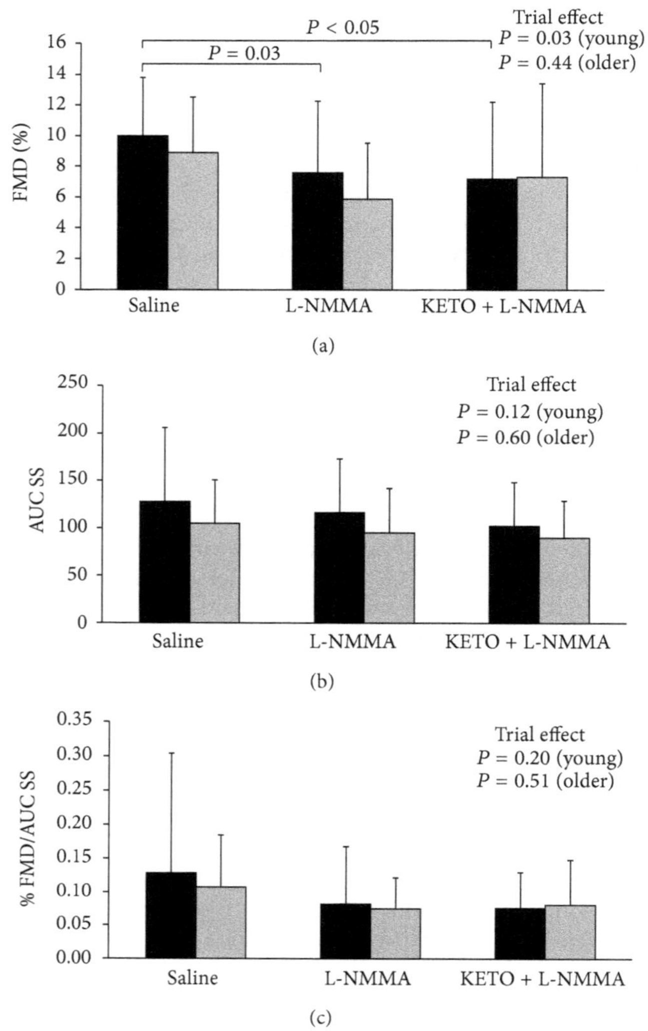

FIGURE 1: Group means ± SD for young (data from young participants have been published previously [8]) (n = 16; black bars) and older (n = 10; grey bars) adults are shown for FMD (a), AUC SS (b), and FMD/AUC SS (c) with P values for trial effects (within each group) and any significant differences between conditions on each graph. n = 9 older adults in the KETO + L-NMMA trial. AUC SS: postocclusion shear stress area under the curve; FMD: flow-mediated dilation; L-NMMA: N(G)-monomethyl-L-arginine; KETO: ketorolac.

TABLE 2: Baseline hemodynamics across infusion trials in young and older adults[a,b].

	Saline	L-NMMA	KETO + L-NMMA	Trial
Young (n = 16)[c]				
RA diameter (mm)	2.09 ± 0.35	2.08 ± 0.34	2.08 ± 0.36	0.68
RBF (mL/min)	16.4 ± 14.2	11.7 ± 7.5	11.7 ± 5.4	0.05
MAP (mmHg)	77.5 ± 9.9	80.6 ± 11.6	84.0 ± 12.6*	0.01
RVC (mL/min/100 mmHg)	20.9 ± 17.7	14.5 ± 9.6*	14.0 ± 6.3*	0.03
Older (n = 10)				
RA diameter (mm)	2.16 ± 0.42	2.12 ± 0.36	2.05 ± 0.46	0.32
RBF (mL/min)	18.0 ± 5.9	13.2 ± 4.0	11.9 ± 6.1	0.01
MAP (mmHg)	82.7 ± 9.4	87.9 ± 11.0	90.3 ± 10.2*	0.01
RVC (mL/min/100 mmHg)	22.9 ± 8.9	15.1 ± 4.4*	13.3 ± 6.9*	0.01

[a]Data are means ± SD.
[b]KETO: ketorolac; L-NMMA: N(G)-monomethyl-L-arginine; MAP: mean arterial pressure; RA: radial artery; RBF: radial artery blood flow; RVC: radial artery vascular conductance.
[c]Data from young participants have been published previously [8].
*Significantly different from saline trial ($P < 0.05$). Trial = P value for trial effect for each variable.

Relative to L-NMMA, ketorolac + L-NMMA infusion increased RA FMD by 1.0 ± 70.1% (trial: $P = 0.68$) and 52.5 ± 101.3% (trial: $P = 0.52$) for young and older adults, respectively (trial ∗ group: $P = 0.38$) (Figure 1(a)). Shear stimulus normalization did not alter the effect of ketorolac infusion in either age group (trial ∗ group: $P = 0.56$) (Figure 1(c)). Similar to the above, absolute RA FMD responses in older adults were no different (trial: $P = 0.24$) from saline (0.20 ± 0.08 mm) following L-NMMA (0.13 ± 0.09 mm) and ketorolac + L-NMMA infusion (0.14 ± 0.13 mm). Individual RA FMD responses to combined infusion in young adults have been reported previously [8] (Figure 2(a)). Compared with L-NMMA, RA FMD in older adults was decreased (n = 2, 83–103% decrease), increased (n = 6, 34–170% increase), or unaffected (n = 1, 2% decrease) following ketorolac + L-NMMA infusion (Figure 2(b)). Absolute RA FMD responses in young adults were decreased (trial: $P = 0.01$) from saline (0.21 ± 0.08 mm) following L-NMMA (0.15 ± 0.07 mm) and ketorolac + L-NMMA infusion (0.14 ± 0.09 mm). There was no difference between age groups in the number of participants who exhibited decreased RA FMD from saline to L-NMMA ($P = 0.11$) and L-NMMA to ketorolac ($P = 0.61$).

Linear regression, comparing the change in RA FMD from saline to L-NMMA with select independent variables (i.e., age, total cholesterol, MAP, SBP, DBP, and BMI), did not reveal any statistically significant relationships when age groups were combined (all $P > 0.15$ for independent variables). The addition of age group into the model did not influence the results (all $P > 0.27$ for independent variables).

4. Discussion

The present findings agree with our previous observation [8] that blocking NO or PN synthesis does not uniformly reduce conduit artery RA FMD in healthy adults. Moreover, in older adults, substantial variability occurred in the magnitude and direction of shear stress-induced vasodilation in response to single and combined blockade of NO and PN synthesis. The present RA data coincide with previous findings in healthy adults [8, 9], including recent data obtained in the brachial artery [10], further questioning the widespread assumption that conduit artery FMD following temporary distal ischemia is primarily NO mediated [2–4, 6].

An age-related decline in FMD has been described in many studies [25–27]. To our knowledge, our study is the first to investigate the impact of healthy aging on the contribution of NO and PN to conduit artery FMD and adds to previous studies investigating the vasodilator pathways contributing to rest and exercise limb hyperemia in aged humans [16–19]. We hypothesized that blocking NO and PN would reduce RA FMD to a greater extent and more uniformly, in older versus younger adults indicating impairment of alternative or redundant vasodilator pathways. However, in contrast to our hypothesis, blocking NO and PN did not consistently reduce RA FMD in older adults. Specifically, only 22% (2 of 9) of older adults exhibited reductions in RA FMD to combined blockade (83–103% decrease). In comparison, 44% (7 of 16) of adults ~40 years younger exhibited reduced RA dilation following ketorolac + L-NMMA infusion (10–115% decrease) [8]. Older adults exhibited substantial variability in the magnitude and direction of RA FMD responses following single and combined blockade of NO and PN suggesting that redundant vasodilator pathways are present in healthy older adults and that aged arteries are able to compensate for loss of specific vasodilators.

We observed that 9 of 16 young and 6 of 9 older adults exhibited an increase in RA FMD in response to combined PN and NO blockade, indicating that non-NO and PN mechanisms are able to compensate for the loss of these two vasodilators and further supporting the existence of redundant vasodilator pathways in humans. Alternatively, our observation of increased FMD in 6 of 9 older adults following combined NO and PN blockade compared to L-NMMA alone might suggest a vasoconstrictor role for PN which is consistent with previous findings [28]. By inhibiting NO and PN synthesis, it is assumed that the remaining dilatory response is attributable to EDHF [29].

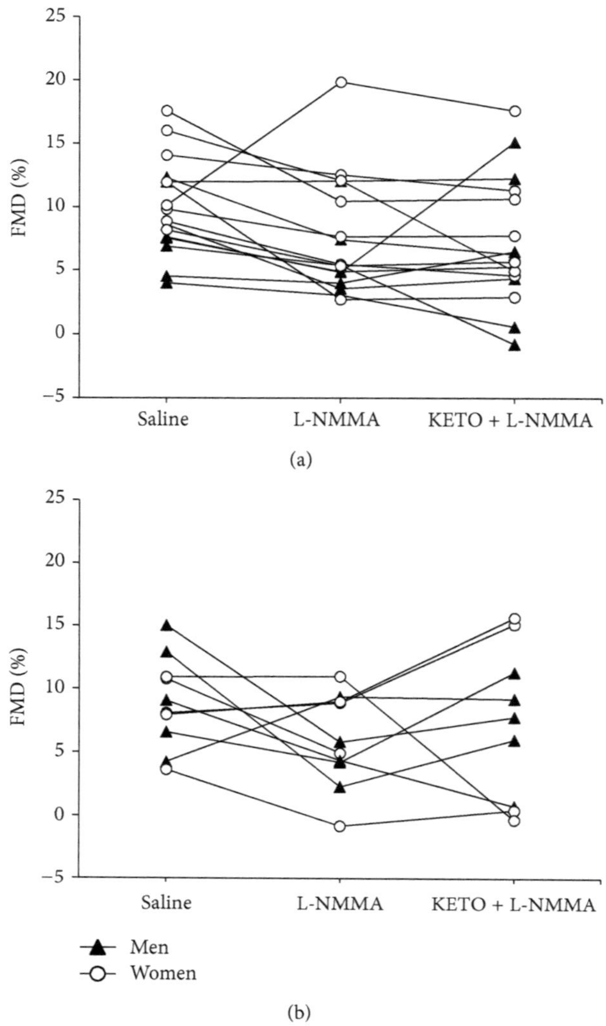

FIGURE 2: Individual FMD responses to saline, L-NMMA, and KETO + L-NMMA infusion are shown for young (data from young participants have been published previously [8]) (a) and older adults (b). FMD: flow-mediated dilation; L-NMMA: N(G)-monomethyl-L-arginine; KETO: ketorolac.

However, the involvement of EDHF was not directly tested in our study design. Furthermore, the contribution of additional vasodilators to endothelial responses in healthy adults, including cytochrome P (CYP)450 epoxygenases [30, 31], cannot be ruled out. Infusion of the specific CYP 2C9 inhibitor sulphenazole reduces RA FMD from 11.5% to 7.4% [31], demonstrating a role for CYP 2C metabolites in the FMD response. Single (L-NMMA) and combined (sulphenazole + L-NMMA) blockade lowered RA FMD to 6.0% and 3.9%, respectively [31], suggesting multiple, redundant pathways underlying shear stress-induced dilation. Redundancy occurs in the pathways contributing to the hyperemic response induced by ischemic exercise in young adults [32] suggesting that redundant vasodilator systems are involved in the adequate delivery of blood to metabolically active tissues during exercise. Further support of the importance of redundant vasodilator pathways to cardiovascular function is demonstrated by the maintenance of resting and exercise-induced increases in coronary blood flow following administration of specific inhibitors of vasodilation in healthy men [14]. The relatively robust RA FMD responses observed in healthy adults following NO and/or PN blockade indicate that redundant vasodilator systems, which are likely beneficial for cardiovascular health [12, 14], compensate for the loss of specific vasodilators and that aging in the absence of additional CVD risk factors does not impair these vasodilator systems.

Further research is warranted to determine if redundant vasodilator systems are impaired in clinical conditions associated with endothelial dysfunction. Currently, limited data exist regarding the mechanisms underlying endothelium-dependent dilation in individuals at increased risk for CVD. Patients with essential hypertension [33] and heart failure [29], conditions characterized by the presence of endothelial dysfunction [34, 35], utilize EDHF to maintain endothelium-dependent dilation through activation of the CYP450 epoxygenase pathway. However, EDHF is insufficient in maintaining dilation to levels seen in healthy adults as evidenced by only partial compensation for impaired NO bioavailability by EDHF [33]. Evidence that inhibition of CYP450 epoxygenases does not affect resistance vessel dilation in healthy older adults [36] or conduit artery dilation in patients with essential hypertension [30] suggests that partial compensation to impaired NO bioavailability [33] is dependent on the vascular bed and/or clinical condition studied. Whether the inability of the vascular system to compensate for the loss of specific vasoactive mediators, as observed in certain chronic disease states, underlies future vascular disease remains to be determined.

We acknowledge that our observation of variable responses within individuals to drug infusion may be explained by factors other than the existence of redundant vasodilator pathways, including individual differences in drug sensitivity/metabolism, drug order effects, and the inherent variability of FMD testing. Furthermore, we cannot exclude the possibility that conduit artery FMD of older subjects may be altered by nonendothelium mediated mechanisms. In the present study, sodium nitroprusside was not infused to exclude potential differences in endothelium-independent dilation due to aging [25, 37], a finding not supported by others following administration of exogenous NO donors [36, 38]. We did not perform an additional catheterization visit in older adults to test the effect of drug order on dilator responses due to a lack of statistically significant effects observed previously in young adults who participated in a reverse drug order trial ($n = 8$) [8]. Our existing data [8] support the efficacy of the NO and PN blockade in the present study. For example, we have previously reported that thromboxane B2, an indicator of platelet cyclooxygenase (COX) activity during whole blood clotting, dramatically decreased in a younger cohort following an identical combined infusion protocol [8] demonstrating effective blockade of PN. Furthermore, doses of ketorolac were infused that equaled or exceeded those used previously to block PN [18, 20, 21]. Future studies should investigate whether infusion of a selective COX-2 inhibitor rather than our use of a nonselective COX inhibitor impacts endothelial function differently, an effect observed previously in hypertensives [39]. Infusing acetylcholine would have directly confirmed the efficacy of NOS inhibition. However, our infusion dose of L-NMMA was equivalent or greater than the dose used in previous studies [4, 6, 18, 20–22] and our observed decrease in RA vascular conductance following L-NMMA infusion was similar to previous reports [4, 8, 9, 22, 40–42] supporting that NO synthesis was effectively blocked by L-NMMA infusion in the present investigation. Future infusion studies are needed utilizing a larger number of participants and multiple trials with each drug to better understand the dependence of conduit artery FMD on specific vasodilators in humans and the impact that cardiovascular risk factors have on these vasoregulatory pathways.

5. Conclusions

Single and combined blockade of NO and PN synthesis did not consistently reduce RA FMD in older adults adding to the existing literature that NO inhibition does not uniformly decrease conduit artery FMD in healthy humans. Rather, there is substantial variability in the individual RA response to NOS inhibition suggesting a variable contribution of NO to conduit FMD. Therefore, the persistent assumption that conduit FMD is primarily a NO-dependent response limits our interpretation of findings regarding mechanisms both underlying and improving blunted FMD. Furthermore, a large proportion of older adults exhibited increased or minimally reduced RA FMD responses following combined NO and PN blockade suggesting the existence of redundant vasodilator pathways and indicating that aging per se does not uniformly impair these pathways. Future studies are warranted to investigate if the collective influence of additional factors such as disease and/or lifestyle impacts the effect of age on conduit vasodilator pathways.

Conflict of Interests

Kevin D. Ballard, Michael E. Tschakovsky, Amanda L. Zaleski, Donna M. Polk, Francis J. Kiernan, and Beth A. Parker declare that they have no conflict of interests. Paul D. Thompson reports receiving research grants from the National Institutes of Health, GlaxoSmithKline, Anthera, B. Braun, Genomas, Roche, Aventis, Novartis, and Furiex; serving as a consultant for Astra Zenica, Furiex, Regeneron, Merck, Takeda, Roche, Genomas, Abbott, Lupin, Runners World, Genzyme, Sanolfi, Pfizer, and GlaxoSmithKline; receiving speaker honoraria from Merck, Pfizer, Abbott, Astra Zenica, GlaxoSmithKline, and Kowa; owning stock in Zoll, General Electric, JA Wiley Publishing, Zimmer, J&J, Sanolfi-Aventis, and Abbott; and serving as a medical legal consultant on cardiac complications of exercise, statin myopathy, tobacco, ezetimibe, and nonsteroids. None of these business relationships pose a conflict of interests for the current study.

Acknowledgments

The authors acknowledge the dedicated participants as well as the assistance of Jeffrey Capizzi, William Roman, Lindsay Lorson, Dr. David Proctor, Candy Johnson, and Nicole Chomek. Financial support was provided by a Hartford Hospital Open Competition Grant, Connecticut Department of Public Health Biomedical Research Award [2010-0089], and a National Heart, Lung, and Blood Institute Grant to BAP [1R01 HL098085-01].

References

[1] J. P. Cooke and V. J. Dzau, "Nitric oxide synthase: role in the genesis of vascular disease," *Annual Review of Medicine*, vol. 48, pp. 489–509, 1997.

[2] S. N. Doshi, K. K. Naka, N. Payne et al., "Flow-mediated dilatation following wrist and upper arm occlusion in humans: the contribution of nitric oxide," *Clinical Science*, vol. 101, no. 6, pp. 629–635, 2001.

[3] B. Jiang, M. Seddon, H. Fok, A. Donald, and P. Chowienczyk, "Flow-mediated dilation of the radial artery is offset by flow-induced reduction in transmural pressure," *Hypertension*, vol. 57, no. 6, pp. 1145–1150, 2011.

[4] R. Joannides, W. E. Haefeli, L. Linder et al., "Nitric oxide is responsible for flow-dependent dilatation of human peripheral conduit arteries in vivo," *Circulation*, vol. 91, no. 5, pp. 1314–1319, 1995.

[5] M. Kooijman, D. H. J. Thijssen, P. C. E. de Groot et al., "Flow-mediated dilatation in the superficial femoral artery is nitric oxide mediated in humans," *Journal of Physiology*, vol. 586, no. 4, pp. 1137–1145, 2008.

[6] M. J. Mullen, R. K. Kharbanda, J. Cross et al., "Heterogenous nature of flow-mediated dilatation in human conduit arteries in vivo: relevance to endothelial dysfunction in hypercholesterolemia," *Circulation Research*, vol. 88, no. 2, pp. 145–151, 2001.

[7] D. J. Green, E. A. Dawson, H. M. Groenewoud, H. Jones, and D. H. Thijssen, "Is flow-mediated dilation nitric oxide mediated?: a meta-analysis," *Hypertension*, vol. 63, no. 2, pp. 376–382, 2014.

[8] B. A. Parker, M. E. Tschakovsky, A. L. Augeri, D. M. Polk, P. D. Thompson, and F. J. Kiernan, "Heterogenous vasodilator pathways underlie flow-mediated dilation in men and women," *American Journal of Physiology—Heart and Circulatory Physiology*, vol. 301, no. 3, pp. H1118–H1126, 2011.

[9] K. Pyke, D. J. Green, C. Weisbrod et al., "Nitric oxide is not obligatory for radial artery flow-mediated dilation following release of 5 or 10 min distal occlusion," *American Journal of Physiology—Heart and Circulatory Physiology*, vol. 298, no. 1, pp. H119–H126, 2010.

[10] D. W. Wray, M. A. Witman, S. J. Ives et al., "Does brachial artery flow-mediated vasodilation provide a bioassay for no?" *Hypertension*, vol. 62, no. 2, pp. 345–351, 2013.

[11] S. J. Duffy, S. F. Castle, R. W. Harper, and I. T. Meredith, "Contribution of vasodilator prostanoids and nitric oxide to resting flow, metabolic vasodilation, and flow-mediated dilation in human coronary circulation," *Circulation*, vol. 100, no. 19, pp. 1951–1957, 1999.

[12] J. Bellien, M. Iacob, L. Gutierrez et al., "Crucial role of NO and endothelium-derived hyperpolarizing factor in human sustained conduit artery flow-mediated dilatation," *Hypertension*, vol. 48, no. 6, pp. 1088–1094, 2006.

[13] J. Bellien, C. Thuillez, and R. Joannides, "Role of endothelium-derived hyperpolarizing factor in the regulation of radial artery basal diameter and endothelium-dependent dilatation in vivo," *Clinical and Experimental Pharmacology and Physiology*, vol. 35, no. 4, pp. 494–497, 2008.

[14] A. Edlund, A. Sollevi, and A. Wennmalm, "The role of adenosine and prostacyclin in coronary flow regulation in healthy man," *Acta Physiologica Scandinavica*, vol. 135, no. 1, pp. 39–46, 1989.

[15] D. J. Green, H. Jones, D. Thijssen, N. T. Cable, and G. Atkinson, "Flow-mediated dilation and cardiovascular event prediction: does nitric oxide matter?" *Hypertension*, vol. 57, no. 3, pp. 363–369, 2011.

[16] A. J. Donato, L. B. Gano, I. Eskurza et al., "Vascular endothelial dysfunction with aging: endothelin-1 and endothelial nitric oxide synthase," *American Journal of Physiology—Heart and Circulatory Physiology*, vol. 297, no. 1, pp. H425–H432, 2009.

[17] W. T. Nicholson, B. Vaa, C. Hesse, J. H. Eisenach, and M. J. Joyner, "Aging is associated with reduced prostacyclin-mediated dilation in the human forearm," *Hypertension*, vol. 53, no. 6, pp. 973–978, 2009.

[18] W. G. Schrage, J. H. Eisenach, and M. J. Joyner, "Ageing reduces nitric-oxide- and prostaglandin-mediated vasodilatation in exercising humans," *Journal of Physiology*, vol. 579, no. 1, pp. 227–236, 2007.

[19] S. Taddei, A. Virdis, L. Ghiadoni et al., "Age-related reduction of NO availability and oxidative stress in humans," *Hypertension*, vol. 38, no. 2, pp. 274–279, 2001.

[20] F. A. Dinenno and M. J. Joyner, "Combined NO and PG inhibition augments α-adrenergic vasoconstriction in contracting human skeletal muscle," *American Journal of Physiology—Heart and Circulatory Physiology*, vol. 287, no. 6, pp. H2576–H2584, 2004.

[21] N. R. Saunders, F. A. Dinenno, K. E. Pyke, A. M. Rogers, and M. E. Tschakovsky, "Impact of combined NO and PG blockade on rapid vasodilation in a forearm mild-to-moderate exercise transition in humans," *American Journal of Physiology—Heart and Circulatory Physiology*, vol. 288, no. 1, pp. H214–H220, 2005.

[22] D. Walter Wray, M. A. H. Witman, S. J. Ives et al., "Progressive handgrip exercise: evidence of nitric oxide-dependent vasodilation and blood flow regulation in humans," *American Journal of Physiology—Heart and Circulatory Physiology*, vol. 300, no. 3, pp. H1101–H1107, 2011.

[23] M. A. Black, N. T. Cable, D. H. J. Thijssen, and D. J. Green, "Importance of measuring the time course of flow-mediated dilatation in humans," *Hypertension*, vol. 51, no. 2, pp. 203–210, 2008.

[24] D. H. J. Thijssen, M. A. Black, K. E. Pyke et al., "Assessment of flow-mediated dilation in humans: a methodological and physiological guideline," *American Journal of Physiology—Heart and Circulatory Physiology*, vol. 300, no. 1, pp. H2–H12, 2011.

[25] L. Lind, N. Fors, J. Hall, K. Marttala, and A. Stenborg, "A comparison of three different methods to evaluate endothelium-dependent vasodilation in the elderly: The Prospective Investigation of the Vasculature in Uppsala Seniors (PIVUS) study," *Arteriosclerosis, Thrombosis, and Vascular Biology*, vol. 25, no. 11, pp. 2368–2375, 2005.

[26] G. F. Mitchell, H. Parise, J. A. Vita et al., "Local shear stress and brachial artery flow-mediated dilation: The Framingham Heart Study," *Hypertension*, vol. 44, no. 2, pp. 134–139, 2004.

[27] E. A. Skaug, S. T. Aspenes, L. Oldervoll et al., "Age and gender differences of endothelial function in 4739 healthy adults: the HUNT3 Fitness Study," *European Journal of Preventive Cardiology*, vol. 20, no. 4, pp. 531–540, 2013.

[28] S. Taddei, A. Virdis, L. Ghiadoni, A. Magagna, and A. Salvetti, "Cyclooxygenase inhibition restores nitric oxide activity in essential hypertension," *Hypertension*, vol. 29, no. 1, part 2, pp. 274–279, 1997.

[29] S. D. Katz and H. Krum, "Acetylcholine-mediated vasodilation in the forearm circulation of patients with heart failure: indirect evidence for the role of endothelium-derived hyperpolarizing factor," *American Journal of Cardiology*, vol. 87, no. 9, pp. 1089–1092, 2001.

[30] J. Bellien, M. Iacob, I. Remy-Jouet et al., "Epoxyeicosatrienoic acids contribute with altered nitric oxide and endothelin-1 pathways to conduit artery endothelial dysfunction in essential hypertension," *Circulation*, vol. 125, no. 10, pp. 1266–1275, 2012.

[31] D. Fischer, U. Landmesser, S. Spiekermann et al., "Cytochrome P450 2C9 is involved in flow-dependent vasodilation of peripheral conduit arteries in healthy subjects and in patients with chronic heart failure," *European Journal of Heart Failure*, vol. 9, no. 8, pp. 770–775, 2007.

[32] M. G. Lopez, B. M. Silva, M. J. Joyner, and D. P. Casey, "Ischemic exercise hyperemia in the human forearm: reproducibility and roles of adenosine and nitric oxide," *European Journal of Applied Physiology*, vol. 112, no. 6, pp. 2065–2072, 2012.

[33] S. Taddei, D. Versari, A. Cipriano et al., "Identification of a cytochrome P450 2C9-derived endothelium-derived hyperpolarizing factor in essential hypertensive patients," *Journal of the American College of Cardiology*, vol. 48, no. 3, pp. 508–515, 2006.

[34] S. D. Katz, L. Biasucci, C. Sabba et al., "Impaired endothelium-mediated vasodilation in the peripheral vasculature of patients with congestive heart failure," *Journal of the American College of Cardiology*, vol. 19, no. 5, pp. 918–925, 1992.

[35] S. Taddei and A. Salvetti, "Endothelial dysfunction in essential hypertension: clinical implications," *Journal of Hypertension*, vol. 20, no. 9, pp. 1671–1674, 2002.

[36] A. J. Donato, I. Eskurza, K. L. Jablonski, L. B. Gano, G. L. Pierce, and D. R. Seals, "Cytochrome P-450 2C9 signaling does not contribute to age-associated vascular endothelial dysfunction in humans," *Journal of Applied Physiology*, vol. 105, no. 4, pp. 1359–1363, 2008.

[37] B. A. Parker, S. J. Ridout, and D. N. Proctor, "Age and flow-mediated dilation: a comparison of dilatory responsiveness in the brachial and popliteal arteries," *American Journal of Physiology—Heart and Circulatory Physiology*, vol. 291, no. 6, pp. H3043–H3049, 2006.

[38] P. E. Gates, M. L. Boucher, A. E. Silver, K. D. Monahan, and D. R. Seals, "Impaired flow-mediated dilation with age is not explained by L-arginine bioavailability or endothelial asymmetric dimethylarginine protein expression," *Journal of Applied Physiology*, vol. 102, no. 1, pp. 63–71, 2007.

[39] D. Bulut, S. Liaghat, C. Hanefeld, R. Koll, T. Miebach, and A. Mügge, "Selective cyclo-oxygenase-2 inhibition with parecoxib acutely impairs endothelium-dependent vasodilatation in patients with essential hypertension," *Journal of Hypertension*, vol. 21, no. 9, pp. 1663–1667, 2003.

[40] K. A. Engelke, J. R. Halliwill, D. N. Proctor, N. M. Dietz, and M. J. Joyner, "Contribution of nitric oxide and prostaglandins to reactive hyperemia in human forearm," *Journal of Applied Physiology*, vol. 81, no. 4, pp. 1807–1814, 1996.

Effect of Posture Training with Weighted Kypho-Orthosis (WKO) on Improving Balance in Women with Osteoporosis

Seyed Ahmad Raeissadat,[1] Leyla Sedighipour,[1] Safura Pournajaf,[1] Reza Vahab Kashani,[2] and Shahram Sadeghi[1]

[1] *Department of Physical Medicine & Rehabilitation, Clinical Research Development Center of Shahid Modares Hospital, Shahid Beheshti University of Medical Sciences, Tehran, Iran*
[2] *Department of Orthotics and Prosthetics, University of Social Welfare and Rehabilitation Science, Kodakyar street, Daneshjo Boulevard, Evin, Tehran 1985713834, Iran*

Correspondence should be addressed to Safura Pournajaf; safurapurnajaf@yahoo.com

Academic Editor: Barbara Shukitt-Hale

Objectives. To determine the effect of weighted kypho-orthosis (WKO) on improving balance in women with osteoporosis. In this nonrandomized controlled clinical trial, 31 patients with osteoporosis were included. The patients were assigned to two groups: (1) control group who received 4-week home-based daily exercise program including weight bearing, back strengthening, and balance exercises and (2) intervention group (WKO) who performed aforementioned exercises and wore WKO for one hour twice a day. Patients were assessed using clinical balance tests (timed up and go test, functional reach test, and unilateral balance test) before and 4 weeks after start of treatment. *Results.* Functional reach and timed up and go test were improved significantly in both groups compared to baseline. The improvement in intervention group was more significant in comparison to control group ($P < 0.05$). *Discussion.* Posture training with WKO together with exercise program improved two clinical balance tests in women with osteoporosis. *Conclusion.* Posture training support (PTS) applied as WKO together with back extension exercises can be prescribed as an intervention in elderly women in order to reduce the risk of falling.

1. Introduction

Osteoporosis is the most common metabolic bone disease in the world [1–3]. The most common clinical consequences are back pain, hyperkyphosis, limitations of physical functioning and activities of daily life, and impaired health-related quality of life in osteoporotic patients [4–6]. It is characterized by low bone mass and microarchitectural deterioration of bone tissue, leading to increased bone fragility and a consequent increase in fracture risk [1, 2, 7]. Vertebral fractures are the main clinical consequences of spinal osteoporosis and constitute a major public health burden. The incidence of spine fracture is estimated to be 20% in postmenopausal women [4]. The weakness of paraspinal extensor muscles noticed in osteoporosis accompanied by repetitive vertebral microfracture results in progressive change in alignment of the spine, mainly hyperkyphosis, in osteoporotic patients [2, 8–10]. The postural changes and vertebral fractures impose additional physical stress on the mechanically less robust vertebral bodies leading to acute and chronic back pain [5]. Furthermore, osteoporosis is associated with deficits of gait and balance, all together resulting in an increased risk of falls and a subsequent aggravation of fracture risk [7]. Falls among the elderly, especially for those with osteoporosis, are associated with high morbidity and mortality and can involve high-cost medical intervention [11]. In fact, falls are responsible for 90% of the growing increase in hip fractures [11] and are the sixth cause of death among patients aged over sixty.

Fall prevention is a necessity to reduce health costs in the senile population [11]. There are studies indicating that almost one-third of falls followed by detrimental consequences are preventable [12]. Apart from environmental modifications, improvements in internal factors such as static and dynamic posture and balance training are among most precious preventive strategies. Beside pharmaceutical therapy, physical rehabilitative measures play a key role in prevention of falls. Muscle reeducations and resistance exercises for strengthening and reduction of kyphosis are key elements for reducing the risk of falls and subsequent fractures [2, 13–15].

The flexed posturing in kyphotic patients caused by osteoporosis places their center of gravity closer to its limits of stability and increases the risk of falling [16, 17]. Therefore, measures that can improve axial stability can decrease disequilibrium and increase the risk of falls.

Previous studies have shown that wearing a spinal orthosis such as osteomed, spinomed, and WKO has a role in reduction of pain as well as improvements of posture and back extensor strength. WKO is among the most known orthosis in osteoporotic patients. In 2005, Sinaki et al. conducted a study to evaluate the effects of WKO on gait disturbances and risk of falls in patients with osteoporosis [18]. In the mentioned study, she indicated the positive effects of WKO together with spinal proprioceptive extension exercise on balance, gait, and risk of falls assessed by computerized dynamic posturography.

Most of the mentioned studies mainly focused on para clinic and laboratory based computerized tests to evaluate the efficacy of WKO on risk of falling. To date, there is no study having evaluated the effects of WKO on balance and gait stability via functional clinical tests in patients with osteoporosis. Therefore the purpose of the present study was to assess the effects of wearing WKO together with spinal exercises on balance via performing functional clinical tests in women with osteoporosis.

2. Methods

This study was conducted between 2010 and 2011 in Shahid Modarres Hospital, Tehran, Iran. The protocol of this experiment was approved by Shahid Beheshti University of Medical Sciences, Human Ethics Research Committee. Participants were patients voluntarily referred to physical medicine and rehabilitation clinic. All patients were screened by experienced clinicians skilled in the evaluation and the management of osteoporotic patients.

Inclusion criteria were as follows: women with osteoporosis documented by low bone mineral densitometry at spine (T-score of <−2.5 aged between 55 and 75 years, thoracic kyphosis angle between 35 and 55 degree (Cobb's angle of thoracic kyphosis was calculated from lateral radiograph of spine)).

The patients with the following criteria were excluded:

history of secondary osteoporosis due to metabolic diseases (such as hyperthyroidism) evaluated by clinical laboratory tests, the presence of neuromuscular disorders, history of vertebral fracture in last 6 months, and history of spinal or lower limb surgical interventions including arthroplasty, vertebroplasty, and discectomy.

Patients who met the above-mentioned criteria were assigned to two groups (intervention and control groups).

2.1. Recruitment. This study was designed a non randomized clinical trial. Patients were recruited by convenient sampling. Patients were screened initially by physiatrists to determine whether they met the inclusion criteria. Those who met inclusion criteria and were willing to participate in the study were scheduled to wear the orthosis as intervention group.

At the same clinic, like orthosis group, matched controls of comparable age and weight and height were enrolled in the study as control group.

Patients in both groups, that is, orthosis and control groups, received medications including 1000 mg calcium citrate or carbonate and 400 IU vitamin E daily and sodium alendronate 70 mg weekly.

Patients in both groups were also instructed to have 30 minutes of daily walking.

Patients were followed via telephone calls to home to make sure that they were sticking to the exercises correctly as prescribed for them.

2.2. Control Group. No orthosis was prescribed for this group, but patients were taught to perform back extensor strengthening exercises at home (including 10 contractions of back extensors without increasing the low back lordosis) based on professor Sinaki program in Mayo clinic [19] as follows.

(1) In supine position, the patient flexes the knees and then abducts and adducts the shoulders, while the elbows are extended and upper limbs are in contact with the floor.

(2) In the supine position, the patient flexes the knees and puts hands over the head. By contracting abdominal muscles the patient tries to draw the lowback to the floor and keep this position for 10 seconds.

(3) In the prone position, the patient puts a pillow under the lower abdomen and gently raises the head and shoulders from the floor as much as possible and keeps this position for 10 seconds.

(4) The patient sits on a chair and puts the hands behind the head. Then he/she moves the elbows behind the head while inhaling. The patient will do the opposite while exhaling.

(5) Sitting on a chair, the patient flexes the elbows while keeping the arms near to the trunk and then moves the arms back to reduce thoracic kyphosis.

All of the exercise programs were taught by an experienced physical therapist. In addition, an illustrated paper describing each exercise was presented to each participant. Besides, each patient was given a paper with a table and was asked to specify every day if he/she would do the exercises and bring it on followup visits. The patients were called by the educating physical therapist every week to assess exercise performance and associated problems. After 4 weeks, patients were called to return to hospital for reevaluations.

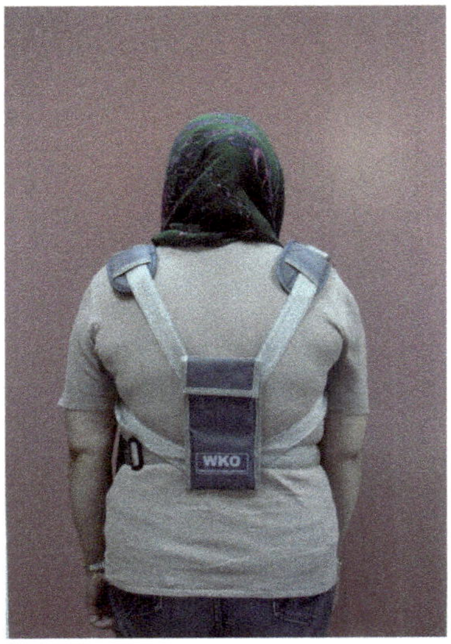

FIGURE 1: Patient wearing WKO (back view).

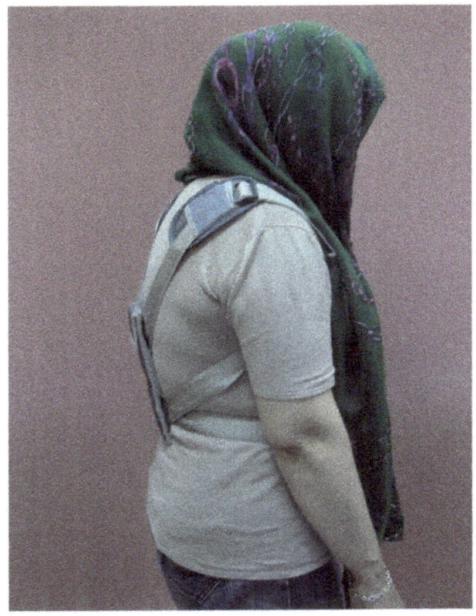

FIGURE 2: Patient wearing WKO (side view).

2.3. Intervention Group (Orthosis Group). Patients in this group were guided to perform exercises the same as control group.

WKO was also administered for the patients in this group.

2.4. Weighted Kypho-Orthosis (WKO). Weighted kypho-orthosis is an especially designed orthosis (made by Techno-Tan company) with a harness and a 2-pound pouch, which centers its weight on the posterior of the spine at T10 to L4 (Figures 1 and 2).

The patients were guided to place the WKO over the thoracic spine and adjust the straps such that the bottom of the pouch is located at the waistline.

Patients were instructed to wear the device when ambulating for one hour a day (30 minutes at the morning and the evening) for 4 weeks. During those 4 weeks, patients were followed by telephone calls to assure that they were using the orthosis correctly.

An experienced orthotist instructed the patient regarding the proper usage of orthosis.

3. Measures

Dual X-ray absorptiometry (DXA) was used for measuring bone mineral density of spine or hip. All patients were referred to one imaging center for bone mineral density.

Cobb's angle of kyphosis is calculated from perpendicular lines drawn on a standard thoracic spine radiograph: a line extends through the superior endplate of the vertebral body, marking the beginning of the thoracic curve, and the inferior endplate of the vertebral body, marking the end of the thoracic curve.

Osteoporotic fractures were ruled out via evaluating X-rays by an experienced radiologist.

Functional tests which were performed at study entry were repeated 4 weeks after initiating therapy in both groups.

The same therapist performed the functional tests before and after therapy.

3.1. Functional Reach Test (FR). Functional reach was tested by placing a yardstick or tape measure on the wall, parallel to the floor, at the height of the acromion of the subject's dominant arm. The subject was asked to stand with the feet in a comfortable distance apart, make a fist, and forward flex the dominant arm to approximately 90 degrees. The subject was asked to reach forward as far as possible without taking a step or touching the wall. The distance between the start and end point was then measured using the head of the metacarpal of the third finger as the reference point [20].

3.2. Timed Up and Go Test (TUG). We asked the patients to wear their usual footwear and be seated in a chair with their back to the chair and their arms resting on the arm rests, and then we asked the patient to stand up from that chair and walk a distance of 10 ft. (3 m), then turn around, walk back to the chair, and sit down again.

Timing began when the person started to rise from the chair and ended when he or she returned to the chair and sits down.

The person was given 1 practice trial and then 3 actual trials. The durations from the three actual trials were averaged.

3.3. Unilateral Stance Test (US). This test was performed in the standing position without foot wear with the patients' arms set by their sides and with open eyes. Timing was started when the subjects raised the appropriate foot off the ground. Timing was stopped if subjects displaced the foot they were standing on, touched the suspended foot to support the weight bearing limb, or reached the maximum balance time of 30 seconds [21, 22]. Third trial was performed if the maximum balance time was not reached in either of the first two trials. The longest trial with eyes open was used for data analysis. The length of each trial was ten seconds.

Table 1: Demographic characteristics including age, height, weight, and body mass indices compared between two groups.

	Case group ($n = 11$) Mean ± SD	Control group ($n = 20$) Mean ± SD	P value
Age (years)	65.63	62.45	0.177
Height (cm)	150.45	152.25	0.47
Weight (Kg)	68.81	68.20	0.89
Body mass index (Kg/M^2)	30.41	29.40	0.58

SD: standard deviation; case group (intervention group): orthosis and exercise; control group: exercise only.

4. Data Analysis

SPSS-18 was used for data analysis. According to kolmogorov-smirnov normality tests, all variables including demographic data and the time of functional tests were normally distributed and therefore parametric tests including independent t-test and paired t-test were conducted to determine if there was a statistically significant change in demographic characteristics between the two groups and improvement in functional tests after therapy.

The assessors including the statistician and the physical therapist who observed the patients during functional tests and recorded the results were blinded to which group the patients belonged to.

5. Ethics

From the ethical point of view, the patients were enrolled after providing informed consent as approved by the institutional review board of Shahid Beheshti Medical University study. The process of treatment was explained completely to the patients and once the physician assured that the patient completely understood the study protocol and became aware of his or her rights during the study, the written consent form was signed or fingerprinted by the patient. The process of treatment had no harm for their health, and they had authority to stop the process of treatment liberally. The control group had also received routine medication and exercise therapy as treatment. Participants of this study were not charged for being involved in the study or using orthosis.

6. Results

The patients' characteristics at the start of study are displayed in Table 1. There were no between-group differences at the baseline in demographic characteristics and functional balance tests (Table 1).

At the beginning, 164 osteoporotic patients (hip and/or spine) were assessed for eligibility to enter the study. From 40 patients with osteoporosis at spine, 31 patients met the inclusion criteria and accepted to participate in the study, and 28 people stayed at the program during the followup (two persons from orthosis and one person from control group were dropped out of the study due to incomplete exercises and not wearing the orthosis completely). The results of 28 patients (19 patients in control and 9 patients in intervention group) who remained in the study were analyzed. (CONSORT flow chart, Figure 3).

The mean of T score in control group was -2.74 ± 0.2 and the mean T-score of the intervention group was -2.99 ± 0.2 and there was no difference between two groups ($P > 0.05$).

Kyphosis angle's mean of the control group was 48.6 ± 5.5 degree and for the intervention group was 45.8 ± 5.7 degree and there was no difference between the two groups ($P > 0.05$).

6.1. Timed Up and Go Test (TUG). As it can be read from Table 2, there was no statistically significant difference in this test scores between the two groups at the start of study; but at the end of study, patients in both intervention and control groups improved significantly regarding the scores of this test. This improvement was significantly more noticeable in intervention group compared to control group ($P = 0.005$).

6.2. Functional Reach Test (FR). The scores of this test was not statistically different between the two groups at baseline, the scores of this test improved in both intervention and control groups significantly at the end of study.

However, patients in intervention group improved more significantly compared to control group ($P = 0.005$) (Table 2).

6.3. Unilateral Stance Test (US). There was not any between-group differences regarding the scores of this test at baseline; but at the end of the study, the scores of this test improved significantly only in control group (Table 2).

7. Discussion

According to the results of the present study, improvement in balance was noticed in patients with osteoporosis after wearing WKO for 4 weeks according to TUG and FR tests.

Functional reach is a valuable tool for identifying those elderly with a high risk of falling. This test is designed to evaluate anteroposterior stability by measuring the maximum distance that a person can reach forward while standing over a fixed base of support. It assesses the ability to remain stable in this plane of movement [23].

TUG test included many components of other functional tests such as sit-to- stand, gait, and turning which requires many aspects of postural control; therefore the predictive value of this test for falling is high [24, 25]. This test was introduced as a basic test for functional mobility evaluation in 1991 [26, 27].

TABLE 2: Functional scores compared between two groups before and after study.

	Case group	Control group	*P* value
TUG			
Before Tx	(n = 11) 9.28 ± 2.25	(n = 20) 9.20 ± 1.80	0.91
After Tx	(n = 9) 7.14 ± 1.10	(n = 19) 8.40 ± 1.03	0.00
P value	0.00	0.01	
FR			
Before Tx	(n = 11) 25.04 ± 2.69	(n = 20) 23.66 ± 3.56	0.91
After Tx	(n = 9) 31.64 ± 2.61	(n = 19) 26.43 ± 2.84	0.00
P value	0.00	0.00	
US			
Before Tx	(n = 11) 16.08 ± 8.20	(n = 20) 18.20 ± 10.01	0.55
After Tx	(n = 9) 18.18 ± 7.74	(n = 19) 18.81 ± 9.06	0.85
P value	0.30	0.00	

TUG: timed up and go test; FR: functional reach test; US: unilateral stance test; A: after trial, B: before trial.

TUG is the simplest and probably the most reliable clinical test in evaluating balance [28]. Additionally, previous studies have found that TUG can discriminate between faller and nonfallers; therefore this test can be considered as a screen measure to predict falling in the elderly [25, 29]. This is mainly due to the fact that TUG is the only measure that includes a gait component which is functionally important because many falls occur during ambulation [25]. It is a valid method for screening of both level of functional mobility and risk of falling in community-dwelling elderly people [30].

TUG and FR both have high specificities (100% and 92%, resp.) [31].

Considering good predictive value of FR and TUG tests for falls, the improvement of these test scores after wearing WKO in our study can be suggestive of decreased risk of fall.

There are few studies evaluating the beneficial impacts of spinal orthosis on gait balance and reducing the risk of fall-in old aged population [9, 18, 32–34].

In 1996, Kaplan and Sinaki [9] evaluated effect of back supports on back strength in patients with osteoporosis in a pilot study. Patients were assigned to three groups (1) postural exercise only, (2) postural exercise and a conventional thoracolumbar support, or (3) postural exercise and a posture training support (PTS) (a WKO). Compliance with the use of the WKO was better than the one with the thoracolumbar support. Back extensor strength increased in patients who complied with the WKO and postural exercise program.

In 2005, Sinaki et al. [18] conducted a study to determine the outcome of intervention with a spinal weighted kypho-orthosis (WKO) and a spinal proprioceptive extension exercise dynamic (SPEED) program on the risk of fall-in osteoporotic patients. After 4 weeks of intervention, balance, gait, and risk of falls assessed by computerized dynamic posturography improved significantly with the 4-week SPEED program.

The role of exercise in the treatment of osteoporosis is to improve axial stability through improvement of muscle strength. Therapeutic exercise should address osteoporosis-related deformities of axial posture, which can increase risk of fall and fracture [35].

In our study, the beneficial effect of exercises was shown as patients in exercise group (control group) improved significantly based on FR, TUG, and US tests compared to baseline, even though this improvement was less than WKO regarding FR and TUG tests.

WKO promotes improvement in posture and increases back extensor strength by two mechanisms: first, the device produces a posterior force below the inferior angle of scapula and reduces anterior compressive forces exerted on the kyphotic spine [10]. Second, application of the WKO increases a patient's perception of spinal joint position, which plays an important role in static and dynamic posture. It creates a preprioceptive input and enhances the patient's ability to sense the position of the spine, which has an important role in strengthening the back extensor muscles and leads to improvement in static and dynamic postural stability [18]. WKO also promotes muscle reeducation and decreases painful contractions of the erector spinae muscles in kyphosis due to decrease in the load over the anterior aspect of the spinal column and vertebral bodies through use of a WKO [36].

Besides WKO, there are some studies investigating other types of spinal orthoses in osteoporosis. In 2008, Vogt et al. [32] investigated the efficacy of a flexible spinal orthosis without any stabilizing components in posture improvement. Forty women were randomized to three treatment groups: (1) osteomed orthosis with paravertebral/lumbosacral air chamber pads; (2) the same orthosis without air chamber pads; and (3) placebo body stocking. Measurements were performed with a 3D real-time ultrasound topometry system (Zebris (R) CMS 70). The posture correction was significantly more marked in the first group as compared to the second and third groups. The orthosis with air chamber pads causes a clinically meaningful trunk support in patients with osteoporotic posture changes. Since the device contains no rigid stabilizing elements, the change in posture was considered

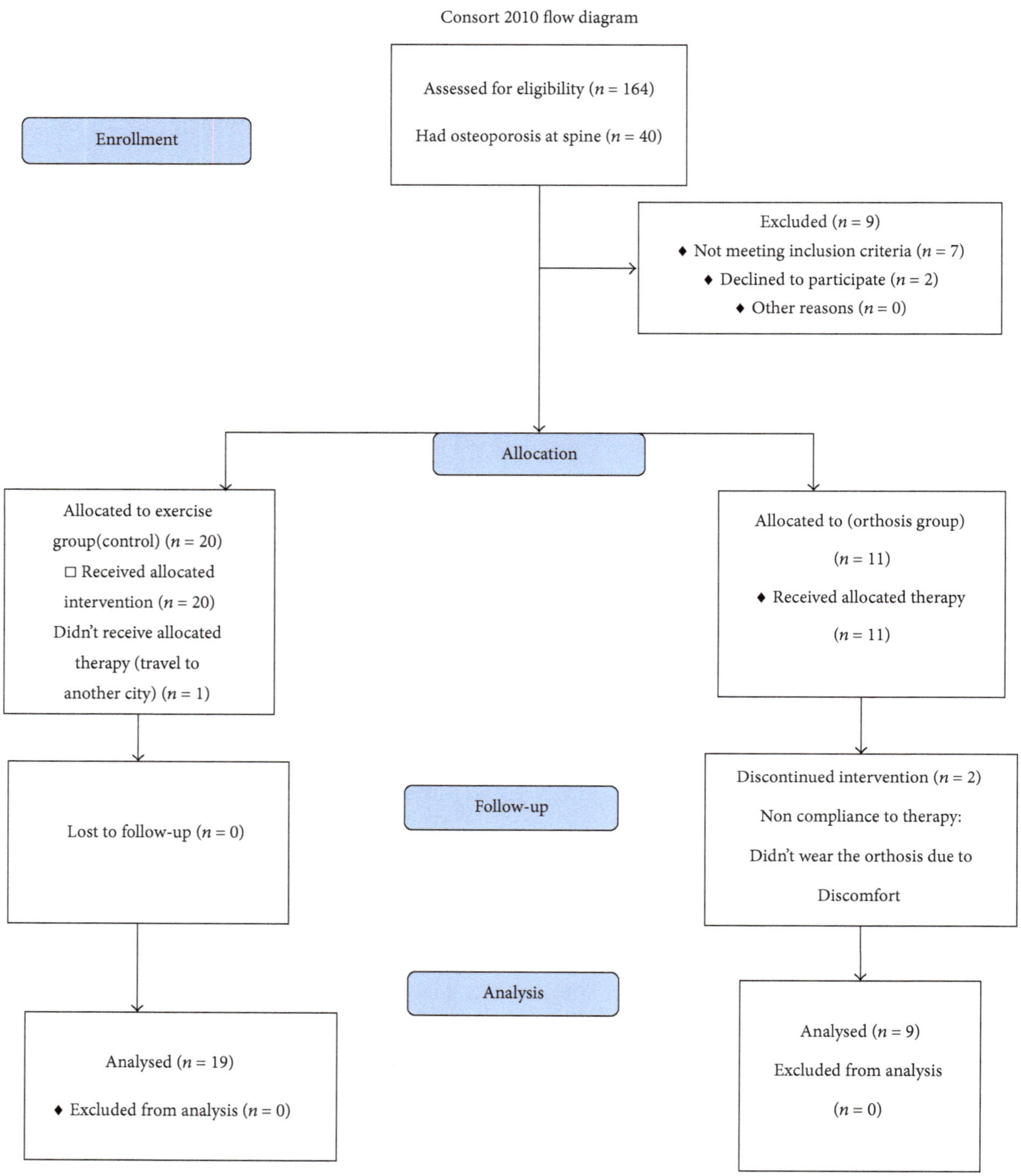

Figure 3: CONSORT 2010 Flow Diagram.

to be a result of muscle activation due to sensorimotor stimulation by the air chamber pads [27].

Another trial was conducted in 2012 evaluating the influence of Thämert Osteo-med spinal orthosis on gait and physical functioning in osteoporotic women with postmenopausal osteoporosis. At a 6-month followup, the study demonstrated that wearing a spinal orthosis reduced double support time associated with improvement on gait stability. Furthermore, there was also positive effect on pain-related restrictions of ADL. Beside reductions in pain and improvements in back extensor strength and correction of posture, the application of a spinal orthosis might induce advantages for gait stability and physical functioning in women with postmenopausal osteoporosis [33]. Pfeifer and his colleagues conducted a randomized study to evaluate the efficacy of two newly developed spinal orthoses in patients with osteoporotic vertebral fractures. Wearing the orthosis Spinomed in that study was associated with increase in back extensor and abdominal flexor strength, decrease in the angle of kyphosis and body sway, and also decrease in average pain. In addition, a better quality-of-life was achieved by pain reduction, decreased limitations of daily living, and improved the well-being [34].

In all above, mentioned studies, spinal orthosis had positive effects on postural balance which is in agreement with the results of our studies indicating improvement in FR and TUG test.

The only test which was not improved in WKO orthosis was unilateral stance test. One explanation can be relative small number of patients in intervention group compared to control group. The other explanation may be the fact that US only tests one aspect of balance-that is maintaining equilibrium on a reduced base of support. However, the greater task constraints and the need to cope with greatly increased postural sway may challenge a particular aspect of balance that is needed in saving a person during potential fall [25]. The US quantifies postural sway velocity with the patient standing on either the right or left foot on the floor. FR and TUG tests assess the aspects of balance that is different from US test. These tests altogether examine several different aspects of balance.

It may be speculated that WKO accompanied by home-based daily exercise program improved the aspects of balance which can be assessed by TUG and FR tests and not US test.

In conclusion, applying WKO together with back extensor strengthening exercises in women with osteoporosis leads to improvement in functional balance test which can be translated to decreased risk of fall-in real life in this population.

The limitations of our study were the relatively small number of cases included and short term follow ups evaluations. Absence of a control group receiving no intervention was another limitation of this study; however, due to ethical considerations we had to consider the least routine interventions including exercise and medications for all patients.

The potential bias which could arise by performing similar exercises in both groups was minimal due to the fact that these exercises needed more time (in comparison to our intervention duration) to cause significant clinical changes [18].

We encourage more randomized controlled clinical trials with larger sample size evaluating the effect of WKO on risk of falls in long term via applying clinical functional and paraclinical tests in the elderly with osteoporosis.

Conflict of Interests

There is no conflict of interests for this paper.

Acknowledgments

The authors would like to thank Mrs. Fatemeh Rahimi Far, the manager of Shahid Modarres hospital's library and Mrs. Mehranz Mehrabi, research assistant at Clinical Research Development Center of Shahid Modarres Hospital for their help and cooperation in this study.

References

[1] J. T. Lin and J. M. Lane, "Rehabilitation of the older adult with an osteoporosis-related fracture," *Clinics in Geriatric Medicine*, vol. 22, no. 2, pp. 435–447, 2006.

[2] A. C. M. Renno, R. N. Granito, P. Driusso, D. Costa, and J. Oishi, "Effects of an exercise program on respiratory function, posture and on quality of life in osteoporotic women: a pilot study," *Physiotherapy*, vol. 91, no. 2, pp. 113–118, 2005.

[3] A. Nordström, T. Tervo, and M. Högström, "The effect of physical activity on bone accrual, osteoporosis and fracture prevention," *Open Bone Journal*, vol. 3, pp. 11–21, 2011.

[4] J. Fechtenbaum, C. Cropet, S. Kolta, S. Horlait, P. Orcel, and C. Roux, "The severity of vertebral fractures and health-related quality of life in osteoporotic postmenopausal women," *Osteoporosis International*, vol. 16, no. 12, pp. 2175–2179, 2005.

[5] N. Miyakoshi, E. Itoi, M. Kobayashi, and H. Kodama, "Impact of postural deformities and spinal mobility on quality of life in postmenopausal osteoporosis," *Osteoporosis International*, vol. 14, no. 12, pp. 1007–1012, 2003.

[6] A. R. Martin, E. Sornay-Rendu, J. M. Chandler, F. Duboeuf, C. J. Girman, and P. D. Delmas, "The impact of osteoporosis on quality-of-life: the OFELY cohort," *Bone*, vol. 31, no. 1, pp. 32–36, 2002.

[7] J. A. Kanis, E. V. McCloskey, H. Johansson, A. Oden, O. Ström, and F. Borgström, "Development and use of FRAX in osteoporosis," *Osteoporosis International*, vol. 21, pp. S407–S413, 2010.

[8] M. Sinaki, "Prevention treatment of osteoporosis," in *Physical Medicine and Rehabilitation*, R. Braddom, Ed., pp. 939–950, Saunders Elsevier, 3 edition, 2007.

[9] R. S. Kaplan and M. Sinaki, "Effect of back supports on back strength in patients with osteoporosis: a pilot study," *Mayo Clinic Proceedings*, vol. 71, no. 3, pp. 235–241, 1996.

[10] M. Sinaki, E. Itoi, J. W. Rogers, E. J. Bergstralh, and H. W. Wahner, "Correlation of back extensor strength with thoracic kyphosis and lumbar lordosis in estrogen-deficient women," *American Journal of Physical Medicine and Rehabilitation*, vol. 75, no. 5, pp. 370–374, 1996.

[11] M. M. Madureira, L. Takayama, A. L. Gallinaro, V. F. Caparbo, R. A. Costa, and R. M. R. Pereira, "Balance training program is highly effective in improving functional status and reducing the risk of falls in elderly women with osteoporosis: a randomized controlled trial," *Osteoporosis International*, vol. 18, no. 4, pp. 419–425, 2007.

[12] S. S. Vaapio, M. J. Salminen, A. Ojanlatva, and S.-L. Kivelä, "Quality of life as an outcome of fall prevention interventions among the aged: a systematic review," *European Journal of Public Health*, vol. 19, no. 1, pp. 7–15, 2009.

[13] Z. Gunendi, O. Ozyemisci-Taskiran, and N. Demirsoy, "The effect of 4-week aerobic exercise program on postural balance in postmenopausal women with osteoporosis," *Rheumatology International*, vol. 28, no. 12, pp. 1217–1222, 2008.

[14] M. Hongo, E. Itoi, M. Sinaki et al., "Effect of low-intensity back exercise on quality of life and back extensor strength in patients with osteoporosis: a randomized controlled trial," *Osteoporosis International*, vol. 18, no. 10, pp. 1389–1395, 2007.

[15] S. A. Raeissadat, P. Mojgani, and S. Pournajaf, "Short-term effect of back extensor strengthening exercises on the quality of Life of patients with primary osteoporosis," *Life Science Journal*, vol. 10, pp. 1060–1065, 2013.

[16] M. Sinaki, R. H. Brey, C. A. Hughes, D. R. Larson, and K. R. Kaufman, "Balance disorder and increased risk of falls in osteoporosis and kyphosis: significance of kyphotic posture and muscle strength," *Osteoporosis International*, vol. 16, no. 8, pp. 1004–1010, 2005.

[17] I. Melzer, N. Benjuya, and J. Kaplanski, "Postural stability in the elderly: a comparison between fallers and non-fallers," *Age and Ageing*, vol. 33, no. 6, pp. 602–607, 2004.

[18] M. Sinaki, R. H. Brey, C. A. Hughes, D. R. Larson, and K. R. Kaufman, "Significant reduction in risk of falls and back pain in osteoporotic-kyphotic women through a spinal proprioceptive extension exercise dynamic (SPEED) program," *Mayo Clinic Proceedings*, vol. 80, no. 7, pp. 849–855, 2005.

[19] M. Sinaki, "Prevention treatment of osteoporosis," in *Physical Medicine and Rehabilitation*, R. Braddom, Ed., pp. 939–950, Saunders Elsevier, 2007.

[20] P. W. Duncan, D. K. Weiner, J. Chandler, and S. Studenski, "Functional reach: a new clinical measure of balance," *Journals of Gerontology*, vol. 45, no. 6, pp. M192–M197, 1990.

[21] R. W. Bohannon, P. A. Larkin, and A. C. Cook, "Decrease in timed balance test scores in aging," *Physical Therapy*, vol. 64, no. 7, pp. 1067–1070, 1984.

[22] R. C. Briggs, M. R. Gossman, R. Birch, J. E. Drews, and S. A. Shaddeau, "Balance performance among noninstitutionalized elderly women," *Physical Therapy*, vol. 69, no. 9, pp. 748–756, 1989.

[23] S. G. Brauer, Y. R. Burns, and P. Galley, "A prospective study of laboratory and clinical measures of postural stability to predict community-dwelling fallers," *Journals of Gerontology A*, vol. 55, no. 8, pp. M469–M476, 2000.

[24] R. Morris, R. H. Harwood, R. Baker, O. Sahota, S. Armstrong, and T. Masud, "A comparison of different balance tests in the prediction of falls in older women with vertebral fractures: a cohort study," *Age and Ageing*, vol. 36, no. 1, pp. 78–83, 2007.

[25] J. I. Thomas and J. V. Lane, "A pilot study to explore the predictive validity of 4 measures of falls risk in frail elderly patients," *Archives of Physical Medicine and Rehabilitation*, vol. 86, no. 8, pp. 1636–1640, 2005.

[26] F. Langley and S. Mackintosh, "Functional Balance assessment of older community dwelling adults: a systematic review of literature," *Journal of Allied Health Science and Practice*, vol. 5, no. 4, pp. 1540–1580, 2007.

[27] L. Thundryke, "Osteoporosis," in *Common Problems in Geriatrics*, Adelman am, Ed., pp. 139–150, McGraw-Hill, New York, NY, USA, 2001.

[28] A. Yelnik and I. Bonan, "Clinical tools for assessing balance disorders," *Neurophysiologie Clinique*, vol. 38, no. 6, pp. 439–445, 2008.

[29] T. S. Alexandre, D. M. Meira, N. C. Rico, and S. K. Mizuta, "Accuracy of timed up and go test for screening risk of falls among community-dwelling elderly," *Revista Brasileira De Fisioterapia*, vol. 16, no. 5, pp. 381–388, 2012.

[30] A. Shumway-Cook, S. Brauer, and M. Woollacott, "Predicting the probability for falls in community-dwelling older adults using the timed up and go test," *Physical Therapy*, vol. 80, no. 9, pp. 896–903, 2000.

[31] D. De Kam, E. Smulders, V. Weerdesteyn, and B. C. M. Smits-Engelsman, "Exercise interventions to reduce fall-related fractures and their risk factors in individuals with low bone density: a systematic review of randomized controlled trials," *Osteoporosis International*, vol. 20, no. 12, pp. 2111–2125, 2009.

[32] L. Vogt, M. Hübscher, K. Brettmann, W. Banzer, and M. Fink, "Postural correction by osteoporosis orthosis (Osteo-med): a randomized, placebo-controlled trial," *Prosthetics and Orthotics International*, vol. 32, no. 1, pp. 103–110, 2008.

[33] K. Schmidt, M. Hübscher, L. Vogt et al., "Influence of spinal orthosis on gait and physical functioning in women with postmenopausal osteoporosis," *Orthopade*, vol. 41, no. 3, pp. 200–205, 2012.

[34] M. Pfeifer, L. Kohlwey, B. Begerow, and H. W. Minne, "Effects of two newly developed spinal orthoses on trunk muscle strength, posture, and quality-of-life in women with postmenopausal osteoporosis: a randomized trial," *American Journal of Physical Medicine and Rehabilitation*, vol. 90, no. 10, pp. 805–815, 2011.

[35] M. Sinaki, M. Pfeifer, E. Preisinger et al., "The role of exercise in the treatment of osteoporosis," *Current Osteoporosis Reports*, vol. 8, no. 3, pp. 138–144, 2010.

[36] M. Sinaki, "Musculoskeletal rehabilitation in patients with osteoporosis—Rehabilitation of Osteoporosis Program-Exercise (ROPE)," *Journal fur Mineralstoffwechsel*, vol. 17, no. 2, pp. 60–65, 2010.

14

A Community-Based, Technology-Supported Health Service for Detecting and Preventing Frailty among Older Adults: A Participatory Design Development Process

Lex van Velsen,[1,2] Maddalena Illario,[3,4] Stephanie Jansen-Kosterink,[1,2] Catherine Crola,[3,4] Carolina Di Somma,[5,6] Annamaria Colao,[5,6] and Miriam Vollenbroek-Hutten[1,2]

[1] *Roessingh Research and Development, Telemedicine Cluster, P.O. Box 310, 7500 AH Enschede, Netherlands*
[2] *University of Twente, Biomedical Signals and Systems Group, P.O. Box 217, 7500 AE Enschede, Netherlands*
[3] *Federico II University, Department of Translational Medical Sciences, Largo S. Marcellino 10, 80138 Naples, Italy*
[4] *Federico II University Hospital, Research & Development, Largo S. Marcellino 10, 80138 Naples, Italy*
[5] *Federico II University Hospital, Department of Clinical Medicine and Surgery, Largo S. Marcellino 10, 80138 Naples, Italy*
[6] *Federico II University Hospital, Department of Gastroenterology, Endocrinology and Surgery, Largo S. Marcellino 10, 80138 Naples, Italy*

Correspondence should be addressed to Lex van Velsen; l.vanvelsen@rrd.nl

Academic Editor: Wojtek Chodzko-Zajko

Frailty is a multifaceted condition that affects many older adults and marks decline on areas such as cognition, physical condition, and nutritional status. Frail individuals are at increased risk for the development of disability, dementia, and falls. There are hardly any health services that enable the identification of prefrail individuals and that focus on prevention of further functional decline. In this paper, we discuss the development of a community-based, technology-supported health service for detecting prefrailty and preventing frailty and further functional decline via participatory design with a wide range of stakeholders. The result is an innovative service model in which an online platform supports the integration of traditional services with novel, Information Communication Technology supported tools. This service is capable of supporting the different phases of screening and offers training services, by also integrating them with community-based services. The service model can be used as a basis for developing similar services within a wide range of healthcare systems. We present the service model, the general functioning of the technology platform, and the different ways in which screening for and prevention of frailty has been localized. Finally, we reflect on the added value of participatory design for creating such health services.

1. Introduction

Aging can be considered a success story for health policies in the modern world. And while living longer is a beautiful thing, it also comes with downsides, such as frailty. Frail older adults are those "who are at increased risk for future poor clinical outcomes, such as development of disability, dementia, falls, hospitalization, institutionalization, or increased mortality" [1]. As such, frailty is a state that consists of many dimensions. Physical and cognitive decline, as well as malnutrition, have been identified as the major dimensions of frailty among older adults [2]. Becoming frail is something that happens gradually. A person starts out robust (or healthy), becomes prefrail (a stage in which components of frailty become manifest), and can then evolve to become frail (which can be observed clinically easily) [3]. In ten European countries, the percentage of prefrail people among community-dwelling older adults have been found to range from 30.4% to 44.9%, and the percentage of frail people among this group ranged from 1.3% to 5.9% [4].

Determining the level of frailty among older adults and offering them interventions to train their health have been found to help them live at home independently for a longer amount of time and to reduce the rate of falls [5]

or helps them to maintain their functional capacity [6]. However, current identification methods for frailty and prefrailty among older adults are resource-intensive and more efficient (but equally reliable) alternatives need to be developed [7]. This need aligns with the great challenges that society has to deal with in organizing its healthcare. Demand is rising due to a population that includes increasingly more older adults that have to be supported by increasingly fewer young people; older adults should be able to function in society independently and without drawing too much on society's resources; increasingly high standards of living lead to higher expectations with regard to the quality of care while budgets are being tightened [8]. Two types of healthcare services have been identified as possible solutions to these problems: community-based services and eHealth [9, 10]. A community-based healthcare service is a form of care that is provided out of medical institutions within a patient's community. This does not mean that healthcare professionals (e.g., a general practitioner) are not involved. Rather, the majority of the service is provided at a location in a patient's neighborhood that is not care-related (e.g., the community house) and involves a collaboration of healthcare professionals, local organizations, and volunteers. For the context of care for older persons, such services are meant to help older people live independently in their own house while maintaining their quality of life [11]. Community-based services can be a method to decrease the pressure on the healthcare system by moving care from medical institutions towards local community services. Collaborations between primary care, volunteers, and community services have been shown, among other things, to be able to predict poor nutrition among older adults [12], to prevent hospitalizations and major disabilities among chronically ill older adults [13], and to prevent the number of falls among older adults with a history of falling or having concerns about falling [14].

eHealth (or "health services and information delivered or enhanced through the internet and related technologies" [15]) has been proposed as a solution for overcoming the aforementioned challenges and is associated with great promises, such as improved access to health information, greater quality of care, and higher adoption of healthy behavior [16]. By means of eHealth services, patients can be empowered to take care of themselves, assisted by technology. This way, the burden on the healthcare system decreases, while patients gain control.

A community-based, technology-supported service model for screening for frailty among older adults and training their health can be a cost-effective alternative for the clinically based services that are currently available. By combining both approaches, care is moved away from care institutions, while it allows older adults to choose which kind of service they prefer (face-to-face in the community or via online self-service technology). But creating such a service means that new working procedures need to be devised. Therefore, involvement from stakeholders and potential end-users is extremely important [17, 18]. In this paper, we discuss the development of a community-based, technology-supported service model that aims to detect and prevent frailty among older adults, by means of a participatory design approach.

2. Materials and Methods

2.1. Participatory Design. We approached the design of the service model by means of participatory design. Participatory design is a design approach that advocates the inclusion of all stakeholders (including potential end-users and/or their representatives) during design activities in order to come to a design solution that aligns with all stakeholders' and end-users' needs and context [19, 20]. We conducted a series of workshops in which stakeholders and end-user (representatives) were gathered with multiple goals. First, we wanted to create awareness of the upcoming services. Second, we gathered direct input from the people that we anticipated to be actually working with the service or were going to be affected by it for service design. And third, as the workshop participants, for a large part, were also going to be the persons working with in the service, providing them input would them a sense of responsibility and ownership that, in turn, leads to higher acceptance [21].

2.2. Project Context. The design of the service model was part of the European FP7 project PERSSILAA (which stands for Personalised Information Communication Technology (ICT) Supported Services for Independent Living and Active Ageing). This project has the goal to develop a health service for detecting and preventing frailty among older adults by offering them innovative eHealth services and has a strong basis in their local community. Within this project, we see frailty as the rate of functional decline, whereby people can be robust (no functional decline), prefrail (some to quite some functional decline), and frail (an amount of functional decline that necessitates immediate medical intervention). eHealth interventions for improving physical and cognitive functioning and a website for educating older adults about healthy nutrition were developed in the project for improving older adults' health. The nutritional intervention educates people about healthier choices and to improve food habits, geared towards older adults. The physical intervention focuses on exercising for strength, endurance, and mobility training. The cognitive intervention, finally, targets improving the main cognitive functions: attention, memory, and executive functions. Those older adults that, during a screening, displayed some decline on the nutritional, cognitive, or physical aspect can then make use of these interventions. The service was initially developed for and implemented in two regions: Campania in Italy and Enschede in Netherlands. At the start of the project, an initial, high-level service model was developed by the project partners (including clinicians and experts in telemedicine) that served as input during the initial workshops (which are described below). In this model, the use of technology was foreseen during screening and prevention, but it still remained unclear how older adults could be guided best to the services, what the role of healthcare professionals was, how older adults should be guided during training, and so forth.

2.3. Setup in Italy. A first meeting was organized to create awareness among relevant stakeholders about the upcoming service for detecting and preventing functional decline and for the activities which would be deployed within its scope. The meeting (and the workshops that followed) also provided the opportunity to identify existing gaps in terms of digital and health literacy so that support could be arranged for overcoming these gaps and to facilitate the adoption of the innovative, ICT-supported services. A set of organizations that were closest to the older adults in the community (i.e., they are key stakeholders) were invited. These key stakeholders were then expected to discuss the proposed service with others in their vicinity. The stakeholders were selected and contacted based on the knowledge and experience of Caritas. Caritas is an international, religious organization that aims to improve the life and possibilities of people, by working closely with local churches. As in the Campania region (where the service model would at first be deployed), religion and spirituality play a large role in the life of older adults, Caritas and the Catholic Church were taken as the starting point for service design. In the end, 60 people attended the meeting. They were representatives from local hospitals, local nonprofit organizations that were interested in collaborating (such as Caritas or a large, local Judo club), local governments, seniors' associations, and the older adults themselves. During this meeting, the following topics were presented and discussed with all representatives and older adults to elicit the background knowledge needed to set-up local activities for detecting and preventing frailty:

(1) the role of older adults within the service and the service design (emphasizing the concept that the older adults are at the same time "object" of the screening, and "partners" in that their feedback was important for optimizing the service design and implementation);

(2) the initial service model;

(3) a comparison with other, highly-esteemed, sociosanitary services in Italy;

(4) making use of voluntary work to support the detection and prevention of functional decline (focusing on health promotion, socialization, and health and ICT literacy);

(5) the use of ICT to offer new services and the integration of the new services with existing medical information systems;

(6) how to provide older adults with an environment that makes it easier to make a life-altering change towards a healthier lifestyle.

This meeting led to an ideal service model that was subsequently detailed during nine meetings with representatives from two local communities where the service would be made available and the other key-stakeholders, like Caritas, general practitioners, the municipal health service, involved nonprofit organizations, and the local hospital. The goal of these workshops was to transform the ideal service model into a model that could easily be implemented locally by modifying it to fit local contexts in terms of opportunities (available resources), needs, and expectations. An ideal model was used as input for these meetings, as such models can aid a discussion on how to set up a service in a local community [22]. The meetings were held over a period of three months. While the first meeting was plenary (and included an overview of the aims of the service and the ideal service model), in-between meetings were focused more on specific topics (such as developing sessions in which the detection of frailty is combined with health literacy classes for older adults). Over time, the following topics about the anticipated service model were discussed with and among all stakeholders:

(1) the current role(s) and task(s) of every stakeholder with regard to detecting, monitoring, and preventing functional decline;

(2) the gain of every stakeholder to participate in and use the service;

(3) the envisioned role(s) and task(s) of every stakeholder within the service;

(4) agreement on the division of role(s) and task(s) among the stakeholders.

2.4. Setup in the Netherlands. A first workshop had the goal to create an "ideal" service model. This was done with a wide range of stakeholders and end-user representatives: a community nurse, a specialist in geriatric medicine, a general practitioner, a manager of a homecare organization, a representative from a municipality, a representative from a seniors' association (who acted as end-user representative), and a representative of a municipal health service. These stakeholders were selected after a brainstorm in which as many relevant stakeholders as possible were listed. Subsequently, they were ranked on three attributes that make up stakeholder salience: power, legitimacy, and urgency [23]. This ranking was used to determine which stakeholders were most needed at the workshop. After an introduction, the following subjects were discussed:

(1) each participant's current roles and tasks regarding detecting and preventing frailty and functional decline;

(2) an inventory of problems with the current way frailty is dealt with in care;

(3) introduction of a conceptual service model (e.g., demonstrating the options technology provides for training health on a distance);

(4) listing the roles and tasks each participant sees for himself/herself in the new service model;

(5) mapping the perfect procedure for a fictitious persona.

This workshop led to an "ideal" service model that was subsequently refined in a set of nine meetings and workshops with representatives from local organizations that resided in the area in which the service would be deployed for the first time. Like we mentioned above, this tactic was used to aid the discussion on how to set up a service in a local community. These nine meetings were held with the municipality, a healthcare center, a healthcare insurer, a physical therapy practice, a healthcare organization for older adults, a community center, the University of Applied Sciences, and the researchers. The goal of these workshops was to transform the ideal service model into one that would fit the stakeholders' and users' contexts and routines. These meetings were also held in a time span of three months. Not all meetings were held with all stakeholders. Where the first and last meeting were plenary, in-between meetings were held to discuss issues affecting mainly a few stakeholders (such as creating a student assignment that allows students of the Applied University to do an internship within the project). The topics that were addressed during these meetings were similar to those in Italy: determining current roles of the stakeholders, assessing their potential gain, determining the role(s) and task(s) each stakeholder would like to have, and reaching consensus over the division of roles and tasks.

2.5. Data Analysis. Both plenary meetings in Italy and Netherlands (where the "ideal" service models were created) were audio-recorded and transcribed. Next, they were analyzed by means of thematic analysis whereby stakeholders' and end-users' interests with respect to frailty care, and their preferred role(s) and task(s) within the process of detecting and preventing frailty were mapped. The ideal service model was mapped by means of an activity diagram. In Italy, the subsequent meetings to refine the service model were documented via minutes of the meetings that were confirmed by all parties present. In Netherlands, after each meeting an improved version of the service model was created that was discussed in a subsequent meeting until all stakeholders agreed that this was a suitable service model. The final service models were also mapped by means of activity diagrams.

3. Results

3.1. The "Ideal" Service Model. The initial meetings that were used to come to an "ideal" service model resulted in two important insights about the way frailty care is currently provided; detection and prevention of frailty is dispersed over many different actors who do not collaborate, and there is currently no shared language for dealing with frailty. These views were shared in both countries. Next, for the to-be-developed service all stakeholders and end-users agreed on the following starting points.

(1) The older adult is responsible for the management of his or her own health and should be the party that takes initiative when health problems should be addressed (urgently).

(2) General practitioners want to be informed about the results of the screening, and there is a need to integrate their routine activities with the novel services for the detection and prevention of frailty and functional decline. Hereby, the aim is not to provide any additional work for them.

Alongside, in Italy it became apparent that there is a need for activities that educate older adults about working with ICT technology (e.g., the internet). Ideally, activities with regard to frailty detection and prevention should be combined with meetings in which older adults learn to work with ICT.

The ideal service models that were discussed resulted in an initial design in which older adults are invited for a two-stage screening process (one consisting of questionnaires, one consisting of physical and cognitive tests and additional questions) that identifies their rate of functional decline and classifies them as either robust, prefrail, or frail. While frail individuals are referred to a medical professional, and robust people receive an invitation for a new screening a year later, the group of prefrail people (those with some functional decline) are offered eHealth interventions for improving their cognitive functioning and physical functioning or for educating them about healthy nutrition for older adults. These services can be accessed at home, or, for the Italian context: at the local church, where the older adults are helped by trained volunteers. During the process, the general practitioner is kept up to date about the results and is only involved when an older adult needs urgent attention. For the two contexts, the ideal service model was mapped by means of activity diagrams (see Figure 1 for an excerpt in which an older adult is invited for and undergoes a first screening). These activity diagrams then served as input for the subsequent meetings in which the service model was further refined.

3.2. Refining the Ideal Service Model. In a series of meetings with local stakeholders in Italy and Netherlands, the ideal service models were refined, so that they could be implemented in practice.

In Italy, the subsequent meetings were used to formalize the division of tasks and to make this official by specific agreements. Next, tasks were divided and new organizations were included as collaborators, like Health Campus, a non-profit organization that involves more than 200 volunteer clinicians and focuses on providing free health screenings and promotes healthy lifestyles. Finally, the need for solving the existing health and ICT literacy gaps was addressed. The solution was found in an interactive "nutrition meeting," where people learned about healthy nutrition, were provided essential information on preventive medicine, and were in parallel taught ICT skills (use of office functionalities, to write down recipes, prepare PowerPoint presentations, access, and navigation on the internet to search for nutritional information, etc.). This way, they could gain the knowledge necessary for making well-informed dietary choices, and could receive additional information from professionals on topics they identified as relevant. At the same time, they could also learn the ICT skills that are needed in today's society and for making use of the service's ICT modules. To support the ICT training, another non-profit organization, Progetto Alpha, collaborated. Support was also provided by general practitioners of "Salute in Collina," by the Campania Regional Center for Urban Veterinary Safety and by the Department of Public Health of Federico II University.

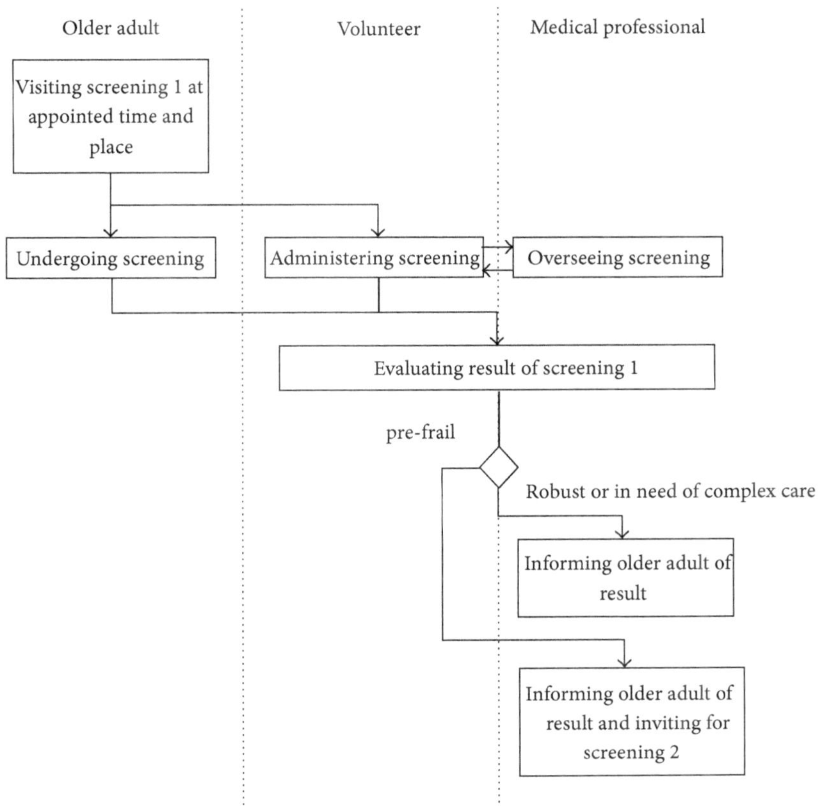

FIGURE 1: Excerpt of the "ideal" service model activity diagram for Italy.

In Netherlands, local general practitioners were doubtful about the feasibility of providing screening and training services via the internet only. They thought many older adults would not have access to the internet. Furthermore, they would like to see older adults leaving their house and mingling with other people, as loneliness is quite a big problem. Therefore, we explored new collaborations for opening up screening and training services in the local community. New partners were happy to be involved and it was agreed upon that kiosks will be opened at a local physical therapy practice, a healthcare organization for older adults, and the local community center. Next, the need for a cost-effective, sustainable business model led to the idea to involve the local University of Applied Sciences, which is always in a need for places for their students to do an internship. The University of Applied Sciences was also willing to collaborate and it was decided upon that their students (physical therapy and nursing) will support the logistics behind the service (e.g., sending out invitations) and will support the older adults during the screening and training, both at home and at a location within the community.

3.3. A Community-Based, Technology-Supported Service Model for Detecting and Preventing Frailty among Older Adults. Figure 2 displays the service model that was created on the basis of the ideal service models and the alterations that were made in the subsequent meetings. In the service model, there are unique routes for entering the screening and training services. In Italy, older adults are invited for the first screening via the church, after which they can complete this screening at the church with the help of a trained volunteer or online. As older adults in Italy frequently visit the church, where many activities take place, this appeared to be the best way to reach them. In Netherlands, older adults are invited by the general practitioner's office (in name only, logistics are handled by the students) after which they can complete the first screening at home on paper, online, or with the help of a trained student. The general practitioner was chosen as the party sending out the invitations as this would yield the highest response from the older adults, due to his or her authority. This first screening consists of a set of questionnaires to assess an individual's general health status and his or her physical and cognitive status, as well as their nutritional habits (by means of questionnaires like the Groningen Frailty Indicator and the Mini Nutritional Assessment). In all cases, the results of the first screening are sent or uploaded to a central database that also determines the outcome for every individual (using cut-off scores for the different survey instruments that classify an individual as frail, (pre)frail, or robust, based on their rate of functional decline). Frail individuals are referred to a medical specialist (e.g., the general practitioner), who will, after personal examination, make a diagnosis and determine a treatment plan. Robust individuals will receive an invitation for

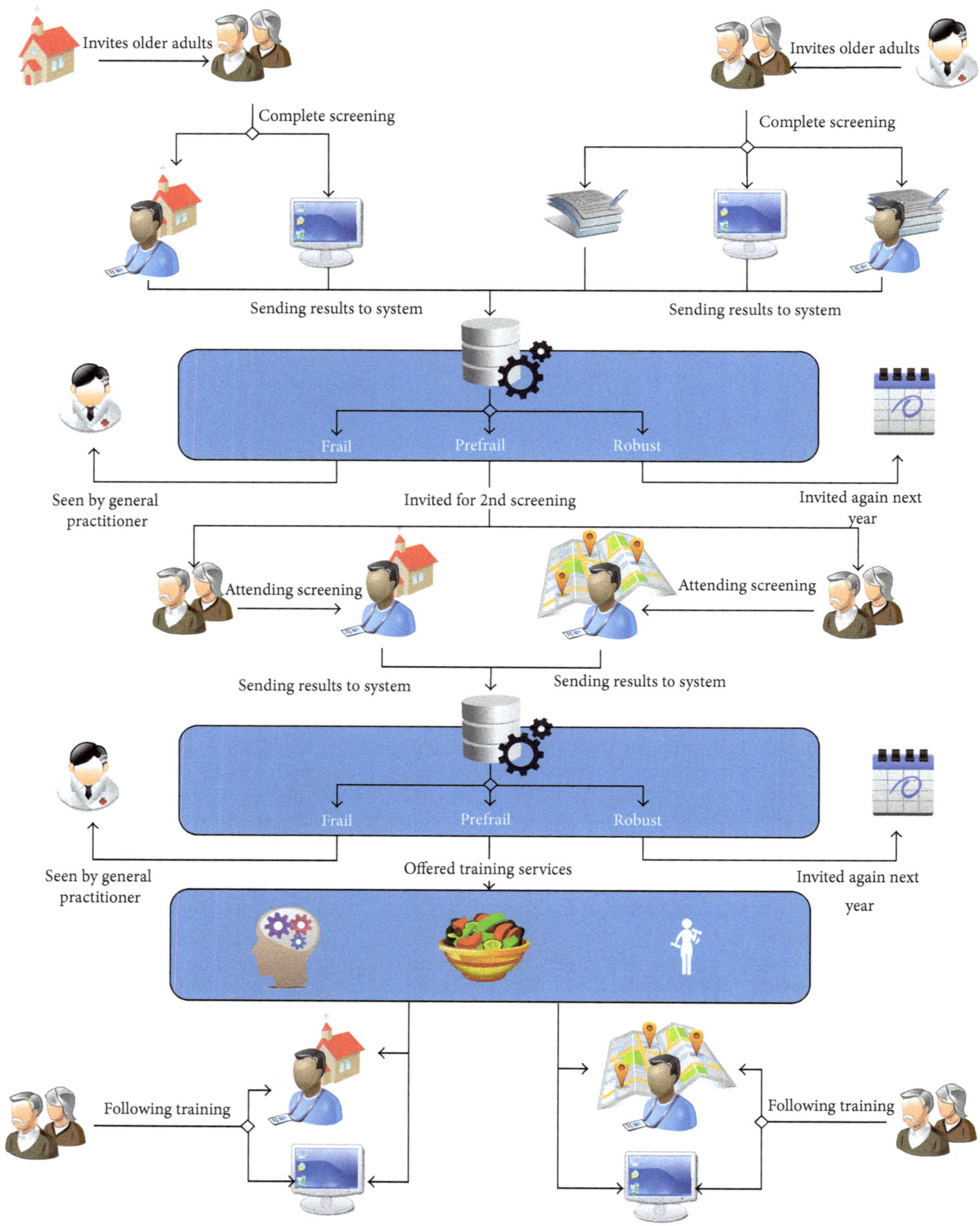

FIGURE 2: Service model.

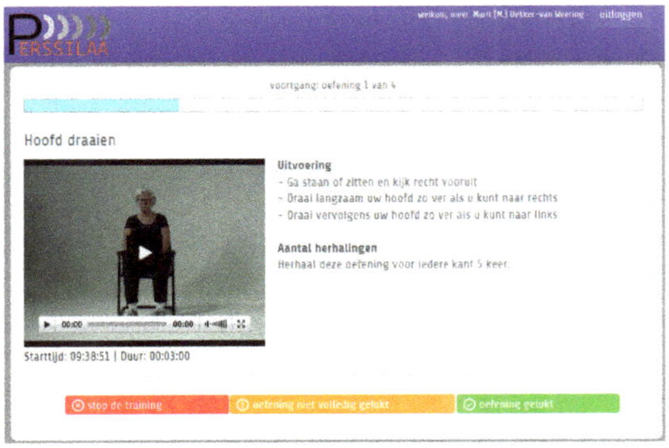

FIGURE 3: Screenshot of the service for training physical functioning.

a new screening a year later. An individual is classified as prefrail when limited decline is identified on at least one of the following three domains: nutrition, cognition, or physical status. These prefrail individuals are invited for a second screening. The second screening is administered by a trained volunteer at the church (Italian context) or by a trained student at different locations in the community (Dutch situation). This second screening consists of physical and cognitive tests, as well as some additional questions. Again, results are sent towards the database that, again, classifies every individual. This time, frail people are sent to a medical professional, robust people receive an invitation for a new screening a year later, and prefrail individuals are offered training services (for training physical or cognitive functioning or to educate people about healthy nutrition for older adults). These training services can be used at home via an online service. See Figure 3 for a screenshot of the service for training physical functioning, where people are instructed to do exercises via video, audio, and text. Alternatively, in Italy older adults can make use of the training services at the church and in Netherlands at the same locations in the community at which they could join the screening.

4. Discussion

In this paper, we have discussed how we have created a community-based, technology-supported service model for the detection and prevention of frailty among older adults. We applied a participatory design approach to come to a useful model that easily aligns with working procedures and the designated context of work. In the service model, older adults are screened via different modalities (online, on paper, or in person at a location in the community) after which they are provided training services for improving their physical or cognitive functioning, or for educating them about healthy nutrition for older adults. These training services are also offered via different modalities (as online, self-service module or at locations in the community). Medical professionals (such as general practitioners and nurse practitioners) are informed about the medical status of each older adult but do not play an active role unless the situation calls for it.

The service model and the technology can be used as a basis for developing a similar service model in a wide range of regions, countries, or healthcare models. But when one embarks on implementing the service model, several steps need to be localized. The way in which older adults are guided towards the screening and training services needs to be adapted to the traditions, possibilities, and stakeholder needs in a specific region. For example, we found that in Italy, the church is one of the most suitable venues for inviting and helping older adults, the general practitioner should invite people, while trained students at different locations in the community can aid older adults in their training efforts. Other assumptions within the service model (how the General Practitioner should be informed about results, and how to integrate the novel services supporting the screening for frailty to the advantage of his routine activity and especially of his patients) should be checked. Ideally, this should be done by conducting stakeholder meetings in which the key players for a setting in which the service is to be implemented gather and discuss the adaptations that need to be made to the service model we presented. It could take a few meetings before consensus is reached, but the investment in terms of time and effort should be quite small. Specifically, we see the following issues that need to be discussed. First, one must assess how the service model can be streamlined with existing working procedures. One should especially determine which actor is most suitable for inviting older adults for a screening, and which actor(s) should host and support the local screenings and training services in the community. Second, as the different medical professionals in a region will want to be kept up-to-date about the results of the screening and progress of training, connections will need to be made between the online frailty service and database and the local medical information system(s). As it differs per country or even region which medical information systems are used, one will need to determine which system to connect to, how to make this connection, and how and to whom to display results from the screening and training in the specific medical information system. For example, in Netherlands, general practitioners stated that they wanted to receive the results of each screening to be incorporated into a patient's electronic health file as an episode with an ICPC code (for overall decline). Third, a business model should be created that specifies how all the different activities are financed and how all the stakeholders are rewarded for their efforts. Without such a business model, the service will not be sustainable beyond the point where seed money runs out.

The setup of the service model (with a special focus on technology-supported, community-based care) has the potential to be cost-effective. It provides easy access for older adults towards healthcare service (as they can access them online or visit them in their local neighborhood). Finally, due to the use of online tools for screening and training, the service can scale up easily. As a result of these advantages, the service model can be a solution for the challenges that healthcare is currently facing: to provide care to a growing number of older adults with fewer resources, all the while ensuring that people retain a good quality of life. Via this service model, care is moved from a reactive, cure-oriented approach that is centered at medical institutions and medical professionals towards a prevention-focused model that takes advantage from patient empowerment, online services, and trained volunteers, in a health-aware, responsible community. Consequently, the demand on the healthcare system decreases, shifting to prevention and health promotion, while citizens take an active role in their health, are empowered in receiving the care they need in the form they want (online, in the community, or as a combination), and improve their overall health outcomes.

The use of participatory design with stakeholders and end-users has resulted in a service model that not only is innovative but also aligns with the context and working routines in which it is to be implemented. Apart from these benefits, their involvement has, as we have experienced, also other advantages. First, as they become not only consumer of the service but also creator, stakeholders and end-users are more willing to adopt the service model and associated technology. After all, it is also partly "theirs." Second, for many end-users, adopting a new service (especially one that is fundamentally different from the traditional healthcare services they are familiar with) requires a paradigm shift. In our study, we saw that the older adults need to realize they should not rely on a doctor to arrange everything for them but should seize control themselves. Involving end-users into design provides them with the opportunity to get used to the idea and to discuss it with their peers. Ultimately, this leads to an implementation context where end-users are more willing to accept a new service's starting points.

5. Limitations

The development of the service model was done in participation with stakeholders and end-users but focused on a hypothetical situation. Existing initiatives for detecting and preventing frailty are scarce, so all participants had to talk about and imagine a future scenario. It might well be that they missed barriers that hinder successful implementation and service delivery and the only way to identify these barriers is to implement, execute, and evaluate the service. Then, with the insights from this evaluation, the service model can be further improved.

As we mentioned before, the service model cannot be copied "as is" to a new region where working procedures and the implementation context are different. Instead, one should adapt the service model to fit a specific region following the steps we have formulated above.

6. Concluding Remarks

The service model that we have developed is unique in that it is the first to detect and prevent frailty by means of community-based, technology-supported services. As such, it marks a step forward in creating healthcare services for older adults that not only include care by professional caregivers to deal with acute problems but also lead to a set of healthcare services that prevent problems by integrating initiatives in the community with online services. Our next steps are to implement the service model in different regions in Italy, in Netherlands, and in EU, taking advantage of the Reference Site Collaborative Network of the European Innovation Partnership on Active and Healthy Ageing (all the while improving the service by taking into account the lessons that the actual deployment provides us) and to evaluate the services in terms of clinical effectiveness and adoption by stakeholders. This way, we can also assess whether the model lives up to its potential.

Conflict of Interests

The authors declare that there is no conflict of interests regarding the publication of this paper.

Acknowledgments

The work was undertaken within the context of the PERSSILAA project (see http://www.perssilaa.eu/) and with financial support from the EU (FP7 Grant no. 610359). The authors would like to thank all members of the PERSSILAA project and those who participated in the workshops and meetings for their valuable input and enthusiasm. They would especially like to thank all older adults that joined, and especially Nunzia Oliviero, the communities Confalone and Pilar and the municipality of Enschede, all volunteers that helped us out, especially Susy Tofanelli (Confalone Community), and Enrico Borrelli (Pilar Community); Health Campus; Pasquale Riccio of Progetto Alpha; Vincenzo Caputo and Annamaria Di Maggio of CRIUV; Paolo Montuori; and Professor Maria Triassi of the Department of Public Health of the University of Naples.

References

[1] European Innovation Partnership on Active and Healthy Ageing, *Action Plan on Prevention and Early Diagnosis of Frailty and Functional Decline, Both Physical and Cognitive in Older People*, European Union, Brussels, Belgium, 2012.

[2] M. I. Gomez, I. García-Sánchez, A. Carta, and J. P. Antunes, *A Collection of Good Practices That Support the Prevention and Early Diagnosis of Frailty and Functional Decline, Both Physically and Cognitive, in Older People*, European Commission, Brussels, Belgium, 2013.

[3] S. A. Sternberg, A. W. Schwartz, S. Karunananthan, H. Bergman, and A. Mark Clarfield, "The identification of frailty: a systematic literature review," *Journal of the American Geriatrics Society*, vol. 59, no. 11, pp. 2129–2138, 2011.

[4] B. Santos-Eggimann, P. Cuénoud, J. Spagnoli, and J. Junod, "Prevalence of frailty in middle-aged and older community-dwelling Europeans living in 10 countries," *The Journals of Gerontology Series A: Biological Sciences and Medical Sciences*, vol. 64, no. 6, pp. 675–681, 2009.

[5] A. D. Beswick, K. Rees, P. Dieppe et al., "Complex interventions to improve physical function and maintain independent living in elderly people: a systematic review and meta-analysis," *The Lancet*, vol. 371, no. 9614, pp. 725–735, 2008.

[6] E. L. Cadore, L. Rodríguez-Mañas, A. Sinclair, and M. Izquierdo, "Effects of different exercise interventions on risk of falls, gait

ability, and balance in physically frail older adults: a systematic review," *Rejuvenation Research*, vol. 16, no. 2, pp. 105–114, 2013.

[7] A. Clegg, J. Young, S. Iliffe, M. O. Rikkert, and K. Rockwood, "Frailty in elderly people," *The Lancet*, vol. 381, no. 9868, pp. 752–762, 2013.

[8] S. Koch, "Ubiquitous care in aging societies—a social challenge," *Studies in Health Technology and Informatics*, vol. 134, pp. 89–95, 2008.

[9] J. Peterson, J. R. Atwood, and B. Yates, "Key elements for church-based health promotion programs: outcome-based literature review," *Public Health Nursing*, vol. 19, no. 6, pp. 401–411, 2002.

[10] D. K. Ahern, J. M. Kreslake, and J. M. Phalen, "What is eHealth (6): perspectives on the evolution of eHealth research," *Journal of Medical Internet Research*, vol. 8, no. 1, article e4, 2006.

[11] L.-F. Low, M. Yap, and H. Brodaty, "A systematic review of different models of home and community care services for older persons," *BMC Health Services Research*, vol. 11, article 93, 2011.

[12] K. B. Yap, M. Niti, and T. P. Ng, "Nutrition screening among community-dwelling older adults in Singapore," *Singapore Medical Journal*, vol. 48, no. 10, pp. 911–916, 2007.

[13] S. G. Leveille, E. H. Wagner, C. Davis et al., "Preventing disability and managing chronic illness in frail older adults: a randomized trial of a community-based partnership with primary care," *Journal of the American Geriatrics Society*, vol. 46, no. 10, pp. 1191–1198, 1998.

[14] L. Clemson, R. G. Cumming, H. Kendig, M. Swann, R. Heard, and K. Taylor, "The effectiveness of a community-based program for reducing the incidence of falls in the elderly: a randomized trial," *Journal of the American Geriatrics Society*, vol. 52, no. 9, pp. 1487–1494, 2004.

[15] G. Eysenbach, "What is e-health?" *Journal of Medical Internet Research*, vol. 3, no. 2, article e20, 2001.

[16] G. L. Kreps and L. Neuhauser, "New directions in eHealth communication: opportunities and challenges," *Patient Education and Counseling*, vol. 78, no. 3, pp. 329–336, 2010.

[17] S. Koch, "Healthy ageing supported by technology—a cross-disciplinary research challenge," *Informatics for Health and Social Care*, vol. 35, no. 3-4, pp. 81–91, 2010.

[18] L. van Velsen, J. Wentzel, and J. E. W. C. van Gemert-Pijnen, "Designing eHealth that matters via a multidisciplinary requirements development approach," *JMIR Research Protocols*, vol. 2, no. 1, article e21, 2013.

[19] S. Kujala, "User involvement: a review of the benefits and challenges," *Behaviour & Information Technology*, vol. 22, no. 1, pp. 1–16, 2003.

[20] K. Bødker, F. Kensing, and J. Simonsen, *Participatory IT Design. Designing for Business and Workplace Realities*, MIT Press, Cambridge, Mass, USA, 2004.

[21] C. Cherry and R. D. Macredie, "The importance of context in information system design: an assessment of participatory design," *Requirements Engineering*, vol. 4, no. 2, pp. 103–114, 1999.

[22] J. Farmer and A. Nimegeer, "Community participation to design rural primary healthcare services," *BMC Health Services Research*, vol. 14, article 130, 2014.

[23] R. K. Mitchell, B. R. Agle, and D. J. Wood, "Toward a theory of stakeholder identification and salience: defining the principle of who and what really counts," *Academy of Management Review*, vol. 22, no. 4, pp. 853–886, 1997.

15

The Propensity for Inducing Atrial Fibrillation: A Comparative Study on Old versus Young Rabbits

Hongliang Li,[1] Benjamin J. Scherlag,[1] David C. Kem,[1] Caitlin Zillner,[1] Shailesh Male,[1] Sorkko Thirunavukkarasu,[1] Xiaohua Shen,[1] Alexandria Benbrook,[1] Jan V. Pitha,[2] Ralph Lazzara,[1] and Xichun Yu[1]

[1] *Heart Rhythm Institute, Department of Medicine, University of Oklahoma Health Sciences Center and Veterans Affairs Medical Center, Oklahoma City, OK 73104, USA*

[2] *Department of Pathology, University of Oklahoma Health Sciences Center and Veterans Affairs Medical Center, Oklahoma City, OK 73104, USA*

Correspondence should be addressed to Xichun Yu; xichun-yu@ouhsc.edu

Academic Editor: F. R. Ferraro

It is well established that atrial fibrillation (AF) is far more common in elderly humans. Autonomic activation is thought to be an operative mechanism for AF propensity. The aim of the study was to investigate the impact of age on atrial tachyarrhythmia induction in a rabbit model. Six old (aged 4–6 years) and 9 young (aged 3-4 months) New Zealand white rabbits were subjected to a catheter-based electrophysiological study. Atrial tachyarrhythmia susceptibility was tested by burst pacing before and after infusion of increasing concentrations of acetylcholine. Both young and old rabbits were in normal sinus rhythm at the beginning of the infusion/burst pacing protocol. The old rabbits had faster heart rates and a marked increase in atrial tachyarrhythmias compared to the young rabbits. Nonsustained and sustained AF events were more frequent in the old rabbits. No significant fibrosis was observed in the atria of either young or old rabbits. In conclusion, the old rabbits have a greater propensity for induction of AF. The significantly faster heart rates in the old rabbits suggest that dominant sympathetic activity may play an important role in the propensity for AF in this group.

1. Introduction

The incidence of atrial fibrillation (AF) in the human population increases with age, particularly in those over the age of 60 [1]. The mechanisms proposed for contributing to this association have ranged from structural [2, 3] and electrophysiological [4, 5] to metabolic issues [6–8]. The well-known association of AF with thyrotoxicosis has long been associated with older age [6–8]. We have previously reported a group of patients with thyrotoxicosis and concurrent AF and confirmed the interaction of increasing age as well as the significant association and effect of autoantibodies that activate the β-adrenergic and M2 muscarinic receptors [9]. In a previous study, we infused the autonomic neurotransmitter acetylcholine (ACh) into rabbits that had been immunized to produce activating autoantibodies to the β2-adrenergic receptor [10]. The results indicated a significantly greater incidence of sustained atrial tachycardia than in the same rabbits prior to immunization. In preliminary studies in selected animals that were older than 4 years of age, we observed a much lower threshold for induction of atrial tachyarrhythmias (unpublished observations). For this reason, we have investigated whether an autonomic mechanism may be the basis for a greater AF propensity in an old (4–6 years) group of rabbits compared to young (3-4 months) rabbits in whom different concentrations of ACh were infused intravenously to test the inducibility of AF with concomitant burst atrial pacing.

2. Materials and Methods

2.1. In Vivo Electrophysiological Assessment of Cardiac Tachyarrhythmia Propensity. This study protocol was approved by the Institutional Animal Care and Use Committee of

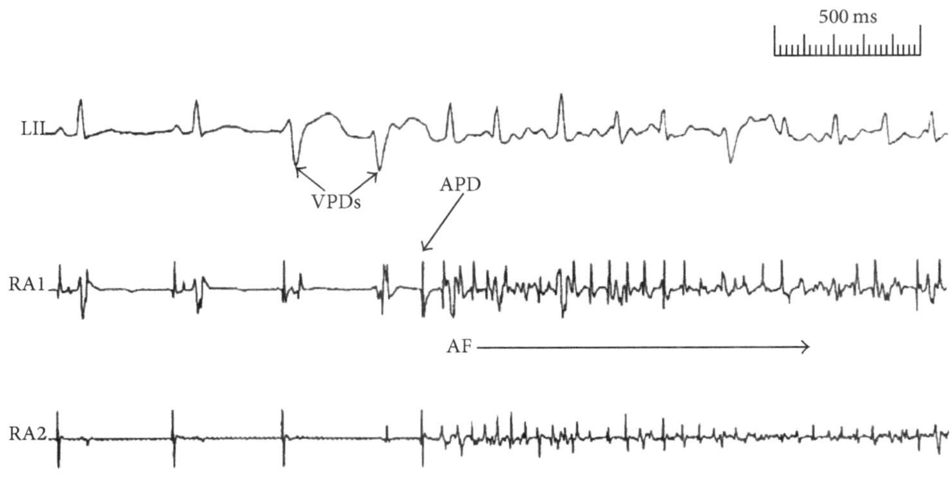

(a) Spontaneous AF (ACh 1 mM)

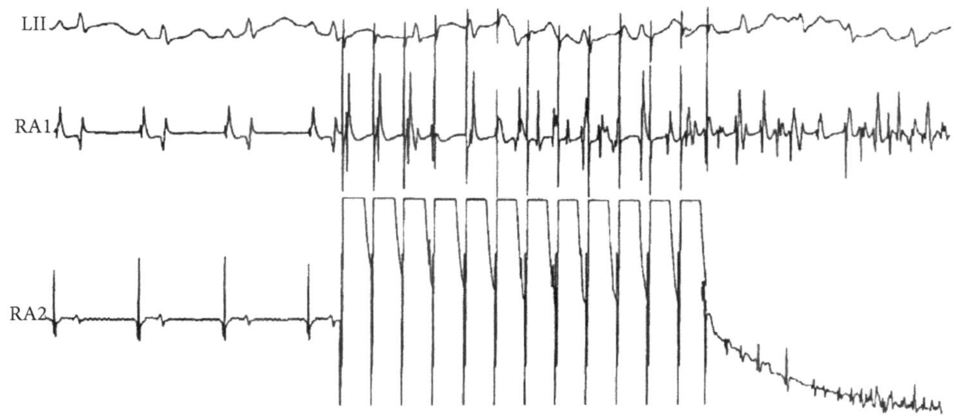

(b) Induced AF (burst pacing, ACh 100 μM)

FIGURE 1: Examples of sustained atrial fibrillation (AF) in the old rabbits. (a) Spontaneously occurring sustained AF initiated by an atrial premature depolarization (APD) following two ventricular premature depolarizations (VPDs). (b) Burst pacing-induced sustained AF.

the Oklahoma City Veterans Affairs Medical Center and University of Oklahoma Health Sciences Center. Six old (aged 4-6 years) and 9 young (aged 3-4 months) New Zealand white rabbits of either sex fed standard rabbit chow were studied. Each animal was anesthetized with ketamine/xylazine (35 mg/5 mg/kg) and subjected to a catheter-based electrophysiologicalstudy [10]. Standard electrocardiograms (Leads 1-aVF) were continuously monitored. After shaving the neck area, the right jugular vein was dissected and cannulated with a 4-French multielectrode catheter. Under electrographic control, the catheter was passed into the right atrium to record atrial potentials in conjunction with the ECG leads. After a 5-minute stabilization and determination of the mean sinus rate, atrial tachyarrhythmia susceptibility was tested by delivering bursts of stimuli (3–5 sec duration) at a high frequency (20 Hz) and voltage that was at least twice the diastolic pacing threshold. Burst pacing was delivered 3–10 times before and after the infusion of ACh in 3 incremental concentrations (10 μM, 100 μM, and 1 mM) at a rate of 1 mL/min. Nonsustained (<10 sec) and sustained (≥10 sec) arrhythmia occurrence was determined in response to burst pacing at baseline and with each of the 3 concentrations of ACh infusions for 2 minutes before initiating burst pacing. Rhythm disturbances were characterized from the ECG by their rate and duration and from the morphology of the recorded atrial electrograms (Figure 1).

2.2. Histological Studies. Portions of the atria and ventricles from the hearts fixed in formalin were prepared for histological study. Specimens were processed in paraffin-embedded histological sections cut along the long axis of the atria and ventricles. Sections were stained with hematoxylin-eosin and Masson's trichrome for detection of fibrosis. The degree of fibrosis was quantified on the basis of the following scale: 0, no fibrosis; 1+, stainable collagen adjacent to capillaries and/or between myocytes (excluding large vessels) less than half of myocyte diameter; 2+, greater than half to equal to myocyte diameter; 3+, greater than myocyte diameter or fibrosis with features of replacement.

2.3. Statistical Analysis. Data are expressed as mean ± standard deviation (SD). A standard t-test was used to compare

TABLE 1: Comparison of atrial fibrillation induction in old versus young rabbits.

Rabbit	Baseline	10 μM ACh	100 μM ACh	1 mM ACh
Old #1	0	0	0	0
Old #2	<1[a]	1 and 4[a]	10	118
Old #3	<1	2	15	11
Old #4	0	0	11	3
Old #5	0	0	<1	681
Old #6	0	0	<2	960
Young #1	<1[a]	0	0	0
Young #2	<1	0	0	0
Young #3	0	0	0	2
Young #4	0	0	0	0
Young #5	0	0	0	0
Young #6	<1[a]	0	0	4
Young #7	<1	0	0	0
Young #8	0	0	0	3
Young #9	0	0	0	0

Numbers represent the duration (in seconds) of atrial fibrillation or atrial tachycardia induced.
[a]Atrial tachycardia.

heart rates between young and old rabbits. Chi-square analysis (2 × 2 contingency table) followed by a two-tailed Fisher's exact was used to determine the difference in occurrence of a sustained arrhythmia (≥10 sec) for each rabbit at all concentrations of ACh infusion. A P value of <0.05 was considered statistically significant.

3. Results

In the baseline state, the mean heart rate for the old rabbits ($n = 6$) was 200 ± 23/min, compared to the young rabbits ($n = 9$) whose heart rate averaged 160 ± 13/min ($P = 0.003$). In addition, there were a significantly greater number of AF events in the old versus young rabbits (Table 1). There were more nonsustained (<10 sec) and sustained (≥10 sec) AF events in the old rabbits than the young rabbits. Specifically, in the old rabbits there were 13 nonsustained or sustained atrial tachyarrhythmias, either atrial tachycardia or AF induced in 24 induction attempts. On the other hand, the young rabbit group had only 4 such events in 36 induction attempts ($P = 0.0004$). As for sustained AF, there were 7 of 24 inductions in the old rabbits and 0 of 36 in the young rabbits ($P = 0.0009$). The average duration of AF in the old rabbits was 258 seconds. Figure 1 shows examples of the occurrence of spontaneous and pacing-induced AF in the old rabbits.

To determine whether atrial fibrosis was a factor in the differences in AF susceptibility between old and young rabbits, we examined histological sections of the atria in both groups. In order to quantitate the degree of fibrosis, a grading system was developed. In the sections evaluated in the young rabbits, fibrosis was graded as 0 in four sections of atria and ventricular tissues, whereas in the old rabbits the grades for the atria ranged from 0 in 4 sections to 1+ in 3 sections. In the ventricles fibrosis was graded as 1+ in one section, 2+ in two sections, and 3+ in 3 sections. Figures 2(a) and 2(b) show representative atrial sections from the young versus old rabbits, respectively. There was no significant fibrosis observed in the atria of either group. However, the old rabbits did demonstrate moderate to severe interstitial fibrosis as well as scar formation in the ventricles (Figure 2(d)). There was no significant fibrosis seen in the ventricular sections made from the young rabbits (Figure 2(c)).

4. Discussion

In the present study, two extraneous factors (ACh infusion and burst pacing) were used to initiate arrhythmias. Previous studies in ambulatory dogs with a propensity for inducing atrial tachyarrhythmias were based on the simultaneous interaction of the neural activity of both arms of the autonomic nervous system [11]. In this rabbit model, there was a significantly greater incidence of AF, particularly of the sustained (≥10 sec) form, in the old rabbits than in the young group. The young rabbits showed no evidence of sustained AF using the same protocol of ACh infusions that were effective in inducing AF in the old rabbits. Lee et al. [12] previously reported that 3-year-old rabbits, fed a standard chow, and a second comparably aged group fed a high cholesterol chow demonstrated a greater atrial tachyarrhythmia response to programmed stimulation and/or rapid atrial pacing than the 3-month-old rabbits fed a standard chow. The maximal duration of the atrial arrhythmias in this study was 30 seconds and consisted predominantly of atrial tachycardias. In the present study, infusion of incremental concentrations of ACh and burst pacing consistently induced sustained AF with a mean uninterrupted duration of 258 seconds (Table 1).

Clinical studies have shown that humans aged 60–80 years have diminished autonomic cardiovascular responses [13, 14]. We hypothesized that the extrinsic autonomic nervous system, including innervation from the brain and spinal cord, exerts inhibitory control of the intrinsic autonomic nervous system preventing the intrinsic nerves and ganglia on the heart from becoming independently hyperactive. On the other hand, denervation [15] or disconnection of the extrinsic from the intrinsic innervation [16] induces a hyperactive state of the intrinsic system with the development of AF. We have demonstrated previously that stimulation of the vagosympathetic trunks to simulate tonic levels of activation can prevent and/or suppress AF induced by hyperactive remodeling of the ganglionated plexi of the intrinsic autonomic nervous system. In the dog heart, AF has been shown to be directly associated with excessive release of cholinergic and adrenergic neurotransmitters, the former shortening the refractory period and the latter inducing triggered firing [17, 18]. In our previous study using ACh infusions in the rabbit with enhanced activation of $\beta 2$-adrenergic receptor, sustained atrial tachycardias were consistently evoked [10]. There is evidence in the present study for an increased level of sympathetic tone in the old rabbits whose mean heart rate was 200/min compared to the young rabbits with a rate of 160/min. As noted from our previous dog

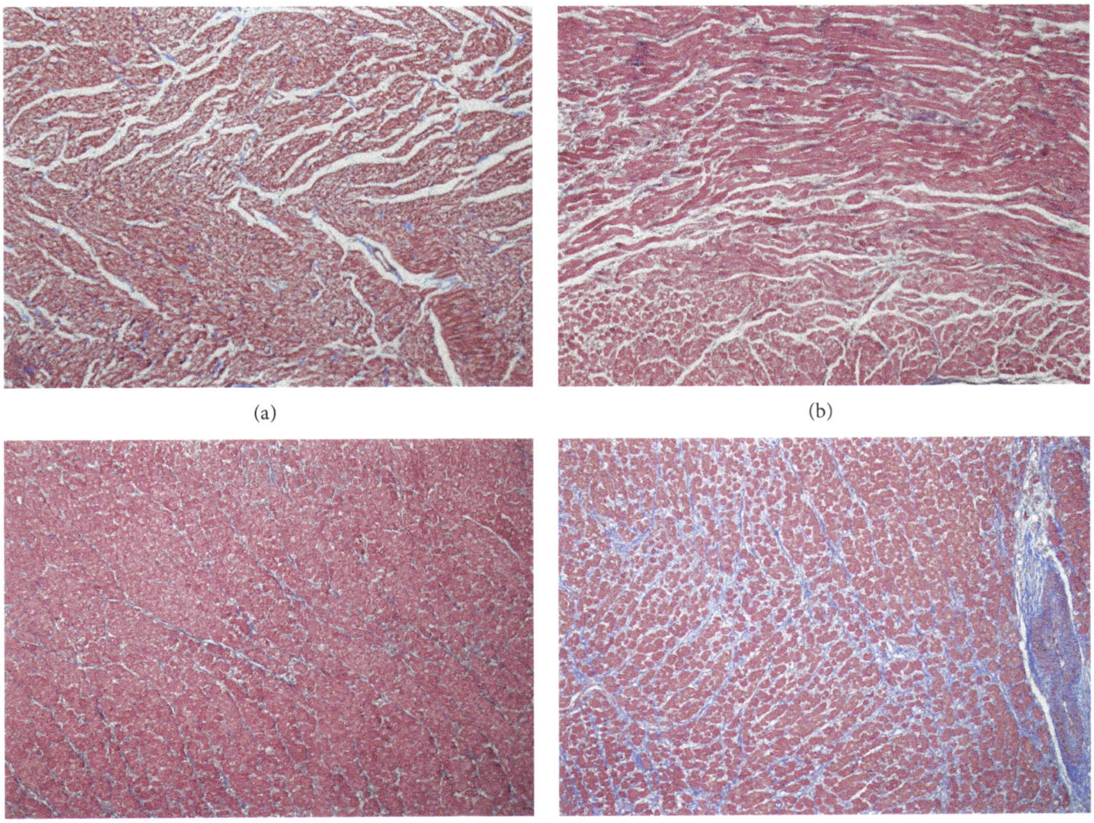

(a) (b) (c) (d)

FIGURE 2: Representative histological sections of atria and ventricles from old and young rabbits. (a) Atrial cross section from a young rabbit (3-4 months). (b) Atrial cross section from an old rabbit (4–6 years). Neither atrial section showed appreciable interstitial fibrosis. (c) Ventricular cross section from a young rabbit. (d) Ventricular cross section from an old rabbit. Note the marked interstitial fibrosis and scar compared to (c).

studies, ACh can activate neurons, which cause release of their neurotransmitters, in ganglionated plexi of the intrinsic autonomic nervous system [19]. These neurons have been shown to colocalize vesicles containing both cholinergic and adrenergic neurotransmitters [20], both of which are the major ingredients for initiation and maintenance of AF.

One of the first questions which arises when considering susceptibility to AF in old animals is the presence of atrial fibrosis. Whether there is a direct cause or effect relationship between atrial fibrosis and AF is still open to question. A histological study of lone AF patients found that 25% of patients did not have atrial fibrosis [21]. On the other hand, both clinical [22] and experimental [23] studies have associated atrial fibrosis development with structural heart disease or changes due to long term rapid ventricular pacing to induce heart failure, respectively. In the present study, we found no significant fibrosis in the atria of either old or young rabbits. However, our histological sections clearly showed moderate to severe interstitial fibrosis in the ventricles of the old rabbits but not in the young rabbits. Similar results were reported by Lee et al. [12] in old rabbit hearts, and, after providing several explanations such as 3-year-old rabbits may not be old enough (our rabbits were 4–6 years of age), they concluded that "atrial fibrosis may not play an important role in the induction of AF in rabbits with no significant structural heart disease. In addition, the increased incidence of AF as age increased may not solely be explained by atrial fibrosis." It should be mentioned that an experimental aged rat model did show AF associated with fibrosis [2]. This difference may be related to species differences.

Appropriate animal models for AF are problematic. Issues include changes in innervation, size of the heart, and differences in aging. Recent pressures in the United States and elsewhere have led to significant restrictions on use of the common canine model. Substitution with small rodents is difficult owing to their small cardiac size and notable differences in biological function from humans. These difficulties are even greater when there is a need to study the effect of aging. The telescoped life span of rodents is advantageous for aging research but may not reflect the pathophysiology of larger mammals. The present study presents evidence that the rabbit may represent a convenient intermediate species wherein such studies of aging are possible within a reasonable time frame and the pathophysiological changes in the heart are not insurmountable.

5. Conclusions

Using a relatively new experimental model, we have demonstrated that rabbits 4–6 years of age have an increased susceptibility to develop AF compared to the young rabbits. This was associated with evidence supportive of increased autonomic activity and was induced by the combination of ACh and burst pacing. Atrial fibrosis was not observed in the atria and could be ruled out as a potential explanation for the greater propensity for AF in the old rabbits. This rabbit model presents several advantages for the study of immunological issues that affect atrial or ventricular tachyarrhythmias.

Conflict of Interests

The authors have no conflict of interests to disclose.

Acknowledgments

This work was supported in part by grants from the Heart Rhythm Institute at the University of Oklahoma Health Sciences Center, the Helen and Will Webster Arrhythmia Research Fund of the University of Oklahoma Foundation, the Talley Research Award of the Harold Hamm Diabetes Center at the University of Oklahoma, an American Heart Association Postdoctoral Fellowship, and Veterans Affairs Merit Award.

References

[1] W. M. Feinberg, J. L. Blackshear, A. Laupacis, R. Kronmal, and R. G. Hart, "Prevalence, age distribution, and gender of patients with atrial fibrillation: analysis and implications," *Archives of Internal Medicine*, vol. 155, no. 5, pp. 469–473, 1995.

[2] H. Hayashi, C. Wang, Y. Miyauchi et al., "Aging-related increase to inducible atrial fibrillation in the rat model," *Journal of Cardiovascular Electrophysiology*, vol. 13, no. 8, pp. 801–808, 2002.

[3] T. Luo, C. X. Chang, X. Zhou, S. K. Gu, T. M. Jiang, and Y. M. Li, "Characterization of atrial histopathological and electrophysiological changes in a mouse model of aging," *International Journal of Molecular Medicine*, vol. 31, no. 1, pp. 138–146, 2013.

[4] E. P. Anyukhovsky, E. A. Sosunov, P. Chandra et al., "Age-associated changes in electrophysiologic remodeling: a potential contributor to initiation of atrial fibrillation," *Cardiovascular Research*, vol. 66, no. 2, pp. 353–363, 2005.

[5] P. M. Kistler, P. Sanders, S. P. Fynn et al., "Electrophysiologic and electroanatomic changes in the human atrium associated with age," *Journal of the American College of Cardiology*, vol. 44, no. 1, pp. 109–116, 2004.

[6] C. T. Sawin, A. Geller, P. A. Wolf et al., "Low serum thyrotropin concentrations as a risk factor for atrial fibrillation in older persons," *The New England Journal of Medicine*, vol. 331, no. 19, pp. 1249–1252, 1994.

[7] L. Frost, P. Vestergaard, and L. Mosekilde, "Hyperthyroidism and risk of atrial fibrillation or flutter: a population-based study," *Archives of Internal Medicine*, vol. 164, no. 15, pp. 1675–1678, 2004.

[8] A. R. Cappola, L. P. Fried, A. M. Arnold et al., "Thyroid status, cardiovascular risk, and mortality in older adults," *Journal of the American Medical Association*, vol. 295, no. 9, pp. 1033–1041, 2006.

[9] S. Stavrakis, X. Yu, E. Patterson et al., "Activating autoantibodies to the beta-1 adrenergic and M2 muscarinic receptors facilitate atrial fibrillation in patients with graves' hyperthyroidism," *Journal of the American College of Cardiology*, vol. 54, no. 14, pp. 1309–1316, 2009.

[10] H. Li, B. J. Scherlag, D. C. Kem et al., "Atrial tachycardia provoked in the presence of activating autoantibodies to beta2-adrenergic receptor in the rabbit," *Heart Rhythm*, vol. 10, no. 3, pp. 436–441, 2013.

[11] M. J. Shen, E.-K. Choi, A. Y. Tan et al., "Patterns of baseline autonomic nerve activity and the development of pacing-induced sustained atrial fibrillation," *Heart Rhythm*, vol. 8, no. 4, pp. 583–589, 2011.

[12] K.-T. Lee, C.-C. Hsieh, W.-C. Tsai et al., "Characteristics of atrial substrates for atrial tachyarrhythmias induced in aged and hypercholesterolemic rabbits," *Pacing and Clinical Electrophysiology*, vol. 35, no. 5, pp. 544–552, 2012.

[13] L. Kaijser and C. Sachs, "Autonomic cardiovascular responses in old age," *Clinical Physiology*, vol. 5, no. 4, pp. 347–357, 1985.

[14] C. Sachs, B. Hamberger, and L. Kaijser, "Cardiovascular responses and plasma catecholamines in old age," *Clinical Physiology*, vol. 5, no. 6, pp. 553–565, 1985.

[15] F. M. Smith, A. S. McGuirt, D. B. Hoover, J. A. Armour, and J. L. Ardell, "Chronic decentralization of the heart differentially remodels canine intrinsic cardiac neuron muscarinic receptors," *American Journal of Physiology*, vol. 281, no. 5, pp. H1919–H1930, 2001.

[16] L. W. Lo, B. J. Scherlag, H. Y. Chang, Y. J. Lin, S. A. Chen, and S. S. Po, "Long term proarrhythmia after parasympathetic denervation between extrinsic and intrinsic cardiac autonomic nervous system," *Heart Rhythm*, vol. 8, no. 5, pp. S264–S265, 2011.

[17] S. S. Po, B. J. Scherlag, W. S. Yamanashi et al., "Experimental model for paroxysmal atrial fibrillation arising at the pulmonary vein-atrial junctions," *Heart Rhythm*, vol. 3, no. 2, pp. 201–208, 2006.

[18] E. Patterson, S. S. Po, B. J. Scherlag, and R. Lazzara, "Triggered firing in pulmonary veins initiated by in vitro autonomic nerve stimulation," *Heart Rhythm*, vol. 2, no. 6, pp. 624–631, 2005.

[19] B. J. Scherlag, Y.-L. Hou, J. Lin et al., "An acute model for atrial fibrillation arising from a peripheral atrial site: evidence for primary and secondary triggers," *Journal of Cardiovascular Electrophysiology*, vol. 19, no. 5, pp. 519–527, 2008.

[20] A. Y. Tan, H. Li, S. Wachsmann-Hogiu, L. S. Chen, P.-S. Chen, and M. C. Fishbein, "Autonomic innervation and segmental muscular disconnections at the human pulmonary vein-atrial junction. Implications for catheter ablation of atrial-pulmonary vein junction," *Journal of the American College of Cardiology*, vol. 48, no. 1, pp. 132–143, 2006.

[21] A. Frustaci, C. Chimenti, F. Bellocci, E. Morgante, M. A. Russo, and A. Maseri, "Histological substrate of atrial biopsies in patients with lone atrial fibrillation," *Circulation*, vol. 96, no. 4, pp. 1180–1184, 1997.

[22] T. D. Pham and J. J. Fenoglio Jr., "Right atrial ultrastructure in chronic rheumatic heart disease," *International Journal of Cardiology*, vol. 1, no. 3-4, pp. 289–304, 1982.

[23] K. Shinagawa, Y.-F. Shi, J.-C. Tardif, T.-K. Leung, and S. Nattel, "Dynamic nature of atrial fibrillation substrate during development and reversal of heart failure in dogs," *Circulation*, vol. 105, no. 22, pp. 2672–2678, 2002.

16

Does Physical Activity Increase Life Expectancy?

C. D. Reimers,[1] G. Knapp,[2] and A. K. Reimers[3]

[1] *Klinik für Neurologie, Zentralklinik Bad Berka, Robert-Koch-Allee 9, 99438 Bad Berka, Germany*
[2] *Fakultät Statistik, Technische Universität Dortmund, 44221 Dortmund, Germany*
[3] *Sportwissenschaft, Universität Konstanz, Universitätsstraße 10, 78457 Konstanz, Germany*

Correspondence should be addressed to C. D. Reimers, c.d.reimers@t-online.de

Academic Editor: Iris Reuter

Physical activity reduces many major mortality risk factors including arterial hypertension, diabetes mellitus type 2, dyslipidemia, coronary heart disease, stroke, and cancer. All-cause mortality is decreased by about 30% to 35% in physically active as compared to inactive subjects. The purpose of this paper was to synthesize the literature on life expectancy in relation to physical activity. A systematic PubMed search on life expectancy in physically active and inactive individuals was performed. In addition, articles comparing life expectancy of athletes compared to that of nonathletes were reviewed. Results of 13 studies describing eight different cohorts suggest that regular physical activity is associated with an increase of life expectancy by 0.4 to 6.9 years. Eleven studies included confounding risk factors for mortality and revealed an increase in life expectancy by 0.4 to 4.2 years with regular physical activity. Eleven case control studies on life expectancy in former athletes revealed consistently greater life expectancy in aerobic endurance athletes but inconsistent results for other athletes. None of these studies considered confounding risk factors for mortality. In conclusion, while regular physical activity increases life expectancy, it remains unclear if high-intensity sports activities further increase life expectancy.

1. Introduction

The most important causes of death in Western industrialized countries are cardio- and cerebrovascular diseases and malignancies. For instance, in Germany in 2008, 68.6% of all women and 65.9% of all men died from these diseases. In contrast, the third most frequent cause of death are respiratory diseases which cause less than 10% of deaths each year (Table 1). Important risk factors for cardio- and cerebrovascular diseases include smoking, arterial hypertension, obesity, diabetes mellitus, and dyslipidemia along with atrial fibrillation for ischemic strokes [1, 2].

Regular physical activity reduces the risk of and/or improves many diseases and conditions including arterial hypertension, diabetes mellitus type 2, dyslipidemia, obesity, coronary heart disease, chronic heart failure [3, 4], and chronic obstructive pulmonary disease [4]. In addition, the risk of colon [3, 5], breast [4, 5], and possibly endometrial, lung, and pancreatic cancer is reduced [5] (Table 2).

The relative risk of death is approximately 20% to 35% lower in physically active and fit persons compared to that in inactive and unfit persons [6, 7]. Physical inactivity represents a major independent risk factor for mortality accounting for up to 10% of all deaths in the European region [3]. Hence, because a 40% lower mortality rate corresponds to an approximately 5-year higher life expectancy [8], one would expect an approximately 3.5- to 4.0-year higher life expectancy in physically active persons compared to that in inactive persons.

The purpose of this review was to synthesize the literature on life expectancy in relation to physical activity. Specifically, cohort studies on physically active and inactive subjects were reviewed to detect a possible difference in life expectancy between these subject groups. In addition, cohort studies on athletes and non-athletes were reviewed to detect a possible difference in life expectancy between these subject groups.

Table 1: Number of deaths (percentage of total number of deaths) for the three most frequent causes of death for women and men in Germany in 2008 [9].

	Women (per 100,000 persons/y)	Men (per 100,000 persons/y)
Total	467.3 (100.0%)	720.5 (100.0%)
Vascular diseases	186.4 (39.9%)	263.6 (36.6%)
Coronary heart disease	61.8 (13.2%)	117.4 (16.3%)
Strokes	35.8 (7.7%)	41.6 (5.8%)
Malignant tumors	134.0 (28.7%)	210.9 (29.3%)
Respiratory diseases	27.7 (5.9%)	53.3 (7.4%)

2. Method

To identify all relevant articles about cohort studies investigating the life expectancy of physically active versus inactive persons, a systematic literature search was conducted in the electronic bibliographical database PubMed (http://www.ncbi.nlm.nih.gov/pubmed/). We only searched for English-language peer-reviewed journal articles using the search terms "(life expectancy OR longevity) AND (physical activity OR exercise OR sport)" (last update January 3, 2012). A total of 1,932 articles were found. Using the abstracts and/or titles, forty-one of these articles were identified as cohort studies comparing mortality and/or life expectancy of physically active and inactive persons. However, of these, only 13 articles presented detailed data on life expectancy for both groups.

Subsequently, a search was performed using the terms "(life expectancy OR longevity) AND athlete" to find articles on life expectancy in (former) athletes. Sixty-six articles were found. Additional publications were identified using the search term "(life expectancy OR longevity) AND (physical activity OR exercise OR sport)." Of all these articles, 21 articles investigated mortality and/or life expectancy of (former) athletes. Eleven of these articles presented detailed data on life expectancy of athletes compared to that of a control group.

The remaining life expectancy for physically active and inactive individuals or the difference in remaining life expectancy between the two groups, respectively, were reported in the articles. However, the attained ages of subject groups differed between studies. Because the differences of remaining life expectancies cannot be assumed to be independent from the attained age, we report the results stratified for attained age. Within each stratum of attained age, the results were presented for both sexes.

Only five articles [16–20] reported confidence intervals for the difference in remaining life expectancies between groups. In four articles [16, 18–20], a parametric bootstrap procedure was used, and in one publication [17] a nonparametric maximum likelihood approach was used. Consequently, we did not combine the results in a meta-analysis model.

Because a meta-analysis model was not appropriate, all data found in the literature search were reported despite some overlaps between the cohort studies. For instance, Jonker et al. [18] and Nusselder et al. [19] used data from the Framingham Heart Study and Paffenbarger et al. [21–24] used data from the Harvard Alumni cohort. While most studies reported results based on multivariate life-table analysis, the studies by Menotti et al. [25] and Pekkanen et al. [26] only reported the results of gained life expectancies for the cohorts based on classical survival analysis. Additionally, the study of Pekkanen et al. [26] reported the survival rate of men aged 40 to 65 years in the following 20 years and not the total life expectancy.

3. Results

Thirteen cohort studies presented data on life expectancy in physically active individuals compared to that in physically inactive control subjects (Table 3). All studies reported a higher life expectancy in physically active subjects, ranging from 0.43 to 6.9 additional years (mean ± one standard deviation, men: 2.9 ± 1.3 years, women: 3.9 ± 1.8 years). Eleven studies considered confounding factors that could affect life expectancy, such as body mass index, blood pressure, diabetes mellitus, dyslipidemia, cardiovascular and lung diseases, cancer, smoking, or alcohol consumption [16–25, 27]. The additional life expectancy in physically active compared to inactive persons in these studies ranged between 0.43 and 4.21 years (2.7 ± 1.1 years). The physically most active groups, included in the estimations of life expectancy, participated in moderate to high leisure time [16, 27–29] or leisure time and all-day activities [17–25].

The median increase of life expectancy of men and women in the eight studies presenting data on both sexes amounted to 3.7 years each. Physical activity during leisure time seems to increase life expectancy more effectively than total physical activity (all-day, professional, or leisure time activity altogether; professional physical activity alone has not been studied): 3.4 added years due to total activities and 4.7 added years (median values) due to leisure time activities in women, 1.9 and 3.9 added years, respectively, in men. The number of studies, however, is too low for a statistical analysis. Furthermore, the description of the amount of physical activity in the active and inactive groups are too heterogeneous for any statistical correlation between the amount of activity and the added years of life.

The eleven case control studies on life expectancy of athletes, mostly elite athletes (Table 4), reported a mean life expectancy that was between 5.0 years lower and 8.0 years higher than that of the nonathlete control groups. Aerobic endurance sports resulted on average in a 4.3 to 8.0 years higher life expectancy and team sports activities on average in a 5.0 years lower to about 5 years higher life expectancy compared to that for normal physical activity. Only one study presented data on strength sports and reported a slightly higher life expectancy compared to that for normal physical activity. None of these studies considered any confounding factor that could affect life expectancy.

TABLE 2: Preventive effects of regular physical activity on major risk factors for cardio- and cerebrovascular diseases and cancer.

Author(s)	Risk factor	Effect of regular physical activity on the risk factor in healthy subjects
Adami et al. [3], Halle and Schoenberg [10], Warburton et al. [6], Warburton et al. [11]	Colon cancer	Incidence −30% to −40%
Adami et al. [3], Monninkhof et al. [12], Warburton et al. [6]	Breast cancer	Incidence −20% to −50%
Walker et al. [13], Warburton et al. [11]	Type 2 diabetes mellitus	Incidence −28% to −59%
G. A. Kelley and K. S. Kelley [14]	Dyslipidemia	HDL cholesterol +11%
Pedersen and Saltin [4]	Arterial hypertension	Systolic and diastolic blood pressure −3.84/−2.58 mmHg
Pedersen and Saltin [4]	Obesity	Increased chance to maintain body weight
Warburton et al. [11], Reimers et al. [15]	Stroke	Incidence −27% to −40%

4. Discussion

The purpose of this review was to synthesize the literature on life expectancy in relation to physical activity. Being physically active indeed appears to be associated with a higher life expectancy. Samitz et al. [7] as well as Warburton et al. [11] reported a mean reduction of mortality of 31% to 35% in persons who participate in regular leisure-time or daily life physical activity compared to that in inactive persons. Assuming a 40% lower mortality corresponding to a 5-year higher life expectancy [8], regular physical activity should increase mean life expectancy by approximately (31% to 35%)/40% × 5 years or by 3.9 to 4.4 years. Indeed, the few articles that presented data on life expectancy in physically active individuals reported a 0.43- to 6.9-year higher life expectancy. High-quality studies considering confounding factors that could affect mortality reported a 0.43- to 4.21-years higher life expectancy in physically active compared to inactive persons. The wide range of years added cannot be explained based on the published data.

The studies that standardized extended life estimates for confounding factors [16, 18–25, 27] virtually calculated a net gain in life expectancy by being physically active. However, the actual increase in life expectancy should be much higher because of favorable effects of physical activity on other risk factors for mortality such as arterial hypertension, glucose and lipid metabolism, coronary heart disease, stroke, or malignancies (Table 1). In fact, nonsmoking, normal weight, and physically fit men live on average 12 years (95% confidence interval, 8.6 to 14.6 years) longer than smoking, overweight, and physically unfit control subjects [41]. Subjects who never smoked, follow a healthy diet, are adequately physically active, and consume only moderate alcohol have a mean life expectancy that is 11.1 years longer than those who practice none of these healthy life behaviors [42].

The mechanisms underlying the net effect of physical activity are speculative and include reduction of triglyceride and apolipoprotein B concentrations, increase of high-density lipoproteins and tissue plasminogen activator activity, and reduction of coronary artery calcium resulting in reduced risks of vascular diseases, which carry the strongest mortality risk [43]. In addition, regular physical activity increases the endurance of cells and tissues to oxidative stress, vascularization, and energy metabolism [44].

According to the results of the meta-analysis on all-cause mortality in relation to physical activity performed by Samitz et al. [7], vigorous physical activity (>6 metabolic equivalents (MET)) reduces mortality slightly, but this reduction is significantly more pronounced than that for moderate activity (3–6 MET).

A greater life expectancy is not associated with more years of being frail and depending on assistance. In contrary, Nusselder et al. [20] reported a gain of disability-free years of life with a higher life expectancy.

The few data available on life expectancy in athletes who were much more physically active than the average individual are inconclusive. All studies proved an increased life expectancy in endurance athletes ranging between 2.8 to 8.0 added years. This gain is probably higher than that found for persons performing vigorous physical activity in the cohort studies. In team sports and other sports disciplines, life expectancy may fall below or be above that of the control groups. However, data on health behaviors of these athletes other than their physical activity during their active sports career such as smoking, food, and alcohol consumption are not available. Thus, the effect of elite sports activities on life expectancy warrants further investigation.

In summary, as expected from numerous prospective cohort studies on all-cause mortality in physically active and physically inactive persons, estimates on life expectancy in relation to physical activity indicate additional years of life in active subjects: the conservative estimate of the net increase in life expectancy with physical activity is about 2–4 years but presumably even greater because of the positive influence of physical activity on major risk factors for mortality.

TABLE 3: Cohort studies comparing the life expectancy of physically active and inactive persons.

Sex	Age (class) at start of followup	Authors	Country	Number of individuals, duration of follow-up	Estimate additional years of life (95% CI) (years)	Activity of the "active" group	Activity of the "inactive" group	Confounding factors
Women	30	Fraser and Shavlik [17]	USA	#12 y	2.19 (0.92–3.45)*	At least 3 times per week vigorous all-day or sports activities ≥ 15 min.	Less than 3 times per week intensive all-day and sportive activities ≥15 min.	Vegetarian/nonvegetarian, high/low nut consumption, body mass index, never/past smoker, hormone replacement therapy
	30	Wen et al. [27]	Taiwan	216.910 8.05 ± 4.02 y	3.67 84.08 versus 87.75	Very vigorous physical activity (≥25.5 MET·h/week) during leisure time	Inactivity (<3.75 MET·h/week) during leisure time	Age, sex, education, physical work, smoking, alcohol consumption, diabetes mellitus, arterial hypertension, cancer, fasting glucose, systolic blood pressure, total cholesterol, body mass index
	45	Bélanger et al. [28]	Canada	#2 y	6.9 81.7 versus 88.6	≥1.5 kcal/kg/d energy expenditure during leisure time	<1.5 kcal/kg/d energy expenditure during leisure time	
	50	Jonker et al. [18]	USA (Framingham Heart Study)	2.813 12 y	3.7 (2.6–4.9) 82.3 versus 86.0	High physical activity level (>33 METs/d)	Low physical activity level (<30 METs/d)	Age, education, smoking, marital status, cardiovascular and lung diseases, cancer, left ventricular hypertrophy, arthritis, ankle edema, total cholesterol, familial history of diabetes mellitus
	50	Nusselder et al. [20]	The Netherlands	1.447 2 y	1.8 (0.5–2.7) 76.5 versus 78.3	Walking, biking, gardening, sports >17.33 METs/week	Walking, biking, gardening, sports <12 METs/week	Age, sex, education, cardiovascular disease, cancer, COPD, arthritis, back complaints, neurological diseases

Table 3: Continued.

Sex	Age (class) at start of followup	Authors	Country	Number of individuals, duration of follow-up	Estimate additional years of life (95% CI) (years)	Activity of the "active" group	Activity of the "inactive" group	Confounding factors
	50	Nusselder et al. [19]	USA (Framingham Heart Study)	2.873 12 y	3.4 (2.3–4.5) 82.7 versus 86.1	High physical activity level (>33 METs/d)	Low physical activity level (<30 METs/d)	Age, sex, education, marital status, smoking, body mass index, blood pressure, cancer, diabetes mellitus, left ventricular hypertrophy, ankle edema, any pulmonary disease, smoking
	65	Ferrucci et al. [29]	USA	5.215 6 y	Nonsmoker: 5.7 77.7 versus 83.4 Smoker: 4.2 76.1 versus 80.3	High physical activity (gardening, walking, vigorous exercise) each once per week or several times per month *or* one of these activities several times per week and another activity once per week or several times per month	Activities as in the active group at most once per month	
Men	30	Fraser and Shavlik [17]	USA	#12 y	2.1 (0.4–3.9)*	At least 3 times per week vigorous all-day or sports activities ≥15 min.	Less than 3 times per week intense all-day and sportive activities ≥15 min.	Vegetarian/nonvegetarian, high/low nut consumption, body mass index, never/past smoker, hormone replacement therapy
	30	Wen et al. [27]	Taiwan	199.265 8.05 ± 4.02 y	4.21 80.37 versus 84.58	Very vigorous physical activities (≥25.5 MET·h/week) during leisure time	Inactivity (<3.75 MET·h/week) during leisure time	Age, sex, education, physical work, smoking, drinking, diabetes mellitus, arterial hypertension, history of cancer, fasting blood glucose, systolic blood pressure, total cholesterol, body mass index
	35–39	Paffenbarger et al. [21]	USA (Harvard Alumni)	16.936 16 y	1.5*	Physical activities (walking, climbing stairs, sports) ≥2.000 kcal/week	Physical activities (walking, climbing stairs, sports) <2.000 kcal/week	Age, cigarette smoking, arterial hypertension, body mass index, age of parental death

Table 3: Continued.

Sex	Age (class) at start of followup	Authors	Country	Number of individuals, duration of follow-up	Estimate additional years of life (95% CI) (years)	Activity of the "active" group	Activity of the "inactive" group	Confounding factors
	35–39	Paffenbarger et al. [22]	USA (Harvard Alumni)	16.936 12–16 y	2.51*	Physical activities (walking, climbing stairs, sports) ≥2.000 kcal/week	Physical activities (walking, climbing stairs, sports) <500 kcal/week	Age, cigarette smoking, arterial hypertension, body mass index, age of parental death
	40–59	Menotti et al. [25]	Italy	1.712 40 y	1.6*	Physically active	Sedentary	Age, family history of both parents, mean blood pressure, serum cholesterol, mid-arm circumference, forced exspiratory volume, chronic diseases (cardiovascular, diabetes mellitus, cancer), corneal arcus, xanthelasma, body mass index
	45	Bélanger et al. [28]	Canada	#2 y	3.9 76.9 versus 80.8	≥1.5 kcal/kg/d energy expenditure during leisure time	<1.5 kcal/kg/d energy expenditure during leisure time	
	45–54	Paffenbarger et al. [23]	USA (Harvard Alumni)	10.269 8 y	0.43*	Physical activities ≥2.000 kcal/week	Physical activities <2.000 kcal/week	Age, cigarette smoking, arterial hypertension, overweight, early parental death
	45–54	Paffenbarger et al. [24]	USA (Harvard Alumni)	14.785 11 y	1.78*	Physical activity (walking, stair climbing, sports, or recreational activities) increased from <1.500 to ≥1.500 kcal/week	Physical activity (walking, stair climbing, sports, or recreational activities) continuing <1.500 kcal/week	Age, cigarette smoking, arterial hypertension, overweight, alcohol consumption, early parental death, chronic diseases
	50	Jonker et al. [18]	USA (Framingham Heart Study)	2.396 12 y	4.1 (2.8–5.4) 75.3 versus 79.4	High physical activity level (>30 METs/d)	Low physical activity level (<30 METs/d)	Age, education, smoking, marital status, cardiovascular and lung diseases, cancer, left ventricular hypertrophy, arthritis, ankle edema, total cholesterol, familial history of diabetes mellitus

Table 3: Continued.

Sex	Age (class) at start of followup	Authors	Country	Number of individuals, duration of follow-up	Estimate additional years of life (95% CI) (years)	Activity of the "active" group	Activity of the "inactive" group	Confounding factors
	50	Nusselder et al. [20]	The Netherlands	1.519 2 y	2.9 (0.9–4.3) 74.8 versus 76.7	Walking, biking, gardening, sports >17.33 METs/week	Walking, biking, gardening, sports <12 METs/week	Age, sex, education, cardiovascular disease, cancer, chronic obstructive pulmonary disease, arthritis, back complaints, neurological diseases
	50	Nusselder et al. [19]	USA (Framingham Heart Study)	2.336 12 y	3.5 (2.5–4.6) 76.4 versus 80.0	High physical activity level (>33 METs/d)	Low physical activity level (<30 METs/d)	Age, sex, education, marital status, body mass index, blood pressure, cancer, diabetes mellitus, left ventricular hypertrophy, ankle edema, any pulmonary disease, smoking
	50	Byberg et al. [16]	Sweden	2.205 35 y	2.3 (1.3–3.3)*	Regularly hard physical training or competitive sport or any active recreational sports or heavy gardening at least 3 hours every week	Spending most of the time reading, watching TV, going to the cinema, or engaging in other, mostly sedentary activities	Smoking, weight and height, alcohol use, obesity, diabetes mellitus, musculoskeletal, neurological, or psychiatric disorders, blood pressure, antihypertensive drugs, total serum cholesterol, educational level, socioeconomic group
	65	Ferrucci et al. [29]	USA	3.389 6 y	Nonsmoker: 5.2 76.0 versus 81.2 Smoker: 3.4 74.5 versus 77.9	High physical activity (gardening, walking, vigorous exercise) each once per week or several times per month *or* one of these activities several times per week and another activity once per week or several times per month	Activities as in the active group maximally once per month	

*Total life expectancy not presented, #number of individuals not differentiated between men and women.

Table 4: Case control studies presenting life expectancy of (former) athletes compared to that of control subjects.

Author(s)	Type of sports	Reduction/increase in life expectancy (y)
Prout [30]	Endurance sports (college rowers from Harvard and Yale)	+6.3
Sarna et al. [31]	Endurance sports (long distance running, cross-country skiing)	+5.7
Karvonen [32], Karvonen et al. [33]	Endurance sports (cross-country skiing)	+2.8 to +4.3
Sanchis-Gomar et al. [34]	Endurance sports (Tour de France cyclists)	+8.0
Sarna et al. [31], Sarna and Kaprio [35]	Power sports (throwing sports, wrestling, weight lifting, boxing)	+1.6
Sarna et al. [31], Sarna and Kaprio [35]	Team sports (ice hockey, soccer, basketball, other outdoor sports)	+4.0
Abel and Kruger [36]	Team sports (baseball)	−5.0
Abel and Kruger [37]	Team sports (baseball)	+4 to 5
Kuss et al. [38]	Team sports (German international soccer players)	−1.9 J. (+0.6 to −3.2)
Hudec et al. [39]	Various sports disciplines	−0.38
Rook [40]	Various sports disciplines	+1.03

Abbreviations

CI: Confidence interval
COPD: Chronic obstructive pulmanry disease
d: Day
h: Hour(s)
MET: Metabolic equivalent value (1 MET = 1 kcal per h per kg of bodyweight)
Min.: Minute(s)
TV: Television
vs: Versus
y: Year(s).

References

[1] S. E. Straus, S. R. Majumdar, and F. A. McAlister, "New evidence for stroke prevention: scientific review," *Journal of the American Medical Association*, vol. 288, no. 11, pp. 1388–1395, 2002.

[2] S. Ebrahim, F. Taylor, K. Ward, A. Beswick, M. Burke, and G. Davey Smith, "Multiple risk factor interventions for primary prevention of coronary heart disease," *Cochrane Database of Systematic Reviews*, vol. 1, Article ID CD001561, 2011.

[3] P. E. Adami, A. Negro, N. Lala, and P. Martelletti, "The role of physical activity in the prevention and treatment of chronic diseases," *Clinica Terapeutica*, vol. 161, no. 6, pp. 537–541, 2010.

[4] B. K. Pedersen and B. Saltin, "Evidence for prescribing exercise as therapy in chronic disease," *Scandinavian Journal of Medicine and Science in Sports*, vol. 16, no. 1, pp. 3–63, 2006.

[5] C. M. Ulrich, J. Wiskemann, and K. Steindorf, "Physiologic and molecular mechanisms linking physical activity to cancer risk and progression," *Bundesgesundheitsblatt Gesundheitsforschung Gesundheitsschutz*, vol. 55, no. 1, pp. 3–9, 2012.

[6] D. E. R. Warburton, C. W. Nicol, and S. S. D. Bredin, "Health benefits of physical activity: the evidence," *CMAJ*, vol. 174, no. 6, pp. 801–809, 2006.

[7] G. Samitz, M. Egger, and M. Zwahlen, "Domains of physical activity and all-cause mortality: systematic review and dose-response meta-analysis of cohort studies," *International Journal of Epidemiology*, vol. 40, no. 5, Article ID dyr112, pp. 1382–1400, 2011.

[8] B. Farahmand, G. Broman, U. De Faire, D. Vågerö, and A. Ahlbom, "Golf: a game of life and death—reduced mortality in Swedish golf players," *Scandinavian Journal of Medicine and Science in Sports*, vol. 19, no. 3, pp. 419–424, 2009.

[9] E. Gaber and M. Wildner, "Heft 52—Sterblichkeit, Todesursachen und regionale Unterschiede," in *Gesundheitsberichterstattung des Bundes*, E. Gaber and T. Ziese, Eds., Robert Koch-Institut, Berlin, Germany, 2011.

[10] M. Halle and M. H. Schoenberg, "Physical activity in the prevention and treatment of colorectal carcinoma," *Deutsches Ärzteblatt*, vol. 106, no. 44, pp. 722–727, 2009.

[11] D. E. R. Warburton, S. Charlesworth, A. Ivey, L. Nettlefold, and S. S. D. Bredin, "A systematic review of the evidence for Canada's Physical Activity Guidelines for Adults," *International Journal of Behavioral Nutrition and Physical Activity*, vol. 7, article 39, 2010.

[12] E. M. Monninkhof, S. G. Elias, F. A. Vlems et al., "Physical activity and breast cancer: a systematic review," *Epidemiology*, vol. 18, no. 1, pp. 137–157, 2007.

[13] K. Z. Walker, K. O'Dea, M. Gomez, S. Girgis, and R. Colagiuri, "Diet and exercise in the prevention of diabetes," *Journal of Human Nutrition and Dietetics*, vol. 23, no. 4, pp. 344–352, 2010.

[14] G. A. Kelley and K. S. Kelley, "Aerobic exercise and HDL2-C: a meta-analysis of randomized controlled trials," *Atherosclerosis*, vol. 184, no. 1, pp. 207–215, 2006.

[15] C. D. Reimers, G. Knapp, A. K. Reimers, and B. Griewing, "Physical activity and stroke," *Aktuelle Neurologie*. In press.

[16] L. Byberg, H. Melhus, R. Gedeborg et al., "Total mortality after changes in leisure time physical activity in 50 year old men: 35 Year follow-up of population based cohort," *British Journal of Sports Medicine*, vol. 43, no. 7, artice 482, 2009.

[17] G. E. Fraser and D. J. Shavlik, "Ten years of life is it a matter of choice?" *Archives of Internal Medicine*, vol. 161, no. 13, pp. 1645–1652, 2001.

[18] J. T. Jonker, C. De Laet, O. H. Franco, A. Peeters, J. Mackenbach, and W. J. Nusselder, "Physical activity and life expectancy with and without diabetes: life table analysis of the Framingham Heart Study," *Diabetes Care*, vol. 29, no. 1, pp. 38–43, 2006.

[19] W. J. Nusselder, O. H. Franco, A. Peeters, and J. P. MacKenbach, "Living healthier for longer: comparative effects of three heart-healthy behaviors on life expectancy with and without cardiovascular disease," *BMC Public Health*, vol. 9, article 487, 2009.

[20] W. J. Nusselder, C. W. N. Looman, O. H. Franco, A. Peeters, A. S. Slingerland, and J. P. Mackenbach, "The relation between non-occupational physical activity and years lived with and without disability," *Journal of Epidemiology and Community Health*, vol. 62, no. 9, pp. 823–828, 2008.

[21] R. S. Paffenbarger, R. T. Hyde, C. C. Hsieh, and A. L. Wing, "Physical activity, other life-style patterns, cardiovascular disease and longevity," *Acta Medica Scandinavica*, vol. 220, no. 711, pp. 85–91, 1986.

[22] R. S. Paffenbarger, R. T. Hyde, A. L. Wing, and C. C. Hsieh, "Physical activity, all-cause mortality, and longevity of college alumni," *The New England Journal of Medicine*, vol. 314, no. 10, pp. 605–613, 1986.

[23] R. S. Paffenbarger, R. T. Hyde, A. L. Wing, I. M. Lee, D. L. Jung, and J. B. Kampert, "The association of changes in physical-activity level and other lifestyle characteristics with mortality among men," *The New England Journal of Medicine*, vol. 328, no. 8, pp. 538–545, 1993.

[24] R. S. Paffenbarger, J. B. Kampert, I. M. Lee, R. T. Hyde, R. W. Leung, and A. L. Wing, "Changes in physical activity and other lifeway patterns influencing longevity," *Medicine and Science in Sports and Exercise*, vol. 26, no. 7, pp. 857–865, 1994.

[25] A. Menotti, M. Lanti, G. Maiani, and D. Kromhout, "Determinants of longevity and all-cause mortality among middle-aged men. Role of 48 personal characteristics in a 40-year follow-up of Italian Rural Areas in the Seven Countries Study," *Aging*, vol. 18, no. 5, pp. 394–406, 2006.

[26] J. Pekkanen, B. Marti, and A. Nissinen, "Reduction of premature mortality by high physical activity: a 20-year follow-up of middle-aged Finnish men," *The Lancet*, vol. 1, no. 8548, pp. 1473–1477, 1987.

[27] C. P. Wen, J. P. M. Wai, M. K. Tsai et al., "Minimum amount of physical activity for reduced mortality and extended life expectancy: a prospective cohort study," *The Lancet*, vol. 378, no. 9798, pp. 1244–1253, 2011.

[28] A. Bélanger, L. Martel, J. M. Berthelot, and R. Wilkins, "Gender differences in disability-free life expectancy for selected risk factors and chronic conditions in Canada," *Journal of Women and Aging*, vol. 14, no. 1-2, pp. 61–83, 2002.

[29] L. Ferrucci, G. Izmirlian, S. Leveille et al., "Smoking, physical activity, and active life expectancy," *American Journal of Epidemiology*, vol. 149, no. 7, pp. 645–653, 1999.

[30] C. Prout, "Life expectancy of college oarsmen," *JAMA*, vol. 220, no. 13, pp. 1709–1711, 1972.

[31] S. Sarna, T. Sahi, M. Koskenvuo, and J. Kaprio, "Increased life expectancy of world class male athletes," *Medicine and Science in Sports and Exercise*, vol. 25, no. 2, pp. 237–244, 1993.

[32] M. J. Karvonen, "Endurance sports, longevity, and health," *Annals of the New York Academy of Sciences*, vol. 301, pp. 653–655, 1977.

[33] M. J. Karvonen, H. Klemola, J. Virkajarvi, and A. Kekkonen, "Longevity of endurance skiers," *Medicine and Science in Sports and Exercise*, vol. 6, no. 1, pp. 49–51, 1974.

[34] F. Sanchis-Gomar, G. Olaso-Gonzalez, D. Corella, M. C. Gomez-Cabrera, and J. Vina, "Increased average longevity among the Tour de France cyclists," *International Journal of Sports Medicine*, vol. 32, no. 8, pp. 644–647, 2011.

[35] S. Sarna and J. Kaprio, "Life expectancy of former elite athletes," *Sports Medicine*, vol. 17, no. 3, pp. 149–151, 1994.

[36] E. L. Abel and M. L. Kruger, "The longevity of baseball hall of famers compared to other players," *Death Studies*, vol. 29, no. 10, pp. 959–963, 2005.

[37] E. L. Abel and M. L. Kruger, "Longevity of major league baseball players," *Research in Sports Medicine*, vol. 13, no. 1, pp. 1–5, 2005.

[38] O. Kuss, A. Kluttig, and K. H. Greiser, "Longevity of soccer players: an investigation of all German internationals from 1908 to 2006," *Scandinavian Journal of Medicine and Science in Sports*, vol. 21, no. 6, pp. e260–e265, 2011.

[39] A. Hudec, E. Mahoney, H. J. Montoye, H. Olson, and W. D. van Huss, "Study of the longevity and morbidity of college athletes," *JAMA*, vol. 162, no. 12, pp. 1132–1134, 1956.

[40] A. ROOK, "An investigation into the longevity of Cambridge sportsmen," *British Medical Journal*, vol. 1, no. 4865, pp. 773–777, 1954.

[41] C. D. Lee, X. Sui, S. P. Hooker, J. R. Hébert, and S. N. Blair, "Combined impact of lifestyle on cancer mortality in men," *Annals of Epidemiology*, vol. 21, no. 10, pp. 749–754, 2011.

[42] E. S. Ford, G. Zhao, J. Tsai, and C. Li, "Low-Risk lifestyle behaviors and all-cause mortality: findings from the national health and nutrition examination survey III mortality study," *American Journal of Public Health*, vol. 101, no. 10, pp. 1922–1929, 2011.

[43] H. M. Ahmed, M. J. Blaha, K. Nasir, J. J. Rivera, and R. S. Blumenthal, "Effects of physical activity on cardiovascular disease," *American Journal of Cardiology*, vol. 109, no. 2, pp. 288–295, 2012.

[44] Z. Radak, N. Hart, L. Sarga et al., "Exercise plays a preventive role against Alzheimer's disease," *Journal of Alzheimer's Disease*, vol. 20, no. 3, pp. 777–783, 2010.

17

Physical Mistreatment in Persons with Alzheimer's Disease

Carla VandeWeerd,[1] Gregory J. Paveza,[2] Margaret Walsh,[3] and Jaime Corvin[4]

[1] *The Harrell Center for The Study of Family Violence, Department of Community and Family Health, College of Public Health, University of South Florida, 13301 Bruce B. Downs Boulevard, MDC 56, Tampa, FL 33612, USA*
[2] *School of Health and Human Services, Southern Connecticut State University, 501 Crescent Street, Lang House, New Haven, CT 06515, USA*
[3] *Department of Community and Family Health, College of Public Health, University of South Florida, 13301 Bruce B. Downs Boulevard, MDC 56, Tampa, FL 33612, USA*
[4] *Department of Global Health, College of Public Health, University of South Florida, 13301 Bruce B. Downs Boulevard, MDC 56, Tampa, FL 33612, USA*

Correspondence should be addressed to Carla VandeWeerd; cvdwe@hotmail.com

Academic Editor: Karl Rosengren

Physical mistreatment has been estimated to affect 2 million older persons each year and dramatically affects health outcomes. While researchers have attempted to examine risk factors for specific forms of abuse, many have been able to focus on only victim or perpetrator characteristics, or a limited number of psychosocial variables at any one time. Additionally, data on risk factors for subgroups such as persons with Alzheimer's disease who may have heightened and/or unique risk profiles has also been limited. This paper examines risk for physical violence in caregiver/patient dyads who participated in the Aggression and Violence in Community-Based Alzheimer's Families Grant. Data were collected via in-person interview and mailed survey and included demographics as well as measures of violence, physical and emotional health, and health behaviors. Logistic regression analysis indicated that caregivers providing care to elders with high levels of functional impairment or dementia symptoms, or who had alcohol problems, were more likely to use violence as a conflict resolution strategy, as were caregivers who were providing care to elders who used violence against them. By contrast, caregivers with high self-esteem were less likely to use violence as a conflict resolution strategy. Significant interaction effects were also noted.

1. Introduction

While child abuse has been recognized and studied in the literature in depth, in the past 30 years researchers have begun to recognize the vulnerability of older adults to this issue and to increase the scope of abuse research to include the study of mistreatment in older persons. Mistreatment of older adults has been associated with age and gender of victim [1–6] with the oldest old and women found to be at significant risk. It has been linked to domestic violence theories with spouses often found to be the most likely perpetrators [7–9]. Heightened risk has been linked to increased stress, with caregivers financial [10–12] or emotional dependence [9, 13–15], marital discord, and financial difficulties [16] increasing the likelihood that abuse will happen.

Caregiver and care receiver isolation have also been associated with elder mistreatment [15, 17–20], as have inadequate exchange issues such as violence by care recipients [21–27] and poor caregiver/care receiver relationships [22, 26, 28–30]. Caregiver psychopathology such as substance abuse, depression [9, 31–36], and caregiver emotional problems [29, 31, 36, 37] have also been linked [36, 38, 39]. Care receiver cognitive impairment has recently received attention as a risk factor for elder mistreatment [23, 26, 40–46].

Physical abuse involves acts of violence that may result in pain, injury, impairment, or disease [22, 47]. Physical mistreatment dramatically affects the lives of older adults and it has been estimated to affect as many as 2 million [48]. Further it is estimated that 2–10% of older adults may be victims of abuse, with only 1 out of every 14 incidents reported [49]. While researchers have attempted to look for risk factors of specific forms of mistreatment such as physical abuse [11, 12, 21, 50–52] many have been able to utilize only victim or perpetrator characteristics, or to focus on a limited number of psychosocial indicators at any one time. The ability to study subgroups of older adults who might be at increased risk for elder mistreatment as a result of special needs has also been limited. While researchers have begun examining subgroups, such as persons with dementia who may have increased risk for physical mistreatment as result of the etiology of their disease [42, 53, 54], the relationship between elder mistreatment and persons with Alzheimer's Disease (AD) has been largely understudied as a result of difficulties in finding and accessing these populations on a large scale. As a result, the ability to study multiple caregiver and care recipient risk factors in these populations simultaneously has often been curtailed.

What is known is that elder mistreatment results in family distress, impaired life functioning [55, 56], and cognitive difficulties [57, 58]. It results in emotional difficulties such as feelings of inadequacy, and self-contempt [37, 59, 60], decreased self-esteem [57, 59–63] and depression [56, 64, 65]. It has also been linked to health problems such as increased mortality [66–68] and immunological dysfunction [56, 57, 63, 65, 69, 70]. As such, it is imperative that we begin to study it not only in older adults in general, but also in specific subgroups who may have unique characteristics that result in a differing risk profile.

This paper will look at risk factors for physical mistreatment in a sample of community dwelling older adults with Alzheimer's Disease in the state of Florida using the risk and vulnerability model of Elder Mistreatment (see Figure 1). The Risk and Vulnerability model proposed by Rose and Killian (1983) [71] was first applied to elder mistreatment in 1994 by Frost and Willette, and then to neglect by Fulmer and Paveza [72]. While many studies conducted to date focus only on victim or perpetrator characteristics, what is unique about this model is its ability to see both as contributing to the likelihood that abuse will happen. Risk under the model refers to hazards or stressors in the environment external to the elder that contribute to likelihood of mistreatment, while vulnerability refers to characteristics within an elder that may influence the likelihood that abuse happens. For a person with Alzheimer's disease, vulnerability may stem from factors such as decreased cognitive status, increased levels of functional impairment, as well as behavioral difficulties, which stem from the etiology of their disease and result in the need for a primary caregiver, and add "risk" in the form of caregiver burden, poor functional and psychological health, and difficulties in coping. This model postulates that abuse may stem from several areas in which AD persons might be susceptible and offers a framework to test several risk factors for mistreatment simultaneously (Figure 1).

2. Methods

2.1. The Data Set. This study represents a secondary analysis of data collected as part of the Aggression and Violence in Community Based Alzheimer's families grant (AV_CAD) described in detail in VandeWeerd and Paveza (2006) [73]. Potential subjects were enrolled though solicitation via membership in one of 3 local chapters of the Alzheimer's Association located in Tampa, Orlando, and Miami, or through their participation with the 5 state funded memory disorder clinics (Tampa, Central Florida, North Broward, Miami, and Miami Beach) over a 3 step procedure (see Box 1). In step one, all older adults diagnosed with AD who were receiving treatment from one of the memory disorder clinics ($n = 1,781$), or who were members of Alzheimer's Associations during the studies enrollment period ($n = 5,648$) were mailed an introductory pamphlet explaining the study. Pamphlet packages included a response card indicating a person's interest in the study and their consent to have their information released from their enrollment site to the study team. In step two, all interested persons were contacted by the USF study team who explained the study in detail and verified whether the elder and caregiver met the inclusion criteria. If inclusion criteria were met, staff collected address information for mailing the in-home questionnaire and scheduled an appointment for an in-home interview. In step three of the study, in-home interviews were completed with caregivers and elders where eligible, using a computer assisted live interview technique.

Inclusion criteria for the study required that: (1) elders be 60 years of age or older, (2) have a diagnosis of AD according to the NINCDS/ADRDA criteria or dementia of Alzheimer's type according to the DSM-III-R or DSM-IV in the 3 years prior to their enrollment in the study, (3) possess the ability to speak English, and (4) achieve a score of 16 or greater on the Folstein Mini Mental Status Exam (MMSE.) Inclusion criteria for caregivers required that: (1) caregivers be a family member, (2) with the ability to speak English, (3) provide 20 hours a week or more of care, and possess a phone.

Persons who did not meet the inclusion criteria were excluded from participating in the study with the exception of elders who met all criteria except requisite MMSE score. In these cases a surrogate was used to provide answers on an elder's behalf providing that the surrogate felt close to the elder, had met at least one time per week with the elder over the past year, and was not the primary caregiver.

Requisite MMSE score was lowered from the standard of 18 to 16 or higher, and data collection was limited to persons diagnosed within the 3-year period prior to enrollment to reduce the number of patients who were likely to have surpassed the cognitive decline cut-off. This was also an effort to decrease the response bias that a large number of surrogates might induce. Of the 76 elders who participated, only 17 required the inclusion of surrogate information.

2.2. Tests and Measures. The selection of measures used to determine the characteristics that place a family at risk for, or are protective against physical violence were based on formal criteria. The selection of measures had to: (1) reflect proposed theoretical risk factors for the increased risk or prevention of violence and aggression as based on previous work on elder abuse in the general population, or specific work on violence

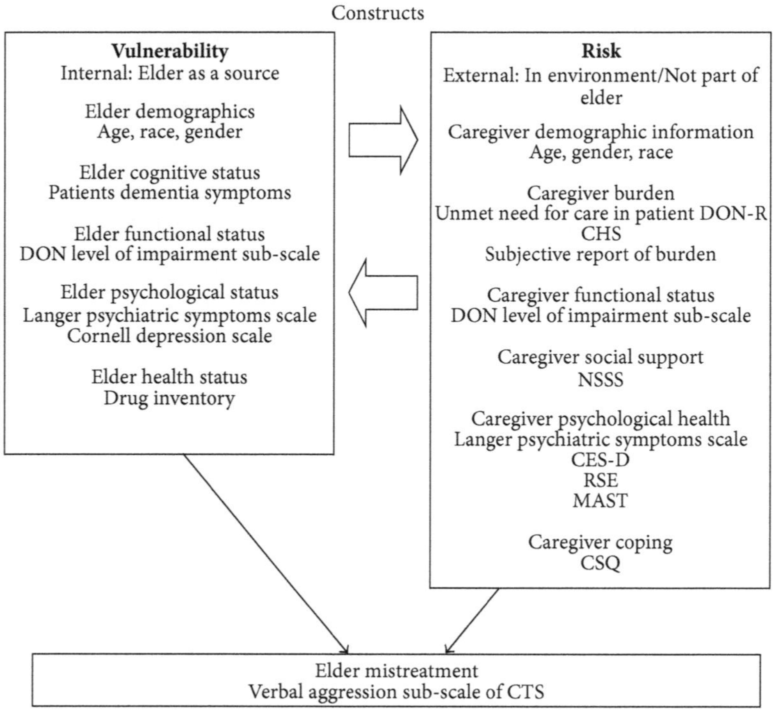

CES-D: Center for epidemiological studies depression inventory
CHS: Caregiver Hassle scale
CSQ: Coping styles questionnaire
CTS: Conflict tactics scale
DON: Determination of need scale
DON-R: Determination of need scale revised
MAST: Michigan alcohol screening test
NSSS: Norbeck social support scale
RSE: Rosenberg self esteem scale

FIGURE 1: A Risk Vulnerability Model of Elder Mistreatment.

(i) Step One:
Mass mailing of introductory pamphlet to all persons who were members of a Florida State Alzheimer's Association in the year 1998 (n = 5,648) or who were members of a state-funded memory disorder clinic (MDC) diagnosed with AD (n = 1,781) during study enrollment

(ii) Step Two:
Phone interview to ensure interested subjects (n = 1, 011) met eligibility criteria, confirm address for the mailing of questionnaire and scheduling of in-home interview.
Of the interested subjects, 65% (n = 657) met inclusion criteria, and 254 agreed to participate once the study was explained in detail.

(iii) Step Three:
In-home interview conducted with caregivers (n = 254) and patients who were cognitively eligible (n = 60), or who had a surrogate available to provide responses on their behalf (n = 16)

Box 1: Data collection.

and aggression in family members with AD; (2) represent a conceptual and logical indicator of the construct being assessed; (3) exhibit strong to moderate reliability and validity as evidenced by formal testing; (4) be relatively short and easy to administer with an economy of time; and (5) have a history of use with diverse samples.

The Conflict Tactic Scale (CTS) was the principal measure of elder mistreatment in the AV_CAD, and the violence subscale served as the principal outcome measure of this study. The CTS was originally developed by Straus and his colleagues for use in their seminal study on violence in the American family [74]. This instrument was chosen because of its frequency of use in the study of violence in families [9], as well as by studies that have looked at violence in AD families on a smaller scale [23]. It includes items in compliance with the definition for physical abuse such as "pushed, shoved, or grabbed" and "slapped, and spanked", as measured through caregivers' reports of their own behavior and caregivers' reports of elders behavior, and it offers a dichotomous way to measure the presence or absence of physical mistreatment.

Independent variables included measures of risk and vulnerability as outlined in Figure 1. Measures of vulnerability on the part of the caregiver included elder's demographic information such as age, gender and race; elder's cognitive status as measured by the number of dementia symptoms present; elder's functional status as measured by the "Elders Level of Impairment" subscale of the DON-R; psychological status as measured by the Langer Psychiatric Symptoms Scale [75] and the Cornell Depression Scale, CDS [76]; and the elders health status by the number of drugs prescribed for the treatment of health conditions. Measures of risk included caregiver's demographic information such as age, gender, and race; caregiver's cognitive status as measured by the Folstein Mini Mental Status exam, MMSE [77]; caregiver burden as measured by the "Patients unmet need for care" subscale of the Determination of Need Scale Revised, DON-R [78], the Caregiver Hassle Scale, CHS [79], and subjective report of caregiver burden; and caregiver functional status as measured by the level of impairment subscale of the DON-R. Additional measures of caregiver risk included the presence of social support as measured by the Norbeck Social Support Scale, NSSS [80]; caregiver psychological health as measured by the Langer Psychiatric Symptoms Scale [75], the Center for Epidemiological Studies depression scale, CES-D [81], the Rosenberg Self Esteem Scale, RSE [82], and the Michigan Alcohol Screening Test, MAST [83]; and caregiver coping as measured by the Coping Styles Questionnaire, CSQ [84].

2.3. Data Analysis. Data were collected through mailed questionnaire and in-home interview. Data collected during the in-home interview were entered immediately into an Epi-Info database format via laptop computer, and later transformed into an SPSS useable format using Stat Transfer 6.0 software. Data collected via mailed questionnaire were entered directly into an SPSS 11.0 database for data analysis.

For the purpose of this analysis, demographics of the overall sample were computed, and a step-wise logistic regression model was used to test for variables significantly associated with physical mistreatment of elders. All independent variables were entered into the model on step one. Variables were considered to be significant protective or risk factors if they were found significant on step one, and if they remained significant when tested against all other significant variables in the model on step two. All variables were tested for multicollinearity prior to the running of the regression models.

3. Results

In all, 254 caregivers (see Table 1) and 76 elders (See Table 2) participated in the study. Caregivers had a mean age of 63.84 years (±13.07 years) and were primarily wives (34.2%) and children (33.3%), followed by husbands (18.5%). Care-recipients had a mean age of 78.57 years (±8.41 years) and 59% were female. Both care-recipients and caregivers were 85% Caucasian, 10.3% Hispanic, and approximately 4.5% African American. Forty-four percent of caregivers were non-Roman Catholic Christians, as were 43.2% of elders. An additional 26.1% of caregivers and elders were Roman Catholics. Of those, 21.7% had household incomes between \$20,000 and \$29,000. For care-recipients who do not live with their caregivers, many are living in poverty. Thirty-five percent have incomes less than \$20,000 a year. Forty-nine percent of caregivers were providing care to someone with 11–15 dementia symptoms, 84.3% reported a subjective feeling that providing care to the elder was a burden, and 41.9% were seriously considering the need for nursing home placement in the future. Only 17.4% of caregivers and 25.9% of patients reported no level of depression. Twenty-six percent of caregivers were mildly depressed, 37% were moderately depressed, and 20% reported severe depression as measured by the self-report CES-D. Interestingly, only 7% of caregivers reported low self-esteem as measured by the Rosenberg self esteem scale. Minor depression was reported in 29.6% of elders, possible major depression in 16.2% of elders, probable major depression in 19.9% of elders, and definite major depression was reported in 8.3% of elders as measured by the Cornell Depression Scale, which identifies depression in elders based on caregivers responses.

The use of violence was self-reported by 17.2% of caregivers, and was reported as a technique used against them by 26.1% of elders. Upon comparison of caregivers who used violence as a conflict resolution strategy with those who did not (see Table 3), logistic regression analyses indicated that caregivers who were providing care to elders with high levels of functional impairment (P = .034; OR = 2.049; CI = 1.093–4.912) were twice as likely to be violent with their care recipient than those who were not. Caregivers with alcohol problems were 3 times as likely to be violent with elders for whom they were providing care (P = .041; OR = 3.217; CI = 2.382–4.775), and those providing care to elders with greater numbers of dementia symptoms (P = .019; OR = 4.817; CI = 3.509–12.518), or to elders who used violence (P = .010; OR = 4.168; CI = 2.176–8.399) were four times as likely to be violent with the elder in their care. Caregivers with high self-esteem were significantly less likely to engage in violent behavior (P = .046; OR = .662; CI = .591–.748). Additionally, the interaction effect of risk and vulnerability was found to result in greater likelihood for physical mistreatment. The interactions between dementia symptoms displayed on the part of elders and depression in caregivers (P = .007; OR = 5.483; CI = 3.217–7.075), and dementia symptoms and violent behavior on the part of elders, and alcoholism on the part of caregivers (P = .052; OR = 6.176; CI = 4.511–9.706), were significantly related to the likelihood of physical mistreatment. Depressed caregivers providing care to elders with more dementia symptoms were five times as likely to engage in violent behavior as those who were not. Caregivers who abused alcohol, and who were providing care to violent elders with high levels of dementia symptoms were six times as likely to engage in violent behavior as those who did not. The model accounted for 48.3% of the variance (Nagelkerke R square = .483). The Homer-Lemeshow goodness of fit test

Table 1: Caregiver demographics (N = 254).

Mean age	63.84 (±13.07)
Age by group	
21–30	0.5%
31–40	5%
41–50	9.9%
51–60	27%
61–70	19.8%
71–80	28.8%
81–90	8.6%
90+	0.5%
Gender	
Female	74.8%
Male	25.2%
Ethnicity	
Caucasian	85.1%
African American	4.6%
Hispanic	10.3%
Religion	
Roman Catholic	26.1%
Other Christian	44.1%
Jewish	15.8%
Other	14.0%
Relationship to patient	
Wife	34.2%
Husband	18.5%
Child	33.2%
Other	14.0%
Income[1]	
Under $19,999	10.9%
$20,000–$29,999	18.6%
$30,000–$39,999	13.2%
$40,000–$49,999	12.3%
$50,000+	45.0%
Subjective feeling of burden	
Yes	84.3%
No	15.7%
Psychiatric symptoms	
0-1	24.9%
2-3	19.2%
4-5	23.2%
6+	32.5%
Level of depression	
Non-depressed	17.4%
Mildly depressed	25.7%
Moderately depressed	36.7%
Severely depressed	20.2%
Level of Self Esteem	
Moderately low	0.9%
Low	6.0%
High	18.1%
Moderately high	30.2%
Very high	44.7%

Table 1: Continued.

Considering nursing home	
Not really considering	31.4%
Considering	26.7%
Seriously considering	41.9%
Physically violent[2]	
Yes	17.2%
No	82.8%

[1]Figures represent combined household income.
[2]As measured by the Violence sub-scale of the CTS.

was not significant ($\chi^2 = 9.628$; df = 8; P = .365) and indicates that the model is a good fit.

4. Discussion

This paper has revealed several factors such as self-esteem and alcohol abuse in caregivers, and violence, dementia symptoms, and functional impairment in elders, that increase the likelihood of physical mistreatment. That cognitive impairment is a factor in elder mistreatment has been suggested by other researchers [23, 26, 36, 41, 43–45, 85] and is clearly supported by this research in light of the increased numbers of persons in this group who report physical violence (43 in 254) compared to persons in the population at large (20 in 1000) [9]. While persons may be protected from mistreatment at the onset of their disease when they show few symptoms, AD is a progressive dementing disorder, which gradually results in more cognitive difficulties. As a result, it is likely that as their disease progresses their risk goes up. In addition as a direct result of the etiology of the disease, as it progresses, persons with AD become more functionally impaired, may fail to recognize loved ones, lose their social filters, and become more verbally and physically combative. As a consequence, they may become more physically abusive and receive more physical abuse. This pattern exemplifies cases of reciprocal violence and may explain the largest of what is likely two subgroups of persons who are mistreating: those who are engaging in violent behavior as a direct result of having violence used against them, and those who are engaging in violent behavior unprovoked. While this data set did not contain sufficient numbers of persons engaging in non-reciprocal violence to examine this population with scientific certainty (N = 17), future research should separate cases of caregiver violence in which elders are physically violent and those cases in which elders are not, as it is likely that they represent two differing risk profiles. With a larger sample gathered from several geographic regions it is likely that sufficient cases could be gathered to examine this question.

Psychological health of the perpetrator was also found to be a significant predictor of physical violence in caregivers. Those with who abused alcohol were three times more likely to engage in physical violence than those who did not. This research supports other research findings that substance abuse increases risk of elder mistreatment [31, 33, 36, 38] and suggests that screening for this condition by health

TABLE 2: Elder demographics ($N = 76$).

Mean age	78.57 (±8.41)
Age by group	
60–70	14.5%
71–80	43.4%
81–90	36.7%
90+	5.4%
Gender	
Female	59%
Male	41%
Ethnicity	
Caucasian	84.8%
African American	4.5%
Hispanic	9.4%
Other	1.3%
Religion	
Roman Catholic	26.1%
Other Christian	43.2%
Jewish	15.8%
Other	14.9%
Income[1]	
Under \$19,999	35.5%
\$20,000–\$29,999	15.7%
\$30,000–\$39,999	11.4%
\$40,000–49,999	8.5%
\$50,000+	28.9%
Income[2]	
Under \$19,999	15.2%
\$20,000–29,999	21.7%
\$30,000–\$39,999	11.6%
\$40,000–49,999	13.8%
\$50,000+	37.6%
Dementia Symptoms	
1–5 symptoms noticed	1.3%
6–10 symptoms noticed	24.1%
11–15 symptoms noticed	49.1%
16–20 symptoms noticed	25.4%
Depression	
No depression	25.9%
Minor depression	29.6%
Possible major depression	16.2%
Probable major depression	19.9%
Definite major depression	8.3%
Number of drugs taken	
None reported	79.2%
1-2	5.0%
3-4	5.4%
5-6	3.5%
Verbally Aggressive[3]	
No	25.2%
Yes	74.2%
Violent[4]	
Yes	73.9%
No	26.1%

[1]Represents household income when not living with caregiver.
[2]Represents household income when living with caregiver.
[3]As measured by the Verbal Aggression sub-scale of the CTS.
[4]As measured by the Violence sub-scale of the CTS.

professionals may contribute to an avenue of prevention. Additionally, since higher levels of functional impairment resulted in twice the risk for physical mistreatment, avenues for prevention may lie in increased physical, occupational, and assistive device therapies for older adults, as studies have shown that many older adults are significantly below their functional capacity despite the presence of physical impairment [67].

That many of these factors contribute to physical mistreatment in older adults is not altogether surprising. It makes intuitive sense that those least able to defend themselves as a result of functional impairment, or those least able to report as a result of factors such as cognitive impairment will have the greatest likelihood of mistreatment. The unique aspect of this research is the theoretically supported decision to look at risks and vulnerabilities in older adults with AD and their caregivers simultaneously, and to discover in doing so that the interaction of elders "vulnerabilities" and caregiver "risk" results in an even greater likelihood abuse will happen. Elders with high levels of dementia symptoms being cared for by caregivers with low self-esteem were five times more likely to be victims of physical mistreatment than those who were not. Additionally, violent elders with dementia being cared for by a caregiver with alcohol problems were six times more likely to be physically mistreated compared with the fourfold risk of dementia symptoms on its own. While determining whether or not alcoholism stems from caring for someone who is violent, or whether alcoholism in caregivers contributes to violence in elders is beyond the scope of this paper, what this research demonstrates is the need for models that account for both victim and perpetrator characteristics, as well as the interaction between them such as that posited by the Risk and Vulnerability model used here.

Future research should include other risk factors such as familial history, behavioral acculturation, and state-trait anger which may also contribute to physical mistreatment and should include, if possible, a random sample of older adults over a larger, more diverse, geographic region. This would generate larger samples which would allow for the testing of cases of physical mistreatment versus those who do not verbally or physically mistreat, as well as for the testing of differences within mistreatment subgroups (i.e., those who involve instances of reciprocal violence and those that do not). Additionally, while the consequences of elder mistreatment have been found to include emotional difficulties such as depression [56, 64, 65], feelings of inadequacy and self-contempt [37, 59, 60], impaired life functioning [55, 56], and health problems such as immunological dysfunction [56, 57, 63, 65, 69, 70], and increased mortality [66–68], no study has examined the long term consequences of physical mistreatment in persons with Alzheimer's disease specifically. While elder mistreatment may result in a threefold increase in mortality in persons over the age of 65 as a whole [66, 68] it may result in even greater effects for persons with AD.

5. Conclusion

Caring for a loved one with Alzheimer's disease is a difficult job. Alzheimer's disease is a progressive dementing disorder that lasts from 5 to 15 years. It starts with difficulties in cognition and ends with a complete loss of ability to complete

TABLE 3: Logistic regression analysis: violent caregivers versus all others (n = 254).

Variable	B	S.E.	Sig.	EXP(B)	95% C.I. for EXP(B)	
					Lower	Upper
Patient vulnerability						
Age	.564	.555	.309	1.758	.593	5.214
Gender	−.202	.972	.048	.817	.422	.949
Race	9.569	27.669	.999	14.274	.437	8.453
Number of dementia symptoms	2.470	1.050	.019	4.817	3.509	12.518
Level of functional impairment	1.231	.581	.034	2.049	1.093	4.912
Depression	−.634	.423	.134	.530	.231	1.216
Number of drugs taken	.463	.538	.390	1.589	.553	4.563
Verbal aggression	2.129	1.450	.142	.119	.007	2.841
Violence	3.185	1.228	.010	4.168	2.176	8.399
Caregiver risk						
Age	.355	.382	.352	1.426	.675	3.013
Sex	−1.497	1.471	.309	.224	.013	3.998
Race	−8.897	27.669	.999	1.010	.653	8.976
Hassle experienced by caregiving	.173	.234	.460	1.189	.751	1.880
Level of impairment sub-scale	−14.523	54.843	.996	4.962	.655	9.877
Cognitive status	.953	.800	.233	2.594	.541	12.435
Level of social support	.023	.418	.956	1.023	.451	2.322
Psychiatric symptoms	.249	.486	.608	1.283	.495	3.326
Depression	.872	.535	.103	2.391	.837	6.825
Self esteem	−.472	.514	.046	.662	.591	.748
Alcoholism	3.562	2.308	.041	3.217	2.382	4.775
Coping style	−17.491	33.673	.999	2.534	.544	5.436
Interaction of risk and vulnerability						
Pt dementia ∗ cg depression	1.728	.408	.007	5.483	3.217	7.075
Pt depression ∗ cg hassle ∗ Cg psychiatric symptoms	.162	.425	.052	6.176	4.511	9.706
Constant	−38.572	26.066	.139	.000		

(a) Step wise logistic regression model: variables were considered significant risk factors if they were found significant on step one and if they remained significant when tested against all other significant variables in the model onstep two. All variables found significant on step 1 remained significant at step 2.
(b) Model accounts for 48.3% of the variance. Nagelkerke R square = .483.
(c) Homer-Lemeshow goodness of fit test (X^2 = 9.628, df = 8, P = .365).

most activities of daily living unassisted. As health care professionals, we have a duty to monitor the quality of life in these persons to prevent abuse where possible. The closer we come to a risk profile, the easier this task will be. This study also suggests that continued funding for research at this level of detail, as suggested by the National Research Council report on elder abuse [48], is imperative if useful, specific interventions are to be implemented.

Acknowledgment

This research was funded by a grant from the National Institute on Aging (1RO1-AG14412).

References

[1] A. B. Amstadter, J. M. McCauley, M. A. Hernandez, and R. Acierno, "Do incident and perpetrator characteristics of elder mistreatment differ by gender of the victim? Results from the national elder mistreatment study," *Journal of Elder Abuse and Neglect*, vol. 23, no. 1, pp. 43–57, 2011.

[2] M. Block and J. Sinnott, Eds., *The Battered Elderly Syndrome: An Exploratory Study*, University of Maryland, Center on Aging, College Park, Md, USA, 1979.

[3] A. C. Coyne, W. E. Reichman, and L. J. Berbig, "The relationship between dementia and elder abuse," *The American Journal of Psychiatry*, vol. 150, no. 4, pp. 643–646, 1993.

[4] M. Lithwick, "The mistreatment of older adults: perpetrator-victim relationships and interventions," *Journal of Elder Abuse and Neglect*, vol. 11, no. 4, pp. 95–112, 2000.

[5] M. C. Sengstock and M. Hwalek, "Sources of information used in measures for the identification of elder abuse," in *Proceedings the Annual Meeting of the Gerontological Society of America*, November 1983.

[6] T. Tatara, "Understanding the nature and scope of domestic elder abuse with the use of state aggregate data: summaries of key findings of a national survey of state APS and aging agencies," *Journal of Elder Abuse and Neglect*, vol. 5, pp. 35–57, 1993.

[7] R. Acierno, M. A. Hernandez, A. B. Amstadter et al., "Prevalence and correlates of emotional, physical, sexual, and financial abuse and potential neglect in the United States: the national elder mistreatment study," *The American Journal of Public Health*, vol. 100, no. 2, pp. 292–297, 2010.

[8] C. A. Field and R. Caetano, "Longitudinal model predicting partner violence among white, black, and Hispanic couples in the United States," *Alcohol and Clinical Experimental Research*, vol. 27, no. 9, pp. 1451–1458, 2003.

[9] K. Pillemer and D. Finkelhor, "The prevalence of elder abuse: a random sample survey," *The Gerontologist*, vol. 28, no. 1, pp. 51–57, 1988.

[10] M. S. Lachs and K. Pillemer, "Elder abuse," *The Lancet*, vol. 364, no. 9441, pp. 1263–1272, 2004.

[11] L. B. Schiamberg and D. Gans, "Elder abuse by adult children: an applied, ecological framework for understanding contextual risk factors and the intergenerational character of quality of life," *International Journal of Aging and Human Development*, vol. 50, no. 4, pp. 329–359, 2000.

[12] R. S. Wolf and K. A. Pillemer, "The older battered woman: wives and mothers compared," *Journal of Mental Health and Aging*, vol. 3, no. 3, pp. 325–336, 1997.

[13] T. T. Fulmer, "The debate over dependency as a relavant predisposing factor in elder abuse and neglect with commentary," *Journal of Eler Abuse and Neglect*, vol. 2, no. 1-2, pp. 51–72, 1990.

[14] C. J. Hildreth, A. E. Burke, and R. M. Glass, "Elder abuse," *The Journal of the American Medical Association*, vol. 302, no. 5, pp. 1–2, 2009.

[15] J. Kosberg and J. Garcia, "Common and unique themes on elder abuse from a world wide perspective," *Journal of Elder Abuse and Neglect*, vol. 6, no. 3-4, pp. 183–197, 1995.

[16] A. Mowlam, R. Tennant, J. Dixon, and C. McCreadie, "UK study of abuse and neglect of older people: qualitative findings," Tech. Rep., National Centre for Social Research, Comic Relief and Department of Health, http://www.jipeast.org/attachments/527_ComicRelief-ElderAbuse-Full-Stage21%20UK%20study-%20of%20abuse%20%20neglect.pdf.

[17] B. M. Barer, "The relationship between homebound older people and their home care worker," *The Journal of Gerontological Social Work*, vol. 19, pp. 129–147, 1992.

[18] M. Bendik, "Reaching the breaking point: dangers of the mistreatment in elder caregiving situations," *Journal of Elder Abuse and Neglect*, vol. 4, no. 3, pp. 39–59, 1992.

[19] R. Harrell, C. H. Toronjo, J. Mclaughlin, N. Valory, D. J. Hyman, and C. Bitondo Dyer, "How geriatricians identify elder abuse and neglect," *The American Journal of the Medical Sciences*, vol. 323, no. 1, pp. 34–38, 2002.

[20] S. Vida, R. C. Monks, and P. Des Rosiers, "Prevalence and correlates of elder abuse and neglect in a geriatric psychiatry service," *Canadian Journal of Psychiatry*, vol. 47, no. 5, pp. 459–468, 2002.

[21] S. R. Beach, R. Schulz, G. M. Williamson, L. S. Miller, M. E. Weiner, and C. E. Lance, "Risk factors for potentially harmful informal caregiver behavior," *Journal of the American Geriatrics Society*, vol. 53, no. 2, pp. 255–261, 2005.

[22] C. Cooper, A. Selwood, and G. Livingston, "The prevalence of elder abuse and neglect: a systematic review," *Age and Ageing*, vol. 37, no. 2, pp. 151–160, 2008.

[23] G. J. Paveza, D. Cohen, C. Eisdorfer et al., "Severe family violence and Alzheimer's disease: prevalence and risk factors," *The Gerontologist*, vol. 32, no. 4, pp. 493–497, 1992.

[24] R. J. Eastley, R. Macpherson, H. Richards, and I. H. Main, "Assaults on professional carers of elderly people," *British Medical Journal*, vol. 307, no. 6908, article 845, 1993.

[25] L. R. Phillips, E. Torres de Ardon, and G. S. Briones, "Abuse of female caregivers by care recipients: another form of elder abuse," *Journal of Elder Abuse and Neglect*, vol. 12, no. 3-4, pp. 123–143, 2001.

[26] M. Hamel, D. P. Gold, D. Andres et al., "Predictors and consequences of aggressive behavior by community-based dementia patients," *The Gerontologist*, vol. 30, no. 2, pp. 206–211, 1990.

[27] M. B. Ryden, "Aggressive behavior in persons with dementia who live in the community," *Alzheimer Disease and Associated Disorders*, vol. 2, no. 4, pp. 342–355, 1988.

[28] G. M. Williamson and D. R. Shaffer, "Relationship quality and potentially harmful behaviors by spousal caregivers: how we were then, how we are now," *Psychology and Aging*, vol. 16, no. 2, pp. 217–226, 2001.

[29] G. Gioglio and P. Blakemore, *Elder Abuse in New Jersey: The Knowledge and Experience of Abuse among Older New Jerseyans*, New Jersey Division on Aging, Trenton, NJ, USA, 1982.

[30] M. Reis and D. Nahmiash, "Abuse of seniors: personality, stress and other indicators," *Journal of Mental Health and Aging*, vol. 3, no. 3, pp. 337–356, 1997.

[31] N. G. Choi and J. Mayer, "Elder abuse, neglect, and exploitation: risk factors and prevention strategies," *Journal of Gerontological Social Work*, vol. 33, no. 2, pp. 5–25, 2000.

[32] A. Flaherty and P. Raia, "Beyond risk protection and Alzheimer's disease," *Journal of Elder Abuse and Neglect*, vol. 6, no. 2, pp. 75–93, 1994.

[33] T. Fulmer, L. Guadagno, C. B. Dyer, and M. T. Connolly, "Progress in elder abuse screening and assessment instruments," *Journal of the American Geriatrics Society*, vol. 52, no. 2, pp. 297–304, 2004.

[34] D. Gallagher, A. Wrabetz, S. Lovett, S. Del Maestro, and J. Rose, "Depression and other negative affects in family caregivers," in *Alzheimer's Disease Treatment and Family Stress: Directions for Research*, Light and Lebowitz, Eds., pp. 218–244, Hemisphere, New York, NY, USA, 1990.

[35] W. E. Haley, E. G. Levine, S. Brown, and g. Hughes, "Psychological, social, and health consequences of caring for a relative with senile dementia," *Journal of the American Geriatrics Society*, vol. 35, no. 5, pp. 405–411, 1987.

[36] G. J. Anetzberger, *The Etiology of Elder Abuse by Adult Offspring*, Springfield Publishing, Chicago, Ill, USA, 1987.

[37] T. Fulmer, G. Paveza, C. VandeWeerd et al., "Dyadic vulnerability and risk profiling for elder neglect," *The Gerontologist*, vol. 45, no. 4, pp. 525–534, 2005.

[38] E. Bristowe and J. Collins, "Family mediated abuse of non-institutionalized frail elderly men and women living in British Colombia," *Journal of Elder Abuse and Neglect*, vol. 1, no. 1, pp. 45–64, 1989.

[39] M. Cohen, S. Halevi-Levin, R. Gagin, and G. Friedman, "Development of a screening tool for identifying elderly people at risk of abuse by their caregivers," *Journal of Aging and Health*, vol. 18, no. 5, pp. 660–685, 2005.

[40] G. Anetzberger, J. Korbin, and C. Austin, "Alcoholism and elder abuse," *Journal of Interpersonal Violence*, vol. 9, no. 2, pp. 184–193, 1994.

[41] A. M. Campbell Reay and K. D. Browne, "Risk factor characteristics in carers who physically abuse or neglect their elderly dependants," *Aging and Mental Health*, vol. 5, no. 1, pp. 56–62, 2001.

[42] A. Coyne, "The relationship between cognitive impairment and elder abuse," in *Findings of Five Elder Abuse Studies*, T. Tatara, Ed., pp. 23–50, National Agency Resource Center on Elder Abuse, Washington, DC, USA, 1991.

[43] W. Haley and J. Coleton, "Alzheimer's disease: special issues in elder abuse and neglect," *Journal of Elder Abuse and Neglect*, vol. 4, no. 4, pp. 71–85, 1992.

[44] D. Jamuna, "Issues of elder care and elder abuse in the Indian context," *Journal of Aging and Social Policy*, vol. 15, no. 2-3, pp. 125–142, 2003.

[45] L. S. Miller, M. S. Lewis, G. M. Williamson et al., "Caregiver cognitive status and potentially harmful caregiver behavior," *Aging and Mental Health*, vol. 10, no. 2, pp. 125–133, 2006.

[46] L. R. Shugarman, B. E. Fries, R. S. Wolf, and J. N. Morris, "Identifying older people at risk of abuse during routine screening practices," *Journal of the American Geriatrics Society*, vol. 51, no. 1, pp. 24–31, 2003.

[47] E. R. Welfel, P. R. Danzinger, and S. Santoro, "Mandated reporting of abuse/maltreatment of older adults: a primer for counselors," *Journal of Counseling and Development*, vol. 78, no. 3, pp. 284–292, 2000.

[48] National Research Council (US), "Panel to review risk and prevalence of elder abuse and neglect," in *Elder Mistreatment: Abuse, Neglect and Exploitation in an Aging America*, J. Richard Bonnie and B. Robert Wallace, Eds., National Academies Press, Washington, DC, USA, 2003.

[49] National Center on Elder Abuse, "Fact Sheet: elder abuse prevalence and incidence," http://www.ncea.aoa.gov/ncearoot/Main_Site/index.aspx, 2005.

[50] H. C. Comijs, C. Jonker, W. van Tilburg, and J. H. Smit, "Hostility and coping capacity as risk factors of elder mistreatment," *Social Psychiatry and Psychiatric Epidemiology*, vol. 34, no. 1, pp. 48–52, 1999.

[51] K. Pillemer and J. J. Suitor, "Violence and violent feelings: what causes them among family caregivers?" *Journals of Gerontology*, vol. 47, no. 4, pp. S165–S172, 1992.

[52] E. Pittaway and A. Westhues, "The prevalence of elder abuse and neglect of older adults who access health and social services in London, Ontario, Canada," *Journal of Elder Abuse and Neglect*, vol. 5, no. 4, pp. 77–93, 1993.

[53] G. J. Anetzberger, B. R. Palmisano, M. Sanders et al., "A model intervention for elder abuse and dementia," *The Gerontologist*, vol. 40, no. 4, pp. 492–497, 2000.

[54] A. Wiglesworth, L. Mosqueda, R. Mulnard, S. Liao, L. Gibbs, and W. Fitzgerald, "Screening for abuse and neglect of people with dementia," *Journal of the American Geriatrics Society*, vol. 58, no. 3, pp. 493–500, 2010.

[55] C. VandeWeerd, G. J. Paveza, and T. Fulmer, "Abuse and neglect in older adults with Alzheimer's disease," *Nursing Clinics of North America*, vol. 41, no. 1, pp. 43–55, 2006.

[56] S. H. Zarit, P. A. Todd, and J. M. Zarit, "Subjective burden of husbands and wives as caregivers: a longitudinal study," *The Gerontologist*, vol. 26, no. 3, pp. 260–266, 1986.

[57] B. M. Barer, "The secret shame of the very old: 'I've never told this to anyone else'," *Journal of Mental Health and Aging*, vol. 3, no. 3, pp. 365–375, 1997.

[58] L. M. Gibbs and L. Mosqueda, "Confronting elder mistreatment in long-term care," *Annals of Long-Term Care*, vol. 12, no. 4, pp. 30–36, 2004.

[59] Metge, *In and Out of Touch: Whakamaa in Cross Cultural Perspective*, Victoria University Press, Wellington, New Zealand, 1986.

[60] M. Lewis, *Shame: The Exposed Self*, The Free Press, New York, NY, USA, 1992.

[61] H. C. Comijs, A. M. Pot, J. H. Smit, L. M. Bouter, and C. Jonker, "Elder abuse in the community: prevalence and consequences," *Journal of the American Geriatrics Society*, vol. 46, no. 7, pp. 885–888, 1998.

[62] E. Podnieks, "Social inclusion: an interplay of the determinants of health—new insights into elder abuse," *Journal of Gerontological Social Work*, vol. 46, no. 3-4, pp. 57–79, 2006.

[63] B. Saverman, *Formal Carers in Healthcare and the Social Services Witnessing the Abuse of Elderly in Their Homes*, Umea University, Umea, Sweden, 1994.

[64] J. M. Heath, F. A. Kobylarz, M. Brown, and S. Castaño, "Interventions from home-based geriatric assessments of adult protective service clients suffering elder mistreatment," *Journal of the American Geriatrics Society*, vol. 53, no. 9, pp. 1538–1542, 2005.

[65] E. Light and B. Lebowitz, *Alzheimer's Disease Treatment and Family Stress: Direction for Research*, National Institute of Mental Health, Rockville, Md, USA, 1994.

[66] M. W. Baker, "Elder mistreatment: risk, vulnerability, and early mortality," *Journal of the American Psychiatric Nurses Association*, vol. 12, no. 6, pp. 313–321, 2007.

[67] C. A. Helfrich, M. J. Lafata, S. L. MacDonald, A. Aviles, and L. Collins, "Domestic abuse across the lifespan: definitions, identification and risk factors for occupational therapists," *Occupational Therapy in Mental Health*, vol. 16, no. 3, pp. 5–34, 2001.

[68] M. S. Lachs, C. S. Williams, S. O'Brien, K. A. Pillemer, and M. E. Charlson, "The mortality of elder mistreatment," *Journal of the American Medical Association*, vol. 280, no. 5, pp. 428–432, 1998.

[69] K. A. Collins and S. E. Presnell, "Elder neglect and the pathophysiology of aging," *The American Journal of Forensic Medicine and Pathology*, vol. 28, no. 2, pp. 157–162, 2007.

[70] L. K. George and L. P. Gwyther, "Caregiver well-being: a multidimensional examination of family caregivers of demented adults," *The Gerontologist*, vol. 26, no. 3, pp. 253–259, 1986.

[71] M. H. Rose and M. Killien, "Risk and vulnerability: a case for differentiation," *Advances in nursing science*, vol. 5, no. 3, pp. 60–73, 1983.

[72] T. Fulmer and G. Paveza, "Neglect in the elderly patient," *The Nursing Clinics of North America*, vol. 33, no. 3, pp. 457–466, 1998.

[73] C. VandeWeerd and G. J. Paveza, "Verbal mistreatment in older adults: a look at persons with Alzheimer's disease and their caregivers in the State of Florida," *Journal of Elder Abuse and Neglect*, vol. 17, no. 4, pp. 11–30, 2006.

[74] M. A. Straus, R. J. Gelles, and S. K. Steinmetz, *Behind Closed Doors: Violence in the American Family*, Anchor Books, New York, NY, USA, 1980.

[75] T. S. Langer, "A twenty-two item screening score of psychiatric symptoms indicating impairment," *Journal of Health and Human Behavior*, vol. 12, pp. 269–276, 1973.

[76] G. S. Alexopoulos, R. C. Abrams, R. C. Young, and C. A. Shamoian, "Cornell scale for depression in dementia," *Biological Psychiatry*, vol. 23, no. 3, pp. 271–284, 1988.

[77] M. F. Folstein, S. E. Folstein, and P. R. McHugh, "'Mini mental state': a practical method for grading the cognitive state of patients for the clinician," *Journal of Psychiatric Research*, vol. 12, no. 3, pp. 189–198, 1975.

[78] G. J. Paveza, D. Cohen, C. J. Blaser, and M. Hagopian, "A brief form of the mini-mental state examination for use in community settings," *Behavior, Health and Aging*, vol. 1, pp. 133–139, 1990.

[79] J. M. Kinney and M. A. Stephens, "Caregiving hassles scale: assessing the daily hassles of caring for a family member with dementia," *The Gerontologist*, vol. 29, no. 3, pp. 328–332, 1989.

[80] J. S. Norbeck, A. M. Lindsey, and V. L. Carrieri, "Further development of the norbeck social support questionnaire: normative data and validity testing," *Nursing Research*, vol. 32, no. 1, pp. 4–9, 1983.

[81] L. S. Radloff and L. Teri, "Use of the center for epidemiological studies-depression scale with older adults," *Clinical Gerontologist*, vol. 5, no. 1-2, pp. 119–136, 1986.

[82] M. Rosenberg, *Society and the Adolescent Self-Image*, Princeton University Press, Princeton, NJ, USA, 1965.

[83] M. L. Selzer, "The Michigan alcoholism screening test: the quest for a new diagnostic instrument," *The American Journal of Psychiatry*, vol. 127, no. 12, pp. 1653–1658, 1971.

[84] H. A. Kiyak, "Coping with Alzheimer's disease: patient and family responses," in *Proceedings of the Gerontological Society of America Symposium: Aging and Adaptation in Chronic Illnesses*, Chicago, Ill, USA, November 1986.

[85] T. T. Fulmer, "Elder mistreatment," *Annual Review of Nursing Research*, vol. 12, pp. 51–64, 1992.

Evaluation of Potential Drug-Drug Interactions with Medications Prescribed to Geriatric Patients in a Tertiary Care Hospital

Varsha Shetty, Mukta N. Chowta, Nithyananda Chowta K, Ashok Shenoy, Ashwin Kamath, and Priyanka Kamath

Department of Medicine and Pharmacology, Kasturba Medical College, Mangalore, Manipal Academy of Higher Education, Mangalore, India

Correspondence should be addressed to Mukta N. Chowta; mukta.chowta@manipal.edu

Academic Editor: F. R. Ferraro

Background and Objectives. The drugs most commonly implicated in major potential interactions are those used in the day-to-day clinical management of elderly patients with chronic diseases. This study is planned to evaluate the profile of drug-drug interactions in the medications prescribed to elderly population and also to identify the possible predictors for potential drug-drug interactions in the elderly. *Methods*. This cross-sectional study included patients aged above 60 years with a minimum of two drugs in the prescriptions. Data were collected from medical prescriptions and patients' medical records. The data collected included demographic characteristics such as age, gender, height, weight, educational status, socioeconomic status, medical history, and medications prescribed. The prescriptions were analyzed for the potential drug interactions using Lexi-Interact™ Online, an online software to check drug-drug interactions. *Results*. A total of 209 patients were included in the study, among them 104 (49.8%) were males and 105 (50.2%) were females. The mean number of medications received was 6.53 ± 2.15 per prescription. Around 138 (66%) patients received more than six medications. The mean number of potential drug interactions seen in the prescription of these patients was 3.17 ± 2.78. Around 18.2% patients had more than five drug interactions. Major drug interactions were observed in 21.42% of cases. Around 3.02% of drug interactions belonged to risk category X, i.e., to be avoided. Logistic regression analysis showed that age above 70 years was associated with the presence of drug interactions. Increased number of medication was independently associated with the occurrence of drug interactions. The presence of drug interactions was not associated with increased number of comorbidities. *Conclusion*. A significant number of potential drug-drug interactions were seen in the prescriptions of elderly patients. Increasing age and polypharmacy were identified as the predictors of potential drug interactions.

1. Introduction

Alteration in the efficacy or toxicity of one drug due to the presence of another simultaneously administered drug is termed as drug-drug interactions (DDIs). This alteration is mostly quantitative, i.e., the response to a drug is either increased or decreased in intensity. DDIs may occur due to pharmacokinetic processes, i.e., the delivery of a drug to its site of action is altered by a second drug or due to pharmacodynamic processes, i.e., when the two drugs act on same or interrelated target resulting in synergistic or antagonistic activity. Clinically relevant drug-drug interactions may occur with drugs exhibiting steep dose-response curve/narrow therapeutic index, drugs causing microsomal enzyme induction/inhibition, drugs following zero-order elimination kinetics, severely ill patients, in the presence of significant renal/hepatic impairment and elderly patients receiving multiple drugs [1].

Drug therapy is an integral part of patient management. Though the use of multiple drugs may be required either to manage a single disease or comorbidities, harmful interactions may occur between these drugs. The enthusiasm to use new drugs may lead to DDIs that are yet to be identified. Adverse drug reactions may occur as the consequence of DDIs and clinicians may be unaware of the clinical risks of some drug combinations. Drug-drug interactions are a significant cause of hospital admissions and hospital visits, thereby contributing to a huge economic burden. Gathering more and more information on DDIs could help to reduce such adverse effects from DDIs [2–4]. The drugs most commonly implicated in major potential interactions are those used in the day-to-day clinical management of elderly patients with chronic diseases [5]. Few cross-sectional studies involving elderly patients have been conducted to evaluate DDIs, especially in India. Hence, this study is planned to assess the profile of drug-drug interactions in the medications prescribed to elderly population and also to identify the possible predictors for potential drug-drug interactions in the elderly.

2. Methods

This cross-sectional study included male and female patients aged above 60 years who attended the Medicine outpatient department of a tertiary care hospital and were prescribed a minimum of two drugs. The study was performed after the approval from the Institutional Ethics Committee, Kasturba Medical College, Mangalore (Ref no. IEC KMC MLR02-16/26). Data were collected for a duration of 6 months, from medical prescriptions and patients' medical records. The data collected included the age of the patient, gender, height, weight, educational status, socioeconomic status, and medical history. Data regarding renal function tests and liver function tests, if available, were recorded. The medications prescribed to the patients were noted and analyzed for potential DDIs.

A sample size of 367 was calculated considering confidence interval of 95% and absolute precision of 5% and the prevalence of DDIs as 45% [6].

The prescriptions were analyzed for the potential drug interactions using Lexi-Interact™ Online, an online software to check drug-drug interactions (http://www.uptodate.com/crlsql/interact/frameset.jsp) [7] available on the website www.uptodate.com. This software provides the severity, risk rating, and the summary of drug-drug interactions.

The risk rating is categorized as A, B, C, D, or X. The progression from A to X is accompanied by increased urgency in the action to be taken. In general, A and B are of academic, but not of clinical concern where as C, D, or X always require attention. Risk category "A" corresponds to no evidence of drug interaction while category "B" denotes the presence of evidence for potential interactions but with little evidence for clinical concern. Hence, for both these categories, no action is required. Monitoring of therapy is recommended for category "C" where there is evidence of potential interaction which is clinically significant. However, the benefits usually outweigh the risks. Dosage adjustments are rarely needed. Therapy modification is to be considered for category "D," which may involve dose adjustment, considering alternative therapy, aggressive monitoring to minimize toxicity. Drug combinations in the risk category "X" are to be avoided since the risks usually outweigh the benefits. Such drug combinations are considered contraindicated.

DDI can also be categorized by its mechanism, as pharmacokinetic and pharmacodynamic.

2.1. Statistical Analysis. For categorical variables, frequencies/percentages were calculated, and continuous variables were expressed as mean ± SD. Comparisons among subgroups were performed using Fisher exact test/Student "*t*" test. The binary logistic regression model was used to analyze the association of occurrence of potential drug-drug interactions with specified risk factors, including gender, age, comorbidities and the number of drugs prescribed. The output of the logistic regression was expressed as adjusted odds ratios with 95% confidence intervals. All tests were performed using a two-tailed test at a significance level of 0.05. SPSS for Windows version 20 (SPSS, Inc., Chicago, IL, USA) was employed for all statistical analyses.

3. Results

A total of 209 patients were included in the study. Among them, 104 (49.8%) were males and 105 (50.2%) were females. The mean age of study population was 71.22 ± 7.91 years. The mean number of comorbidities was 2.56 ± 0.94 per patient and the mean number of medications received was 6.53 ± 2.15 per prescription. Table 1 shows the category-wise number of drug interactions among all patients; 18.2% of patients having more than 5 drug interactions in their prescription. Around 138 (66%) patients received more than six medications. The mean number of potential drug interactions seen in the prescription of these patients was 3.17 ± 2.78 per prescription.

There was a statistically significant difference in the mean age of males and females (males 69.89 ± 7.81 years versus females 72.52 ± 7.83 years, $t = 2.43$, $p = 0.016$). There were no significant differences with regard to the number of comorbidities, number of medications, and number of drug interactions between males and females.

The common comorbidities present in the study population were diabetes mellitus (78%), hypertension (73.2%), CVA (26.8%), CAD (10.5%), and dyslipidemia (7.2%). Hypertension was more prevalent in females ($p = 0.013$, X^2 test).

A total of 663 potential drug interactions were seen in 209 patients, with males having 340 and females having 323 encounters. Majority of the drug interactions were pharmacokinetic in nature (Table 2).

Among the total drug interactions, 68.33% belonged to the risk category C, 15.84% were risk category B, and 12.82% were category D. Around 3.02% of drug interactions belonged to risk category X, i.e., to be avoided. There were no differences between males and females with regard to distribution of drug interactions, based on risk category (Table 3).

Table 4 shows the comparison of patients with and without polypharmacy. The mean age between the two

Table 1: Number of drug interactions among all patients.

Number of drug interactions	All patients, *n* (%)
0	35 (16.7)
1-2	71 (34)
3–5	65 (31.1)
>5	38 (18.2)

Table 2: Distribution of drug interactions based on mechanism (pharmacokinetic and pharmacodynamic interactions).

D/Is	All patients	Male	Female	*p* value
Overall	663	340	323	0.24
Pharmacokinetic, *n* (%)	241 (36.35)	117 (34.41)	124 (38.39)	0.055
Pharmacodynamic, *n* (%)	422 (63.65)	223 (65.59)	199 (61.61)	0.296

X^2 test.

Table 3: Distribution of drug interactions based on risk category.

Risk category of D/Is	All patients	Males	Females	*p* value
B, *n* (%)	105 (15.84)	47 (13.82)	58 (17.96)	0.14
C, *n* (%)	453 (68.33)	247 (72.65)	206 (63.78)	0.53
D, *n* (%)	85 (12.82)	34 (10)	51 (15.79)	0.26
X, *n* (%)	20 (3.02)	12 (3.53)	8 (2.48)	0.28

X^2 test.

Table 4: Comparison of comorbidities between patients with and without polypharmacy.

Variables	Number of medications >6	Number of medications <6	*t* value	*p* value
Age (years)	71.36 ± 7.36	70.93 ± 8.93	0.35	0.73
Number of comorbidities	2.7 ± 0.97	2.28 ± 0.83	3.12	0.002*

Values are expressed as mean ± SD. Student "*t*" test. *Significant.

groups was comparable. The differences between two groups with regard to the mean number of comorbidity were statistically significant ($p < 0.002$). Patients with polypharmacy (number of medications >6) had a higher number of comorbidity.

There were significant correlations of the frequency of drug interactions with age, the number of medications, and the number of comorbidities (Pearson correlation, $p < 0.05$). Among the comorbidities, hypertension was significantly correlated with the frequency of drug interactions.

Logistic regression analysis showed that age above 70 years is associated with the presence of drug interactions (OR = 1.05; CI: 1.00–1.097; $p = 0.02$). Increased number of medication was independently associated with the occurrence of drug interactions (OR = 10.37; CI: 3.35–32.11; $p < 0.001$). The presence of drug interactions was not associated with increased number of comorbidities (Table 5).

Table 6 shows the drug pairs involved in risk X category of drug interactions. The clopidogrel-esomeprazole combination was used in 4 patients.

4. Discussion

Elderly patients are the largest consumers of medication. As the elderly patients are more likely to receive multiple medications, potential drug-drug interactions are more likely in this population. Various methods were used to identify and categorize drug-drug interactions. The present study used LexiComp® to evaluate potential drug interactions [7]. Our study showed the mean number of medications per prescription as 6.53 ± 2.15. Earlier studies have also shown the same findings, with a study done at Taiwan [8] showing the mean number medications as 5.8 ± 2.4 and the study done by Teka et al. [9] showing the mean number medication prescribed to elderly patients as 6 ± 4 per patient. Two Indian studies reported a slightly higher values for the mean number of medication received by the patient (7.61 ± 3.37 and 9.15 ± 0.03) [10, 11]. Differences in study settings, number and type of comorbidity as well as the prescribing culture may explain the discrepancy in the findings. In our study, 66% of patients had more than six medications in their prescription. Teka et al. also reported that 42.2% patients had <5 prescribed drugs and 62.2% were exposed to at least one potential DDI [9]. Salwe et al. have reported 52.69% of potential drug interactions with 761 medicines prescribed on admission and 52.91% of drug interactions with 548 medicines prescribed on discharge. Potentially severe drug interactions are 6.98% of total potential drug-drug interactions [11]. Björkman et al. reported potential drug interactions in 46% of elderly patients [12]. Girre et al. studied the potential drug interactions in elderly cancer patients and shown that mean number of medications per patient as 4.7 and identified 45 potential interactions, occurring in 32 patients [13]. In a questionnaire-based study, Loya et al. reported the prevalence of polypharmacy as 72.3% and 46.2% were at risk of having at least one potential drug-drug interaction [14]. Turner et al identified 398 potential drug interactions in 300 patients [15]. Chavda et al. found that 58.27% patients had at least one pDDI and the most common pDDIs were pharmacodynamic in nature and of moderate severity. They observed that the number of pDDI increased with the increase in the age of patients and the number of drugs prescribed [16].

Our study has noted that 83.25% had at least one drug interactions. It is of concern to note that 18.2% patients had more than five drug interactions. The total number of drug interactions identified in the present study is 663, which is sufficiently high to warn us to have a careful monitoring for potential drug interactions in the prescriptions of the elderly. It is gratifying to note that most of these interactions were of moderate intensity. It is unfortunate to observe that a small percentage of patients (3.02%) received drug combinations considered as to be avoided (risk category X).

Hypertension and diabetes were the most common comorbidities. Among the comorbidities, hypertension was more prevalent in females. Obviously, patients with more

Table 5: Predictors of D/Is (multivariate logistic regression analysis).

Variables	Groups	Patients with D/Is	Patients without D/Is	Wald	Odds ratio (95% CI)	p value
Age	<70	75	22	4.04	1.05 (1.00–1.097)	0.04
	>70	99	13			
Gender	Male	89	15	0.18	0.86(0.42–1.75)	0.67
	Female	85	20			
Number of comorbidities	1	22	7	0.31	0.87 (0.54–1.42)	0.58
	2	52	15			
	3	75	10			
	4	21	2			
	>4	4	1			
Type of comorbidity	Diabetes	136	27	0.20	0.81 (0.31–2.11)	0.66
	Hypertension	130	23	1.71	1.92 (0.72–5.09)	0.19
	CAD	21	1	0.60	1.56 (0.51–4.82)	0.44
	Dyslipidemia	14	1	0.05	1.17 (0.31–4.46)	0.82
	CVA	51	7	0.38	0.76 (0.32–1.81)	0.54
Number of medications	<6	48	23	16.47	10.37 (3.35–32.11)	<0.001
	>6	126	12			

Table 6: Medication pairs involved in risk X category drug interactions (to be avoided).

Medication pairs	Number of D/Is	Effect of drug interaction
Azithromycin-silodosin	1	Increased serum concentration of silodosin
Domperidone-escitalopram	2	Enhanced QTc-prolonging effect
Domperidone-quetiapine	2	Enhanced QTc-prolonging effect
Escitalopram-quetiapine	1	Enhanced QTc-prolonging effect
Atorvastatin-silodosin	2	Increased serum concentration of silodosin
Clopidogrel-esomeprazole	4	Diminished antiplatelet effect of clopidogrel
Ciprofloxacin-domperidone	1	Enhanced QTc-prolonging effect
Domperidone-fluconazole	1	Increased serum concentration of domperidone
Nifedipine-phenytoin	1	Increased serum concentration of phenytoin
Prazosin-tamsulosin	1	Enhanced antihypertensive effect
Domperidone-granisetron	1	Enhanced QTc-prolonging effect
Escitalopram-flupentixol	1	Enhanced QTc-prolonging effect
Bambuterol-salmeterol	1	Enhanced adverse/toxic effects
Amitriptyline-salbutamol + ipratropium	1	Enhanced anticholinergic effect

than five drug interactions had a higher number of comorbidities when compared to patients with less than five drug interactions. Univariate analysis showed significant correlations between the frequency of drug interactions and the age, the number of medications, and number of comorbidities. Among the comorbidities, hypertension was significantly correlated with the frequency of drug interactions. However, the multivariate (logistic regression) analysis showed significant association of occurrence of potential drug interactions only with age and number of medications. Patients with age above 70 years had the higher risk of having drug interactions. Delafuente also reported that the older age and the number of drugs prescribed are more likely to lead to major drug interactions [17]. Similar to our findings, earlier studies also identified polypharmacy as one of the predictors for the occurrence of potential drug interactions [18–22].

The risk of potential drug interaction increases from 39% to 100% when patients are on more than six medications compared to when they are on 2-3 medications [23]. Many elderly patients take one or more medications that are not medically required [21]. However, multiple medications may be needed to cure, to slow the progression of the disease, to prevent its complications and to reduce the symptoms of the disease, thereby improving the quality of life in elderly patients. Hence, balancing the risks and benefits of multiple drug therapies, thereby avoiding harmful drug-drug interactions, in geriatrics is a major challenge for health care providers. Management of drug interactions in the elderly may pose difficulty due to frailty, interindividual variation, and disturbed homeostasis. Better prescribing practices in the elderly can reduce the adverse drug reactions to a great extent [24]. Identifying patient characteristics, as the predictors of potential drug-drug interactions, may help to suggest preventive practices and policies to avoid such interactions.

There were 20 encounters of use of to be avoided drug combinations. The clopidogrel-esomeprazole combination was the most commonly used to be avoided drug combination. Many of the drug interactions can be minimized by using alternative medications or congeners that are not associated with drug interactions. For example, instead of omeprazole, pantoprazole can be used in patients receiving clopidogrel, as pantoprazole do not interfere with the activation of clopidogrel. Balanced use of multiple medications to avoid drug interactions requires the wide knowledge of the pharmacology of drugs.

Apart from prescribed medication, patients may also consume nonprescription medications, further adding to the risk of drug interactions. Age-related alterations in pharmacokinetics also pose them to increased risk of clinically significant drug interactions. The quality of life in elderly may be affected by the presence of drug interactions and morbidity may be increased by clinically unrecognized drug interactions. Hence, careful use of medications and strict monitoring is required to avoid drug-drug interactions. Medications given to treat most common comorbidities like diabetes and hypertension should be screened for potential drug interactions. Patient education and counseling by clinicians are essential to avoid improper use of nonprescription drugs.

Limitation of our study needs to be mentioned. This study is a medical record-based study wherein patient's data were collected from the patient's files without direct interaction with the patients and drug interactions identified were potential or theoretical. Studies based on clinical evaluation of the patients for the possibility of drug interactions may be more valid as it provides real-time data. This study is done at a tertiary care hospital, where the prescription pattern may be different, compared with primary care settings. Many elderly patients are treated in primary care settings and hence generalizations of our findings may not be appropriate. Another limitation is that, being a record-based study, nonprescription drugs were not taken into account. However, this study being the first in our settings provides the baseline data that can be used in finding the prevalence of potential drug-drug interactions in elderly patients.

5. Conclusion

A significant number of prescriptions of elderly patients had more than five potential drug-drug interactions. A small percentage of drug interactions were belonging to the risk category X (i.e., to be avoided drug combination), which could be easily avoided by using alternative medications or congeners that are not associated with drug interactions. Increasing age and polypharmacy were identified as the predictors of potential drug interactions.

Conflicts of Interest

The authors declare that there are no conflicts of interest regarding the publication of this article.

Authors' Contributions

All authors have contributed significantly to the research concept, literature review, objectives, and design of the study. They all are in agreement with the content of the manuscript. All authors approved the manuscript and this submission.

References

[1] K. D. Tripathi, *Drug interaction. Essentials of Medical Pharmacology*, pp. 928–934, 7 edition, Jaypee, Delhi, 2013.

[2] S. Dechanont, S. Maphanta, B. Butthum, and C. Kongkaew, "Hospital admissions/visits associated with drug-drug interactions: a systematic review and meta-analysis," *Pharmacoepidemiology and Drug Safety*, vol. 23, no. 5, pp. 489–497, 2014.

[3] B. Mannheimer, J. Ulfvarson, S. Eklof, M. Bergqvist, E. Andersen-Karlsson et al., "Drug-related problems and pharmacotherapeutic advisory intervention at a medicine clinic," *European Journal of Clinical Pharmacology*, vol. 62, no. 12, pp. 1075–1081, 2006.

[4] J. J. V. Teixeira, M. T. L. Crozatti, C. A. dos Santos, and N. S. Romano-Lieber, "Potential drug-drug interactions in prescriptions to patients over 45 years of age in primary care, Southern Brazil," *PLoS One*, vol. 7, no. 10, Article ID e47062, 2012.

[5] R. M. Seymour and P. A. Routledge, "Important drug-drug interactions in the elderly," *Drugs and Aging*, vol. 12, no. 6, pp. 485–494, 1998.

[6] N. Fokter, M. Možina, and M. Brvar, "Potential drug-drug interactions and admissions due to drug-drug interactions in patients treated in medical departments," *Wiener klinische Wochenschrift*, vol. 122, no. 3-4, pp. 81–88, 2010.

[7] Lexi-Interact™ online, http://www.uptodate.com/crlsql/interact/frameset.jsp.

[8] C. F. Lin, C. Y. Wang, and C. H. Bai, "Polypharmacy, aging and potential drug–drug interactions in outpatients in Taiwan: a retrospective computerized screening study," *Drugs and Aging*, vol. 28, no. 3, pp. 219–225, 2011.

[9] F. Teka, G. Teklay, E. Ayalew, and T. Teshome, "Potential drug-drug interactions among elderly patients admitted to medical ward of Ayder Referral Hospital, Northern Ethiopia: a cross sectional study," *BMC Research Notes*, vol. 9, no. 1, p. 431, 2016.

[10] M. Kashyap, S. D'Cruz, A. Sachdev, and P. Tiwari, "Drug–drug interactions and their predictors: results from Indian elderly inpatients," *Pharmacy Practice*, vol. 11, no. 4, pp. 191–195, 2013.

[11] K. J. Salwe, D. Kalyansundaram, and Y. Bahurupi, "A study on polypharmacy and potential drug–drug interactions among elderly patients admitted in Department of Medicine of a Tertiary Care Hospital in Puducherry," *Journal of Clinical and Diagnostic Research*, vol. 10, pp. FC06–FC10, 2016.

[12] I. K. Björkman, J. Fastbom, I. K. Schmidt, and C. B. Bernsten, "Pharmaceutical care of the elderly in Europe research (PEER) group. Drug-drug interactions in the elderly," *Annals of Pharmacotherapy*, vol. 36, pp. 1675–1681, 2002.

[13] V. Girre, H. Arkoub, M. T. E. Puts, C. Vantelon, F. Blanchard, and J. P. Droz, "Potential drug interactions in elderly cancer patients," *Critical Reviews in Oncology and Hematology*, vol. 78, no. 3, pp. 220–226, 2011.

[14] A. M. Loya, A. González-Stuart, and J. O. Rivera, "Prevalence of polypharmacy, polyherbacy, nutritional supplement use and potential product interactions among older adults living on the United States-Mexico border: a descriptive, questionnaire-based study," *Drugs and Aging*, vol. 26, no. 5, pp. 423–436, 2009.

[15] L. R. Tulner, S. V. Frankfort, G. J. Gijsen, J. P. van Campen, C. H. Koks, and J. H. Beijnen, "Drug-drug interactions in a geriatric outpatient cohort: prevalence and relevance," *Drugs and Aging*, vol. 25, no. 4, pp. 343–355, 2008.
[16] N. B. Chavda, P. P. Solanky, H. Baria, R. Naik, and K. Bharti, "Study of potential drug–drug interaction between prescribed drugs in patients attending outpatient department of medicine at tertiary-care hospital in south Gujarat region," *National Journal of Physiology, Pharmacy and Pharmacology*, vol. 5, no. 3, pp. 236–242, 2015.
[17] J. C. Delafuente, "Understanding and preventing drug interactions in elderly patients," *Critical Reviews in Oncology and Hematology*, vol. 48, no. 2, pp. 133–143, 2003.
[18] P. R. Obreli Neto, A. Nobili, S. Marusic et al., "Prevalence and predictors of potential drug-drug interactions in the elderly: a cross-sectional study in the Brazilian primary public health system," *Journal of Pharmacy and Pharmaceutical Sciences*, vol. 15, no. 2, pp. 344–354, 2012.
[19] P. R. Obreli-Neto, A. Nobili, A. de Oliveira Baldoni et al., "Adverse drug reactions caused by drug-drug interactions in elderly outpatients: a prospective cohort study," *European Journal of Clinical Pharmacology*, vol. 68, no. 12, pp. 1667–1676, 2012.
[20] P. Mibielli, S. Rozenfeld, G. C. Matos, and A. Fde Acurcio, "Potential drug–drug interactions among elderly using antihypertensives from the Brazilian list of essential medicines," *Cadernos de Saúde Pública*, vol. 30, no. 9, pp. 1947–1956, 2014.
[21] R. L. Maher, J. T. Hanlon, and E. R. Hajjar, "Clinical consequences of polypharmacy in elderly," *Expert Opinion on Drug Safety*, vol. 13, no. 1, pp. 57–65, 2014.
[22] M. Bogetti-Salazar, C. González-González, T. Juárez-Cedillo, S. Sánchez-García, and O. Rosas-Carrasco, "Severe potential drug–drug interactions in older people with dementia and associated factors," *Clinics*, vol. 71, no. 1, pp. 17–21, 2016.
[23] R. S. Mendes-Nett, C. Q. Silva, A. D. Oliveira-Filbo, C. E. Rocha, and D. P. Lyra-Junior, "Assessment of drug interactions in elderly patients of a family healthcare unit in Aracaju (Brazil): a pilot study," *African Journal of Pharmacy Pharmacology*, vol. 5, no. 7, pp. 812–818, 2011.
[24] A. Spinewine, K. E. Schmader, N. Barber, C. Hughes, K. L. Lapane, and C. Swine, "Appropriate prescribing in elderly people: how well can it be measured and optimised?," *Lancet*, vol. 370, no. 9582, pp. 173–184, 2007.

19

Factors Associated with Women's Chronic Disease Management: Associations of Healthcare Frustrations, Physician Support, and Self-Care Needs

Matthew Lee Smith,[1,2] Marcia G. Ory,[2] SangNam Ahn,[3] and Toni P. Miles[4]

[1] *The University of Georgia, College of Public Health, Department of Health Promotion and Behavior, 330 River Road, 315 Ramsey Center Athens, GA 30602, USA*
[2] *Texas A&M Health Science Center, School of Rural Public Health, Department of Health Promotion and Community Health Sciences, TAMU 1266, College Station, TX 77843, USA*
[3] *The University of Memphis, School of Public Health, Division of Health Systems Management and Policy, Robison Hall 133, Memphis, TN 38152-3530, USA*
[4] *The University of Georgia, College of Public Health, Department of Epidemiology and Biostatistics, 255 E. Hancock Avenue, Athens, GA 30602, USA*

Correspondence should be addressed to Matthew Lee Smith; matthew.smith@srph.tamhsc.edu

Academic Editor: Wojtek Chodzko-Zajko

Previous research emphasizes the importance of reducing healthcare frustrations and enhancing physician supports to help patients engage in recommended healthcare regimens. However, less is known about how these factors are associated with aging women's knowledge about self-care behavior. This study examined the sociodemographics, health indicators, healthcare-related frustrations, and perceptions of physician support associated with middle-aged and older adult females' self-reported need for help to learn how to take better care of their health. Data were analyzed from 287 females with one or more chronic conditions who completed The National Council on Aging (NCOA) Chronic Care Survey. A logistic regression model was developed. Women who were non-White (OR = 2.26, $P = 0.049$) were more likely to need help learning how to better manage their health. Those who had some college education or more (OR = 0.55, $P = 0.044$) and lower healthcare-related frustrations (OR = 0.44, $P = 0.017$) and perceived to have more physician support (OR = 0.49, $P = 0.033$) were less likely to need help learning how to better manage their health. Findings can inform the planning, implementation, assessment, and dissemination of evidence-based self-management programs for middle-aged and older women within and outside of clinical settings.

1. Introduction

Over the next several decades, the number of Americans living to advanced ages will increase substantially. Although many individuals will age in relatively good health, a growing number will encounter challenges associated with the burdens of chronic conditions and associated disabilities [1–3]. This is especially so for the large numbers of women who will continue to outlive their male counterparts and likely live those additional years with chronic illnesses requiring day-to-day management [4, 5]. Further, with a dramatic increase of female "baby boomers" with obesity-related chronic conditions, accompanied by reduced fertility rates among this rapidly aging cohort, the additive or multiplicative effects of living with one or more chronic conditions are likely to result in a diminution of (1) individuals' capacity to adequately care for themselves, (2) caregivers to serve as efficient resources, and (3) healthcare providers to give adequate attention and guidance to complex patients with multiple chronic conditions (MCCs) [6].

In line with the millions of older women struggling to manage the symptoms associated with chronic disease, there is growing recognition about the importance of self-care behavior, which is supported by strong epidemiological documentation regarding the positive association of self-care and health outcomes [7–10]. However, this issue transcends women's exposure to and understanding of pertinent information and their development of self-care skills. Older women with chronic conditions also need to assess their surrounding resources to develop the confidence and efficacy necessary to initiate and maintain self-care behavior [11–13]. Self-care behavior are intended to draw upon one's physical, social, and healthcare environments to compensate for, or delay, physical limitations and chronic conditions from progressing into more severe disabilities [14]. Further, self-care skills include (1) identifying strategies that enable older women to adopt and institute appropriate self-care behavior such as getting adequate exercise, eating healthy, or managing medications [15, 16]; (2) interacting with healthcare providers to obtain resources and referrals necessary to manage the progression of chronic conditions [10, 17, 18]; and (3) locating social and community resources to become more educated about their conditions and alleviate the stressors and frustration acting as barriers to self-care behavior [6, 19].

While a growing literature has identified general disparities related to self-care among women with chronic conditions based on their race/ethnicity [20–22], socioeconomic status [22–24], and residential rurality [22, 25], the extent to which self-care disparities exist based on these and other sociodemographics requires further investigation. Similarly, the role of education an indicator of socioeconomic status, healthcare access, and health behavior engagement emphasizes its importance when assessing disparities issues [26, 27]. Additional efforts are needed to examine the influence of sociodemographics on self-care skills and behavior among aging women, especially in the presence of perceptions about healthcare-related factors.

Healthcare provider-patient interactions can foster self-care behavior [17] although such interactions can also have a less-recognized negative effect on disease self-management. Women can feel frustrated and helpless when their physicians do not fully explain or clarify the causes of their disease or ways how to best manage their illness [28]. Some patients report not having enough time to address their concerns, or that their physicians simply would not listen to them. Conversely, among patients with diabetes, those who have good communication with their physicians report feeling more involved in decision-making efforts to manage their condition more effectively. Also, patients who report their physicians provided adequate information about their conditions were more likely to better self-manage their illnesses [29].

Healthcare professionals often encounter challenges to address their female patients' MCC alongside existing barriers to self-care behavior in their home or community environments. Regardless of the source or cause of these barriers, competing demands on the side of either the patient or provider have potential to create a recursive relationship resulting in disconnect, miscommunication, frustration, and fewer self-care practices [30]. These occurrences may inevitably contribute to decreased health outcomes and rapid chronic disease progression, which highlights the importance of support mechanisms available to the patient.

Women with chronic conditions receive self-care support from various channels. Effective self-care support mechanisms and resources identified to promote self-care behavior include traditional in-person, familial, and community support systems (e.g., support groups and faith-based organizations) [6, 31–35]; however, an emergence in technology-based support mechanisms has been shown to enable individuals with chronic conditions to access and utilize self-care information, despite traditional barriers [18, 36–39]. Further, the active seeking of self-care support and resources has been shown to enhance self-care behavior among individuals with chronic conditions [12, 38, 40]. The preferred and/or utilized support mechanisms differ by population subgroup and type of chronic condition. Evidence shows that racial/ethnic minorities with chronic conditions report increased in-person support mechanisms compared to their non-Hispanic white counterparts [41, 42]. Conversely, those residing in rural areas have shown improvement in their self-care behavior through the use of internet-based support mechanisms [43], which may be critical to overcome traditional challenges associated with geographic isolation, less healthcare resources, and longer travel distances to healthcare services [25, 44].

The advancing study of self-care behavior has identified factors influencing the adoption and maintenance of self-care behavior for different populations and people of all ages, with more recent attention paid to lifestyle relative to disease self-care behavior [17, 45, 46]. To advance the translation of research to practice, this secondary data analysis assesses issues surrounding self-care barriers, healthcare-related frustrations, and perceived supports among middle-aged and older adults with one or more chronic conditions. In an effort to further understand the multilevel influences on perceived barriers to self-care, this study will examine the roles of healthcare frustrations and doctor-patient interactions alongside other simultaneously occurring contextual factors (see Figure 1). More specifically, the purposes of this study were to (1) describe sociodemographic variables, health indicators, healthcare-related frustrations, and perceptions of physician support among middle-aged and older adult women with one or more chronic conditions and (2) identify these factors' association with reporting the need to help learning how to take better care of their health among this female population.

2. Materials and Methods

2.1. Study Participants and Procedures. The National Council on Aging (NCOA), with support from Atlantic Philanthropies and the California HealthCare Foundation (CHCF), commissioned the NCOA Chronic Care Survey, which offers unique insight into the lives of Americans with chronic health conditions [47]. The NCOA Chronic Care Survey is a nationally representative probability survey of 960 community-dwelling men and women aged 44 years and older with at least one chronic condition. Lake Research Partners utilized telephone-based interviewing to collect data using random digit dialing (RDD) sampling techniques, which oversampled those aged 65 and older and Hispanics/Latinos. Telephone interviews were conducted in both English and Spanish. The

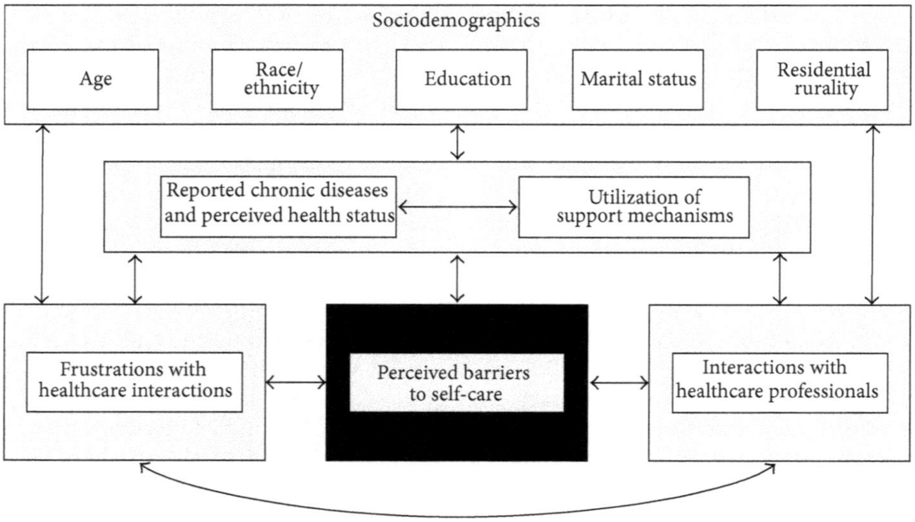

FIGURE 1: Conceptual framework indicating influences on women's perceived barriers to self-care.

dataset was weighted by age, race, and region to reflect the overall population of Americans 44+ with chronic condition(s). The margin of sampling error for the total results was ±2.9 percentage points. Margin of error is greater when analyzing smaller subgroups within the sample.

To be eligible for inclusion in The NCOA Chronic Care Survey, participants had to report having at least one chronic condition at the time of the study. Participants were screened for chronic condition(s) with the following question(s): "Have you ever been told by a doctor, nurse, or other health professional that you have (name of chronic condition)?" Chronic conditions included in the screening process included heart disease, cancer, stroke, diabetes, arthritis, asthma, hypertension or high blood pressure, emphysema, chronic bronchitis, depression, anxiety, and others. Only participants who reported "yes" to at least one of these items were included in the survey.

Of the 960 adults age 44 years and older in this sample, only women were included in study analyses ($n = 427$; 44.5%). Of these women, an additional 140 cases (32.8%) were omitted for incomplete data on variables of interest. More specifically, cases were omitted for incomplete data on rurality ($n = 48$), frustration with the healthcare system ($n = 25$), perceived physician support ($n = 18$), self-reported chronic conditions ($n = 17$), marital status ($n = 8$), using the Internet for general support ($n = 7$), race/ethnicity ($n = 6$), education ($n = 4$), perceived barriers to self-care ($n = 4$), and activity limitations ($n = 3$). The analytic sample for this study contained 287 community-dwelling women, aged 44 years and older who self-reported having at least one chronic condition. When comparing characteristics of women omitted from the study ($n = 140$) with those in the analytic sample ($n = 287$), a significantly larger proportion of the analytic sample was younger ($\chi^2 = 4.98$, $P = 0.026$), non-Hispanic white ($\chi^2 = 4.60$, $P = 0.032$), and married ($\chi^2 = 11.78$, $P = 0.001$). No significant differences were observed based on education or residential rurality.

2.2. Data and Measures

2.2.1. Dependent Variable. Participants were asked to self-report their perceived barriers to self-care using an item intended to measure their need for help to *learn how* to take better care of their health. More specifically, participants were asked to rate their level of agreement to the following statement: "I need help learning how to take better care of my health in a way that works for me and my life." Responses were scored on a 5-point Likert-type scale ranging from "strongly disagree" to "strongly agree." Based on the frequency distribution, participant responses were then dichotomized into two categories: "disagree" (scored 0) and "agree" (scored 1).

2.2.2. Healthcare Frustrations. Participants were asked to report their frustrations with healthcare interactions using items intended to measure their feelings about repeatedly having to describe their conditions at each doctor visit, the self-care instructions they received from the healthcare provider, the time spent interacting with the healthcare provider, and having a friend or family member attend physician's visits with them. For example, participants were asked to rate their level of agreement to statements like "How often do you feel tired of describing your same conditions and problems every time you go to a hospital or doctor's office?" and "How often do you wish you had a friend or family member who could go to the doctor with you?" Responses were scored using a 3-point Likert-type scale with categories of "never" (scored 0), "occasionally" (scored 1), and "frequently" (scored 2). The Healthcare-Related Frustration Scale (ranging from 0 to 12) was created using these six items. Factor analysis with Varimax rotation was performed to generate this scale. All items loaded on one factor and the items were summed into a single-composite score ($\alpha = 0.766$). Higher scores for the Healthcare-Related Frustration Scale indicate a higher level of frustration with healthcare interactions. Based on the frequency distribution, this scale was converted into tertiles for the analytic purposes. The highest tertile (i.e., representing the highest frustration levels) served as the referent group.

2.2.3. Perceived Physician Support. Participants were asked to self-report the degree to which their physician engages them in treatment-related problem-solving/decision-making, refers them to other healthcare services and professionals, and asks if they understand their medications and associated regimens. For example, participants were asked to rate their level of agreement to statements like "How often does your physician ask for your ideas about how you can take care of your health problems?" and "How often does your physician talk to other doctors and nurses who are taking care of you?" Responses were scored using a 5-point Likert-type scale with categories of "never" (scored 1), "rarely" (scored 2), "occasionally" (scored 3), "frequently" (scored 4), and "always" (scored 5). The Perceived Physician Support Scale (ranging from 6 to 30) was created using these six items. Factor analysis with Varimax rotation was performed to generate this scale. All items loaded on one factor and the items were summed into a single-composite score (α = 0.776). Higher scores for the Perceived Physician Support Scale indicate a higher level of perceived physician support. Based on the frequency distribution, this scale was converted into tertiles for the analytic purposes. The lowest tertile (i.e., representing the lowest perceived support levels) served as the referent group.

2.2.4. Health Status Indicators. Participants were asked to self-report aspects of their current health status using items intended to measure activity limitations, the number of prescription medications taken regularly each day, and the number of physician visits in the previous 12 months. Participants were asked "Are you limited in any way in any activities because of physical, mental, or emotional problems?" Responses were scored as "no" (scored 0) or "yes" (scored 1). Participants were asked "How many different prescription medications do you regularly take each day?" Responses ranged from 0 to 26 for this open-ended item. Participants were also asked "In the past 12 months, how many times have you, yourself made a doctor visit?" Responses ranged from 0 to 10 for this open-ended item.

2.2.5. General Support Perceptions. Participants were asked to self-report their perceptions about their use of the Internet for general support related to managing their health problems. Participants were asked "How much do you rely on the Internet for ongoing help and support with your health problems?" Responses were scored on a 4-point Likert-type scale with categories of "not at all" (scored 0), "a little" (scored 1), "some" (scored 2), and "a lot" (scored 3). Based on the frequency distribution, participant responses were then dichotomized into two categories: "no" (scored 0; indicating that they do not rely on the internet at all) and "yes" (scored 1; indicating that they rely on the internet at least a little). Participants were also asked "How often do you feel you get the help and support you need to improve your health and manage your health problems?" Responses were scored using a 5-point Likert-type scale with categories of "never" (scored 0), "rarely" (scored 1), "occasionally" (scored 2), "frequently" (scored 3), and "always" (scored 4).

2.2.6. Sociodemographic Characteristics. To identify personal characteristics of these women, sociodemographic variables in this study included age (i.e., 44–64 years, 65+ years); race/ethnicity (i.e., non-Hispanic white, non-White); education level (i.e., high school or less, some college or more); marital status (i.e., unmarried, married); and residential rurality (i.e., urban, suburban, and rural).

2.3. Data Analysis. All statistical analyses were performed using IBM SPSS (version 20). Frequencies were calculated for all major study variables, which were initially examined in relationship to participants' age group (44–64 years, 65+ years) and whether they reported needing help learning how to take better care of their health (yes or no). Pearson's χ^2 tests were performed to assess the independence between the dependent variable and categorized independent variables. *t*-tests were used to examine mean differences for continuous variables. Logistic regression was performed to examine how sociodemographics, health indicators, perceived support, and frustrations were associated with reporting the need to help learning how to take better care of their health (i.e., not needing help served as the referent group). Odds ratios (OR) with 95% confidence intervals are displayed.

3. Results

3.1. Sample. Sample characteristics of study participants are presented in Table 1. Of the 287 females participating in this study, 34.5% reported needing help learning how to better care for their health. Over 65% of participants were between the ages of 44 and 64 years and 34.4% were aged 65 years and older. Respondents were disproportionately non-Hispanic white (88.5%), married (69.0%), and had an education level of some college or more (61.7%). Fifty percent of the study population resided in suburban areas, 25.2% resided in urban areas, and 24.8% resided in rural areas. Approximately 33% of participants reported being limited from activities because of physical, mental, or emotional problems. On average, participants reported taking 3.67 (±3.83) medications daily and visiting a physician 3.07 (±1.94) times in the previous 12 months. Over 45% of participants reported relying on the Internet for ongoing help and support to manage their health problems, and 67% of participants reported frequently or always getting the help and support they need to improve their health and manage their health problems.

Compared to women aged 65 years and older, a significantly larger proportion of participants aged 44–64 years had some college education or more (χ^2 = 7.14, P = 0.008) and relied on the Internet for ongoing support to manage their health problems (χ^2 = 21.15, P < 0.001). A significantly larger proportion of participants who reported needing help learning how to better care for their health problems were

TABLE 1: Sample characteristics by age and needing help learning HOW to take better care of own health.

	Total (n = 287)	Age group 44 to 64 (n = 189)	65+ (n = 98)	χ^2 or t	P	Need help learning How to care for health No (n = 188)	Yes (n = 99)	χ^2 or t	P
Age									
44 to 64 years	65.6%	—	—	—	—	64.4%	68.0%	0.38	0.536
65+	34.4%	—	—			35.6%	32.0%		
Race/ethnicity									
Non-Hispanic white	88.5%	86.8%	91.8%	1.63	0.202	91.5%	82.8%	4.78	0.029
Non-White	11.5%	13.2%	8.2%			8.5%	17.2%		
Education									
High school or less	38.3%	32.8%	49.0%	7.14	0.008	34.0%	46.5%	4.23	0.040
Some college or more	61.7%	67.2%	51.0%			66.0%	53.5%		
Marital status									
Unmarried	31.0%	28.0%	36.7%	2.28	0.131	27.8%	37.0%	2.57	0.109
Married	69.0%	72.0%	63.3%			72.2%	63.0%		
Residential rurality									
Urban	25.2%	17.4%	8.0%			23.5%	28.3%		
Suburban	50.0%	48.9%	52.0%	0.33	0.847	49.2%	51.5%	1.95	0.376
Rural	24.8%	24.7%	24.5%			27.3%	20.2%		
Limited activities for any reason (physically/mentally/emotionally)									
No	67.4%	64.7%	72.4%	1.75	0.186	71.3%	60.0%	3.78	0.052
Yes	32.6%	35.3%	27.6%			28.7%	40.0%		
Get help and support to improve health and manage health problems									
Never	5.6%	6.3%	4.0%			5.9%	5.0%		
Rarely	9.7%	9.5%	10.1%			9.0%	11.0%		
Occasionally	17.7%	11.8%	5.9%	1.27	0.866	14.9%	23.0%	7.98	0.092
Frequently	31.9%	21.5%	10.4%			29.8%	36.0%		
Always	35.1%	33.3%	38.4%			40.4%	25.0%		
Rely on internet for ongoing support to manage health problems									
No	54.7%	45.0%	73.5%	21.15	<0.001	53.7%	56.6%	0.21	0.646
Yes	45.3%	55.0%	26.5%			46.3%	43.4%		
Number of medications taken daily	3.67 (±3.83)	3.64 (±4.18)	3.73 (±3.08)	−0.20	0.843	3.58 (±3.77)	3.84 (±3.96)	−0.56	0.574
Number of physician visits in the previous 12 months	3.07 (±1.94)	3.10 (±2.00)	3.00 (±1.83)	0.41	0.684	3.00 (±1.97)	3.18 (±1.89)	−0.75	0.452

non-White (χ^2 = 4.78, P = 0.029) and had a high school education or less (χ^2 = 4.23, P = 0.040).

3.2. Healthcare-Related Frustrations. Healthcare-Related Frustration Scale characteristics are presented in Table 2. Of those who reported healthcare-related frustrations, 16.4% reported frequently wishing their doctor had more time to spend talking to them; 16.0% reported frequently feeling tired of describing their same conditions and problems every time they go to a hospital or doctor's office; 8.7% reported frequently wishing they had a friend or family member who could go to the doctor with them; and 8.3% reported frequently being tired of feeling on their own when it comes to taking care of their health problems. Fewer respondents (5.6%) reported frequently feeling their doctor does not realize what it is really like for them at home trying to take care of their health problems or (5.2%) frequently leaving the hospital or doctor's office feeling confused about what they should do. On average, participants scored 2.56 (±2.69) on the Healthcare-Related Frustration Scale. No significant differences were observed when comparing healthcare-related frustrations by age group. Conversely, when comparing frustrations by whether the participant reported needing help learning how to better care for their health problems, those needing help reported significantly

Table 2: Healthcare frustrations by age and needing help learning HOW to take better care of own health.

Healthcare-related frustration scale items ($\alpha = 0.766$)	Total ($n = 287$)	Age group 44 to 64 ($n = 189$)	Age group 65+ ($n = 98$)	χ^2 or t	P	Need help learning how to care for health: No ($n = 188$)	Need help learning how to care for health: Yes ($n = 99$)	χ^2 or t	P
Wish your doctor had more time to spend talking with you									
Never	59.1%	56.8%	62.6%			67.4%	43.4%		
Occasionally	24.5%	24.7%	24.2%	1.47	0.479	21.9%	29.3%	18.54	<0.001
Frequently	16.4%	18.4%	13.1%			10.7%	27.3%		
Feel tired of describing your same conditions and problems every time you go to a hospital or doctor's office									
Never	59.4%	59.8%	59.2%			67.6%	44.0%		
Occasionally	24.7%	22.8%	28.6%	2.01	0.367	21.3%	31.0%	16.42	<0.001
Frequently	16.0%	17.5%	12.2%			11.2%	25.0%		
Wish you had a friend or family member who could go to the doctor with you									
Never	76.0%	76.2%	76.5%			80.9%	66.7%		
Occasionally	15.3%	14.8%	15.3%	0.06	0.969	11.7%	22.2%	7.40	0.025
Frequently	8.7%	9.0%	8.2%			7.4%	11.1%		
Tired of feeling on your own when it comes to taking care of your health problems									
Never	68.1%	66.8%	70.7%			72.9%	59.0%		
Occasionally	23.6%	25.8%	19.2%	1.93	0.381	20.2%	30.0%	5.80	0.055
Frequently	8.3%	7.4%	10.1%			6.9%	11.0%		
Feel that your doctor does not realize what it is really like for you at home trying to take care of your health problems									
Never	71.4%	70.4%	72.7%			78.2%	58.6%		
Occasionally	23.0%	22.8%	24.2%	1.84	0.398	14.9%	38.4%	20.81	<0.001
Frequently	5.6%	4.5%	1.0%			6.9%	3.0%		
Leave the hospital or a doctor's office and feel confused about what you should do									
Never	71.0%	70.9%	70.7%			79.7%	54.5%		
Occasionally	23.8%	23.8%	24.2%	0.01	0.994	16.6%	37.4%	19.86	<0.001
Frequently	5.2%	5.3%	5.1%			3.7%	8.1%		
Healthcare-related frustration tertiles (higher scores indicate more frustration)									
Lowest tertile	30.30%	30.00%	30.60%			38.30%	15.20%		
Middle tertile	47.00%	44.70%	51.00%	1.89	0.388	30.70%	16.40%	25.94	<0.001
Highest tertile (referent group)	22.60%	25.30%	18.40%			14.90%	37.40%		
Healthcare-related frustration scale (ranging from 0 to 12)	2.55 (±2.69)	2.64 (±2.79)	2.39 (±2.50)	0.75	0.452	2.00 (±2.47)	3.60 (±2.80)	−4.79	<0.001

higher scores on the Healthcare-Related Frustration Scale ($t = -4.79$, $P < 0.001$) and higher frustration levels for five of the six individual scale items ($t = 25.94$, $P < 0.001$).

3.3. Perceived Physician Support. Perceived Physician Support Scale characteristics are presented in Table 3. Of those who reported receiving physician support, 50.9% reported their physician always helped them get an appointment they needed; 46.5% reported their physician always asked if they understood their medications when their doctor prescribed them; 15.7% reported their physician always talked to other doctors and nurses who were taking care of them; and another 15.7% reported their physician always made plans to contact them after a visit to see how they were doing. Fewer respondents (13.3%) reported their physician always

TABLE 3: Perceived physician support by age and needing help learning HOW to take better care of own health.

Perceived physician support scale items ($\alpha = 0.776$)	Total ($n = 287$)	Age group				Need help learning how to care for health			
		44 to 64 ($n = 189$)	65+ ($n = 98$)	χ^2 or t	P	No ($n = 188$)	Yes ($n = 99$)	χ^2 or t	P
Help you get appointments that you need									
Never	12.9%	14.3%	10.2%			16.0%	7.1%		
Rarely	5.9%	3.8%	2.1%			4.8%	8.1%		
Occasionally	12.9%	9.1%	3.8%	4.66	0.324	10.1%	18.2%	8.50	0.075
Frequently	17.4%	12.9%	4.5%			17.6%	17.2%		
Always	50.9%	30.7%	20.2%			51.6%	49.5%		
Ask if you understand your medications when your doctor prescribes them									
Never	15.3%	15.8%	14.1%			17.6%	11.0%		
Rarely	6.6%	7.4%	5.1%			6.4%	7.0%		
Occasionally	14.2%	9.7%	4.5%	1.85	0.763	10.6%	21.0%	7.30	0.121
Frequently	17.4%	10.4%	7.3%			18.6%	15.0%		
Always	46.5%	46.3%	46.5%			46.8%	46.0%		
Talk to other doctors and nurses who are taking care of you									
Never	25.4%	25.4%	25.5%			28.3%	20.0%		
Rarely	15.0%	11.5%	3.5%			12.3%	20.0%		
Occasionally	26.8%	24.3%	31.6%	4.08	0.395	26.2%	28.0%	4.79	0.309
Frequently	17.1%	11.8%	5.2%			16.6%	18.0%		
Always	15.7%	9.8%	5.9%			16.6%	14.0%		
Make plans to contact you after a visit to see how you are doing									
Never	26.8%	28.6%	24.5%			28.3%	24.0%		
Rarely	15.3%	10.8%	4.5%			13.4%	19.0%		
Occasionally	25.1%	16.4%	8.7%	2.80	0.591	27.8%	20.0%	4.25	0.373
Frequently	17.1%	9.4%	7.3%			16.0%	19.0%		
Always	15.7%	10.5%	5.2%			14.4%	18.0%		
Tell you about other people who can help you with your health problems									
Never	30.1%	19.4%	10.4%			30.5%	29.3%		
Rarely	11.5%	6.6%	5.2%			12.3%	10.1%		
Occasionally	30.1%	18.7%	11.1%	5.06	0.282	30.5%	29.3%	3.56	0.469
Frequently	15.0%	11.8%	3.5%			12.3%	20.2%		
Always	13.3%	9.7%	3.8%			14.4%	11.1%		
Ask for your ideas about how you can take care of your health problems									
Never	29.2%	19.2%	9.8%			33.0%	22.0%		
Rarely	13.2%	9.8%	3.5%			11.7%	16.0%		
Occasionally	23.6%	14.3%	9.4%	2.66	0.616	18.6%	33.0%	10.48	0.033
Frequently	20.8%	14.7%	6.3%			22.3%	18.0%		
Always	13.2%	12.2%	14.4%			14.4%	11.0%		

TABLE 3: Continued.

Perceived physician support scale items ($\alpha = 0.776$)	Total ($n = 287$)	Age group: 44 to 64 ($n = 189$)	Age group: 65+ ($n = 98$)	χ^2 or t	P	Need help learning how to care for health: No ($n = 188$)	Need help learning how to care for health: Yes ($n = 99$)	χ^2 or t	P
Perceived physician support tertiles (higher scores indicate more support)									
Highest tertile	25.40%	27.50%	21.40%			27.10%	22.20%		
Middle tertile	41.50%	41.80%	40.80%	1.93	0.381	41.50%	41.40%	1.10	0.577
Lowest tertile (referent group)	33.10%	30.70%	37.80%			31.40%	36.40%		
Perceived physician support scale (ranging from 6 to 30)	18.70 (±5.84)	18.52 (±5.83)	19.03 (±5.87)	−0.70	0.482	18.53 (±6.06)	19.01 (±5.43)	−0.67	0.505

TABLE 4: Factors associated with needing help learning HOW to take better care of own health.

	OR	P	95% CI Lower	95% CI Upper
Age 44 to 64 years	1.00	—	—	—
Age 65+	0.79	0.437	0.43	1.43
Non-Hispanic white	1.00	—	—	—
Non-White	2.26	0.049	1.00	5.09
High school or less	1.00	—	—	—
Some college or more	0.55	0.044	0.31	0.98
Married: no	1.00	—	—	—
Married: yes	0.96	0.889	0.53	1.74
Urban	1.00	—	—	—
Suburban	1.72	0.178	0.78	3.79
Rural	1.87	0.074	0.94	3.73
Limited activities for any reason: no	1.00	—	—	—
Limited activities for any reason: yes	1.07	0.847	0.56	2.02
Get help and support to manage health problems: never	1.00	—	—	—
Get help and support to manage health problems: rarely	1.23	0.765	0.32	4.64
Get help and support to manage health problems: occasionally	2.11	0.156	0.75	5.90
Get help and support to manage health problems: frequently	1.61	0.260	0.70	3.66
Get help and support to manage health problems: always	1.62	0.171	0.81	3.23
Rely on internet for ongoing support to manage health problems: no	1.00	—	—	—
Rely on internet for ongoing support to manage health problems: yes	0.94	0.848	0.52	1.70
Number of medications taken daily	0.98	0.695	0.91	1.07
Number of physician visits in the previous 12 months	0.93	0.428	0.79	1.11
Healthcare-related frustration scale: highest tertile	1.00	—	—	—
Healthcare-related frustration scale: middle tertile	0.17	<0.001	0.07	0.41
Healthcare-related frustration scale: lowest tertile	0.44	0.017	0.22	0.86
Perceived physician support scale: lowest tertile	1.00	—	—	—
Perceived physician support scale: middle tertile	0.50	0.081	0.23	1.09
Perceived physician support scale: highest tertile	0.49	0.033	0.25	0.94

told them about other people who could help them with their health problems or (13.2%) their physician always asked for their ideas about how they can take care of their health problems. On average, participants scored 18.70 (±5.84) on the Perceived Physician Support Scale. No significant differences were observed when comparing perceived physician support by age group. Conversely, when comparing support by whether the participant reported needing help learning how to better care for their health problems, a significantly smaller proportion of those needing help reported asked for their ideas about how they can take care of their health problems ($\chi^2 = 10.48$, $P = 0.033$).

3.4. Factors Explaining Needing Help Learning How to Take Better Care of Own Health. Table 4 displays the results of the logistic regression analysis explaining factors associated with participants reporting they need help learning how to better care for their health problems (i.e., not needing help served as the referent group). Participants who were non-White were significantly more likely to report needing help learning how to better care for their health problems (compared to non-Hispanic whites, OR = 2.26, $P = 0.049$), whereas those with some college or more were significantly less likely to report needing help learning how to better care for their health problems (compared to those with high school or less education, OR = 0.55, $P = 0.044$). Compared to participants with the highest level (tertile) of healthcare-related frustrations, those with middle (OR = 0.17, $P < 0.001$) and lowest (OR = 0.44, $P = 0.017$) frustration levels were significantly less likely to report needing help learning how to better care for their health problems, respectively. Compared to participants with the lowest level (tertile) of perceived physician support, those with the highest level of perceived support were significantly less likely to report needing help learning how to better care for their health problems (OR = 0.49, $P = 0.033$).

4. Discussion

Despite our concerns that the majority of older women would likely experience self-care problems [48–50], our analyses revealed that only about one-third of the women in our sample reported needing help learning how to take better care of their chronic conditions. But consistent with health disparities in the epidemiology of chronic illnesses [22, 24], persistent health disparities related to self-care behavior were noted among minorities and those with less education. The rural healthcare disparity often reported in other studies [25, 51–53] was not observed in this study, nor were unmarried women disadvantaged relative to their married counterparts. These findings suggest middle-aged and older women in this sample were comparable in terms of having a variety of social supports for learning how to take care of their health.

Additionally, despite the previous assumption that older women might be disadvantaged relative to younger baby-boomers, no significant differences in help needed based on age group were reported. Similarly, our proxy measures for disease magnitude and severity (i.e., number of medications, physician visits, and limitations in activities) did not differentiate those needing help. However, the existence of an age-based digital divide was observed [54–56], with older women less likely to use online/technology as a resource for chronic condition self-management. Further investigation is needed to examine differences in the types of methods/strategies in which these older women engage when caring for their health conditions outside of the healthcare setting.

This study helps elucidate the complex relationships among contextual factors, healthcare frustrations, and patient-provider interactions and support and points to potential opportunities for intervention. The lack of a significant relationship between age and healthcare-related frustrations or perceptions about physician support may be attributed to the fact that the sample was selected based on the presence of chronic conditions. However, the lack of a significant relationship is consistent with the fact that participation in community-based disease self-management programs is not limited to those of only older ages; rather, program enrollment is based on the participant's chronic disease status [57].

This study reveals two strong modifiable correlates of women needing help learning how to care for their chronic conditions, even after controlling for sociodemographic and health status indicators in multivariate analyses: healthcare-related frustrations and perceived physician support. The majority of identified frustrations were significantly related to middle-aged and older women's perceptions of needing help learning how to care for their health, which is supported in other studies [8, 16, 58, 59]. The recent emphasis on patient-centered care and medical homes [60] is designed to help reduce such frustrations and hence can be expected to help boost women's self-efficacy to care for their own health conditions. Additionally, perceived physician support was another significant factor for knowing how to self-manage chronic conditions, especially in terms of patient activation as exemplified by wanting physicians to "ask for your ideas about how you can take care of your health problems." This reinforces previous research about the importance of perceived physician support for motivating patients to engage in healthier lifestyles and recommended medical regimens [9, 31, 61, 62]. From the health professional point of view, fostering beliefs of patient support can be accomplished through continuing education units (CEUs) or expanded emphasis during medical school training to develop strategies in which clinicians can engage and implement to be supportive, listen to their patients, and solicit their patients' thoughts so they have an active role in their healthcare team [29, 63]. From the patient point of view, widely available evidence-based self-management programs include elements within their curricula to teach older women how they can more effectively communicate with their healthcare providers [64]. Considering perspectives from each side of the healthcare interaction is essential to improve self-management both within and outside of the healthcare setting, which has implications for reducing disease mismanagement, unnecessary healthcare utilization (e.g., emergency room use), and medical costs.

5. Limitations

This secondary dataset did not contain all variables necessary to fully contextualize barriers and challenges associated with chronic disease self-care behavior among this aging population. However, this national study contained many variables of interest to address the current research gaps in knowledge about associations of healthcare frustrations, physician support, and self-care needs to chronic disease management.

Substantial numbers of participants were lost due to incomplete data on particular scale items, resulting in an analytical sample that was systematically different from the full sample (e.g., younger, married, and more white) and potentially limited the generalizability of study findings. This is especially true in that the reduction of cases in the analytic sample reduced the potential proportion of older adults in the study from 42.1% to 33.4%, which may especially influence generalizability of findings to populations aged 65 years and older. Study participants reported a variety of chronic conditions, but subanalyses based on disease type were not performed because the sample size was inadequate to make such comparisons. Recognizing that needed self-care behavior may differ based on women's particular condition diagnoses, disease stage, and the number of comorbidities in which they are diagnosed, future studies should strive to compare about barriers to self-care, perceived physician support, and frustrations with the healthcare system by their chronic condition profile. Further, because women's ability to cope with and adjust to their disease self-care may differ based on their available resources and socioeconomic status, future studies should examine such variables to determine their relationship with self-care disparities.

Another study limitation reducing the ability to widely generalize findings to the greater female community was the self-report and cross-sectional nature of these data. However, the sample was derived from random digit dialing and included items that deeply explore the challenges and frustrations with chronic condition self-management, which are not typically seen in other studies that investigate correlations between self-care behavior and other healthcare or physical health indicators. Thus, this study contributes to a fuller understanding of the complex interrelationships that exist between self-care strategies, provider-patient interactions, and policies/programs in community contexts.

6. Conclusion

The current study adds to the existing science base by examining barriers to self-care with a new lens, exploring healthcare-related frustrations and perceptions of physician support, and how these perceptions relate to various life domains, including diverse health status and sociodemographic contexts. Identifying these common and unique challenges and correlates of these challenges, with a representative national population, advance our current knowledge about self-care issues among middle-aged and older women. Learning more about healthcare-related frustrations of and self-management supports utilized by middle-aged and older women has the potential to help program deliverers, healthcare providers, and health agencies provide the services and resources that women with chronic conditions want and think are helpful. Findings from this investigation has potential to inform and guide modifications in the implementation and dissemination of evidence-based programs for older women to better match individuals with programs that meet their needs.

Acknowledgment

This study was made possible by the vast contributions and leadership of the National Council on Aging (NCOA), with support from Atlantic Philanthropies and the California Healthcare Foundation (CHCF). The authors recognize support from the Center for Community Health Development which is a member of the Prevention Research Centers Program, supported by the Centers for Disease Control and Prevention cooperative agreement no. 5U48 DP000045. The findings and conclusions in this paper are those of the author(s) and do not necessarily represent the official position of the Centers for Disease Control and Prevention or the National Council on Aging.

References

[1] R. Amara and Robert Wood Johnson Foundation, *Health and Health Care 2010: The Forecast, the Challenge*, Jossey-Bass, San Francisco, Calif, USA, 2nd edition, 2003.

[2] L. G. Martin, V. A. Freedman, R. F. Schoeni, and P. M. Andreski, "Trends in disability and related chronic conditions among people ages fifty to sixty-four," *Health Affairs*, vol. 29, no. 4, pp. 725–731, 2010.

[3] T. E. Seeman, S. S. Merkin, E. M. Crimmins, and A. S. Karlamangla, "Disability trends among older Americans: National Health and Nutrition Examination surveys, 1988–1994 and 1999–2004," *American Journal of Public Health*, vol. 100, no. 1, pp. 100–107, 2010.

[4] U.S. Census Bureau, "Table 10. Projected Life Expectancy at Birth by Sex, Race, and Hispanic Origin for the United States: 2010 to 2050," Population Division NP2008-T10, 2008.

[5] C. Vogeli, A. E. Shields, T. A. Lee et al., "Multiple chronic conditions: prevalence, health consequences, and implications for quality, care management, and costs," *Journal of General Internal Medicine*, vol. 22, no. 3, pp. 391–395, 2007.

[6] K. R. Lorig, D. S. Sobel, P. L. Ritter, D. Laurent, and M. Hobbs, "Effect of a self-management program on patients with chronic disease," *Effective Clinical Practice*, vol. 4, no. 6, pp. 256–262, 2001.

[7] D. W. Baker, S. M. Asch, J. W. Keesey et al., "Differences in education, knowledge, self-management activities, and health outcomes for patients with heart failure cared for under the chronic disease model: the improving chronic illness care evaluation," *Journal of Cardiac Failure*, vol. 11, no. 6, pp. 405–413, 2005.

[8] E. A. Bayliss, J. L. Ellis, and J. F. Steiner, "Barriers to self-management and quality-of-life outcomes in seniors with multimorbidities," *Annals of Family Medicine*, vol. 5, no. 5, pp. 395–402, 2007.

[9] S. Du and C. Yuan, "Evaluation of patient self-management outcomes in health care: a systematic review," *International Nursing Review*, vol. 57, no. 2, pp. 159–167, 2010.

[10] U.S. Department of health and Human Services, "Healthy People 2020 Topics and Objectives: Older adults," 2012, http://www.healthypeople.gov/2020/topicsobjectives2020/overview.aspx?topicid=31.

[11] E. H. Wagner, "Chronic disease management: what will it take to improve care for chronic illness?" *Effective Clinical Practice*, vol. 1, pp. 2–4, 1998.

[12] T. Bodenheimer, K. Lorig, H. Holman, and K. Grumbach, "Patient self-management of chronic disease in primary care," *Journal of the American Medical Association*, vol. 288, no. 19, pp. 2469–2475, 2002.

[13] K. Farrell, M. N. Wicks, and J. C. Martin, "Chronic disease self-management improved with enhanced self-efficacy," *Clinical Nursing Research*, vol. 13, no. 4, pp. 289–308, 2004.

[14] M. G. Ory and G. H. DeFriese, Eds., *Self-Care in Later Life: Research, Program, and Policy Issues*, Springer, New York, NY, USA, 1998.

[15] A. Kennedy, A. Rogers, C. Sanders, C. Gately, and V. Lee, "Creating 'good' self-managers?: facilitating and governing an online self care skills training course," *BMC Health Services Research*, vol. 9, article 93, 2009.

[16] J. Nagelkerk, K. Reick, and L. Meengs, "Perceived barriers and effective strategies to diabetes self-management," *Journal of Advanced Nursing*, vol. 54, no. 2, pp. 151–158, 2006.

[17] M. G. Ory, B. M. Peck, C. Browning, and S. N. Forjuoh, "Lifestyle discussions during doctor-older patient interactions: the role of time in the medical encounter," *MedGenMed Medscape General Medicine*, vol. 9, no. 4, article 48, 2007.

[18] J. Hou and M. Shim, "The role of provider-patient communication and trust in online sources in internet use for health-related activities," *Journal of Health Communication*, vol. 15, no. 3, pp. 186–199, 2010.

[19] B. Riegel and B. Carlson, "Facilitators and barriers to heart failure self-care," *Patient Education and Counseling*, vol. 46, no. 4, pp. 287–295, 2002.

[20] M. Lopez-Class and J. Jurkowski, "The limits of self-management: community and health care system barriers among latinos with diabetes," *Journal of Human Behavior in the Social Environment*, vol. 20, no. 6, pp. 808–826, 2010.

[21] Y. Song, H.-J. Song, H.-R. Han, S.-Y. Park, S. Nam, and M. T. Kim, "Unmet needs for social support and effects on diabetes self-care activities in Korean Americans with type 2 diabetes," *Diabetes Educator*, vol. 38, no. 1, pp. 77–85, 2012.

[22] Agency for Healthcare Research and Quality, *2009 National Healthcare Disparities Report*, U.S. Department of Health and Human Services, Rockville, Md, USA, 2010.

[23] S. Kim, F. Love, D. A. Quistberg, and J. A. Shea, "Association of health literacy with self-management behavior in patients with diabetes," *Diabetes Care*, vol. 27, no. 12, pp. 2980–2982, 2004.

[24] Interagency Workgroup on Multiple Chronic Conditions, *Strategic Plan 2010–2015: Optimum Health & Quality of Life for Individuals with Multiple Chronic Conditions*, U.S. Department of Health and Human Services, Washington, DC, USA, 2010.

[25] L. D. Gamm, L. L. Hutchison, B. J. Dabney, and A. M. Dorsey, Eds., *Rural Healthy People 2010: A Companion Document to Healthy People 2010*, The Texas A&M University System Health Science Center, School of Rural Public Health, Southwest Rural Health Research Center, College Station, Tex, USA, 2003.

[26] A. J. Karter, M. R. Stevens, A. F. Brown et al., "Educational disparities in health behaviors among patients with diabetes: the Translating Research into Action for Diabetes (TRIAD) Study," *BMC Public Health*, vol. 7, article 308, 2007.

[27] M. A. Winkleby, D. E. Jatulis, E. Frank, and S. P. Fortmann, "Socioeconomic status and health: how education, income, and occupation contribute to risk factors for cardiovascular disease," *American Journal of Public Health*, vol. 82, no. 6, pp. 816–820, 1992.

[28] A. F. Jerant, M. M. Von Friederichs-Fitzwater, and M. Moore, "Patients' perceived barriers to active self-management of chronic conditions," *Patient Education and Counseling*, vol. 57, no. 3, pp. 300–307, 2005.

[29] M. Heisler, R. R. Bouknight, R. A. Hayward, D. M. Smith, and E. A. Kerr, "The relative importance of physician communication, participatory decision making, and patient understanding in diabetes self-management," *Journal of General Internal Medicine*, vol. 17, no. 4, pp. 243–252, 2002.

[30] C. R. Jaen, K. C. Stange, and P. A. Nutting, "Competing demands of primary care: a model for the delivery of clinical preventive services," *Journal of Family Practice*, vol. 38, no. 2, pp. 166–171, 1994.

[31] S. J. Loeb, J. Penrod, S. Falkenstern, S. H. Gueldner, and L. W. Poon, "Supporting older adults living with multiple chronic conditions," *Western Journal of Nursing Research*, vol. 25, no. 1, pp. 8–23, 2003.

[32] B. Riegel, V. V. Dickson, L. Kuhn, K. Page, and L. Worrall-Carter, "Gender-specific barriers and facilitators to heart failure self-care: a mixed methods study," *International Journal of Nursing Studies*, vol. 47, no. 7, pp. 888–895, 2010.

[33] A.-M. Rosland, M. Heisler, H.-J. Choi, M. J. Silveira, and J. D. Piette, "Family influences on self-management among functionally independent adults with diabetes or heart failure: do family members hinder as much as they help?" *Chronic Illness*, vol. 6, no. 1, pp. 22–33, 2010.

[34] S. Combs, *Counting Costs and Calories: Measuring the Cost of Obesity to Texas Employers*, Texas Comptroller of Public Accounts, 2007.

[35] M. P. Gallant, G. Spitze, and J. G. Grove, "Chronic illness self-care and the family lives of older adults: a synthetic review across four ethnic groups," *Journal of Cross-Cultural Gerontology*, vol. 25, no. 1, pp. 21–43, 2010.

[36] N. Kaufman, "Internet and information technology use in treatment of diabetes," *International Journal of Clinical Practice*, no. 166, pp. 41–46, 2010.

[37] N. Nijland, J. Van Gemert-Pijnen, H. Boer, M. F. Steehouder, and E. R. Seydel, "Evaluation of internet-based technology for supporting self-care: problems encountered by patients and caregivers when using self-care applications," *Journal of Medical Internet Research*, vol. 10, no. 2, article e13, 2008.

[38] J. D. Piette, "Interactive behavior change technology to support diabetes self-management: where do we stand?" *Diabetes Care*, vol. 30, no. 10, pp. 2425–2432, 2007.

[39] C. Kerr, E. Murray, F. Stevenson, C. Gore, and I. Nazareth, "Internet interventions for long-term conditions: patient and caregiver quality criteria," *Journal of Medical Internet Research*, vol. 8, no. 3, article e13, 2006.

[40] K. E. Flynn, M. A. Smith, and J. Freese, "When do older adults turn to the internet for health information? Findings from the Wisconsin Longitudinal Study," *Journal of General Internal Medicine*, vol. 21, no. 12, pp. 1295–1301, 2006.

[41] N. Peña-Purcell, "Hispanics' use of Internet health information: an exploratory study," *Journal of the Medical Library Association*, vol. 96, no. 2, pp. 101–107, 2008.

[42] C. A. Rees, A. J. Karter, and B. A. Young, "Race/ethnicity, social support, and associations with diabetes self-care and clinical outcomes in NHANES," *Diabetes Educator*, vol. 36, no. 3, pp. 435–445, 2010.

[43] C. Weinert, S. Cudney, and E. Kinion, "Development of my health companion to enhance self-care management of chronic health conditions in rural dwellers," *Public Health Nursing*, vol. 27, no. 3, pp. 263–269, 2010.

[44] R. J. W. Cline and K. M. Haynes, "Receiving social support online: implications for health education," *Health Education Research*, vol. 16, no. 6, pp. 693–707, 2001.

[45] C. Centers for Disease and Prevention, *Guide to Community Preventive Services. Behavioral and Social Approaches to Increase Physical Activity: Individually-Adapted Health Behavior Change Programs*, Atlanta, Ga, USA, 2010.

[46] M. E. Cress, D. M. Buchner, T. Prohaska et al., "Best practices for physical activity programs and behavior counseling in older

adult populations," *Journal of Aging and Physical Activity*, vol. 13, no. 1, pp. 61–74, 2005.

[47] National Council on the Aging and Lake Research Partners, "Re-forming healthcare: Americans speak out about chronic conditions and challenges to self-care, Findings from a national survey of Americans 44 and older with chronic conditions," 2009, http://www.ncoa.org/improve-health/chronic-conditions/healthier-lives- a.html.

[48] P. M. Chriss, J. Sheposh, B. Carlson, and B. Riegel, "Predictors of successful heart failure self-care maintenance in the first three months after hospitalization," *Heart and Lung*, vol. 33, no. 6, pp. 345–353, 2004.

[49] S. Heo, D. K. Moser, T. A. Lennie, B. Riegel, and M. L. Chung, "Gender differences in and factors related to self-care behaviors: a cross-sectional, correlational study of patients with heart failure," *International Journal of Nursing Studies*, vol. 45, no. 12, pp. 1807–1815, 2008.

[50] E. A. Bayliss, J. F. Steiner, D. H. Fernald, L. A. Crane, and D. S. Main, "Descriptions of barriers to self-care by persons with comorbid chronic diseases," *Annals of Family Medicine*, vol. 1, no. 1, pp. 15–21, 2003.

[51] M. S. Eberhardt and E. R. Pamuk, "The importance of place of residence: examining health in rural and nonrural areas," *American Journal of Public Health*, vol. 94, no. 10, pp. 1682–1686, 2004.

[52] D. Hartley, "Rural health disparities, population health, and rural culture," *American Journal of Public Health*, vol. 94, no. 10, pp. 1675–1678, 2004.

[53] M. Meit, *Bridging the Health Divide: the Rural Public Health Research Agenda*, University of Pittsburgh Center for Rural Health Practice, Bradford, Pa, USA, 2004.

[54] M. L. Ybarra and M. Suman, "Help seeking behavior and the Internet: a national survey," *International Journal of Medical Informatics*, vol. 75, no. 1, pp. 29–41, 2006.

[55] N. Selwyn, S. Gorard, J. Furlong, and L. Madden, "Older adults' use of information and communications technology in everyday life," *Ageing and Society*, vol. 23, no. 5, pp. 561–582, 2003.

[56] M. Lemire, G. Paré, C. Sicotte, and C. Harvey, "Determinants of Internet use as a preferred source of information on personal health," *International Journal of Medical Informatics*, vol. 77, no. 11, pp. 723–734, 2008.

[57] K. R. Lorig, D. S. Sobel, A. L. Stewart et al., "Evidence suggesting that a chronic disease self-management program can improve health status while reducing hospitalization a randomized trial," *Medical Care*, vol. 37, no. 1, pp. 5–14, 1999.

[58] J. A. Gazmararian, D. C. Ziemer, and C. Barnes, "Perception of barriers to self-care management among diabetic patients," *Diabetes Educator*, vol. 35, no. 5, pp. 778–788, 2009.

[59] J. S. Austrian, R. D. Kerns, and M. C. Reid, "Perceived barriers to trying self-management approaches for chronic pain in older persons," *Journal of the American Geriatrics Society*, vol. 53, no. 5, pp. 856–861, 2005.

[60] K. C. Stange, P. A. Nutting, W. L. Miller et al., "Defining and measuring the patient-centered medical home," *Journal of General Internal Medicine*, vol. 25, no. 6, pp. 601–612, 2010.

[61] C. Beasley, "Supported self care and care planning for patients with long-term conditions," *British Journal of Community Nursing*, vol. 14, no. 9, pp. 394–397, 2009.

[62] M. T. Coleman and K. S. Newton, "Supporting self-management in patients with chronic illness," *American Family Physician*, vol. 72, no. 8, pp. 1503–1510, 2005.

[63] M. Jay, C. Gillespie, S. Schlair, S. Sherman, and A. Kalet, "Physicians' use of the 5As in counseling obese patients: is the quality of counseling associated with patients' motivation and intention to lose weight?" *BMC Health Services Research*, vol. 10, article 159, 2010.

[64] A. National Council, *A New Vision on Aging*, Center for Advancement of Health, 2006.

20

Patient Perspectives on Engagement in Recovery after Hip Fracture

Joanie Sims-Gould,[1,2] Sarah Stott-Eveneshen,[1] Lena Fleig,[3] Megan McAllister,[1] and Maureen C. Ashe[1,2]

[1] *Centre for Hip Health and Mobility, Robert H.N. Ho Research Centre, 2635 Laurel Street, Vancouver, BC, Canada V5Z 1M9*
[2] *Department of Family Practice, University of British Columbia, Vancouver, BC, Canada*
[3] *Freie Universität Berlin, AB Gesundheitspsychologie, Habelschwerdter Allee 45, PF 10, 14195 Berlin, Germany*

Correspondence should be addressed to Joanie Sims-Gould; joanie.sims-gould@hiphealth.ca

Academic Editor: Arshad Jahangir

Purpose. To understand older adults' engagement in their recovery experience and rehabilitation after a fall-related hip fracture. *Method.* 50 community-dwelling older adults recovering from a recent (3–12 months) hip fracture (32 women, 18 men) participated in telephone interviews using a semistructured format at 6 and 12 months after recruitment into the study. Interviews were conducted as part of a mixed-methods study designed to test the effect of a postoperative hip fracture management program (B4 Clinic). *Results.* Three substantive themes were identified in the qualitative data: (1) managing expectations; (2) engaging in physical activity; and (3) there is life after fracture. Participants shared valuable insight into how their expectations for their recovery period compared to their lived experience and the role of physical activity in their ability to return to their prefracture activities. *Conclusions.* Our findings reflect older adults' expectations for recovery from hip fracture. Encouraging engagement in rehabilitative exercises and addressing expectations prior to hospital discharge may improve patients' adherence to rehabilitation programs, functional outcomes, and postoperative quality of life. Implications for rehabilitation include the necessity for early and ongoing engagement of rehabilitation professionals.

1. Introduction

A universal finding in health care research is that patients report difficulty navigating health care systems and that a major factor is a lack of information at the right time, in the right place, from the right person [1, 2]. The Change Foundation (2008) [3] reported that over 40% of surveyed Canadian patients discharged from hospital either did not know who to contact with questions about their condition or treatment or did not receive instructions about symptoms to watch or had no follow-up arrangements made by their hospital. Information is not often shared between health care providers and their patients [4, 5].

Patient engagement is a goal for health care systems, yet full participation in care requires a multitude of actions to ensure that one has the information they need and can experience the highest form of patient engagement: empowerment [6]. Patient engagement is defined by the Centre for Advancing Health [7] as the actions individuals must take to obtain the greatest benefit from the health care services available to them and, as such, places an emphasis on the patients' role in their own care. Specifically, behaviors that contribute to patient engagement include patient participation in making decisions, asking questions, and seeking information. Patient engagement is important because patients who are prepared to manage their symptoms, engage in health promoting behaviors, engage in decision-making, engage with providers, understand quality of care, and navigate the health care system tend to have better health outcomes [6, 8–10]. Patient engagement is particularly important in those circumstances where care needs are high and often complex like in the case of a hip fracture. This is particularly true for those who become patients very suddenly as is the case with those who fracture a hip. Not only must patients and their families become engaged in their care very quickly, they must maintain engagement over time and across changes to their health situation. Central to understanding engagement in care is an understanding of patient experiences [11]. Our research examines the experiences of patients after hip fracture. We focus specifically on patient's perceptions of their recovery experience and their engagement in rehabilitation after hip fracture.

2. Methodology

2.1. Design. This qualitative substudy was part of a larger single-centre randomized control trial (RCT) (Clinical Trials Registration NCT01254942) testing a specialized postoperative hip fracture management program (B4 Clinic) with usual care compared with only usual care (UC) [10]. The primary aim of the study was to test the effect of the B4 Clinic on mobility (operationalized as the Short Physical Performance Battery). For both the RCT and the qualitative substudy we obtained university and hospital ethics approval, and all study participants provided informed written consent. All participants randomized to the intervention group received usual care as above, plus a comprehensive assessment by a geriatrician based on the clinical practice guidelines from the American and British Geriatrics societies. In addition, all participants were assessed by a physiotherapist (PT) and occupational therapist (OT). The geriatrician referred participants to other health professionals (e.g., continence nurse) and/or specialists (ophthalmologist) as deemed appropriate by the initial assessment. As needed, participants attended PT and/or OT sessions on an outpatient basis and/or were given a home exercise program.

2.2. Participants. Participants were community-dwelling older adults age 65 years and older living in Metro Vancouver, who had a hip fracture (proximal, middle, or distal femur) in the 12 months before data collection. All study participants, from both the intervention and control groups, were invited to participate in this qualitative substudy. Participant's demographics are described in Table 1.

2.3. Data Collection. Three trained interviewers completed over-the-phone interviews of approximately 20 minutes (range 5–30 minutes) with 50 participants at 6 months (midpoint) and 12 months (final) after recruitment. Interviewers took extensive notes during the interviews. These notes were then transcribed by the interviewer verbatim. At each point of data collection, 48 participants agreed to complete the interview, with 45 participants participating in both interviews. Those who declined to participate in both qualitative interviews are not included in the described results. The questions asked at each interview are outlined in Table 2. As per our ethics all of our data has been deidentified and pseudonyms have been used.

2.4. Data Analysis. All data were deidentified and organized into a question-and-answer format prior to importing into

Table 1: Frequencies of participant demographics (n = 50).

Sex	
Women	32 (64%)
Men	18 (36%)
Marital status	
Married	27 (54%)
Widowed	8 (16%)
Separated/divorced	5 (10%)
Single	10 (20%)
Age	
65–74 years	14 (28%)
75–84 years	22 (44%)
85+ years	14 (28%)
Living arrangement	
Living alone	21 (42%)
Living with someone (spouse, friend, or family member)	29 (58%)
Completed high school	
Yes	45 (90%)
Education	
Completed postsecondary	33 (66%)
Comorbidity (2+ chronic condition diagnoses)	
No chronic conditions	11 (22%)
2–4 chronic conditions*	26 (52%)
5-6 chronic conditions	10 (20%)
7+ chronic conditions	3 (6%)

*Common chronic conditions include (in order of prominence): arthritis, visual impairment, osteoporosis, asthma, COPD, angina, heart disease, neurological, stroke, vascular disease, diabetes, gastrointestinal, depression, anxiety, hearing, degenerative, and obesity.

NVivo 10®, a computer-assisted data analysis program (QSR International, 2015). A deductive approach was used for initial structural coding to create a broad coding framework a priori based on the aim of each interview question, such as participants' expectations and goals for their recovery, their ability to resume their prefracture activities, and their reasons for joining in the study. Following this first cycle of coding, we used an inductive approach to conduct a second cycle of descriptive coding and a third cycle of line-by-line coding to ensure the assigned codes (i.e., short, descriptive headings assigned to a portion of a transcript) were representative of participant responses [11]. We recorded notes on the procedures and decisions made during data analysis and reflections on emerging themes in a reflexive journal. The study team met to discuss the coding and preliminary findings after each cycle of coding. These discussions informed the following cycle of coding and generated questions to be examined using investigative queries in NVivo 10, such as, "What factors supported participants who reached their recovery goals?" and "What were the difficulties participants encountered during their recovery?" The use of queries was valuable for analyzing the intersections between codes, frequency of responses, and the role of select variables in participants'

TABLE 2: Interview guide questions at 6 and 12 months after study onset.

6 months	12 months
What was your original expectation of your hip fracture recovery process?	Why did you decide to join this study after you broke your hip?
Have you been able to resume all of your pre-fracture activities?	Have you been able to achieve your goals regarding your recovery and return to your pre-fracture activities?
Do you have any goals for returning to your usual activities?	What, if any, benefit did you get out of your involvement in the study?
Related to your participation in the study, what can we do better moving forward?	Related to your participation in the study, what could we have done better?

recovery experiences. The final codebook and the results of these queries were discussed among the research team until consensus was met on the substantive themes in the data. The researchers are in agreement that saturation was obtained in the data, as no new themes were emerging in the last interviews.

3. Results

Three main themes were found to describe the recovery experience of patients: (1) managing expectations, (2) engaging in physical activity, and (3) there is life after fracture. While distinct, the themes share important intersections that cross the patient experience of recovering from hip fracture, from preoperative expectations for their recovery to the processes that support or hinder engagement in rehabilitation.

3.1. Managing Expectations. Participants were asked to describe their expectations for their recovery from hip fracture. For 16% ($n = 8$) of participants, the recovery period was what they had expected. However, for 62% of participants ($n = 31$) the recovery experience was not what they had expected, often because of the length of time required to recover and the onset of unexpected postoperative complications, described by 18% ($n = 9$) of participants as being the most unanticipated event in their recovery. Most participants expected to be fully recovered within 6 months or less after their surgery for hip fracture, as told by their surgeon.

> "The doctor said in 3 weeks I'd be feeling fine and in 6 weeks I'd be back to everything, and I'm not. It's a bit depressing. It's been a long time". *Ella, female, aged 80.*

The source and type of information patients receive preoperatively has an important role in the formation of realistic expectations for their recovery. Those who had high levels of engagement and had sought the perspectives of friends and family members who had personal experience with postoperative recovery from hip fracture or read the advice of past patients on Internet message boards managed their expectations better than those who had not. One participant commented on not knowing what to expect preoperatively and the difficulty in obtaining enough information to manage their expectations. They indicated that "it is hard when information is scare [sic] or incorrect."

> "As a patient we are at huge disadvantage because we don't know what questions to ask. ... I didn't know ... to ask what side effects or residual problems there might be. And I don't know how to get around it, because the surgeons are excellent and capably answer all the questions I did ask, but I can't expect them to tell me everything they know. I tried googling information, but there wasn't the type of discussion I was looking for online. In speaking with another person who had a hip fracture, I recognize that the experience can be quite different". *Robert, male, aged 87.*

Holding unrealistic expectations increases the risk of feeling disappointed and dissatisfied when the level of functional ability recovered does not meet the expectations initially set.

> "I thought I would be 100% or more or less as I was before... I was very optimistic... It is taking much longer than I thought. I guess you could say I'm disappointed. But I look at the stats for people like me and I think I'm doing well. I can live with it when I look at what happens to other people". *Margaret, female, aged 81.*

For three participants, not meeting their expectations discouraged them from continuing to engage in rehabilitative exercises, feeling as though little to no progress was being made.

3.2. Engaging in Physical Activity. The theme of "engaging in physical activity" describes the role of staying engaged and active after hip fracture surgery. For several participants, staying active was a means of regaining autonomy and taking control over the recovery by engaging in behaviors they believed/expected directly contributed to their recovery, such as walking outside and attending exercise classes or physiotherapy sessions. Several participants attributed their ability to return to their prefracture activities to their self-determined motivation; for example, Doreen stated, "because I wanted to" and Ester indicated: "I was determined I would."

For some, their continued belief that you have to keep moving during recovery from hip fracture stems from their optimism and emphasis on keeping a positive attitude (e.g., anticipation of future positive outcomes) as well as their confidence to persevere in the face of challenges, such as pain or slow progress.

> "I would say the attitude mentally is very important. When talking to other people about the study and why I am involved, some don't want to . . . they say it hurts, but I don't say that, I just work at it. It's what the physio says is for your own good, and that positive mental attitude is important". *Ethel, female, aged 90.*

Others reported disengaging from their recovery and ceasing continuation of their exercises after months of not seeing progress and feeling discouraged and dissatisfied. At 6 months after recruitment into the study, one participant commented,

> "I wouldn't say I have a real goal [for recovery] because it [mobility] isn't going to change". *Clara, female, aged 80.*

Clara's comment is a stark contrast to those made by Doreen and Esther, reflecting her perceived lack of control over her ability to change her functional outcome. Those who participated in a progressive exercise program, either through the B4 Clinic or their own home exercises, commented on how doing daily exercises provided a means for them to assess their progress throughout the recovery period:

> "I can see I still have a long way to go. It's good, it [exercises] shows me how I can improve". *Julius, male, aged 93.*

For most participants, exercise and other physical activities were an important part of their recovery. Within the intervention group, this was expressed by 60% (n = 15) of participants compared to 52% (n = 13) of those in the control group. While the control group did not have any formal activity program during the study, many still engaged in physical activity through their own physiotherapy or home exercise program. For several participants, keeping active was an important factor for pain management.

> "When I don't do exercises, my hip hurts and I say to myself it serves you right, you're not doing your exercises". *Vera, female, aged 90.*

Among participants who were not actively involved in exercises, some would comment that they knew they should be doing more or expressed an intention to start getting involved in activities pending the outcome of another ailment or condition in their life. Reasons for not exercising included medication side effects, complications from other health conditions, pain, lethargy, poor weather, and a lack of rehabilitation support (i.e., wanting more physiotherapy services than was offered to them). Several participants expressed feeling that they needed to wait for their body to heal more before they could safely exercise and were, therefore, less likely to engage in exercise activities.

3.3. There Is Life after Fracture. This theme captures participants' perspectives on their return to their prefracture life and activities. Participants predominantly fell into two categories of recovery: those who resumed their prefracture activities or an adapted version of them (N = 33) and those who felt they will never recover to their prefracture functional ability (N = 12). Those who resumed their prefracture activities were more likely to have more engagement in their postfracture care and rehabilitation. This perspective led them to take up participation in new activities (e.g., physiotherapy, home exercise program, or regular walking outside) or modify their prefracture activities to accommodate their changed level of functional capacity (i.e., flexible goal adjustment).

> ". . . there was some pain during the 6 months before the screws were removed, but it was not an impediment [to my activity]. I found ways to hike without pain. [What was that?] Oh, well when I went up steep inclines I would walk on my toes". *Robert, male, aged 87.*

Those who described a return to their prefracture activities often emphasized the importance of keeping a positive perspective throughout their recovery to mitigate feelings of disappointment or depression over a slow progression. This was implemented in their daily lives by consciously appreciating the small gains made and creating a flexible timeline for their recovery goals.

> "I've changed a bit what I do, and I guess I do it all but much slower. I do all other things I did before . . . I walked a lot better [before]. Now I don't know if I will ever be able to, I concentrate and it is a chore". *Margaret, female, aged 81.*

When participants discussed their progress made, it was often qualified that while they are better than they were at the beginning of their recovery period, they are still not back to where they were before hip fracture.

> "Still working towards better balance, better strength, better speed. I tell other people about it and they say I am doing well and perhaps I am for my age, but I am not where I was before. . . . Biking is better and back country skiing is alright, but I'm not as graceful going down stairs – I hold on tight when no one is there and am hesitant. And I don't thinks it's just mental. . . . I'm more fatigued, I think it might have to do with aerobic strength and endurance. . . . I'm just not where I used to be". *Ella, female, aged 80.*

Some participants described their recovery in terms of a percentage of what their abilities were before hip fracture.

> "I had quite extensive physiotherapy . . . after my hip [surgery] and I came out feeling 95%". *Martin, male, aged 80.*

Participants were asked at their final interview if they had achieved the recovery goals that they set for themselves. One participant responded that, "there is life after fracture," and although she did not meet her mobility goals, she sees her recovery as a long-term journey requiring long-term engagement in her rehabilitation activities (e.g., home exercise routine, regularly walking outdoors). For participants who described having had a history of being physically active, this perspective reflects a continuation of their prefracture activities. For others, particularly those over age 85, "life after fracture" is obtained through the ability to engage in activities that bring enjoyment to their life, such as visiting with family members (i.e., social participation). Among all participants, those over age 85 ($N = 12$) more frequently expressed feelings of acceptance over their loss of functional ability than younger participants. This was often attributed to the progression of other chronic conditions or their age-related expectations. To pursue and maintain personally relevant activity goals, individuals appeared to adjust their goals in response to (perceived) losses in their functional ability.

> "I'm realistic about my goals. I know at my age I can't go back to all the activities I used to do". *Stanley, male, aged 93.*

Participants also discussed the importance of social support during their postoperative recovery period. For those living with a spouse or other family member, family was often described as being instrumental for support with daily activities and encouragement to engage in rehabilitative exercises. While caring health care staff was important to most participants, those who lived alone express the greatest appreciation for this source of support. Study-related monthly phone calls to check in on participants' progress was also described as an important source of social support and motivation among some participants.

> "I felt safe and secure knowing that you and other [research assistant] girls were following my progress and that if anything went very wrong I could call – I don't' know if it would do any good, but it gave me a good feeling". *Dorothy, female, aged 93.*

4. Discussion

Hip fracture is a serious life event that has important implications for older adults' personal identity [12], mortality risk [13], and collective health care costs [14]. The theme of "managing expectations" highlights participants' expectations for their recovery and their lived experiences. Participants often described being told by their surgeon to expect a recovery period of 6 months before being able to return to their usual, prefracture activities. It is common for people to underestimate the length of time required to recover from hip fracture [15], particularly when the risk of complications is not taken into account [16]. While some studies suggest that the majority of recovery occurs in the first 6 months after surgery [16], others suggest that recovery can take up to a year or longer [12], with up to a 25% loss of prefracture functional ability remaining for some patients [15, 17]. In one study, only 39% of patients with hip fracture were fully back to their prefracture levels of mobility after one year [16]. Rehabilitation outcomes may be even worse among patients who reside in long-term care, as they often do not obtain the same level of access to rehabilitation services as those residing in the community [18].

As a result, many patients go into their recovery uncertain or misinformed about the length of time required to recover and the activities that would best support their recovery. This issue is compounded by a lack of information provided to patients [19], either as a result of limited resources or a lack of understanding of what is needed by patients for recovery or lack of patient engagement (or some combination). As demonstrated in our results misinformation can further exacerbate disengagement from one's recovery [20, 21]. Providing patients with a more realistic timeline for their recovery has its difficulties given the heterogeneity of those experiencing hip fracture.

This issue highlights a need for increased information sharing and preoperative counselling on the aims of the surgical intervention, risk of complications, expected length of recovery given patients' fracture type, and the importance of early mobilisation and integration of balance and strength exercises for recovery [15]. The use of a preoperative classification system has been suggested as a way to assess patients' characteristics as a means of supporting practitioners to obtain a more personalized projection of the expected recovery timeline for their patients; therefore improving their ability to engage patients appropriate and plan rehabilitative services accordingly [22]. This approach serves to manage patients' expectations and empower them to increase adherence to a rehabilitation program, even when progress may be slower than anticipated [19, 23]. An enhanced understanding of the patient experience may further increase the capacity of health care practitioners to address questions patients do not know to ask, increasing the likelihood that the information they receive is accurate and applicable to their specific condition and fracture.

Staying active and engaging in balance and strength exercise is one of the most effective postoperative measures for patients' return to their prefracture level of functional ability and independent ambulation [20, 24]. Engaging in physical activity was discussed by participants, who emphasized the importance of rehabilitation services, such as physiotherapy, in not only teaching patients what exercises they can do to improve their functional outcomes, but also in motivating them to keep up with their exercises if progress is not initially realized. One participant in our study described the advice of her physician to simply walk more after she asked about participating in physiotherapy; however, exercises prescribed by physiotherapists can better utilize the movements required to perform daily life activities and, as such, better prepare patients to return to these activities than solely walking [21].

Consistent with previous research, the most commonly reported barriers by study participants for engaging in physical activity were pain from complications during recovery [21, 25], lack of information on what they could physically do without hindering their recovery [26], and low motivation or acceptance of their changed level of functional ability [25, 27]. Intrapersonal, psychosocial factors (e.g., positive attitudes, optimism, expectations, motivation, self-efficacy, and outcome experience) and the reception of social support from family, friends, and health care providers can also play an important facilitating role in recovery [12, 21].

In our study, three participants reported discontinuing their exercise activities after not seeing the progress they had expected by 6 months after their surgical intervention. This is in line with previous behavior change theory and research which suggests that (unrealistic) expectations that do not match lived experiences result in dissatisfaction and ultimately disengagement (e.g., [28]). Other participants ($N = 6$) continued with their prescribed physiotherapy but expressed feeling that the exercises were not making a difference to their recovery. For these participants, their disengagement from exercise may not only reflect a lack satisfaction with expected recovery but also a lack of perceived control over their ability to effect change on their functional outcome. However, the majority of participants described seeing noticeable gains in their functional ability over time as a result of their continued participation in exercise activities, such as those prescribed by their physiotherapist. For these participants, exercise had a vital role in their recovery, with many participants expressing their appreciation for the physiotherapy services received.

For those participants who attributed their recovery to their own desire to participate in physical activity which served as a way for them to exert control over the recovery of their functional ability. Comments made by these participants also reflect high level of perceived confidence in their ability (i.e., self-efficacy) to participate in exercise programs and progress in their exercises as they advance in their recovery. Studies show that improvements in patients' level of self-efficacy can effectively increase adherence to exercise activities and improve functional outcomes [8, 29–31], particularly in the first 6 months after surgical intervention [32, 33]. Adherence further increases when exercise is integrated into patients' daily routines [21], and improvements to ambulation and functional ability begin to be realized [21, 28]. Besides self-efficacy, attributing progress in recovery to one's own efforts (e.g., through continued engagement in activity)/having an internal locus of control has been associated with greater independence in performing activities of daily living and lower levels of disability [34].

Studies have shown that between 6 and 12 months after hip fracture, older adults are more likely to experience a decline in their adherence to exercise programs as a result of increased fear of falling, experiencing pain attributed to the onset of complications or new health problems [31], low self-efficacy, or the lack of accountability from the cessation of group or in-home exercise sessions [35]. Therefore, it is important that rehabilitation interventions include components that postoperatively address patients' level of self-efficacy by continued engagement with rehabilitation professionals.

The research on the appropriate location and length of delivery of a rehabilitation program to older adults recovering from hip fracture is mixed. While some studies suggest that short-term programs reduce the risk of dependency on health care professionals and better facilitate functional independence [36] and increase self-efficacy [20], others suggest that functional gains made during the initial recovery period may be lost following program cessation [37], making an extended outpatient rehabilitation program with progressive training more ideal [32]. Participation in extended outpatient programs for at least 6 months has been found to offer measureable improvements in patients' muscle strength, balance, and gait speed, compared to participation in only a low-intensity home exercise program [32]. When measured at one year after hip fracture, those who participated in extended outpatient rehabilitation programs also had a greater level of perceived health [32], walking confidence [33], self-efficacy [33], and quality of life [38], likely a result of the gains made in their functional ability during their extended rehabilitation [39].

Some researchers have argued that longer-term programs are unnecessary given that most improvements to functional ability are made in the initial 4–6 months after hip fracture before plateauing [16], to which others assert that this can be overcome by increasing the intensity of exercise therapy and targeting improvements to patient balance, knee strength, and gait speed throughout the recovery period [24]. It is well understood that the integration of ambulatory and progressive rehabilitation programming into a postfracture care plan is necessary for improving patient strength, balance, and functional independence in completing activities of daily living [16, 33]. Programs that utilize elements of both types of rehabilitation programs, such as coupling the delivery of a short-term, inpatient program with a long-term, progressive outpatient program for up to 4–6 months with an integrated balance, and strength component, may offset declines in patient adherence and produce the best functional outcomes [16, 20, 24, 40, 41]. We support a model that includes sustained engagement.

The final theme in our study highlighted participant's view of life after hip fracture. Three participants in our study described feeling depressed after their hip fracture, which is not uncommon for patients recovering from such a health event [42]. It is also common for patients to have a heightened fear of falling after hip fracture [36] which may hinder their participation in physical activities that would support their recovery (e.g., walking outdoors, balance and strength activities) [37, 38]. By limiting their engagement in these activities, patients place themselves at greater risk of a subsequent fracture [24] for at least 10 years after their initial fracture [43].

Factors found to support or enhance recovery from hip fracture include staying motivated and determined to participate in exercise activities (in hospital and after discharge at home), self-regulatory strategies such as goal-setting and planning, social support, positive attitude, participation in health promoting behaviors (e.g., good nutrition, regular exercise, and taking appropriate medications), and a supportive physical environment conducive of physical activity (e.g., a walkable neighborhood) [44]. Receiving good quality care from health care providers (e.g., surgeon, physiotherapist, and family physician) can also affect patients' recovery. When care providers operate with a positive and friendly demeanor and provide adequate communication of information about the recovery process and address patient questions, recovery outcomes may improve [44].

Previous research has shown that patients with a more positive outlook on their recovery tend to show more signs of resiliency [45] and have better functional outcomes [46]. In our study, some participants attributed their positive attitude to the gains made in their recovery. It may be that those with a more positive perspective on their recovery experience are more likely to engage the rehabilitation supports available to them and keep up with their exercise activities for a longer period of time than those who get discouraged if not fully recovered after doing their exercises activities [47]. In our study, having social support through the encouragement of family members and research staff helped facilitate this positive thinking and keep them motivated to continue the rehabilitation journey.

Four participants who had not reached their original recovery goals in our study discussed the importance of not giving up, adjusting their goals, and continuing with the activities they could within their capacity (i.e., accommodative coping tendency, flexible goal adjustment in response to loss/physical constraints). This ability to accept their circumstances has been related to expressions of resilience in older adult participants in other qualitative studies [48, 49]. For others, their alignment with the theme, "there is life after fracture" is meant in the literal sense, as described by their appreciation for being alive after such as traumatic health event. Participants' discussion of their recovery from hip fracture as a long-term process highlights their continuation with life activities under the adoption of a new perspective. Studies have shown that life after fracture encapsulates a breadth of considerations that extend beyond the rehabilitation of independent ambulation and functional rehabilitation [12, 50]. Similar to findings of previous studies, adapting travel patterns, engaging in everyday activities, signing up for exercises classes at a local community center, and being more cognizant of fall risks are merely some of the ways that participants moved on with their life after fracture [12, 28].

Study Limitations. The aim of our study was to explore the patient experience of recovering from hip fracture among those who participated in the randomized controlled trial. While the themes identified in this study encapsulate the patient experience from the pre- to postoperative periods, several limitations have been identified. The first being that the interviews were not audio recorded. While vigorous notes and verbatim quotes were transcribed by the interviewers during the phone interviews, the transcripts do not reflect a verbatim account of participants' responses. This may have resulted in a recorder bias, where the decision by the interviewer as to what information is deemed important may affect what is recorded. The length of the interviews were also shorter than is typical for a semistructured interview and may reflect the timing of the phone call. Another limitation is that participants were overall a very physically active group. As such, their experience may not reflect the "typical" older adult undergoing surgery for hip fracture. However, similarities have been found between the themes identified in this study and those of other studies using qualitative methods to describe older adults' recovery from hip fracture [12, 51, 52]. These consistencies enhance the body of knowledge in this area and provide a stronger foundation from which to propose recommendations for practice. We also note that the study size of 50 participants at a single center and almost 2 : 1 ratio of women to men limits the generalizability of our findings.

5. Conclusion

Our study captured the experiences of a group of participants who were fairly active during their recovery from hip fracture. While the recovery period was not what participants had expected, most were able to return to some of their prefracture activities, albeit with the necessary adaptions made to the activity in order to do so. By managing expectations, keeping active, and maintaining participation in activities that bring quality to one's life (e.g., exercise, social participation) older adults can resume their life after hip fracture.

Conflicts of Interest

The authors report no conflicts of interest.

Acknowledgments

This work was supported by the Canadian Institute of Health Research (CIHR) operating grant, Demonstration Projects in Mobility and Aging [99051], and the Vancouver General Hospital (VGH) and University of British Columbia (UBC) Hospital Foundation. Dr. Sims-Gould is supported by a Canadian Institutes of Health Research New Investigator Award and a Michael Smith Foundation for Health Research Scholar Award. Dr. Ashe is supported by Tier 2 Canada Research Chair. The authors gratefully acknowledge the study participants for their time and willingness to share their experiences and insights on hip fracture. They would also like to acknowledge the support of the Centre for Hip Health and Mobility, Vancouver, BC, Canada.

References

[1] G. Hesselink, M. Flink, M. Olsson et al., "Are patients discharged with care? A qualitative study of perceptions and experiences of patients, family members and care providers," *BMJ Quality & Safety*, vol. 21, supplement 1, pp. i39–i49, 2012.

[2] M. A. Lamantia, L. P. Scheunemann, A. J. Viera, J. Busby-Whitehead, and L. C. Hanson, "Interventions to improve transitional care between nursing homes and hospitals: a systematic review," *Journal of the American Geriatrics Society*, vol. 58, no. 4, pp. 777–782, 2010.

[3] Who is the puzzle maker? Patient/caregiver perspectives on navigating health services in Ontario, 2008, http://www.change-foundation.ca/who-is-the-puzzle-maker/.

[4] E. A. Coleman, "Falling through the cracks: challenges and opportunities for improving transitional care for persons with continuous complex care needs," *Journal of the American Geriatrics Society*, vol. 51, no. 4, pp. 549–555, 2003.

[5] E. A. Coleman, J. D. Smith, J. C. Frank, S.-J. Min, C. Parry, and A. M. Kramer, "Preparing patients and caregivers to participate in care delivered across settings: the care transitions intervention," *Journal of the American Geriatrics Society*, vol. 52, no. 11, pp. 1817–1825, 2004.

[6] A. Coulter and J. Ellins, "Effectiveness of strategies for informing, educating, and involving patients," *British Medical Journal*, vol. 335, no. 7609, pp. 24–27, 2007.

[7] Centre for Advancing Health, *Engagement: What Is Patient Engagement?*, 2014, http://www.cfah.org/engagement/.

[8] J. H. Hibbard and J. Greene, "What the evidence shows about patient activation: better health outcomes and care experiences; fewer data on costs," *Health Affairs*, vol. 32, no. 2, pp. 207–214, 2013.

[9] R. Voss, R. Gardner, R. Baier, K. Butterfield, S. Lehrman, and S. Gravenstein, "The care transitions intervention: translating from efficacy to effectiveness," *Archives of Internal Medicine*, vol. 171, no. 14, pp. 1232–1237, 2011.

[10] W. L. Cook, K. M. Khan, M. H. Bech et al., "Post-discharge management following hip fracture—get you back to B4: a parallel group, randomized controlled trial study protocol," *BMC Geriatrics*, vol. 11, no. 1, article 30, 2011.

[11] J. Saldana, *The Coding Manual for Qualitative Researchers*, Sage Publications, Thousand Oaks, Calif, USA, 2009.

[12] L. Zidn, M. H. Scherman, and C.-G. Wenestam, "The break remains Elderly people's experiences of a hip fracture 1 year after discharge," *Disability and Rehabilitation*, vol. 32, no. 2, pp. 103–113, 2010.

[13] B. Sobolev, K. J. Sheehan, L. Kuramoto, and P. Guy, "Excess mortality associated with second hip fracture," *Osteoporosis International*, vol. 26, no. 7, pp. 1903–1910, 2015.

[14] K. Alzahrani, R. Gandhi, A. Davis, and N. Mahomed, "In-hospital mortality following hip fracture care in southern Ontario," *Canadian Journal of Surgery*, vol. 53, no. 5, pp. 294–298, 2010.

[15] P. A. E. Rosell and M. J. Parker, "Functional outcome after hip fracture: a 1-year prospective outcome study of 275 patients," *Injury*, vol. 34, no. 7, pp. 529–532, 2003.

[16] V. C. M. Koot, P. H. M. Peeters, J. R. De Jong, G. J. Clevers, and C. Van Der Werken, "Functional results after treatment of hip fracture: a multicentre, prospective study in 215 patients," *European Journal of Surgery*, vol. 166, no. 6, pp. 480–485, 2000.

[17] S. Boonen, P. Autier, M. Barette, D. Vanderschueren, P. Lips, and P. Haentjens, "Functional outcome and quality of life following hip fracture in elderly women: a prospective controlled study," *Osteoporosis International*, vol. 15, no. 2, pp. 87–94, 2004.

[18] M. Crotty, M. Miller, C. Whitehead, J. Krisnan, and T. Hearn, "Hip fracture treatments—what happens to patients from residential care?" *Journal of Quality in Clinical Practice*, vol. 20, no. 4, pp. 167–170, 2000.

[19] S. Klemetti, H. Leino-Kilpi, E. Cabrera et al., "Difference between received and expected knowledge of patients undergoing knee or hip replacement in seven European countries," *Clinical Nursing Research*, vol. 24, no. 6, pp. 624–643, 2015.

[20] M. Crotty, C. H. Whitehead, S. Gray, and P. M. Finucane, "Early discharge and home rehabilitation after hip fracture achieves functional improvements: a randomized controlled trial," *Clinical Rehabilitation*, vol. 16, no. 4, pp. 406–413, 2002.

[21] E. Gorman, A. M. Chudyk, C. A. Hoppmann et al., "Exploring older adults' patterns and perceptions of exercise after hip fracture," *Physiotherapy Canada*, vol. 65, no. 1, pp. 86–93, 2013.

[22] E. A. Eastwood, J. Magaziner, J. Wang et al., "Patients with hip fracture: subgroups and their outcomes," *Journal of the American Geriatrics Society*, vol. 50, no. 7, pp. 1240–1249, 2002.

[23] M. V. Mondloch, D. C. Cole, and J. W. Frank, "Does how you do depend on how you think you'll do? A systematic review of the evidence for a relation between patients' recovery expectations and health outcomes," *Canadian Medical Association Journal*, vol. 165, no. 2, pp. 174–179, 2001.

[24] M. A. Auais, O. Eilayyan, and N. E. Mayo, "Extended exercise rehabilitation after hip fracture improves patients' physical function: a systematic review and meta-analysis," *Physical Therapy*, vol. 92, no. 11, pp. 1437–1451, 2012.

[25] G. Archibald, "Patients' experiences of hip fracture," *Journal of Advanced Nursing*, vol. 44, no. 4, pp. 385–392, 2003.

[26] T. J. McBride, S. Panrucker, and J. C. Clothier, "Hip fractures: public perceptions," *Annals of the Royal College of Surgeons of England*, vol. 93, no. 1, pp. 67–70, 2011.

[27] B. Rasmussen and L. Uhrenfeldt, "Lived experiences of self-efficacy and wellbeing in the first year after hip fracture: a systematic review protocol of qualitative evidence," *The JBI Database of Systematic Reviews and Implementation Reports*, vol. 12, no. 10, pp. 73–84, 2014.

[28] S. B. Robinson, "Transitions in the lives of elderly women who have sustained hip fratures," *Journal of Advanced Nursing*, vol. 30, no. 6, pp. 1341–1348, 1999.

[29] R. H. Fortinsky, R. W. Bohannon, M. D. Litt et al., "Rehabilitation therapy self-efficacy and functional recovery after hip fracture," *International Journal of Rehabilitation Research*, vol. 25, no. 3, pp. 241–246, 2002.

[30] B. H. Marcus, D. M. Williams, P. M. Dubbert et al., "What we know and what we need to know: a scientific statement from the American Heart Association council on nutrition, physical activity, and metabolism (subcommittee on physical activity); council on cardiovascular disease in the young; and the interdisciplinary working group on quality of care and outcomes research," *Circulation*, vol. 114, no. 24, pp. 2739–2752, 2006.

[31] B. Resnick, C. D'Adamo, M. Shardell et al., "Adherence to an exercise intervention among older women post hip fracture," *Journal of Clinical Sport Psychology*, vol. 2, no. 1, pp. 41–56, 2008.

[32] E. F. Binder, M. Brown, D. R. Sinacore, K. Steger-May, K. E. Yarasheski, and K. B. Schechtman, "Effects of extended outpatient rehabilitation after hip fracture: a randomized controlled trial," *The Journal of the American Medical Association*, vol. 292, no. 7, pp. 837–846, 2004.

[33] K. Hauer, N. Specht, M. Schuler, P. Bärtsch, and P. Oster, "Intensive physical training in geriatric patients after severe falls and hip surgery," *Age and Ageing*, vol. 31, no. 1, pp. 49–57, 2002.

[34] C. Shaw, E. Mccoll, and S. Bond, "The relationship of perceived control to outcomes in older women undergoing surgery for fractured neck of femur," *Journal of Clinical Nursing*, vol. 12, no. 1, pp. 117–123, 2003.

[35] E. McAuley, J. F. Konopack, R. W. Motl, K. S. Morris, S. E. Doerksen, and K. R. Rosengren, "Physical activity and quality of life in older adults: Influence of health status and self-efficacy," *Annals of Behavioral Medicine*, vol. 31, no. 1, pp. 99–103, 2006.

[36] L. Zidén, K. Frandin, and M. Kreuter, "Home rehabilitation after hip fracture. A randomized controlled study on balance confidence, physical function and everyday activities," *Clinical Rehabilitation*, vol. 22, no. 12, pp. 1019–1033, 2008.

[37] P. C. Fletcher and J. P. Hirdes, "Restriction in activity associated with fear of falling among community-based seniors using home care services," *Age and Ageing*, vol. 33, no. 3, pp. 273–279, 2004.

[38] G. J. Wijlhuizen, R. de Jong, and M. Hopman-Rock, "Older persons afraid of falling reduce physical activity to prevent

outdoor falls," *Preventive Medicine*, vol. 44, no. 3, pp. 260–264, 2007.

[39] E. McAuley, S. L. Mihalko, and K. Rosengren, "Self-efficacy and balance correlates of fear of falling in the elderly," *Journal of Aging and Physical Activity*, vol. 5, no. 4, pp. 329–340, 1997.

[40] H. H. Handoll, C. Sherrington, and J. C. Mak, "Interventions for improving mobility after hip fracture surgery in adults," *Cochrane Database of Systematic Reviews*, vol. 3, Article ID CD001704, 2011.

[41] J. Zhang, M. L. Ang, and E. B. K. Kwek, "Who will walk again? Effects of rehabilitation on the ambulatory status in elderly patients undergoing hemiarthroplasty for femoral neck fracture," *Geriatric Orthopaedic Surgery & Rehabilitation*, vol. 6, no. 3, pp. 168–172, 2015.

[42] E. J. Lenze, M. C. Munin, E. R. Skidmore et al., "Onset of depression in elderly persons after hip fracture: implications for prevention and early intervention of late-life depression," *Journal of the American Geriatrics Society*, vol. 55, no. 1, pp. 81–86, 2007.

[43] B. Sobolev, K. J. Sheehan, L. Kuramoto, and P. Guy, "Risk of second hip fracture persists for years after initial trauma," *Bone*, vol. 75, pp. 72–76, 2015.

[44] Y. Young and B. Resnick, "Don't worry, be positive: improving functional recovery 1 year after hip fracture," *Rehabilitation Nursing*, vol. 34, no. 3, pp. 110–117, 2009.

[45] J. L. Wiles, K. Wild, N. Kerse, and R. E. S. Allen, "Resilience from the point of view of older people: 'there's still life beyond a funny knee'," *Social Science & Medicine*, vol. 74, no. 3, pp. 416–424, 2012.

[46] L. Fredman, W. G. Hawkes, S. Black, R. M. Bertrand, and J. Magaziner, "Elderly patients with hip fracture with positive affect have better functional recovery over 2 years," *Journal of the American Geriatrics Society*, vol. 54, no. 7, pp. 1074–1081, 2006.

[47] N. F. Taylor, C. Barelli, and K. E. Harding, "Community ambulation before and after hip fracture: a qualitative analysis," *Disability & Rehabilitation*, vol. 32, no. 15, pp. 1281–1290, 2010.

[48] B. M. Janssen, T. Van Regenmortel, and T. A. Abma, "Identifying sources of strength: resilience from the perspective of older people receiving long-term community care," *European Journal of Ageing*, vol. 8, no. 3, pp. 145–156, 2011.

[49] B. Resnick, "Resilience in older adults," *Topics in Geriatric Rehabilitation*, vol. 30, no. 3, pp. 155–163, 2014.

[50] L. Zidén, C.-G. Wenestam, and M. Hansson-Scherman, "A life-breaking event: early experiences of the consequences of a hip fracture for elderly people," *Clinical Rehabilitation*, vol. 22, no. 9, pp. 801–811, 2008.

[51] F. Griffiths, V. Mason, F. Boardman et al., "Evaluating recovery following hip fracture: a qualitative interview study of what is important to patients," *BMJ Open*, vol. 5, no. 1, Article ID e005406, 2015.

[52] C. Schiller, T. Franke, J. Belle, J. Sims-Gould, J. Sale, and M. C. Ashe, "Words of wisdom—patient perspectives to guide recovery for older adults after hip fracture: a qualitative study," *Patient Preference and Adherence*, vol. 9, pp. 57–64, 2015.

Personality and Perceived Health in Spousal Caregivers of Patients with Lung Cancer: The Roles of Neuroticism and Extraversion

Michael Hoerger,[1] Maria Coletta,[2] Silvia Sörensen,[3] Benjamin P. Chapman,[3] Kim Kaukeinen,[4] Xin Tu,[4] and Paul R. Duberstein[3]

[1] *Departments of Psychology, Psychiatry, and Medicine, Tulane Cancer Center, 3070 Stern Hall, New Orleans, LA 70118, USA*
[2] *Main Line Health, Newtown Square, PA 19073, USA*
[3] *Department of Psychiatry, University of Rochester Medical Center, 300 Crittenden Boulevard, Rochester, NY 14642, USA*
[4] *Department of Biostatistics, University of Rochester Medical Center, 300 Crittenden Boulevard, Rochester, NY 14642, USA*

Correspondence should be addressed to Michael Hoerger; mhoerger@tulane.edu

Academic Editor: Elke Bromberg

Purpose. Family members' responsibilities for patients with cancer have increased dramatically over the past decade and will likely continue to rise. Given that caregiving is associated with declines in self-care, there is a need for research on caregivers' perceptions of their own health. The purpose of this study was to examine whether personality is associated with four self-report perceived health items from the SF-36. *Methods.* The sample consisted of 114 spouses of lung cancer patients who completed cross-sectional measures as part of a larger cohort study on adjustment to the diagnosis and treatment of lung cancer. Predictors of interest were Neuroticism and Extraversion scores from the NEO-FFI. Covariates were age, gender, conscientiousness, depressive symptoms, and objective illness burden. *Results.* Multivariate analyses revealed that caregivers with higher Extraversion scores were less likely to respond affirmatively to the item "I expect my health to get worse" (OR = 0.90, $p < 0.05$). Neuroticism was associated with poorer perceived health (ORs from 1.11 to 1.12, p's < 0.05). *Conclusions.* The present cross-sectional findings suggest that personality is associated with responses to SF-36 perceived health items beyond what can be accounted for by objective illness burden and other covariates. The potential overestimation of health among extraverted caregivers may have implications for their health outcomes.

1. Introduction

Family members' caregiving responsibilities for patients with cancer have increased dramatically over the past decade and will likely continue to rise as care is now routinely administered on an outpatient basis and patients are living longer [1]. Understanding the psychological factors that contribute to morbidity among these "hidden patients" [2] may help improve the clinical assessment process and mitigate some of the adverse consequences of caregiving.

Perceived health is an important predictor of morbidity and mortality across various cultural contexts [3–7]. Subjective rating scales are often used to assess perceived health and are straightforward and quick to administer in busy clinical settings. Given the widespread use of these rating scales and their constituent items, it is important to identify influences on responses. In this study, we sought to examine whether personality is associated with perceived health in spouses of patients with lung cancer.

Although the term "caregiving" was initially used to refer to the provision of dementia care by family members, it is applicable to cancer care as well. Family members are not merely bystanders in treatment but also actual or potential cousers of services [8–10]. Family caregivers frequently accompany the patient to appointments, administer medications, and provide other critical day-to-day functions. For patients with lung cancer, where the 5-year survival rate is only 17% [11], spouses often provide in-home care. Recognizing that many caregivers derive psychological benefit from the provision of care [10, 12, 13], up to 30% of cancer caregivers experience significant psychological distress [10, 14–16]. Caregivers of patients diagnosed with lung cancer report more depressive symptoms than other caregivers [17].

Research also suggests that caregivers' physical health diminishes over time [18]. Meta-analyses have found that caregivers have poorer physical health [18, 19], which may result from self-neglect due to caregiving demands and the belief that responding to the health needs of one's spouse is more important than attending to one's own. In particular, caregivers may implicitly compare their health needs with those of their sick spouses [20], leading to a response shift [21, 22] in how they evaluate their own health. This shift might lead caregivers to care for their ill family members at the expense of their own health because they are "healthier" [20].

Personality and Perceived Health. Individual differences in how spouses respond to caregiving demands are now well documented [10, 20, 23, 24], and several studies have examined the personality correlates of perceived health [25–29]. To the best of our knowledge, only one study [2] has examined the personality correlates of health-related quality of life in the caregiving context, and that study did not examine specific perceived health items. Moreover, that study did not control for objective illness burden, so it was unclear whether personality was related to biased health perceptions or merely illness burden. In the current study, we controlled for objective illness burden [30] while examining caregivers' responses to four self-report perceived health items from the SF-36 [31]. These items were as follows: "I am as healthy as anybody I know," "My health is excellent," "I seem to get sick a little easier than other people," and "I expect my health to get worse."

Based on previous research from Chapman and colleagues [26], we derived two sets of hypotheses. The first concerns Neuroticism, a personality dimension involving negative affectivity and emotional instability, which has been associated with more health complaints in general samples [32, 33]. We hypothesized that caregiver Neuroticism would be associated with reports of poorer perceived health on all four items, above and beyond the effects of covariates. The second hypothesis concerns Extraversion, a personality dimension marked by positive affect and sociability. Individuals high in Extraversion tend to have positive views about the future [34, 35] and higher levels of emotional well-being, which may lead to more optimistic health assessments [33, 36]. People who are high in Extraversion may underestimate their symptoms and report overly positive health [37]. Consistent with findings from Chapman et al. [26] we hypothesized that Extraversion would be associated with the item tapping future expectations ("I expect my health to get worse") but not with the other three items.

2. Methods

2.1. Participants and Procedures. The study was approved by the IRB at the University of Rochester. The sample consisted of spouses of patients with lung cancer who completed cross-sectional measures as part of a larger cohort study conducted in the Rochester, New York, region [14, 38]. As a nonintervention study, the parent investigation examined the natural course of adjustment to the diagnosis and treatment of lung cancer. Spouses of patients who had been diagnosed with and treated for lung cancer were eligible to participate.

A member of the research team identified eligible spouses, through introduction by the surgeon or oncologist. The research team member explained the nature of the study and invited the spouse to participate. Of the 340 spouses of lung cancer patients who were approached, 159 (47%) provided written consent for participation, and complete data were available for 114 (72% of those who consented). Informed consent was obtained at the time of the research interview; spouse participants also agreed to allow the research team to review their primary care medical chart. Researcher training sessions were conducted throughout the study to monitor rater drift and ensure the methodological integrity of the data collection process. Trained research assistants administered self-report questionnaires and observer-rated assessment instruments.

2.2. Measures. Personality was assessed with the NEO-Five Factor Inventory (NEO-FFI) [39]. From the NEO-FFI, we selected two specific indicators of personality: Neuroticism and Extraversion. Because it is consistently associated with both health behaviors and objective health indicators [40–42] we controlled for the personality dimension conscientiousness. Internal consistency in this study was good for Neuroticism (Cronbach's $\alpha = 0.84$) and conscientiousness ($\alpha = 0.83$), while being lower for Extraversion ($\alpha = 0.63$). The NEO inventories have been used in prior research on spouses of chronically ill patients [23, 42, 43] and their validity has been well documented [39].

The Cumulative Illness Rating Scale (CIRS) [44] was used to ensure that any relationships between personality and subjective health were not confounded by objective illness burden. The CIRS is a validated [30, 45] physician-rated objective health index derived by means of patient history as well as physical examination and laboratory findings and quantifies the amount of physical disease in each organ system at the time of study entry. A physician-researcher reviewed the spouses' medical charts. Higher scores indicate greater disease burden.

Depressive symptoms were controlled for by using the 24-item observer-rated Hamilton Depression Rating Scale (HDRS) [46], which assesses the presence and severity of depressive symptoms over the past week. Symptoms measured on the HDRS include depressed mood, feelings of worthlessness, helplessness, hopelessness, loss of interest in pleasurable activities, fatigue, and somatic complaints. Higher scores reflect greater depressive symptoms. Scores were based on self-report and nonverbal presentation. In the present study, the HDRS had excellent internal consistency (Cronbach's $\alpha = 0.81$).

To measure subjective health, we dichotomized four items from the General Health Perceptions Scale of the SF-36 [31]. Following Chapman and colleagues [26], we used two positively valenced items ("I am as healthy as anybody I know" and "My health is excellent") and two negatively valenced questions ("I seem to get sick a little easier than other people" and "I expect my health to get worse"). Respondents who endorsed "neutral," "definitely true," or "mostly true" in response to the positive items and "definitely false" and "mostly false" to the negative items were categorized as reporting good perceived health. Respondents who endorsed "neutral," "definitely true," or "mostly true" in response to the negative items and "definitely false" and "mostly false" to the positive items were categorized as having poor perceived health. We dichotomized the item scores because binary scores have more practical utility for health care practitioners, but we also conducted sensitivity analyses on ordinal scores.

2.3. Data Analysis. For each of the outcome variables, we conducted a logistic regression model [47]. Predictors included Neuroticism and Extraversion. Given that perceived health is influenced by sociodemographic factors [48], objective health [33], and depressive symptoms [25, 26], the analyses controlled for age, gender, conscientiousness, CIRS, and HDRS. We also ran the regression models using ordinal logits for perceived health with the following ordered categories: good, neutral, and poor.

3. Results

3.1. Participant Characteristics. Descriptive statistics are summarized in Table 1. Caregivers had a mean age of 63 and were predominantly female (71%), Caucasian (97%), and living with patients (98%). Their mean level of education was 13 years, and the median income bracket was $25,000–34,999 (USD). Patients were distributed among cancer stages, and most of the patients (79%) had completed some form of treatment at the time of the spouse's participation, with surgery being the most common form of treatment, followed by combination therapy (surgery, radiation, and chemotherapy).

Table 2 shows the mean Neuroticism and Extraversion scores of those who endorsed good versus poor perceived health for each of the four SF-36 questions. The means and standard deviations for Neuroticism and Extraversion were comparable to those observed in large samples of healthy US adults [49].

Table 1: Descriptive statistics.

Variable	M (SD) or N (%)
Age, years	63.4 (9.9)
Gender, female	81 (71.1%)
Education, years	13.0 (2.1)
Income	
< $10,000	2 (1.8%)
$10,000–24,999	24 (21.1%)
$25,000–34,999	31 (27.2%)
$35,000–49,999	31 (27.2%)
$50,000 or higher	26 (22.8%)
Race, Caucasian	111 (97.3%)
Residing with patient	112 (98.2%)
Cancer stage	
I	54 (47.4%)
II	14 (12.3%)
III	28 (24.6%)
IV	18 (15.8%)
Cancer treatments	
Surgery only	50 (43.9%)
Radiation only	5 (4.4%)
Chemotherapy only	3 (2.6%)
Combination therapy	32 (28.1%)
No treatments	24 (21.1%)

Note. $N = 114$. Percentages may not sum to 100.0% due to rounding.

3.2. Hypothesis Testing. Table 3 shows the significant predictors in the multiple regression analysis. Higher Neuroticism was significantly associated with poor perceived health measured by the item "I seem to get sick a little easier than other people" ($p < 0.05$). Higher Neuroticism was also a significant predictor for the endorsement of "I expect my health to get worse" ($p < 0.05$). Spouses who reported being more extraverted were less likely to endorse the item "I expect my health to get worse" ($p < 0.05$).

Among the control variables, the CIRS objective illness burden scores ($p < 0.01$) and age ($p < 0.05$) were associated negatively with "My health is excellent." Older respondents were more likely to endorse "I expect my health to get worse" compared to younger respondents ($p < 0.05$). Conscientiousness and HDRS (depressive symptoms) were not significantly associated with responses to any of the perceived health items. Results did not significantly change when the analyses were conducted using ordinal logits.

4. Discussion

The purpose of this study was to test hypotheses about the relationship between two personality dimensions—Neuroticism and Extraversion—and responses to individual items tapping perceived health. Support for our hypotheses about Neuroticism was mixed. Neuroticism was found to be significantly associated with poor perceived health on the negatively worded items ("I seem to get sick a little easier than other people" and "I expect my health to get worse"), but not on the positively worded items ("My health is excellent" and "I am as healthy as anybody I know"). Findings for the negatively worded items are consistent with previous research [26, 32, 50]. Whereas Chapman and colleagues [26] reported significant associations between Neuroticism and the positively valenced items, there are at least four possible explanations for our failure to do so [51]. First, responses to the positively valenced items "My health is excellent" and "I am as healthy as anybody I know" may implicitly require caregiver respondents to make a judgment about their health in comparison to their ill spouse. A second and related point is that very few people reported poor perceived health on the item "I am as healthy as anybody I know," reducing statistical power. Third, the Chapman et al. sample was older, and some of Neuroticism's effects on perceived health may not become

TABLE 2: Personality dimensions associated with good and poor perceived health.

SF-36 item	Perceived health	Neuroticism M (SD)	Extraversion M (SD)
"I seem to get sick a little easier than other people"	Good ($n = 107$)	16.8 (5.39)	28.1 (5.34)
	Poor ($n = 5$)	20.0 (5.57)	27.2 (6.14)
"I am as healthy as anybody I know"	Good ($n = 88$)	16.9 (5.23)	28.4 (4.73)
	Poor ($n = 24$)	16.9 (6.19)	27.1 (7.23)
"I expect my health to get worse"	Good ($n = 99$)	17.1 (5.37)	28.3 (5.44)
	Poor ($n = 13$)	15.6 (5.80)	26.2 (4.36)
"My health is excellent"	Good ($n = 89$)	16.3 (5.14)	28.7 (4.76)
	Poor ($n = 23$)	19.1 (6.00)	25.9 (6.86)

Note. Perceived health responses were dichotomized.

TABLE 3: Personality dimensions and covariates associated with poor perceived health.

SF-36 item	Significant predictor	OR (95% CI)	p
"I seem to get sick a little easier than other people"	Neuroticism	1.11 (1.00–1.23)	0.05
"I am as healthy as anybody I know"	—		
"I expect my health to get worse"	Age	1.06 (1.01–1.13)	0.04
	Neuroticism	1.12 (1.02–1.23)	0.02
	Extraversion	0.90 (0.80–0.99)	0.05
"My health is excellent"	Age	0.94 (0.88–0.99)	0.05
	CIRS	1.51 (1.17–2.02)	0.003

Note. Categorical regression models are reported. Regression model using ordinal logits did not significantly change results. Covariates were age, gender, conscientiousness, Cumulative Illness Rating Scale (CIRS), and Hamilton Depression Rating Scale (HDRS).

observable until later adulthood [25, 52]. Finally, Neuroticism may confer a greater sensitivity to the presence of negative affect and negatively valenced items as opposed to the absence of positive affect [53]. This hypothesis could be examined in future clinical research. If it is supported, it would underscore for clinicians and researchers the importance of language, word choice, and item framing [54].

As hypothesized, people with higher Extraversion scores are less likely to endorse the item "I expect my health to get worse," controlling for physician assessment of actual health status based on medical records. Extraversion may be particularly relevant in the caregiving context because extraverted people tend to be optimistic and feel comfortable in the presence of others. People who are higher in Extraversion tend to have a more positive outlook on life. A factor termed "optimistic control," characterized by optimistic expectation for life outcomes, positive self-esteem, hope, and internal control, is positively correlated with Extraversion [34]. Additionally, positive affect has been shown to underlie thoughts about the future more than negative affect [53, 55, 56], which may impact how individuals higher in Extraversion judge the possibility of future health declines.

Assuming that middle-aged and older adults can expect their health to deteriorate over time and that caregivers are at increased risk for such deterioration, caregivers lower in Extraversion may make more accurate judgments about their health. In contrast, those higher in Extraversion may overlook important signs and symptoms of disease and fail to report these to a physician. Although a positive outlook on life has many physical and mental health benefits [57], some studies suggest that unrealistic optimism about the future in the face of vulnerability to health issues may undermine specific risk reduction behaviors [58, 59]. Extraverted individuals may be identifiable in the consulting room [60]. For example, extraverts often dominate conversations, speak loudly, are gregarious, and are physically animated and enthusiastic [61]. Health care providers are advised to attend to more subtle cues for physical illness among extraverted caregivers and regard with empathy and skeptical curiosity the extravert's appraisals of their own health.

Patient-reported outcomes (PROs) are increasingly being integrated into clinical research, care, accreditation standards, and reimbursement rates [62–65], so studies evaluating the psychometrics of commonly used measures, such as the SF scales, are timely. We found, unsurprisingly, that control variables of objective illness burden and age were associated with perceived health, which underscores the importance of controlling for these variables in research aiming to understand biased health perceptions. One prior study has linked personality to perceived health in a caregiver sample [2], and ours is the first to do so while controlling for objective illness burden. If personality can shape responses to self-reported health items, independent of objective illness burden, clearly more research is needed aimed at understanding psychosocial factors that may bias scores on self-reports of health status and other PROs, such as patient satisfaction with care.

Several study strengths and weaknesses should be noted. This is the first study of which we are aware to examine personality and perceived health in a caregiving context while controlling for objective illness burden. Additional strengths include rigorous controls for other potential confounders like depression and careful analysis of specific SF-36 questions, a level of detail seldom pursued, despite the fact that the wording of the questions varies greatly and that clinical interviews typically assess health through a few such individual questions, rather than a formal composite score. The main limitation is the correlational design. Causal inferences cannot be drawn. Also, the internal consistency reliability of the Extraversion measure was lower than desirable, so the observed effects may have underestimated the association between Extraversion and perceived health. Finally, although levels of Neuroticism and Extraversion in this sample were comparable to those reported in national samples [49] and we have personality data on more than 70 percent of the cohort, generalizability to the entire cohort of consenting participants cannot be guaranteed.

The goal of the present investigation was to examine the association between personality and perceived health in caregivers of patients with lung cancer. An important next step would be to extend these findings by examining moderators of the association, such as demographic and health characteristics. For example, we did not examine health behaviors, such as smoking, drinking, and drug use, and it is possible that the association between Extraversion and optimistic reports of health is stronger among individuals who avoid these behaviors and consequently experience fewer daily reminders of ill health (e.g., coughing and hangovers). Additionally, the association between Neuroticism and poorer perceived health could be stronger for caregivers who have fewer economic resources, whose care receiver has a worse prognosis, or who spend more time providing care.

In closing, the present findings suggest that personality is associated with how spouses of cancer patients think about their health. Given that perceived health has prognostic implications for a variety of health outcomes and the mounting evidence for the role of personality in health and longevity [66, 67], it is important to explore ways to assess personality in clinical settings in order to target and tailor efforts to modify potentially inflated or deflated misperceptions of one's own health. Understanding the factors that contribute to perceived health threats among caregivers can help prevent the commonly observed negative effects of caregiving. This information is of value to the health care providers who care for cancer patients or their spouses.

Competing Interests

None of the authors has any competing interests in conducting or reporting this research.

Acknowledgments

This work was supported by the Roadmap Scholars Award from the Louisiana Clinical and Translational Science (LA CaTS) Center (U54GM104940) from the National Institutes of General Medical Sciences, as well as K07MH01135, R25MH074898, and K24MH072712 from the National Institute of Mental Health.

References

[1] V. Roche, "The hidden patient: addressing the caregiver," *American Journal of the Medical Sciences*, vol. 337, no. 3, pp. 199–204, 2009.

[2] C. E. Löckenhoff, P. R. Duberstein, B. Friedman, and P. T. Costa, "Five-factor personality traits and subjective health among caregivers: the role of caregiver strain and self-efficacy," *Psychology and Aging*, vol. 26, no. 3, pp. 592–604, 2011.

[3] Y. Benyamini and E. L. Idler, "Community studies reporting association between self-rated health and mortality: additional studies, 1995 to 1998," *Research on Aging*, vol. 21, no. 3, pp. 392–401, 1999.

[4] E. L. Idler and Y. Benyamini, "Self-rated health and mortality: a review of twenty-seven community studies," *Journal of Health and Social Behavior*, vol. 38, no. 1, pp. 21–37, 1997.

[5] J. Mackenbach, J. G. Simon, C. W. N. Looman, and I. M. A. Joung, "Self-assessed health and mortality: could psychosocial factors explain the association?" *International Journal of Epidemiology*, vol. 31, no. 6, pp. 1162–1168, 2002.

[6] K. B. DeSalvo, N. Bloser, K. Reynolds, J. He, and P. Muntner, "Mortality prediction with a single general self-rated health question," *Journal of General Internal Medicine*, vol. 21, no. 3, pp. 267–275, 2006.

[7] K. B. DeSalvo, M. Jones, J. Peabody et al., "Health care expenditure prediction with a single item, self-rated health measure," *Medical Care*, vol. 47, no. 4, pp. 440–447, 2009.

[8] C. Thomas and S. M. Morris, "Informal carers in cancer contexts," *European Journal of Cancer Care*, vol. 11, no. 3, pp. 178–182, 2002.

[9] A. J. Applebaum and W. Breitbart, "Care for the cancer caregiver: a systematic review," *Palliative and Supportive Care*, vol. 11, no. 3, pp. 231–252, 2013.

[10] F. Romito, G. Goldzweig, C. Cormio, M. Hagedoorn, and B. L. Andersen, "Informal caregiving for cancer patients," *Cancer*, vol. 119, no. 11, pp. 2160–2169, 2013.

[11] R. Siegel, J. Ma, Z. Zou, and A. Jemal, "Cancer statistics, 2014," *CA: A Cancer Journal for Clinicians*, vol. 64, no. 1, pp. 9–29, 2014.

[12] K. Boerner, R. Schulz, and A. Horowitz, "Positive aspects of caregiving and adaptation to bereavement," *Psychology and Aging*, vol. 19, no. 4, pp. 668–675, 2004.

[13] T. Cassidy, "Benefit finding through caring: the cancer caregiver experience," *Psychology & Health*, vol. 28, no. 3, pp. 250–266, 2013.

[14] M. Pinquart and P. R. Duberstein, "Optimism, pessimism, and depressive symptoms in spouses of lung cancer patients," *Psychology and Health*, vol. 20, no. 5, pp. 565–578, 2005.

[15] M. W. Haun, H. Sklenarova, M. Villalobos et al., "Depression, anxiety and disease-related distress in couples affected by advanced lung cancer," *Lung Cancer*, vol. 86, no. 2, pp. 274–280, 2014.

[16] Y.-H. Lee, Y.-C. Liao, W.-Y. Liao et al., "Anxiety, depression and related factors in family caregivers of newly diagnosed lung cancer patients before first treatment," *Psycho-Oncology*, vol. 22, no. 11, pp. 2617–2623, 2013.

[17] B. Given, G. Wyatt, C. Given et al., "Burden and depression among caregivers of patients with cancer at the end of life," *Oncology Nursing Forum*, vol. 31, no. 6, pp. 1105–1117, 2004.

[18] M. Pinquart and S. Sörensen, "Correlates of physical health of informal caregivers: a meta-analysis," *Journals of Gerontology B: Psychological Sciences and Social Sciences*, vol. 62, no. 2, pp. P126–P137, 2007.

[19] P. P. Vitaliano, J. Zhang, and J. M. Scanlan, "Is caregiving hazardous to one's physical health? A meta-analysis," *Psychological Bulletin*, vol. 129, no. 6, pp. 946–972, 2003.

[20] R. D. Adelman, L. L. Tmanova, D. Delgado, S. Dion, and M. S. Lachs, "Caregiver burden: a clinical review," *JAMA: Journal of the American Medical Association*, vol. 311, no. 10, pp. 1052–1059, 2014.

[21] M. A. G. Sprangers and C. E. Schwartz, "Integrating response shift into health-related quality of life research: a theoretical model," *Social Science & Medicine*, vol. 48, no. 11, pp. 1507–1515, 1999.

[22] P. K. Gandhi, L. D. Ried, I.-C. Huang, C. L. Kimberlin, and T. L. Kauf, "Assessment of response shift using two structural equation modeling techniques," *Quality of Life Research*, vol. 22, no. 3, pp. 461–471, 2013.

[23] K. Hooker, D. J. Monahan, S. R. Bowman, L. D. Frazier, and K. Shifren, "Personality counts for a lot: predictors of mental and physical health of spouse caregivers in two disease groups," *The Journals of Gerontology, Series B: Psychological Sciences and Social Sciences*, vol. 53, no. 2, pp. 73–85, 1998.

[24] M. Hoerger, B. P. Chapman, H. G. Prigerson et al., "Personality change pre- to post-loss in spousal caregivers of patients with terminal lung cancer," *Social Psychological and Personality Science*, vol. 5, no. 6, pp. 722–729, 2014.

[25] P. R. Duberstein, S. Sörensen, J. M. Lyness et al., "Personality is associated with perceived health and functional status in older primary care patients," *Psychology and Aging*, vol. 18, no. 1, pp. 25–37, 2003.

[26] B. P. Chapman, P. R. Duberstein, S. Sörensen, and J. M. Lyness, "Personality and perceived health in older adults: the five factor model in primary care," *Journals of Gerontology Series B: Psychological Sciences and Social Sciences*, vol. 61, no. 6, pp. P362–P365, 2006.

[27] X.-N. Yu, Z. Chen, J. Zhang, and X. Liu, "Coping mediates the association between type D personality and perceived health in Chinese patients with coronary heart disease," *International Journal of Behavioral Medicine*, vol. 18, no. 3, pp. 277–284, 2011.

[28] P. M. C. Mommersteeg, I. Pot, W. Aarnoudse, J. Denollet, and J. W. Widdershoven, "Type D personality and patient-perceived health in nonsignificant coronary artery disease: The TWeesteden mIld STenosis (TWIST) study," *Quality of Life Research*, vol. 22, no. 8, pp. 2041–2050, 2013.

[29] J. K. Hirsch, A. R. Floyd, and P. R. Duberstein, "Perceived health in lung cancer patients: the role of positive and negative affect," *Quality of Life Research*, vol. 21, no. 2, pp. 187–194, 2012.

[30] Y. Conwell, N. T. Forbes, C. Cox, and E. D. Caine, "Validation of a measure of physical illness burden at autopsy: the cumulative illness rating scale," *Journal of the American Geriatrics Society*, vol. 41, no. 1, pp. 38–41, 1993.

[31] J. E. Ware and C. D. Sherbourne, "The MOS 36-item short-form health survey (Sf-36): I. conceptual framework and item selection," *Medical Care*, vol. 30, no. 6, pp. 473–483, 1992.

[32] R. Goodwin and G. Engstrom, "Personality and the perception of health in the general population," *Psychological Medicine*, vol. 32, no. 2, pp. 325–332, 2002.

[33] C. E. Löckenhoff, A. R. Sutin, L. Ferrucci, and P. T. Costa Jr., "Personality traits and subjective health in the later years: the association between NEO-PI-R and SF-36 in advanced age is influenced by health status," *Journal of Research in Personality*, vol. 42, no. 5, pp. 1334–1346, 2008.

[34] G. N. Marshall, C. B. Wortman, R. R. Vickers Jr., J. W. Kusulas, and L. K. Hervig, "The five-factor model of personality as a framework for personality-health research," *Journal of Personality and Social Psychology*, vol. 67, no. 2, pp. 278–286, 1994.

[35] M. Hoerger, B. Chapman, and P. Duberstein, "Realistic affective forecasting: therole of personality," *Cognition and Emotion*, 2015.

[36] C. Moor, D. Zimprich, M. Schmitt, and M. Kliegel, "Personality, aging self-perceptions, and subjective health: a mediation model," *International Journal of Aging and Human Development*, vol. 63, no. 3, pp. 241–257, 2006.

[37] C. E. Löckenhoff and L. L. Carstensen, "Socioemotionol selectivity theory, aging, and health: the increasingly delicate balance between regulating emotions and making tough choices," *Journal of Personality*, vol. 72, no. 6, pp. 1395–1424, 2004.

[38] Y. Kim, P. R. Duberstein, S. Sörensen, and M. R. Larson, "Levels of depressive symptoms in spouses of people with lung cancer: effects of personality, social support, and caregiving burden," *Psychosomatics*, vol. 46, no. 2, pp. 123–130, 2005.

[39] P. Costa and R. McCrae, *Revised NEO Personality Inventory and NEO Five Factor Inventory: Professional Manual*, Psychological Assessment Resources, Odessa , Fla, USA, 1992.

[40] B. P. Chapman, S. Hampson, and J. Clarkin, "Personality-informed interventions for healthy aging: conclusions from a National Institute on Aging Work Group," *Developmental Psychology*, vol. 50, no. 5, pp. 1426–1441, 2014.

[41] T. Bogg and B. W. Roberts, "Conscientiousness and health-related behaviors: a meta-analysis of the leading behavioral contributors to mortality," *Psychological Bulletin*, vol. 130, no. 6, pp. 887–919, 2004.

[42] B. P. Chapman, J. M. Lyness, and P. Duberstein, "Personality and medical illness burden among older adults in primary care," *Psychosomatic Medicine*, vol. 69, no. 3, pp. 277–282, 2007.

[43] J. H. Patrick and J. M. Hayden, "Neuroticism, coping strategies, and negative well-being among caregivers," *Psychology and Aging*, vol. 14, no. 2, pp. 273–283, 1999.

[44] B. S. Linn, M. W. Linn, and L. Gurel, "Cumulative illness rating scale," *Journal of the American Geriatrics Society*, vol. 16, no. 5, pp. 622–626, 1968.

[45] M. Fortin, G. Bravo, C. Hudon et al., "Relationship between multimorbidity and health-related quality of life of patients in primary care," *Quality of Life Research*, vol. 15, no. 1, pp. 83–91, 2006.

[46] J. B. W. Williams, "A structured interview guide for the Hamilton depression rating scale," *Archives of General Psychiatry*, vol. 45, no. 8, pp. 742–747, 1988.

[47] C.-Y. J. Peng, K. L. Lee, and G. M. Ingersoll, "An introduction to logistic regression analysis and reporting," *The Journal of Educational Research*, vol. 96, no. 1, pp. 3–14, 2002.

[48] P. Svedberg, C. Bardage, S. Sandin, and N. L. Pedersen, "A prospective study of health, life-style and psychosocial predictors of self-rated health," *European Journal of Epidemiology*, vol. 21, no. 10, pp. 767–776, 2006.

[49] R. R. McCrae and P. T. Costa Jr., "A contemplated revision of the NEO five-factor inventory," *Personality and Individual Differences*, vol. 36, no. 3, pp. 587–596, 2004.

[50] C. Monden and G. Kraaykamp, "Neuroticism, education and self-assessed health in the general population of the United States. Can smoking behaviour explain the associations?" *Social Indicators Research*, vol. 78, no. 2, pp. 271–285, 2006.

[51] A. Tellegen, "Structures of mood and personality and their relevance to assessing anxiety, with an emphasis on self-report," in *Anxiety and the Anxiety Disorders*, T. Hussain and J. D. Maser, Eds., pp. 681–706, Erlbaum, Hillsdale, NJ, USA, 1985.

[52] B. Canada, Y. Stephan, A. Jaconelli, and P. R. Duberstein, "The moderating effect of chronological age on the relation between neuroticism and physical functioning: cross-sectional evidence from two french samples," *The Journals of Gerontology—Series B: Psychological Sciences and Social Sciences*, vol. 71, no. 1, pp. 35–40, 2015.

[53] C. L. Rusting and R. J. Larsen, "Extraversion, neuroticism, and susceptibility to positive and negative affect: a test of two theoretical models," *Personality and Individual Differences*, vol. 22, no. 5, pp. 607–612, 1997.

[54] C. E. Löckenhoff, A. Terracciano, L. Ferrucci, and P. T. Costa, "Five-factor personality traits and age trajectories of self-rated health: the role of question framing," *Journal of Personality*, vol. 80, no. 2, pp. 375–401, 2012.

[55] P. R. Duberstein, K. R. Conner, Y. Conwell, and C. Cox, "Personality correlates of hopelessness in depressed inpatients 50 years of age and older," *Journal of Personality Assessment*, vol. 77, no. 2, pp. 380–390, 2001.

[56] M. A. Young, L. F. Fogg, W. Scheftner, J. Fawcett, H. Akiskal, and J. Maser, "Stable trait components of hopelessness: baseline and sensitivity to depression," *Journal of Abnormal Psychology*, vol. 105, no. 2, pp. 155–165, 1996.

[57] C. Cloninger, *Feeling Good: The Science of Well Being*, Oxford University Press, New York, NY, USA, 2004.

[58] N. D. Weinstein, "Unrealistic optimism about susceptibility to health problems," *Journal of Behavioral Medicine*, vol. 5, no. 4, pp. 441–460, 1982.

[59] J. A. Shepperd, W. M. P. Klein, E. A. Waters, and N. D. Weinstein, "Taking stock of unrealistic optimism," *Perspectives on Psychological Science*, vol. 8, no. 4, pp. 395–411, 2013.

[60] S. Sörensen, J. K. Hirsch, and J. M. Lyness, "Optimism and planning for future care needs among older adults," *GeroPsych*, vol. 27, no. 1, pp. 5–22, 2014.

[61] D. C. Funder and C. D. Sneed, "Behavioral manifestations of personality: an ecological approach to judgmental accuracy," *Journal of Personality and Social Psychology*, vol. 64, no. 3, pp. 479–490, 1993.

[62] Methodology Committee of the Patient-Centered Outcomes Research Institute (PCORI), "Methodological standards and patient-centeredness in comparative effectiveness research: the PCORI perspective," *The Journal of the American Medical Association*, vol. 307, no. 15, pp. 1636–1640, 2012.

[63] K. H. Sheetz, S. A. Waits, M. E. Girotti, D. A. Campbell Jr., and M. J. Englesbe, "Patients' perspectives of care and surgical outcomes in Michigan: an analysis using the CAHPS hospital survey," *Annals of Surgery*, vol. 260, no. 1, pp. 5–9, 2014.

[64] E. D. Kinney, "The affordable care act and the medicare program: linking medicare payment to quality performance," *New York University Annual Survey of American Law*, vol. 68, pp. 567–673, 2013.

[65] L. I. Wagner, D. Spiegel, and T. Pearman, "Using the science of psychosocial care to implement the New American College of Surgeons Commission on Cancer distress screening standard," *Journal of the National Comprehensive Cancer Network*, vol. 11, no. 2, pp. 214–221, 2013.

[66] B. P. Chapman, B. Roberts, and P. Duberstein, "Personality and longevity: knowns, unknowns, and implications for public health and personalized medicine," *Journal of Aging Research*, vol. 2011, Article ID 759170, 24 pages, 2011.

[67] B. P. Chapman, A. Weiss, K. Fiscella, P. Muennig, I. Kawachi, and P. Duberstein, "Mortality risk prediction: can comorbidity indices be improved with psychosocial data?" *Medical Care*, vol. 53, no. 11, pp. 909–915, 2015.

22

Potential Moderators of Physical Activity on Brain Health

Regina L. Leckie,[1] Andrea M. Weinstein,[1,2] Jennifer C. Hodzic,[1] and Kirk I. Erickson[1,2]

[1] *Department of Psychology, University of Pittsburgh, Sennott Square 3417, 210 S. Bouquet Street, Pittsburgh, PA 15260, USA*
[2] *Center for the Neural Basis of Cognition, Department of Psychology, University of Pittsburgh, Sennott Square 3417, 210 S. Bouquet Street, Pittsburgh, PA 15213, USA*

Correspondence should be addressed to Regina L. Leckie, regina.leckie@gmail.com

Academic Editor: Louis Bherer

Age-related cognitive decline is linked to numerous molecular, structural, and functional changes in the brain. However, physical activity is a promising method of reducing unfavorable age-related changes. Physical activity exerts its effects on the brain through many molecular pathways, some of which are regulated by genetic variants in humans. In this paper, we highlight genes including apolipoprotein E (APOE), brain derived neurotrophic factor (BDNF), and catechol-O-methyltransferase (COMT) along with dietary omega-3 fatty acid, docosahexaenoic acid (DHA), as potential moderators of the effect of physical activity on brain health. There are a growing number of studies indicating that physical activity might mitigate the genetic risks for disease and brain dysfunction and that the combination of greater amounts of DHA intake with physical activity might promote better brain function than either treatment alone. Understanding whether genes or other lifestyles moderate the effects of physical activity on neurocognitive health is necessary for delineating the pathways by which brain health can be enhanced and for grasping the individual variation in the effectiveness of physical activity interventions on the brain and cognition. There is a need for future research to continue to assess the factors that moderate the effects of physical activity on neurocognitive function.

1. Introduction

One in every eight US seniors over the age of 65 has been diagnosed with Alzheimer's disease (AD), amounting to more than 5.4 million people. With the aging baby boomers, this number is predicted to double by 2050 [1]. Unfortunately, pharmaceuticals have had limited success in preventing or treating age-related cognitive dysfunction, such as AD or even normal cognitive aging. Fortunately, physical activity appears to be a promising nonpharmaceutical method to attenuate cognitive dysfunction in late life [2, 3]. Yet, there remain many unanswered questions about the effectiveness of physical activity to improve brain health, prevent dementia, and reduce age-related cognitive decline.

"Physical activity" is an umbrella term defined by the Center for Disease Control (CDC) as any activity that increases heart rate and energy expenditure from one's basal level [4]. Examples of physical activities are walking, gardening, or even household chores such as cleaning. In turn, "exercise" is defined as a subcategory of physical activity, being any structured or repetitive activity that aims to improve fitness, endurance, or health such as strength training, purposefully running, or swimming. Both exercise and physical activity are often measured through self-report questionnaires; however, they can be assessed by identifying "fitness," which is comprised of one's cardiorespiratory and skeletal muscle endurance, flexibility, and balance [4]. Fitness is objectively measured by an assessment of the maximum amount of oxygen consumption by carbon dioxide expulsion or VO_2 max, as this is an objective measure of cardiorespiratory strength [5]. An individual who has a very low VO_2 max or reports very low levels of physical activity or exercise is considered "inactive" or sometimes referred to as "sedentary," but precise definitions of "sedentary" has become a matter of debate [6]. As a result, cross-sectional studies compare inactive or sedentary subjects to those with greater amounts of physical activity or higher fitness levels. In contrast, intervention studies usually recruit inactive individuals with the goal of improving fitness levels by increasing physical activity through engagement in exercise.

Numerous studies, reviews, and meta-analyses have documented that greater amounts of physical activity and higher fitness levels and are associated with greater gray matter volume [7–10], greater white matter integrity [8, 11–13], elevated functional dynamics including heightened connectivity of fronto-parieto-hippocampal circuits [14–17], and enhanced cognitive performance [12, 18]. Yet, despite the favorable effects of physical activity and cardiorespiratory fitness on brain health and cognitive function, there remains significant individual variability in the extent to which any individual benefits from physical activity. For example, randomized controlled trials of physical activity indicate that a subset of individuals often show little cognitive or neural benefit even after spending 12 months in an intervention [19]. On the other hand, others in the intervention show little improvement in cardiorespiratory fitness, while still demonstrating significant improvements in cognitive and brain function [20]. These results suggest that there might be factors moderating the effects of physical activity. Moderating factors could act by either attenuating or augmenting the effects of physical activity on neurocognitive function. For example, it is possible that if greater physical activity is accompanied by an increase in cognitive stimulation that the favorable effects of physical activity on cognitive and brain function could be magnified. On the other hand, if increased physical activity is accompanied by a poor diet, then the benefits of activity might be significantly attenuated. For this reason, it is important for studies to reflect on the factors that are contributing to variation in the effectiveness of physical activity to influence neurocognitive health. Indeed, instead of simply considering individual differences as noise in the analysis they could be considered as (1) an important source for understanding the effectiveness of interventions, (2) a method for identifying potential mechanisms by which physical activity exerts its effects on the brain, and (3) a way to tailor physical-activity-based treatments to more successfully enhance cognitive function for the greatest number of people.

One of the challenges facing researchers in this field is that the list of possible moderating factors is virtually endless, making it difficult to identify which factors might be the most immediately relevant and the most important to study. However, there are several moderating factors that share characteristics with physical activity or have similar putative mechanisms or pathways underlying the effects that provide researchers with a theoretical platform to begin their investigation. Along these lines, pertinent moderators of the effects of physical activity on brain health include (1) genotypes, such as apolipoprotein E (APOE) [21], brain derived neurotrophic factor (BDNF) [22], and catechol-O-methyltransferase (COMT) [23] because these genes influence molecular pathways thought to be regulated by physical activity and (2) dietary variables, such as omega-3 fatty acids [24] that share molecular mechanisms and behavioral outcomes with physical activity. Although there are clearly other factors that are moderating the effects of physical activity on neural outcomes, we will focus this paper on these few moderators for which there is empirical support for their effects. Therefore, in this paper we first review current literature on physical activity and the aging brain (see Table 1 for select studies' characteristics) in an effort to reveal the brain circuits influenced by physical activity. Secondly, we focus on several factors that might moderate the effects of physical activity on brain health and use this evidence to recommend future research directions with the hope of more comprehensively understanding the factors that influence cognitive and brain aging.

2. Physical Activity and Gray Matter (GM) Volume

There is increasing evidence that the brain remains plastic throughout the lifespan and that a greater amount of physical activity or higher fitness levels take advantage of this natural characteristic of the brain. For example, individuals reporting greater amounts of physical activity or who are more physically fit have greater GM volume than individuals reporting less activity [7] or are less physically fit [39–41]. The effect of greater amounts of physical activity on GM volume can be found throughout the brain; however, the prefrontal cortex [8, 41–43] and hippocampus [9, 19, 40, 44] appear to be especially sensitive to these effects. The prefrontal cortex is associated with executive functions, a group of goal-oriented tasks that involve working memory, verbal fluency, and multitasking. The hippocampus, on the other hand, is involved in memory consolidation, spatial learning, and other memory processes. What makes the prefrontal cortex and hippocampus of particular interest is that these regions are some of the earliest regions to atrophy in late adulthood [45–48].

A technique called voxel-based morphometry (VBM) is one way to measure GM volume using high-resolution brain images from magnetic resonance imaging (MRI). This technique uses an automated segmentation algorithm to demarcate gray matter, white matter, and cerebrospinal fluid. Then, on a point-by-point basis throughout the brain the volume or density of gray matter can be examined as a function of any variable of interest (e.g., fitness levels). Studies using VBM have shown widespread age-related atrophy in frontal brain regions [45, 49, 50]. For example, Good et al. [49] examined GM volume in 465 adults as a function of age using VBM and demonstrated significant GM volume loss in several frontal and parietal regions. These results, along with many others, confirm the age sensitive nature of frontal GM volume and highlight the frontal lobe as an area of interest in aging research.

Fortunately, physical activity appears to increase GM volume in the frontal cortex [8]. In a 6-month intervention, older adults were randomly assigned to either a moderate intensity aerobic walking group or to a stretching and toning control group. The walking group was monitored by exercise coordinators and exercised 3 days per week. The control group received similar amounts of social contact with the exercise coordinators, but partook in stretching exercises instead of walking. After the 6-month intervention, the aerobic walking group showed an increase in gray matter volume in the frontal cortex, along the medial wall near the

Table 1: Characteristics of selecting reviewed studies.

First author (citation no.)	Experimental method	Measure(s)	Population mean age (standard deviation)	N	Significant finding(s)
APOE as variable of interest					
Honea et al. [25]	Cross sectional: APOE ε4 carrier status, dementia status × global connectivity, GM volume, cognitive performance, and fitness Nondemented ($n = 56$) Early-stage AD ($n = 61$)	APOE ε4 carrier status VO_2 peak WMS III WAIS MMSE Voxel-based morphometry Diffusion tensor imaging	Older adults aged 73.4 (6.3)	117	Higher aerobic fitness levels were related to greater brain volume in the medial temporal lobe in early AD patients.
Liang et al. [26]	Cross sectional: APOE ε4 carrier status × fitness, biomarker risk status	Walking, running, and jogging questionnaire PIB APOE ε4 carrier status	Healthy older adults aged 55–88	56	Physical activity was associated with reduced plaque deposition in APOE ε4 carriers.
Nichol et al. [27]	Control 1: nontransgenic mice Control 2: Tg2576 mice Experimental group 1: nontransgenic mice with 3 weeks access to running wheel Experimental group 2: Tg2576 mice with 3 weeks access to running wheel	IL-1β TNA-α Aβ	Tg2576 transgenic mice ($n = 29$) C57Bl6/SJL nontransgenic mice ($n = 27$)	56	IL-β and Aβ fibrils are significantly lower in transgenic mice with access to running wheel than transgenic control mice.
Parachikova et al. [28]	Control 1: nontransgenic mice ($n = 6$) Control 2: Tg2576 mice ($n = 6$) Experimental group 1: nontransgenic mice with 3 weeks access to running wheel ($n = 6$) Experimental group 2: Tg2576 mice with 3 weeks access to running wheel ($n = 6$)	Morris water maze latency Aβ mRNA expression CXCL1 and CXCL12 protein	Tg2576 transgenic mice C57Bl6/SJL nontransgenic mice	24	Transgenic mice with voluntary exercise performed significantly better on Morris water maze than control transgenic mice showed no increase in inflammatory markers and increased mRNA production of CXCL1.
Podewils et al. [29]	Cross sectional: APOE ε4 carrier status × onset of dementia × physical activity	Minnesota leisure time activity questionnaire APOE ε4 carrier status	Adults aged >65	3,375	Adults who engaged in regular physical activity had significantly reduced risk of developing AD after a 5-year follow-up than those who were sedentary. ε4 carriers showed no significant changes in risk associated with increased participation in physical activity.
Reinvang et al. [30]	Cross sectional: APOE ε4 ($N = 69$) carriers versus non-ε4 carriers ($N = 117$)	AX-Continuous Performance Task WAIS II Color-Word Interference Task CVLT-II	Healthy adults mean age 64.5	186	There is a negative relationship between ε4 carrier status and performance on working memory tasks where ε4 carriers performed worse than noncarriers.
Schuit et al. [21]	Cross sectional: activity status × APOE ε4 carrier status, cognition Inactive group: self-report less than 1 hr/day physical activity Active group: more than 1 hr/day physical activity	MMSE APOE ε4 allele carrier status	Healthy older adult males 74.6 (4.3)	347	Inactive group showed significant decrease in MMSE score over 3 years. APOE ε4 carriers showed significantly steeper decline than ε4 noncarriers.

Table 1: Continued.

First author (citation no.)	Experimental method	Measure(s)	Population mean age (standard deviation)	N	Significant finding(s)
Smith et al. [15]	Cross sectional: APOE $\varepsilon 4$ carrier status × fitness, cognitive function, fMRI connectivity, and grey matter volume	APOE $\varepsilon 4$ carrier status Stanford Brief Activity Survey MMSE Mattis Dementia Rating Scale 2 Rey auditory verbal learning test Geriatric depression scale Whole-brain event-related fMRI Voxel-based morphometry	Healthy older adults aged 65–85	68	Effects of PA on task-related activation were reliably more pronounced in APOE-$\varepsilon 4$ carriers with no significant differences in grey matter volume.
BDNF as variable of interest					
Erickson et al. [31]	Cross sectional: BDNF serum levels × grey matter volume, spatial memory performance	BDNF serum levels MRI first segmentation Spatial memory task	Healthy older adults mean age 66.5	142	BDNF levels mediated the relationship between the significant decline in hippocampal volume as a function of age.
Mu et al. [32]	Experimental group: rats treated with BDNF antibody ($n = 7$) Control group: IgG treated rats ($n = 6$)	Morris water maze latency Place navigation test Spatial probe test	Male Sprague-Dawley rats	13	BDNF antibody treated rats had longer learning latencies and spatial memory performance.
Neeper et al. [22]	Cross sectional: 0, 2, 4, or 7 days of running wheel access	BDNF mRNA levels in cortical regions	Sprague-Dawley rats	39	2, 4 and 7 days of exercise significantly increased BDNF mRNA levels in the hippocampus and caudate.
Stranahan et al. [33]	Control 1: nontransgenic mice ($n = 12$) Control group 2: nontransgenic mice with access to running wheel ($n = 12$) Experimental group 1: leptin receptor mutant (db/db) transgenic mice ($n = 12$) Experimental group 2: leptin receptor mutant (db/db) transgenic mice with access to running wheel ($n = 12$)	Open field activity Hippocampal BDNF protein levels	Male db/db transgenic mice Male C57Bl6/SJL nontransgenic mice	48	Access to a running wheel increased hippocampal BDNF levels in both wild type and transgenic mice.
COMT as variable of interest					
de Frias et al. [34]	Longitudinal: COMT genotype (Met/Met ($n = 26$); Val/Met ($n = 46$); Val/Val ($n = 23$)) × cognitive performance over 5-year period with 2 time points (0 and 5 years)	COMT genotype Verbal fluency Working memory task Tower of Hanoi task WAIS block design task	Healthy adult males aged 58.1 (12.86)	292	At baseline, COMT Met/Met group performed better than the Val/Val and Val/Met variants on executive function tasks and block design. Greater executive function decline after a 5-year follow-up in Val/Val individuals.
Stroth et al. [23]	Control: nonintervention (Met $n = 19$; Val $n = 9$) participants Experimental group: group running session 3x per week for 4 months (Met $n = 33$; Val $n = 14$)	2-back working memory task Stroop task Dots-mixed task Maximal field track fitness test COMT genotype	Healthy adults aged 22.7 (5.7)	75	Val/Val individuals in running intervention showed increased cognitive performance compared to Met carriers.

Table 1: Continued.

First author (citation no.)	Experimental method	Measure(s)	Population mean age (standard deviation)	N	Significant finding(s)
Wishart et al. [35]	Cross sectional: COMT genotype (Met/Met ($n = 26$); Val/Met ($n = 46$); Val/Val ($n = 23$)) × cognitive performance	COMT genotype Trail making task	Healthy adults aged 18–85	95	COMT Met/Met participants showed increased performance on trails B task than Val/Val or Val/Met genotypes.
Omega-3 fatty acid as variable of interest					
Chytrova et al. [24]	Control: regular diet, no access to running wheel Experimental group 1: regular diet, access to running wheel Experimental group 2: DHA-enriched diet, no access to running wheel Experimental group 3: DHA-enriched diet, access to running wheel	Morris water maze latency Hippocampal levels of STX-3, STX-1, NR2B, and GAP-43	Male Sprague-Dawley rats	24	Both DHA and access to running wheel increased levels of NR2B, STX-3, and Morris water maze learning.
Muldoon et al. [36]	Cross sectional: serum omega-3 fatty acid levels × cognitive performance	Serum omega-3 levels WMS-III WASI Stroop task	Healthy middle aged adults aged 44.6 (6.7)	280	Higher levels of DHA correlated to increased performance on several cognitive measures, specifically working memory.
Oksman et al. [37]	Control: standard diet Experimental group 1: high omega-6 diet Experimental group 2: high omega-3 diet	Morris water maze latency Aβ42 levels and plaques	Female F3 or F4 generation Transgenic mice (APPswe/PS1dE9)	21	Omega-3 enriched diet decreased Aβ42 levels compared to the two control diets.
van Gelder et al. [38]	Longitudinal: omega-3 fatty acid levels × cognitive function over 5 year period with 2 time points (0 and 5 years)	Dietary questionnaire MMSE	Healthy older Dutch males aged 70–89	228	Increased omega-3 fatty acid consumption was associated with smaller decline in cognitive function at 5-year followup.

Citation, experimental procedures, subject information, sample size, and main significant findings, are outlined for studies that have been highlighted as exemplary in text.
Weschler Memory Scale III (WMSIII), Weschler Abbreviated Scale of Intelligence (WASI), California Verbal Learning Test II (CVLTII), and Pittsburgh Compound B (PIB).

anterior cingulate cortex (ACC) and increased white matter volume in the genu of the corpus callosum, whereas the control group showed typical reductions in volume in these same regions. The results from this study indicate that only 6 months of moderate intensity physical activity is sufficient for increasing volume in brain areas that usually shrink during this period of life.

The hippocampus, on the other hand, is involved in spatial navigation and memory. Located in the medial temporal lobe, the hippocampus is also prone to age-related atrophy [40, 46]. Important for memory formation and recall, hippocampal decay may be responsible for many of the symptoms associated with AD [19, 51], but even normal aging is associated with reduced hippocampal volume [52]. Rodent models of AD have shown decreased learning and memory performance accompanied by significant atrophy or even absence of hippocampal tissue [53–55]. Fortunately, the hippocampus is highly sensitive to exercise. In a study by van Praag et al. [56], mice that had access to a running wheel showed a significant increase in hippocampal cell proliferation and survival of new cells when compared to nonrunning mice. These and many other studies [57–59] indicate that exercise affects both the morphology and physiology of the hippocampus, including neurogenesis in the dentate gyrus.

Participation in moderate intensity exercise also appears to affect the hippocampus in humans. In an intervention extending for 1 year, participants were randomly assigned to either a moderate intensity aerobic walking group or to a stretching and toning control group, similar to the 6-month study described above [19]. Over the year, the control group experienced normal age-related atrophy of the hippocampus. However, the walking group experienced a 2% increase in hippocampal volume over this same period. In addition, hippocampal atrophy rates within the control group were inversely related to preintervention fitness levels, indicating that higher fitness levels were protective against hippocampal atrophy. This study provides some key insights into the effects of exercise on the hippocampus: first, only moderate intensity physical activity for 1 year is sufficient for increasing the volume of the hippocampus during a time period of life when the hippocampus tends to decline in size and increasing the risk for dementia. Second, higher fitness levels could reduce the rate of hippocampal decay over a 1 year period. While this study was conducted using healthy adults, these results identify aerobic exercise as a potentially effective method for preventing and treating diseases, such as Alzheimer's disease and dementia, that are associated with hippocampal atrophy.

Recent evidence has also linked the associations between higher fitness levels and greater GM volume with improvements in cognitive function. For example, Erickson et al. [40] found that higher cardiorespiratory fitness levels were associated with increased hippocampal volumes, which in turn mediated the relationship between fitness and spatial memory performance. A similar relationship was found between higher fitness levels, greater prefrontal cortex volume, and better performance on measures of executive control [41]. Thus, increased GM resulting from exercise and associated with higher fitness levels appears to have a significant association with improved cognitive function.

3. Genetic Moderators of Physical Activity on Brain Health

Many different factors may moderate the effect of physical activity on brain health. By including these variables as statistical interaction terms (i.e., physical activity × genotype), the effect of moderation on cognitive or neural outcomes can be quantified. In this way, genetic variants such as APOE, BDNF, and COMT may explain some of the individual differences in the extent to which physical activity augments brain health [60]. Effect sizes in these studies are often difficult to directly compare mainly because of the variation in samples, designs, and candidate genes studied. The genes in this paper have been chosen based on animal literature as well as some supporting human research.

3.1. Apolipoprotein E (APOE). The APOE gene has three different allele variations: ε2, ε3, and ε4. The majority of the population carries the ε3 allele, whereas the ε2 and ε4 alleles are less common [61]. The gene APOE creates the lipoprotein of the same name, abbreviated ApoE. ApoE is found throughout the body and is linked to cardiovascular functions such as the transport of fats and cholesterol from the blood stream to the liver for processing. There have now been numerous studies linking the APOE gene to cognitive performance and risk for dementia [62, 63]. In particular, the APOE ε4 allele is considered a potent risk factor for AD [64]. The APOE ε4 variant also influences cognition in healthy adults without dementia. For example, Reinvang et al. [30] examined whether memory and executive functioning varied by APOE genotype in a group of healthy adults. APOE ε4 carriers performed more poorly on letter and digit span tasks as well as the Stroop color-word task than noncarriers.

β-amyloid (Aβ) plaques are also biomarkers and putative causes of AD and are closely linked to APOE genotype [65–68]. The ApoE protein produced by APOE ε4 can bind to Aβ more efficiently than the other allele variants, increasing the number of plaques, which are thought to lead to AD symptoms [65]. Rodent studies reveal APOE ε4 knockout mice have reduced Aβ deposition [66], further confirming APOE genotype as a risk factor for impaired clearance of Aβ and susceptibility for AD. While Aβ plaque deposition is a putative cause of AD, voluntary physical activity effectively reduces amyloid plaque deposits in rodents [27, 28, 69, 70]. Exercise may have this effect by promoting the expression of growth factors that are associated with reduced amyloid and changes in inflammatory pathways that alter Aβ plaque deposition. For example, a study by Parachikova et al. [28] used transgenic (Tg2576) mice as a model for AD where the particular mutation produces an abundance of amyloid precursor protein (APP), a protein that gets cleaved to produce amyloid. The results revealed a significant decrease in mRNA for inflammatory biomarkers in Tg2576 mice with 3 weeks access to a running wheel when compared to Tg2576 mice without access to running wheels. Nichol et al. [27] extended this to show that reduced mRNA for inflammatory biomarkers coincided with decreased Aβ plaque deposition. Whether participation in physical activity moderates plaque deposition in humans has only recently been studied.

Consistent with the rodent literature, several epidemiological studies have also reported that the association between greater amounts of physical activity and reduced risk of dementia might be dependent on APOE genotype. For example, Podewils et al. [29] examined 3,375 individuals in the United States, measuring physical activity levels with a modified Minnesota Leisure Time Activity Questionnaire. From this measure the authors categorized the activities into groups based on metabolic equivalents, creating a calculation of energy expenditure for each individual. Adults aged 65 and over who engaged in regular physical activity had a markedly reduced risk of developing AD after a 5-year follow-up than those who were sedentary. Interestingly, these results were enhanced in APOE ε4 noncarriers, such that ε4 carriers showed no significant changes in risk associated with increased participation in physical activity. Although one strength of this study is its large sample size, the self-reported nature of physical activity along with its observational design make it difficult to conclude the direction and strength of the association.

In contrast, several other studies have found that APOE ε4 carriers benefit more from exercise than do non-ε4 carriers. Schuit et al. [21] examined the relationship between levels of physical activity and cognitive decline in late adulthood as a function of the presence or absence of the ε4 allele in 347 elderly Dutch men. The infrequent exercising group, defined as those being physically active less than one hour per day, had a twofold increased risk of cognitive decline over the three-year period as measured by the Mini Mental State Exam, but this risk was mitigated in the more frequent exercising APOE ε4 carriers. Hence, this epidemiological study suggests that participation in regular exercise could offset genetic risk factors for dementia. Consistent with this finding, a study of nondemented middle-aged adults found that greater amounts of physical activity was associated with faster performance on a memory task and greater brain activation in APOE ε4 carriers compared to their more sedentary APOE ε4 peers [71]. Again, although provocative, the results from these studies need to be interpreted within the context that physical activity was assessed using self-reported measures, and these studies were observational in nature and not stemming from randomized controlled trials.

Evidence in AD patients shows a slightly different pattern than that described above. For instance, Honea et al. [25] examined whether the association between fitness and brain volume in 61 individuals with early-stage AD would be moderated by the APOE polymorphism. Consistent with previous findings of a cross-sectional study examining VO_2 peak in dementia and early AD patients [10], higher aerobic fitness levels (VO_2 peak) were related to greater brain volume in the medial temporal lobe in early AD patients, as measured using voxel-based morphometry. Surprisingly, APOE ε4 status did not moderate the relationship between fitness and brain volume in either the AD patients or in the 56 healthy control participants. Contrary to this finding, Smith et al. [15] examined the effect of physical activity and APOE ε4 on brain activity during memory processing in older (65–85) cognitively intact adults. They found that physical activity increased semantic memory-related brain activation in cognitively intact older adults who carry the APOE ε4 allele. However, the authors included only 17 subjects per group and assessed physical activity through the self-report Stanford Brief Activity Survey (SBAS), rather than an objective measure such as VO_2 peak. Finally, in a study of amyloid deposition in older adults (55–88), greater amounts of self-reported physical activity were associated with reduced plaque deposition in APOE ε4 carriers [26]. Hence, despite some variability in the literature, there is a growing consensus that the harmful effects of the APOE ε4 allele are mitigated by greater amounts of physical activity. Yet, despite this preliminary conclusion, there is a need for more research to determine if APOE ε4 carriers who were randomly assigned to receive exercise could benefit more from an intervention than their non-ε4 counterparts. There is also a great need for larger sample sizes, as the costly nature of neuroimaging has limited the number of participants assessed in previous studies.

3.2. Brain-Derived Neurotrophic Factor (BDNF). BDNF is another gene that could be moderating the effectiveness of physical activity on brain health. Similar to APOE, BDNF refers to both the gene and its resulting protein. There is a valine to methionine substitution in the BDNF gene at codon 66 resulting in several natural occurring variants of this gene in the human population. The Val/Met and Met/Met genotypes have been associated with decreased cognitive performance [72–74] and GM volume [75, 76] compared to Val homozygotes. The Met allele is associated with a reduction in the regulated secretion and trafficking of BDNF from the cell, which is thought to impact the role of BDNF in cell proliferation and learning.

While present in all brain areas, BDNF is highly concentrated in the hippocampus and cortex [77], promoting cell proliferation and signaling through several pathways, most notably by binding to the receptor tyrosine kinase B (TrkB). BDNF binding to the TrkB receptor depolarizes glutamatergic cells and results in several intracellular signaling cascades that moderate mRNA transcription [78, 79].

Additionally, TrkB binding phosphorylates the NMDA receptors of the postsynaptic neuron, increasing cyclic-AMP production and promoting long-term potentiation (LTP) [80]. In the hippocampus, LTP is considered a cellular analog of learning and is closely coupled with behavioral indices of learning and memory [81]. Rodent models where BDNF-receptor binding has been blocked or in BDNF knockouts, animals show deficits in acquisition and retrieval on the Morris water maze [82]. Mu et al. [32] observed a decrease in spatial memory retention in rats treated with a BDNF blocking antibody, providing further evidence that BDNF is necessary for the facilitation of learning and memory. These studies suggest that BDNF binding is critical to several cognitive processes.

Interestingly for this discussion, BDNF levels also increase as a function of both immediate [83] and longer-term [33] exercise. In fact, increased BDNF expression is a highly replicated effect in exercise studies [84]. For example, Stranahan et al. [33] examined amounts of voluntary wheel running in mice, finding that hippocampal BDNF levels increased with greater amounts of exercise, and in turn, higher levels of hippocampal BDNF was associated with greater dendritic spine density and hippocampal neurogenesis. Thus, increased BDNF signaling is considered one of the primary molecular pathways by which exercise improves neurocognitive function.

BDNF is also found outside of the central nervous system and can be measured in serum and plasma in humans. While it has been argued that serum levels are not a valid measure of cortical BDNF levels [85], rodent studies have found strong correlations between hippocampal and frontal BDNF levels and peripheral BDNF measures [86]. Human studies report that BDNF levels are a reliable biomarker for depression, where there is a strong negative relationship between peripheral BDNF levels and depression [87] and treatment of depression might result in an increase in serum BDNF [88]. Postmortem studies of individuals who have died from suicide also report that cortical levels of BDNF closely correspond to serum levels in individuals diagnosed with depression [89]. Other studies of serum or plasma BDNF find that levels are correlated with measures of brain integrity including hippocampal volume [31] and cognitive function [90]. Yet, despite these correlations, the translation from peripheral to cortical BDNF levels in humans is still unknown as is the significance of BDNF in the serum. Nonetheless, measuring BDNF in the serum allows for a minimally invasive proxy for examining a biomarker of brain health that is simply mirroring what is happening in the brain. From this perspective, given that animal studies have consistently reported increased BDNF levels after exercise, it has become a molecule of interest in human studies of physical activity and exercise. In fact, several studies have reported that acute bouts of physical activity are effective at increasing BDNF levels in serum [85]. In humans, Yarrow et al. [91] examined BDNF by sampling serum levels 0, 30, and 60 minutes into a physical activity session, where participants rode a stationary bike at a moderate pace, as well as 30 minutes after a brief cooldown. They demonstrated that BNDF levels were significantly elevated during and immediately after the physical activity session. Long-term exercise interventions, however, have not shown elevated levels of serum BDNF at follow-up [19] indicating some differences between the effects of acute and long-term exercise on BDNF pathways. The differences between acute versus long-term effects of exercise on BDNF levels remains a matter of speculation.

BDNF clearly remains one of the primary molecular pathways by which exercise is thought to influence cognitive function. In line with this hypothesis, hippocampal volume is correlated with serum BDNF levels in older adults [31], and exercise-induced increases in hippocampal volume are associated with increased BDNF serum levels [19]. Although there is not a one-to-one association between BDNF protein and the BDNF polymorphism, the link between the Met allele and reduced secretion and trafficking of the protein suggests that physical activity could play an important moderating role. Unfortunately, to date, there have not been published investigations of whether physical activity moderates the effect of the BDNF polymorphism on neurocognitive function. This will be an important avenue for future research.

3.3. Catechol-O-methyltransferase (COMT). COMT is a gene that produces an enzyme of the same name and has been hypothesized to influence cognitive function and brain health. The COMT enzyme works by breaking down the neurotransmitters dopamine, epinephrine, and norepinephrine. COMT is located mainly in the frontal cortex and is necessary for the regulation of the aforementioned neurotransmitters but is predominantly associated with dopamine [92]. Dopamine is concentrated in the prefrontal cortex, where it plays a role in executive control [93, 94]. The COMT enzyme is altered by its genotype where a valine (Val) to methionine (Met) amino acid substitution at the 158/108 locus of the peptide sequence affects the thermostability of the enzyme. The COMT gene therefore has three variants, Val/Val, Val/Met, and Met/Met, where Val carriers show increased enzyme activity, which in turn reduces dopamine levels at a faster rate in the synapse [92]. Wishart et al. [35] found that Val homozygotes displayed decreased performance on executive tasks. Additionally, de Frias et al. [34] revealed reduced cognitive performance and greater cognitive decline after a 5-year follow-up in older adult Val/Val individuals. There have now been numerous studies documenting the association between the COMT gene and cognitive performance; yet several recent reviews and meta-analyses have questioned the robustness and consistency of the effect across populations and tasks [95]. Such variation suggests that there might be factors that are moderating the effect of the COMT gene and influencing the direction and consistency of the effect.

One such moderator might be participation in physical activity. Physical activity influences dopaminergic circuitry in both the prefrontal cortex and basal ganglia in animal models [96–99] suggesting that its effects on cognitive function might be partially mediated by its effects on dopamine. Unfortunately, few studies have examined whether the COMT gene moderates the effect of physical activity on neurocognitive function. In one study, Stroth et al. [23] examined whether variants of the COMT gene would be moderated by participation in a 17-week physical activity intervention in a sample of 75 adults. At the end of the intervention, Val carriers who were in the running group displayed disproportionately faster response times on a working memory paradigm when compared to Met homozygotes, indicating that the benefits associated with physical activity on working memory function were dependent on the COMT genotype. This effect could be happening through the effects of physical activity on the gene itself, through physical activity effects on dopamine, or on dopamine receptors. In other words, the pathways by which this effect occurs remain a matter of speculation.

The evidence outlined above marks the COMT gene as a possible moderator of the effects of physical activity on cognitive function, but more studies are needed to replicate this effect and expand it to larger sample sizes and other populations. However, there is a striking resemblance between the moderating effects of physical activity on APOE and COMT genotypes. In each instance there is speculation or evidence that participation in physical activity might mitigate the effect of the gene on cognitive function.

4. Dietary Moderators of Physical Activity on Brain Health

Omega-3 fatty acids provide many beneficial effects to the body [100] and brain [101], and the pathways by which omega-3 fatty acids work on the body are similar to the pathways thought to be regulated by physical activity. Hence, several human and animal studies have speculated about the additive or multiplicative benefits that might arise from combining omega-3 administration or supplementation with greater amounts of physical activity [102].

There are two distinct types of omega-3 fatty acids: docosahexaenoic acid (DHA) and eicosapentaenoic acid (EPA). DHA is primarily located in the cortex and is linked to a variety of cognitive functions such as attention and memory. EPA, however, is found all over the body and is known for its anti-inflammatory effects on the cardiovascular system. Higher DHA levels in the serum and self-reported dietary intake of DHA have been associated with better performance on measures of executive function [103, 104]; however many of these studies have been either cross sectional in nature or consisting of rather small sample sizes. On a molecular level, DHA is critical to cell membrane structure, fluidity, and ion permeability and is synthesized in small amounts in humans [105, 106]. As a result, humans are required to consume most of their necessary DHA to maintain appropriate levels.

DHA has also been linked to dopamanergic pathways via the D2 dopamine receptor [107–109]. Rodents consuming a DHA deficient diet show significantly fewer D2 receptors in the striatum, mimicking similar pathology to rodent models of depression [110]. Rodent models of Parkinson's disease, where dopamanergic cells and receptors are significantly reduced, demonstrate that DHA supplementation is associated with a greater number of dopamanergic cells in the substantia nigra when compared to mice consuming a DHA deficient diet [111]. DHA is also under investigation as a potential nonpharmaceutical treatment for schizophrenia because of its effect on maintenance and preservation of normal dopaminergic function [112].

While both EPA and DHA are currently being explored as nonpharmaceutical treatments for schizophrenia, Parkinsons' disease, and other psychiatric and neurological conditions, other research is examining its links to cognitive function in middle-aged and geriatric populations. Muldoon et al. [36] tested the association between DHA serum levels and measures of cognitive function in midlife adults. They recruited 280 volunteers between 35 and 54 years of age, free of major neuropsychiatric disorders, who were not taking fish oil supplements. Individuals with higher DHA levels performed better on tasks of nonverbal reasoning and mental flexibility, working memory, and vocabulary. They concluded that DHA is related to cognitive health throughout the lifespan and may influence the prevalence of neuropsychiatric and impaired cognitive function in late life. However, this study was cross sectional, as are many others on DHA, so the directionality of the effects remains questionable.

In fact, some evidence suggests DHA might play an important role in dementia and age-related cognitive decline [113]. Individuals with self-reported diets high in omega-3 fatty acids decline at a slower rate on the MMSE as compared to omega-3 deficient individuals [38]. Several reviews of the literature and epidemiological studies over the past 10–12 years have revealed differing results, however, when conducting randomized trials of DHA supplementation or longitudinal studies following individuals with variation in fatty acid intake [114]. There is some evidence that greater intake of DHA might help to prevent or delay AD by preventing tangles and Aβ plaques [37, 115]. Although some research has hypothesized that DHA may be effective at reducing Aβ plaques, no consistent evidence for the treatment of AD has been found in association with DHA supplementation. Jicha and Markesbery [116] outline both epidemiological and clinical studies and conclude that there is evidence that DHA supplementation may act in cellular preservation but cannot be considered a reliable treatment for AD.

Physical activity, however, may provide an avenue by which the effects of DHA on cellular integrity and cognitive function may be enhanced [102, 106]. Chytrova et al. [24] revealed an additive effect of physical activity and DHA supplementation in a rodent model of synaptic plasticity and membrane structure in the dentate gyrus of the hippocampus. Mice in the DHA condition showed increased levels of membrane-bound synaptic proteins when compared to mice in the regular diet condition; however those mice receiving both DHA supplementation and physical activity showed greater levels of synaptic proteins than their counterparts not receiving physical activity. These results suggest that physical activity potentiated the effects of DHA supplementation on membrane proteins associated with synaptic plasticity. Unfortunately, studies in humans have not yet determined whether the effects of DHA on cognitive function are moderated by participation in physical activity. Given the molecular and cellular associations described above, it would be reasonable to hypothesize that such an interaction might be present.

5. Conclusion

Physical activity is effective at enhancing cognitive and brain function; however, many genetic and behavioral factors may be attenuating or augmenting the effect of physical activity. Genes such as APOE, BDNF, and COMT share molecular pathways with exercise and therefore might have the potential to moderate the effect of physical activity on cognitive function and neuronal health. For example, DHA reduces Aβ plaque build-up, similar to APOE, functions in the cell membrane, targets the synapse, similar to BDNF, and has strong ties to the dopaminergic pathway similar to COMT. Physical activity also affects all of these pathways, further weaving these independent variables together as part of a much larger story.

Unfortunately, many studies only assess one or two variables at a time in relation to cognitive function or physical activity. Therefore, the influence of genes or dietary variables on the effect of physical activity remains largely speculative. In fact, in this paper we highlight the evidence that there might be interactions between these variables, but to date, few studies have formally assessed these associations. Future studies with larger sample sizes and more comprehensive assessments of these variables are needed to move this field forward. Individual variability in prior studies highlights the need to more closely examine the potential moderators described here.

In addition, the way in which each of the genetic variables moderates the effect of physical activity is largely unknown. While there is evidence for physical activity to increase mRNA transcription of BDNF and COMT, the exact promoters targeted, and the way in which they are activated has not been identified. Animal models could provide insight to the pathways involved in the moderating effect of certain genotypes on physical activity and are a critical starting point for understanding these potential moderators of physical activity on neuronal changes, brain health, and cognitive function.

It will be important for new studies to take into consideration the individual variability contributed by dietary variables such as omega-3 levels and genes. These variables are clearly a source of "noise" within the data and could contribute to explaining the effects, or lack thereof, of physical activity on cognitive function. As we stated earlier, it will be important for future research to consider these variables as potential moderators instead of just "noise."

In sum, prior reviews and meta-analyses have focused on the protective and enhancing effects of exercise on neurocognitive function [12]. In this paper we have taken a different approach and have described several potential moderating factors that could be contributing to variation in the effectiveness of physical activity to enhance cognition. Although there is a long list of potential moderators, we have chosen here to focus on three different genes and a single dietary factor. This of course does not preclude other potentially important moderators such as intellectual engagement, other genes, other dietary factors, age, sex, or the combination of different types of physical activities (e.g., resistance training paired with aerobic training). We argue that it will be important for future research to consider these variables when designing studies, analyzing data, and interpreting the results from physical activity studies.

Acknowledgment

All authors contributed to the writing of the paper without any competing interests.

References

[1] Alzheimer's Association, "Alzheimer's disease facts and figures," in *Alzheimer'S & Dementia 2012*, Alzheimer's Association, Chicago, Ill, USA, 2012.

[2] C. H. Hillman, K. I. Erickson, and A. F. Kramer, "Be smart, exercise your heart: exercise effects on brain and cognition," *Nature Reviews Neuroscience*, vol. 9, no. 1, pp. 58–65, 2008.

[3] N. T. Lautenschlager, K. Cox, L. Flicker et al., "Effect of physical activity on cognitive function in older adults at risk for Alzheimer disease: a randomized trial," *Journal of the American Medical Association*, vol. 300, no. 9, pp. 1027–1037, 2008.

[4] C. F. D. C. A. Prevention, "Physical activity: glossary of terms," Division of Nutrition, National Center for Chronic Disease Prevention and Health Promotion, http://www.cdc.gov/, 2011.

[5] G. Godin and R. J. Shephard, "A simple method to assess exercise behavior in the community," *Canadian Journal of Applied Sport Sciences*, vol. 10, no. 3, pp. 141–146, 1985.

[6] R. R. Pate, J. R. O'Neill, and F. Lobelo, "The evolving definition of 'sedentary'," *Exercise and Sport Sciences Reviews*, vol. 36, no. 4, pp. 173–178, 2008.

[7] K. I. Erickson, C. A. Raji, O. L. Lopez et al., "Physical activity predicts gray matter volume in late adulthood: the Cardiovascular Health Study," *Neurology*, vol. 75, no. 16, pp. 1415–1422, 2010.

[8] S. J. Colcombe, K. I. Erickson, P. E. Scalf et al., "Aerobic exercise training increases brain volume in aging humans," *Journals of Gerontology A*, vol. 61, no. 11, pp. 1166–1170, 2006.

[9] J. M. Bugg and D. Head, "Exercise moderates age-related atrophy of the medial temporal lobe," *Neurobiology of Aging*, vol. 32, no. 3, pp. 506–514, 2011.

[10] J. M. Burns, B. B. Cronk, H. S. Anderson et al., "Cardiorespiratory fitness and brain atrophy in early Alzheimer disease," *Neurology*, vol. 71, no. 3, pp. 210–216, 2008.

[11] B. L. Marks, D. J. Madden, B. Bucur et al., "Role of aerobic fitness and aging on cerebral white matter integrity," *Annals of the New York Academy of Sciences*, vol. 1097, pp. 171–174, 2007.

[12] S. Colcombe and A. F. Kramer, "Fitness effects on the cognitive function of older adults: a meta-analytic study," *Psychological Science*, vol. 14, no. 2, pp. 125–130, 2003.

[13] M. W. Voss, S. Heo, R. S. Prakash et al., "The influence of aerobic fitness on cerebral white matter integrity and cognitive function in older adults: results of a one-year exercise intervention," *Human Brain Mapping*. In press.

[14] S. J. Colcombe, A. F. Kramer, E. McAuley, K. I. Erickson, and P. Scalf, "Neurocognitive aging and cardiovascular fitness: recent findings and future directions," *Journal of Molecular Neuroscience*, vol. 24, no. 1, pp. 9–14, 2004.

[15] J. C. Smith, K. A. Nielson, J. L. Woodard et al., "Interactive effects of physical activity and APOE-ε4 on BOLD semantic memory activation in healthy elders," *NeuroImage*, vol. 54, no. 1, pp. 635–644, 2011.

[16] M. W. Voss, K. I. Erickson, R. S. Prakash et al., "Functional connectivity: a source of variance in the association between cardiorespiratory fitness and cognition?" *Neuropsychologia*, vol. 48, no. 5, pp. 1394–1406, 2010.

[17] J. H. Burdette, P. Laurienti, M. A. Espeland et al., "Using network science to evaluate exercise-associated brain changes in older adults," *Frontiers in Aging Neuroscience*, vol. 2, p. 23, 2010.

[18] P. J. Smith, J. A. Blumenthal, B. M. Hoffman et al., "Aerobic exercise and neurocognitive performance: a meta-analytic review of randomized controlled trials," *Psychosomatic Medicine*, vol. 72, no. 3, pp. 239–252, 2010.

[19] K. I. Erickson, M. Voss, R. S. Prakash et al., "Exercise training increases size of hippocampus and improves memory," *Proceedings of the National Academy of Sciences of the United States of America*, vol. 108, no. 7, pp. 3017–3022, 2011.

[20] J. L. Etnier, P. M. Nowell, D. M. Landers, and B. A. Sibley, "A meta-regression to examine the relationship between aerobic fitness and cognitive performance," *Brain Research Reviews*, vol. 52, no. 1, pp. 119–130, 2006.

[21] A. J. Schuit, E. J. M. Feskens, L. J. Launer, and D. Kromhout, "Physical activity and cognitive decline, the role of the apolipoprotein e4 allele," *Medicine and Science in Sports and Exercise*, vol. 33, no. 5, pp. 772–777, 2001.

[22] S. A. Neeper, F. Gómez-Pinilla, J. Choi, and C. W. Cotman, "Physical activity increases mRNA for brain-derived neurotrophic factor and nerve growth factor in rat brain," *Brain Research*, vol. 726, no. 1-2, pp. 49–56, 1996.

[23] S. Stroth, R. K. Reinhardt, J. Thöne et al., "Impact of aerobic exercise training on cognitive functions and affect associated to the COMT polymorphism in young adults," *Neurobiology of Learning and Memory*, vol. 94, no. 3, pp. 364–372, 2010.

[24] G. Chytrova, Z. Ying, and F. Gomez-Pinilla, "Exercise contributes to the effects of DHA dietary supplementation by acting on membrane-related synaptic systems," *Brain Research C*, vol. 1341, pp. 32–40, 2010.

[25] R. A. Honea, G. P. Thomas, A. Harsha et al., "Cardiorespiratory fitness and preserved medial temporal lobe volume in alzheimer disease," *Alzheimer Disease and Associated Disorders*, vol. 23, no. 3, pp. 188–197, 2009.

[26] K. Y. Liang, M. A. Mintun, A. M. Fagan et al., "Exercise and Alzheimer's disease biomarkers in cognitively normal older adults," *Annals of Neurology*, vol. 68, no. 3, pp. 311–318, 2010.

[27] K. E. Nichol, W. W. Poon, A. I. Parachikova, D. H. Cribbs, C. G. Glabe, and C. W. Cotman, "Exercise alters the immune profile in Tg2576 Alzheimer mice toward a response coincident with improved cognitive performance and decreased amyloid," *Journal of Neuroinflammation*, vol. 5, p. 13, 2008.

[28] A. Parachikova, K. E. Nichol, and C. W. Cotman, "Short-term exercise in aged Tg2576 mice alters neuroinflammation and improves cognition," *Neurobiology of Disease*, vol. 30, no. 1, pp. 121–129, 2008.

[29] L. J. Podewils, E. Guallar, L. H. Kuller et al., "Physical activity, APOE genotype, and dementia risk: findings from the Cardiovascular Health Cognition Study," *American Journal of Epidemiology*, vol. 161, no. 7, pp. 639–651, 2005.

[30] I. Reinvang, I. L. Winjevoll, H. Rootwelt, and T. Espeseth, "Working memory deficits in healthy APOE epsilon 4 carriers," *Neuropsychologia*, vol. 48, no. 2, pp. 566–573, 2010.

[31] K. I. Erickson, R. S. Prakash, M. W. Voss et al., "Brain-derived neurotrophic factor is associated with age-related decline in hippocampal volume," *Journal of Neuroscience*, vol. 30, no. 15, pp. 5368–5375, 2010.

[32] J. S. Mu, W. P. Li, Z. B. Yao, and X. F. Zhou, "Deprivation of endogenous brain-derived neurotrophic factor results in impairment of spatial learning and memory in adult rats," *Brain Research*, vol. 835, no. 2, pp. 259–265, 1999.

[33] A. M. Stranahan, K. Lee, B. Martin et al., "Voluntary exercise and caloric restriction enhance hippocampal dendritic spine density and BDNF levels in diabetic mice," *Hippocampus*, vol. 19, no. 10, pp. 951–961, 2009.

[34] C. M. de Frias, K. Annerbrink, L. Westberg, E. Eriksson, R. Adolfsson, and L. G. Nilsson, "Catechol-O-methyltransferase Val158Met polymorphism is associated with cognitive performance in nondemented adults," *Journal of Cognitive Neuroscience*, vol. 17, no. 7, pp. 1018–1025, 2005.

[35] H. A. Wishart, R. M. Roth, A. J. Saykin et al., "COMT Val158met genotype and individual differences in executive function in healthy adults," *Journal of the International Neuropsychological Society*, vol. 17, no. 1, pp. 174–180, 2011.

[36] M. F. Muldoon, C. M. Ryan, L. Sheu, J. K. Yao, S. M. Conklin, and S. B. Manuck, "Serum phospholipid docosahexaenonic acid is associated with cognitive functioning during middle adulthood," *Journal of Nutrition*, vol. 140, no. 4, pp. 848–853, 2010.

[37] M. Oksman, H. Iivonen, E. Hogyes et al., "Impact of different saturated fatty acid, polyunsaturated fatty acid and cholesterol containing diets on beta-amyloid accumulation in APP/PS1 transgenic mice," *Neurobiology of Disease*, vol. 23, no. 3, pp. 563–572, 2006.

[38] B. M. van Gelder, M. Tijhuis, S. Kalmijn, and D. Kromhout, "Fish consumption, n-3 fatty acids, and subsequent 5-y cognitive decline in elderly men: the Zutphen Elderly Study," *American Journal of Clinical Nutrition*, vol. 85, no. 4, pp. 1142–1147, 2007.

[39] S. J. Colcombe, K. Erickson, N. Raz et al., "Aerobic fitness reduces brain tissue loss in aging humans," *Journals of Gerontology A*, vol. 58, no. 2, pp. 176–180, 2003.

[40] K. I. Erickson, R. S. Prakash, M. W. Voss et al., "Aerobic fitness is associated with hippocampal volume in elderly humans," *Hippocampus*, vol. 19, no. 10, pp. 1030–1039, 2009.

[41] A. M. Weinstein, M. Voss, K. Prakash et al., "The association between aerobic fitness and executive function is mediated by prefrontal cortex volume," *Brain, Behavior, and Immunity*, vol. 26, no. 5, pp. 811–819, 2012.

[42] K. B. Walhovd, A. M. Fjell, I. Reinvang et al., "Effects of age on volumes of cortex, white matter and subcortical structures," *Neurobiology of Aging*, vol. 26, no. 9, pp. 1261–1270, 2005.

[43] R. A. Honea, E. Vidoni, A. Harsha, and J. M. Burns, "Impact of APOE on the healthy aging brain: a voxel-based MRI and DTI study," *Journal of Alzheimer's Disease*, vol. 18, no. 3, pp. 553–564, 2009.

[44] A. N. Szabo, E. Mcauley, K. Erickson et al., "Cardiorespiratory fitness, hippocampal volume, and frequency of forgetting in older adults," *Neuropsychology*, vol. 25, no. 5, pp. 545–553, 2011.

[45] R. I. Scahill, C. Frost, R. Jenkins, J. L. Whitwell, M. N. Rossor, and N. C. Fox, "A longitudinal study of brain volume changes in normal aging using serial registered magnetic resonance imaging," *Archives of Neurology*, vol. 60, no. 7, pp. 989–994, 2003.

[46] A. T. Du, N. Schuff, X. P. Zhu et al., "Atrophy rates of entorhinal cortex in AD and normal aging," *Neurology*, vol. 60, no. 3, pp. 481–486, 2003.

[47] N. Raz, U. Lindenberger, K. M. Rodrigue et al., "Regional brain changes in aging healthy adults: general trends, individual differences and modifiers," *Cerebral Cortex*, vol. 15, no. 11, pp. 1676–1689, 2005.

[48] A. Pfefferbaum, D. H. Mathalon, E. V. Sullivan, J. M. Rawles, R. B. Zipursky, and K. O. Lim, "A quantitative magnetic resonance imaging study of changes in brain morphology from infancy to late adulthood," *Archives of Neurology*, vol. 51, no. 9, pp. 874–887, 1994.

[49] C. D. Good, I. S. Johnsrude, J. Ashburner, R. N. A. Henson, K. J. Friston, and R. S. J. Frackowiak, "A voxel-based

morphometric study of ageing in 465 normal adult human brains," *NeuroImage*, vol. 14, no. 1, pp. 21–36, 2001.

[50] J. T. Lehmbeck, S. Brassen, W. Weber-Fahr, and D. F. Braus, "Combining voxel-based morphometry and diffusion tensor imaging to detect age-related brain changes," *NeuroReport*, vol. 17, no. 5, pp. 467–470, 2006.

[51] C. R. Jack Jr, R. C. Petersen, Y. Xu et al., "Rates of hippocampal atrophy correlate with change in clinical status in aging and AD," *Neurology*, vol. 55, no. 4, pp. 484–489, 2000.

[52] J. Golomb, M. J. De Leon, A. Kluger, A. E. George, C. Tarshish, and S. H. Ferris, "Hippocampal atrophy in normal aging: an association with recent memory impairment," *Archives of Neurology*, vol. 50, no. 9, pp. 967–973, 1993.

[53] R. E. Clark, N. J. Broadbent, and L. R. Squire, "Hippocampus and remote spatial memory in rats," *Hippocampus*, vol. 15, no. 2, pp. 260–272, 2005.

[54] P. F. Chapman, G. L. White, M. W. Jones et al., "Impaired synaptic plasticity and learning in aged amyloid precursor protein transgenic mice," *Nature Neuroscience*, vol. 2, no. 3, pp. 271–276, 1999.

[55] Q. Guo, W. Fu, B. L. Sopher et al., "Increased vulnerability of hippocampal neurons to excitotoxic necrosis in presenilin-1 mutant knock-in mice," *Nature Medicine*, vol. 5, no. 1, pp. 101–106, 1999.

[56] H. van Praag, G. Kempermann, and F. H. Gage, "Running increases cell proliferation and neurogenesis in the adult mouse dentate gyrus," *Nature Neuroscience*, vol. 2, no. 3, pp. 266–270, 1999.

[57] H. van Praag, T. Shubert, C. Zhao, and F. H. Gage, "Exercise enhances learning and hippocampal neurogenesis in aged mice," *Journal of Neuroscience*, vol. 25, no. 38, pp. 8680–8685, 2005.

[58] W. Deng, J. B. Aimone, and F. H. Gage, "New neurons and new memories: how does adult hippocampal neurogenesis affect learning and memory?" *Nature Reviews Neuroscience*, vol. 11, no. 5, pp. 339–350, 2010.

[59] C. W. Cotman, N. C. Berchtold, and L. A. Christie, "Exercise builds brain health: key roles of growth factor cascades and inflammation," *Trends in Neurosciences*, vol. 30, no. 9, pp. 464–472, 2007.

[60] A. F. Kramer and K. I. Erickson, "Capitalizing on cortical plasticity: influence of physical activity on cognition and brain function," *Trends in Cognitive Sciences*, vol. 11, no. 8, pp. 342–348, 2007.

[61] D. M. Hallman, E. Boerwinkle, N. Saha et al., "The apolipoprotein E polymorphism: a comparison of allele frequencies and effects in nine populations," *American Journal of Human Genetics*, vol. 49, no. 2, pp. 338–349, 1991.

[62] J. C. S. Breitner, B. W. Wyse, J. C. Anthony et al., "APOE-ε4 count predicts age when prevalence of AD increases, then declines: the cache county study," *Neurology*, vol. 53, no. 2, pp. 321–331, 1999.

[63] A. L. Fitzpatrick, L. H. Kuller, D. G. Ives et al., "Incidence and prevalence of dementia in the cardiovascular health study," *Journal of the American Geriatrics Society*, vol. 52, no. 2, pp. 195–204, 2004.

[64] E. H. Corder, A. M. Saunders, W. J. Strittmatter et al., "Gene dose of apolipoprotein E type 4 allele and the risk of Alzheimer's disease in late onset families," *Science*, vol. 261, no. 5123, pp. 921–923, 1993.

[65] T. Grimmer, S. Tholen, B. H. Yousefi et al., "Progression of cerebral amyloid load is associated with the apolipoprotein E epsilon4 genotype in Alzheimer's disease," *Biological Psychiatry*, vol. 68, no. 10, pp. 879–884, 2010.

[66] D. M. Holtzman, K. R. Bales, S. Wu et al., "Expression of human apolipoprotein E reduces amyloid-β deposition in a mouse model of Alzheimer's disease," *Journal of Clinical Investigation*, vol. 103, no. 6, pp. R15–R21, 1999.

[67] Z. S. Nagy, M. M. Esiri, K. A. Jobst et al., "Influence of the apolipoprotein E genotype on amyloid deposition and neurofibrillary tangle formation in Alzheimer's disease," *Neuroscience*, vol. 69, no. 3, pp. 757–761, 1995.

[68] D. Head, J. M. Bugg, A. M. Goate et al., "Exercise engagement as a moderator of the effects of APOE genotype on amyloid deposition," *Archives of Neurology*, vol. 69, no. 5, pp. 636–643, 2012.

[69] C. M. Yuede, S. D. Zimmerman, H. Dong et al., "Effects of voluntary and forced exercise on plaque deposition, hippocampal volume, and behavior in the Tg2576 mouse model of Alzheimer's disease," *Neurobiology of Disease*, vol. 35, no. 3, pp. 426–432, 2009.

[70] N. P. E. Kadoglou, N. Kostomitsopoulos, A. Kapelouzou et al., "Effects of exercise training on the severity and composition of atherosclerotic plaque in apoE-deficient mice," *Journal of Vascular Research*, vol. 48, no. 4, pp. 347–356, 2011.

[71] S. P. Deeny, D. Poeppel, J. B. Zimmerman et al., "Exercise, APOE, and working memory: MEG and behavioral evidence for benefit of exercise in epsilon4 carriers," *Biological Psychology*, vol. 78, no. 2, pp. 179–187, 2008.

[72] T. E. Goldberg and D. R. Weinberger, "Genes and the parsing of cognitive processes," *Trends in Cognitive Sciences*, vol. 8, no. 7, pp. 325–335, 2004.

[73] M. F. Egan, M. Kojima, J. H. Callicott et al., "The BDNF val66met polymorphism affects activity-dependent secretion of BDNF and human memory and hippocampal function," *Cell*, vol. 112, no. 2, pp. 257–269, 2003.

[74] K. G. Bath and F. S. Lee, "Variant BDNF (Val66Met) impact on brain structure and function," *Cognitive, Affective and Behavioral Neuroscience*, vol. 6, no. 1, pp. 79–85, 2006.

[75] A. R. Hariri, T. E. Goldberg, V. S. Mattay et al., "Brain-derived neurotrophic factor val66met polymorphism affects human memory-related hippocampal activity and predicts memory performance," *Journal of Neuroscience*, vol. 23, no. 17, pp. 6690–6694, 2003.

[76] P. R. Szeszko, R. Lipsky, C. Mentschel et al., "Brain-derived neurotrophic factor val66met polymorphism and volume of the hippocampal formation," *Molecular Psychiatry*, vol. 10, no. 7, pp. 631–636, 2005.

[77] V. Leßmann and T. Brigadski, "Mechanisms, locations, and kinetics of synaptic BDNF secretion: an update," *Neuroscience Research*, vol. 65, no. 1, pp. 11–22, 2009.

[78] G. M. Schratt, E. A. Nigh, W. G. Chen, L. Hu, and M. E. Greenberg, "BDNF regulates the translation of a select group of mRNAs by a mammalian target of rapamycin-phosphatidylinositol 3-kinase-dependent pathway during neuronal development," *Journal of Neuroscience*, vol. 24, no. 33, pp. 7366–7377, 2004.

[79] M. Righi, E. Tongiorgi, and A. Cattaneo, "Brain-derived neurotrophic factor (BDNF) induces dendritic targeting of BDNF and tyrosine kinase B mRNAS in hippocampal neurons through a phosphatidylinositol-3 kinase-dependent pathway," *Journal of Neuroscience*, vol. 20, no. 9, pp. 3165–3174, 2000.

[80] L. Minichiello, "TrkB signalling pathways in LTP and learning," *Nature Reviews Neuroscience*, vol. 10, no. 12, pp. 850–860, 2009.
[81] G. Neves, S. F. Cooke, and T. V. P. Bliss, "Synaptic plasticity, memory and the hippocampus: a neural network approach to causality," *Nature Reviews Neuroscience*, vol. 9, no. 1, pp. 65–75, 2008.
[82] K. Yamada and T. Nabeshima, "Brain-derived neurotrophic factor/TrkB signaling in memory processes," *Journal Pharmacological Sciences*, vol. 91, no. 4, pp. 267–270, 2003.
[83] S. A. Neeper, F. Gomez-Pinilla, J. Choi, and C. Cotman, "Exercise and brain neurotrophins," *Nature*, vol. 373, no. 6510, p. 109, 1995.
[84] C. W. Cotman and C. Engesser-Cesar, "Exercise enhances and protects brain function," *Exercise and Sport Sciences Reviews*, vol. 30, no. 2, pp. 75–79, 2002.
[85] K. Knaepen, M. Goekint, E. M. Heyman, and R. Meeusen, "Neuroplasticity exercise-induced response of peripheral brain-derived neurotrophic factor: a systematic review of experimental studies in human subjects," *Sports Medicine*, vol. 40, no. 9, pp. 765–801, 2010.
[86] F. Karege, M. Schwald, and M. Cisse, "Postnatal developmental profile of brain-derived neurotrophic factor in rat brain and platelets," *Neuroscience Letters*, vol. 328, no. 3, pp. 261–264, 2002.
[87] R. S. Duman and L. M. Monteggia, "A neurotrophic model for stress-related mood disorders," *Biological Psychiatry*, vol. 59, no. 12, pp. 1116–1127, 2006.
[88] S. Sen, R. Duman, and G. Sanacora, "Serum brain-derived neurotrophic factor, depression, and antidepressant medications: meta-analyses and implications," *Biological Psychiatry*, vol. 64, no. 6, pp. 527–532, 2008.
[89] F. Karege, G. Vaudan, M. Schwald, N. Perroud, and R. La Harpe, "Neurotrophin levels in postmortem brains of suicide victims and the effects of antemortem diagnosis and psychotropic drugs," *Molecular Brain Research*, vol. 136, no. 1-2, pp. 29–37, 2005.
[90] J. Gunstad, A. Benitez, J. Smith et al., "Serum brain-derived neurotrophic factor is associated with cognitive function in healthy older adults," *Journal of Geriatric Psychiatry and Neurology*, vol. 21, no. 3, pp. 166–170, 2008.
[91] J. F. Yarrow, L. J. White, S. C. McCoy, and S. E. Borst, "Training augments resistance exercise induced elevation of circulating brain derived neurotrophic factor (BDNF)," *Neuroscience Letters*, vol. 479, no. 2, pp. 161–165, 2010.
[92] A. Meyer-Lindenberg, T. Nichols, J. H. Callicott et al., "Impact of complex genetic variation in COMT on human brain function," *Molecular Psychiatry*, vol. 11, no. 9, pp. 867–877, 2006.
[93] J. Savitz, M. Solms, and R. Ramesar, "The molecular genetics of cognition: dopamine, COMT and BDNF," *Genes, Brain and Behavior*, vol. 5, no. 4, pp. 311–328, 2006.
[94] T. W. Robbins and A. F. T. Arnsten, "The neuropsychopharmacology of fronto-executive function: monoaminergic modulation," *Annual Review of Neuroscience*, vol. 32, pp. 267–287, 2009.
[95] J. H. Barnett, L. Scoriels, and M. R. Munafò, "Meta-analysis of the cognitive effects of the catechol-O-methyltransferase gene Val158/108Met polymorphism," *Biological Psychiatry*, vol. 64, no. 2, pp. 137–144, 2008.
[96] P. G. MacRae, W. W. Spirduso, and T. J. Walters, "Endurance training effects on striatal D2 dopamine receptor binding and striatal dopamine metabolites in presenescent older rats," *Psychopharmacology*, vol. 92, no. 2, pp. 236–240, 1987.
[97] A. M. Knab, R. S. Bowen, A. T. Hamilton, A. A. Gulledge, and J. T. Lightfoot, "Altered dopaminergic profiles: implications for the regulation of voluntary physical activity," *Behavioural Brain Research*, vol. 204, no. 1, pp. 147–152, 2009.
[98] B. E. Fisher, G. M. Petzinger, K. Nixon et al., "Exercise-induced behavioral recovery and neuroplasticity in the 1-methyl-4-phenyl-1,2,3,6-tetrahydropyridine-lesioned mouse basal ganglia," *Journal of Neuroscience Research*, vol. 77, no. 3, pp. 378–390, 2004.
[99] G. M. Petzinger, J. P. Walsh, G. Akopian et al., "Effects of treadmill exercise on dopaminergic transmission in the 1-methyl-4-phenyl-1,2,3,6-tetrahydropyridine-lesioned mouse model of basal ganglia injury," *Journal of Neuroscience*, vol. 27, no. 20, pp. 5291–5300, 2007.
[100] C. H. S. Ruxton, S. C. Reed, M. J. A. Simpson, and K. J. Millington, "The health benefits of omega-3 polyunsaturated fatty acids: a review of the evidence," *Journal of Human Nutrition and Dietetics*, vol. 17, no. 5, pp. 449–459, 2004.
[101] S. C. Dyall and A. T. Michael-Titus, "Neurological benefits of omega-3 fatty acids," *NeuroMolecular Medicine*, vol. 10, no. 4, pp. 219–235, 2008.
[102] F. Gómez-Pinilla and C. Feng, "Molecular mechanisms for the ability of exercise supporting cognitive abilities and counteracting neurological disorders," *Functional Neuroimaging in Exercise and Sport Sciences*, pp. 25–43, 2012.
[103] S. Kalmijn, M. P. J. Van Boxtel, M. Ocké, W. M. M. Verschuren, D. Kromhout, and L. J. Launer, "Dietary intake of fatty acids and fish in relation to cognitive performance at middle age," *Neurology*, vol. 62, no. 2, pp. 275–280, 2004.
[104] C. Dullemeijer, J. Durga, I. A. Brouwer et al., "n-3 Fatty acid proportions in plasma and cognitive performance in older adults," *American Journal of Clinical Nutrition*, vol. 86, no. 5, pp. 1479–1485, 2007.
[105] P. M. Kidd, "Omega-3 DHA and EPA for cognition, behavior, and mood: clinical findings and structural-functional synergies with cell membrane phospholipids," *Alternative Medicine Review*, vol. 12, no. 3, pp. 207–227, 2007.
[106] A. Wu, Z. Ying, and F. Gomez-Pinilla, "Docosahexaenoic acid dietary supplementation enhances the effects of exercise on synaptic plasticity and cognition," *Neuroscience*, vol. 155, no. 3, pp. 751–759, 2008.
[107] S. Delion, S. Chalon, D. Guilloteau, J. C. Besnard, and G. Durand, "α-Linolenic acid dietary deficiency alters age-related changes of dopaminergic and serotoninergic neurotransmission in the rat frontal cortex," *Journal of Neurochemistry*, vol. 66, no. 4, pp. 1582–1591, 1996.
[108] A. J. Sinclair, D. Begg, M. Mathai, and R. S. Weisinger, "Omega 3 fatty acids and the brain: review of studies in depression," *Asia Pacific Journal of Clinical Nutrition*, vol. 16, supplement 1, pp. 391–397, 2007.
[109] N. Shioda, Y. Yamamoto, Y. Owada, and K. Fukunaga, "Dopamine D2 receptor as a novel target molecule for heart-type fatty acid binding protein," *Japanese Journal of Neuropsychopharmacology*, vol. 31, no. 3, pp. 125–130, 2011.
[110] P. F. Davis, M. K. Ozias, S. E. Carlson et al., "Dopamine receptor alterations in female rats with diet-induced decreased brain docosahexaenoic acid (DHA): interactions with reproductive status," *Nutritional Neuroscience*, vol. 13, no. 4, pp. 161–169, 2010.
[111] M. Bousquet, M. Saint-Pierre, C. Julien, N. Salem, F. Cicchetti, and F. Calon, "Beneficial effects of dietary omega-3 polyunsaturated fatty acid on toxin-induced neuronal degeneration in an animal model of Parkinson's disease," *FASEB Journal*, vol. 22, no. 4, pp. 1213–1225, 2008.

[112] K. Akter, D. A. Gallo, S. A. Martin et al., "A review of the possible role of the essential fatty acids and fish oils in the aetiology, prevention or pharmacotherapy of schizophrenia," *Clinical Pharmacology & Therapeutics*, vol. 37, no. 2, pp. 132–139, 2012.
[113] G. M. Cole and S. A. Frautschy, "DHA may prevent age-related dementia," *Journal of Nutrition*, vol. 140, no. 4, pp. 869–874, 2010.
[114] A. M. Issa, W. A. Mojica, S. C. Morton et al., "The efficacy of omega-3 fatty acids on cognitive function in aging and dementia: a systematic review," *Dementia and Geriatric Cognitive Disorders*, vol. 21, no. 2, pp. 88–96, 2006.
[115] M. Fotuhi, P. Mohassel, and K. Yaffe, "Fish consumption, long-chain omega-3 fatty acids and risk of cognitive decline or Alzheimer disease: a complex association," *Nature Clinical Practice Neurology*, vol. 5, no. 3, pp. 140–152, 2009.
[116] G. A. Jicha and W. R. Markesbery, "Omega-3 fatty acids: potential role in the management of early Alzheimer's disease," *Clinical Interventions in Aging*, vol. 5, no. 1, pp. 45–61, 2010.

23

Caregivers' Experience of Decision-Making regarding Diagnostic Assessment following Cognitive Screening of Older Adults

Jamie J. Y. Lee[1], **Joanna Barlas**[1], **Claire L. Thompson**[2] **and Yan Hong Dong**[3]

[1]*School of Psychology, James Cook University, Singapore*
[2]*School of Psychology, Central Queensland University, Rockhampton, Australia*
[3]*Centre for Healthy Brain Ageing (CHeBA) and Dementia Collaborative Research Centre—Assessment and Better Care, School of Psychiatry, UNSW Medicine, The University of New South Wales, Sydney, Australia*

Correspondence should be addressed to Jamie J. Y. Lee; jiayanjamie.lee@my.jcu.edu.au

Academic Editor: Barbara Shukitt-Hale

Targeted screening for dementia among older adults in primary healthcare has potential benefits such as better clinical outcomes and the opportunity to access services. Cognitive screening can be followed up by further diagnostic assessment to determine a diagnosis of dementia. Unfortunately, the rates of accepting further diagnostic assessment following cognitive screening are low. The objective of this study was to explore the caregivers' decision-making process regarding uptake of diagnostic assessment following positive screening results. A qualitative design was employed, and interpretative phenomenological analysis was used to analyze the data. Three major themes in caregiver decision-making were identified: gathering information, protecting the patient, and balancing obligation and convenience in caregiving. These findings suggest that the decision-making process involved effort to process information through observations of the patient and that caregivers emphasized quality of life.

1. Introduction

Dementia is a general term that describes cognitive impairment severe enough to impair daily functioning and results in significant cognitive decline and disability among older adults. It is a public health priority that has high economic costs and contributes to caregiver burden and reduced quality of life for both patients and caregivers [1]. Prevalence rates indicate that 47.5 million people worldwide currently have dementia, with a projection that 75.6 million people by 2030 and 135.5 million people by 2050 will have the disease [1]. The prevalence of dementia among older adults aged 60 and above in Singapore is 10%. In 2012, 28,000 older adults over 60 in Singapore were diagnosed with dementia; this figure is projected to increase to 80,000 by 2030 [2]. Despite high prevalence rates, dementia is often undetected by physicians in primary healthcare [3, 4].

Targeted screening of older adults in primary healthcare has the potential benefits of higher detection rates and early commencement of treatment. Early treatment results in better clinical outcomes and more opportunities for access to services and advanced care planning [5–7]. Patients with a positive screen result are asked to follow up with further diagnostic assessment which could include neuropsychological testing, laboratory testing, and physical examinations [8, 9]. Unfortunately, there are low rates of follow-up with further diagnostic assessment following screening [10, 11], and without sufficient follow-up, patients are exposed to the risks associated with a false-positive or false-negative screening result. False-positive results may lead to unnecessary psychological distress and stigma associated with dementia [7, 12]. False-negative results are problematic as the benefits of early treatment are denied, and undetected cognitive impairment may lead to difficulties undertaking activities of daily living that place the older adult at risk of harm [13]. It is therefore important for patients to attend further diagnostic assessment following a positive screen. A previous research identified the low rates of follow-up after cognitive screening in Singapore [14]. The current study sheds light on low follow-up rates through exploration of caregiver decision-making regarding the uptake of further diagnostic assessment.

Individuals with dementia may lose decision-making capacity [15], and caregivers often play an increasingly large role in decision-making regarding medical, legal, and financial matters [16]. Caregiver and patient participation in decision-making ranges from patients' direct involvement [17–19] to patients' refusal to participate in decision-making to avoid fears about future cognitive decline [20, 21]. Caregivers play a bigger role in substitute decision-making; this usually occurs when patients have greater cognitive impairment and reduced decision-making capacity [22]. Early detection of cognitive impairment facilitates decisions regarding use of dementia care services and planning of caregiver duties, which benefits both people with dementia and their caregivers [6]. Furthermore, early detection allows caregivers to access psychosocial support such as support groups and caregiver training programs that have been found to improve morale and ameliorate stress [23, 24].

Fowler et al. [25] examined the association between attitudes and uptake of screening among patients and found that patients' attitudes about benefits of dementia screening have an impact on the acceptance of dementia screening. Persons with dementia have cited benefits to knowing their diagnosis such as having the opportunity to address memory problems, settle financial and legal matters, and understand behavioural changes [26]. Several other factors such as perceived benefits of dementia screening, age, need for future planning in the event of dementia, and gender have been associated with acceptance of dementia screening in primary care [27, 28].

Research evidence sheds some light on the reasons why people reject diagnostic assessment or disclosure of a dementia diagnosis [7, 29, 30]. Boustani et al. [29] found that barriers to screening identified by two groups of participants, those with dementia caregiving experience and those without, were emotional suffering by the family, loss of driving privileges, and becoming depressed. Research on the characteristics of patients who received a positive screen for dementia but refused further diagnostic assessment indicated that greater perceived stigma and living alone were associated with greater odds for refusing diagnostic assessment [31].

Stigma of having a dementia diagnosis has resulted from the disease's association with negative outcomes like a lack of cure, loss of dignity and autonomy, and being excluded and discriminated against by family and healthcare professionals [32]. Stigma has influenced the minimization and concealment of symptoms that leads to late presentation to services, delays in obtaining a diagnosis after presentation due to therapeutic nihilism (belief that no effective intervention or treatment is available for dementia) and pessimism about prognosis, and medical professionals' reluctance to provide a diagnosis of dementia [32, 33].

Lee et al. [34] surveyed the caregivers of participants who had completed screening and preliminary neuropsychological testing to examine uptake of further diagnostic evaluation and the predictors of uptake. Of 140 participants, 33 were identified at screening to have moderate or severe risk of cognitive impairment and were asked to follow up with further diagnostic assessment [34]. The current study is a follow-up to the previous study [34] and explores how caregivers participated in the decision-making for further diagnostic assessment. This is the first study to explore the subjective experience of decision-making following cognitive screening of older adults using a qualitative methodology.

2. Materials and Methods

This study employed a qualitative design using interpretative phenomenological analysis (IPA). IPA is a qualitative approach to examine how individuals perceive, reflect on, and make sense of their experiences [35]. Notably, no research has examined the caregivers' decision-making process for patients to follow up with diagnostic assessment following screening, and therefore, the IPA approach was chosen to explore the subjective experience of decision-making. IPA emphasizes in-depth analysis of individual perspectives [36] and recommends a sample size of three to six participants [37].

Of 140 participants in a study by Lee et al. [34], 33 were identified to have moderate or severe risk of cognitive impairment and were asked to follow up with further diagnostic assessment [34]. The caregivers of these 33 participants were invited to participate in the current study. Six caregivers who consented were interviewed, and one caregiver's data were excluded from analysis because he was unable to provide coherent responses. The five remaining participants were all female and were adult children (one daughter-in-law and four daughters) who lived with and cared for the patient. The remaining caregivers of the original 27 people with moderate or severe risk of cognitive impairment declined the current study's invitation. The 27 who declined to participate had a wider variability of age (37 to 77, $M = 57$), gender (70.4% female), and relationship with patient (7.4% husband, 25.9% wife, 22.2% son, and 44.4% daughter) compared to those who participated. However, the mean age, female gender, and daughter/daughter-in-law relationship of the participants suggest they are typical of the wider sample from which they were recruited.

Data were collected via semistructured interviews with caregivers to explore the decision-making process regarding accepting further diagnostic assessment following screening. Interviews were guided by a list of questions such as "How did you and the care recipient decide to accept/decline further diagnostic assessment?" "What helped you during the decision-making?" and "Who was involved in this decision-making process?"

Participant demographics are displayed in Table 1.

Following ethical approval by the National University Hospital and a university's ethics committees, interviews that lasted approximately 40 minutes were conducted in English at caregivers' homes. A member of the research team undertook analysis of the data obtained from verbatim transcripts of interviews.

Using an idiographic IPA approach to data analysis, descriptive (focusing on the content of the narrative),

Table 1: Demographics of participants.

	Gender	Age	Ethnicity	Education	Relationship	Risk of cognitive impairment	Decision
P1	Female	61	Eurasian	16	Daughter	Severe	Refused
P2	Female	60	Chinese	10	Daughter-in-law	Severe	Accepted
P3	Female	54	Chinese	12	Daughter	Severe	Accepted
P4	Female	55	Chinese	10	Daughter	Moderate	Refused
P5	Female	59	Malay	10	Daughter	Severe	Refused

Note. Relationship = caregiver's relationship to the patient. Decision = decision regarding diagnostic assessment.

Table 2: Master themes and subthemes.

Master themes	Subthemes
Gathering information	Observing the patient Making comparisons
Protecting the patient	From distress From futility
Balancing obligation and convenience in caregiving	Duty of caring and advocating Easing caregiver burden

linguistic (focusing on the use of language), and conceptual (focusing on understanding the narrative at an abstract level) comments were identified [35]. The first author mapped interrelationships, connections, and patterns among these comments, and emerging themes were examined. A list of master themes and subthemes was then generated. This process was repeated for all five transcripts, and cross-case analysis was subsequently conducted. Themes from each transcript were analyzed and compared for convergence and divergence, leading to a final list of master themes and subthemes.

An independent audit was conducted by the second author to affirm the validity of research findings. This process examined comments and themes identified, offered additional interpretation, and improved the validity of research findings by ensuring that interpretations were grounded in the data [35].

3. Results

Major themes derived from the current analysis included gathering information, protecting the patient, and balancing obligation and convenience in caregiving. Discussion of results includes a description of the master themes and subthemes (Table 2).

3.1. Theme 1: Gathering Information. Following recommendation from the hospital to undertake further diagnostic assessment, caregivers described a process of gathering information about the patient's current functional status primarily through observation of the patient. They then appeared to process this information by making comparisons between the patient's previous and current functioning. All caregivers engaged in this process of observing the patient and making comparisons irrespective of whether the decision was to accept or refuse diagnostic assessment.

3.1.1. Observing the Patient. Caregivers monitored patients' functional abilities, memory, and social activities, comparing the patient to others and taking note of any decline. The process of observing and acknowledging the relative's cognitive problems appeared to cause caregivers sadness and anxiety. One participant described watching her mother more closely after the initial screening process and was teary-eyed while talking about the changes she observed. Her anxiety over the patient appeared to contribute to her decision to accept further diagnostic assessment:

> *So I, staying with her, I monitor her daily routine, behaviour you see. So I found that she [pause] there were some changes lah, like normally in the evening she will take a shower, she will come down, she will go for her prayer. But I've realised ah, when she go up she never come down. And then she take so long to come down, so I was thinking what happened. [Participant 2]*

Caregivers reflected on their observations of patients during preliminary neuropsychological testing, using that as a means of gauging patients' ability to cope with further diagnostic assessment. The patient's emotional state was an important factor that informed the decision-making process. In one case, the fear and grief observed during this preliminary neuropsychological testing led a caregiver to refuse further assessment:

> *But I didn't realise that the test would be so elaborate. That it would cause her so much grief. So you know, the thought of someone coming to do these tests, had caused her so much fear. [Participant 1]*

3.1.2. Making Comparisons. Caregivers made comparisons between the patient's past and present functioning and the patient's physical versus cognitive difficulties. Comparing the familiar to the unfamiliar appeared to be a means of gauging the patient's deterioration to inform the decision. One caregiver talked about how the patient's abilities for activities of daily living had deteriorated, using this functional deterioration to justify a decision to follow up with diagnostic assessment:

> *And then instead of looking into the mirror and putting on her cream, she'll just put it on without looking and she'll go out with patches on her face, that kind of thing. It's so different from what she used to do. [Participant 3]*

It was noted that caregivers tended to discuss patient's physical difficulties when asked about patient's cognitive difficulties. For example, a caregiver talked about the patient's refusal of a prior leg operation to assess the level of resistance the patient would have towards further diagnostic assessment. This also implies that the patient's consent and views regarding further testing were pertinent to the decision-making process. Refusal from the patient was understood in the context of the patient's character and respected even when it caused distress to the caregiver:

> *I just feel a little bit upset that if she really don't want to go for diagnosis, like maybe it get worse very soon then how to prevent... Because my mother, we know one, that's why my brother did not even want to talk to her. My brother say 'leave it to her, if she want to go you bring, if she really refuse to go then forget it.' Yah, her character [is] that she think that she's alright. [Participant 4]*

In their struggle to determine the extent of patients' cognitive impairment, caregivers talked about patients' cognitive decline in terms of what they were still capable of accomplishing rather than what abilities they had lost. This likely made it easier for the caregiver to acknowledge the cognitive decline and to discuss it openly. Focusing on patients' accomplishments appeared to facilitate the decision to refuse further assessment:

> *But as of this moment, she is still alright lah, not that serious lah. Occasionally, of course, when she talk, always repeating, still repeating, But other than that, like lunch, dinner or taking medicine, this kind of normal daily work, she still can manage lah. [Participant 4]*

3.2. Theme 2: Protecting the Patient. Caregivers' decisions appeared to stem from a position of wanting to protect the patient from perceived harm. Harm was perceived to come from either psychological distress associated with obtaining a dementia diagnosis or from the fatigue associated with changes in the patient's routine or environment during further assessment. As such, consideration of quality of life played a significant role in caregivers' protectiveness of patients. However, the definition of quality of life differed for those who declined versus those who accepted further assessment. Notably, caregivers who accepted diagnostic assessment differed from those who rejected in their perception of what they were protecting the patient from. For caregivers who rejected diagnostic assessment, quality of life represented maintenance of the status quo and avoidance of perceived stigma and distress. For those who accepted, quality of life was associated with access to treatment to slow cognitive decline that would otherwise progressively impair activities of daily living.

3.2.1. Protecting From Distress. Patients' apparent distress during preliminary neuropsychological testing elicited a protective stance from some caregivers. For example, one caregiver described her mother looking at her to stop the test. This caregiver appeared to assume the role of an advocate for her mother, where she was responsible for protecting her by refusing further diagnostic assessment:

> *Actually, she was the one who said 'I don't want [testing] anymore... And when we talked about why [the tester] was coming, she said 'I don't want anything anymore. It's time for me to go.' She didn't want to anymore... [During testing] she said, 'Ah I got headache already' and then she was looking at me, because I sat next to her, she was looking at me to tell him to stop. [Participant 1]*

Caregivers also reflected on the stigma of dementia that led to patients' fears of being abandoned and losing mental control. For some, this meant refusing further diagnostic assessment to avoid exposing the patient to personal distress and negative emotions associated with stigma. Participant 4 described her mother's emotional state when she was asked to attend further testing:

> *Very... Very angry lor. Like, like why you all think that I got problem? So we do not want to insist, since she think she is alright then later on she might think that wah, we treat her like got mental problem, so we just leave it. [Participant 4]*

Other caregivers who recognized the same potential for stigma and distress but chose to proceed with further diagnostic assessment did so by being deliberately vague about the purpose of further assessment:

> *So we try to tell her we are bringing you to a doctor who is seeing old folks problem. We don't want to tell her 'shi zhi zhen' [dementia in Mandarin]. Because we don't want to make her frighten also... she's always talking about who's having dementia, and who behaving like that. That kind of thing you see. She has this fear of that. So we also don't want to put her into that state of shock. [Participant 3]*

They justified this lack of transparency as protecting the patient from the emotional impact of decision-making where the patient would have to consider the possibility that she had dementia.

3.2.2. Protecting From Futility. Caregivers' understanding of dementia was closely related to their differing reasons for protectiveness of the patient. Those who talked about a lack of cure for the disease and the futility of further treatment in view of the patient's age and deterioration chose to refuse further assessment. Caregivers appeared to gauge what the patient would want by reflecting on the type of end-of-life care they preferred for themselves. For example, a caregiver communicated a belief that prolonging life unnecessarily could lead to further impairment in her mother's physical and social functioning:

> *Yah. I feel that life to a certain extent is meant for a certain span. After that, you cannot expect to go on living a good life. Your quality of life will go down. I think to a certain*

extent, putting you on a respirator and things like that is stupid. Nature should take its course. [Participant 1]

Conversely, caregivers who accepted further assessment defined quality of life as slowing deterioration so that the patient preserved the ability for certain activities of daily living and retained a sense of self. In this way, this caregiver was protecting what she believed was important to her mother:

Dementia there's no cure, but you can stop the deterioration... In order to let her be herself, like before, you need some medical help... If you don't follow up, her quality of life will be down. [Participant 2]

3.3. Theme 3: Balancing Obligation and Convenience. Caregivers described a tension between caring for patients and maximizing the convenience of caregiving. Considering further assessment, caregivers thought about both the duty to act in the best interests of the patient and practical considerations like the cost and convenience of further assessment.

3.3.1. Entrusted as Advocate. This subtheme reflected how caregivers perceived a duty to care as being entrusted with the patient's physical and emotional well-being and having the responsibility of representing the patient's views and opinions about assessment and treatment. Caregivers were familiar with patients' values, preferences, and priorities—often, patients preferred to focus on physical problems over cognitive problems in medical treatment. It is therefore likely that more time and resources were allocated to the treatment of physical ailments than investigating cognitive concerns. One participant described how her mother was more concerned with painful corns on her feet than possible cognitive decline, and prioritizing physical care within this family led to the decision to refuse further diagnostic assessment:

Things that are important to her–her corns, she has very painful corns that sometimes leads her to not being able to move and sometimes I can't even get an appointment at the polyclinics. And then it gets worse to walk... To her, these two things matter more than her mind. In her mind, she's fine. [Participant 1]

For one participant, filial piety was associated with gratitude towards her mother. This gratitude and filial piety may have underpinned the decision to refuse further diagnostic assessment via a desire to protect the patient from distress or perhaps a belief that a formal diagnosis is irrelevant to the duty of care; children will look after their elderly parents no matter what the circumstances:

Now my turn to take care of her. That time only, I got three daughters, Primary 5, Secondary 1 [and] Secondary 4. My mother still can walk a little bit. She helped me. I go work. She looked after my daughter. Since my mother like that, I have to take of my mother. [Participant 5]

For participants that rejected diagnostic assessment, duty of care to the patient encompassed taking on the role of decision-maker and was related to the extent the caregiver perceived that the patient lacked capacity for rational or informed decision-making. Caregivers appeared to feel the weight of responsibility associated with decision-making, likely due to a perception that the patient placed absolute trust in them as an advocate and caregiver. Participant 1 elicited her mother's views and used them as a basis to refuse further diagnostic assessment:

Because she knows that of the three children, it's me that cares for her interest. So whatever I'm doing, it's for her best interest. She never doubted it. Because after that I did ask her, did you want to go for more tests [further diagnostic assessment]? She said no, I don't want. [Participant 1]

Conversely, two out of five caregivers who accepted diagnostic assessment overrode patients' preference to reject diagnostic assessment. This was related to a similar duty of care, although in these cases the caregiver decided that the patient lacked capacity to make good decisions and therefore stepped in to make what appeared to be a "best interest" decision:

Because you know, at this point, she cannot make decision anymore. And she doesn't make very rational or she doesn't make good decisions rather... I would say that she leave a lot of the decision to see doctor with us. [Participant 3]

Even when overriding patient's preferences, participants were not transparent in explaining that further assessments were to diagnose dementia. The lack of transparency could stem from a desire to protect the patient (as per Theme 2) or to avoid negative reactions and resistance from the patient. This caregiver expressed frustration over not being able to communicate the purpose of further diagnostic assessment. This could also be due to not knowing how to communicate the purpose of further tests to her mother-in-law who suffered some cognitive impairment and had difficulty understanding information:

I want to tell her, but how to tell her? I think she doesn't understand. And then if she, she heard what I say, next minute she will forget what I say already. [Participant 2]

3.3.2. Easing Caregiver Burden. The burden of caregiving appeared to factor into caregivers' decisions. Caregivers' struggles to manage their own physical ailments, finances, and work schedule added to the burden of caregiving.

Caregivers described family discussions as either an obligatory part of caregiving or a means of receiving support to manage the burden of care. For instance, one participant described regular family discussions about caregiving arrangements as helpful, which may be particularly salient within families where the primary caregiver and the patient have different views about going for further diagnostic assessment:

> *For us, when we see something is wrong, sometimes I will call her [participant's sister]. Sometimes, she will just check with me if everything is ok, and then if I suspect something is wrong, we will just talk about it. It's actually regularly [referred to discussions with sister]. [Participant 3]*

Caregivers considered various factors such as the cost of further assessments and the patient's difficulties with mobility. These factors increased the burden of care and contributed to the decision to refuse further assessment. Participant 1 communicated a desire to reduce the need to impose additional travel on her mother which led to a refusal of further diagnostic assessment:

> *You know, getting in and out of the car, so as much as possible, even now she doesn't want to go for her evening strolls in the wheel chair. She says it makes her giddy. So you can see that more movement is causing her to get this [giddy]. She gets like a vertigo attack, and she starts throwing up. So as much as possible I don't want much change in her life. [Participant 1]*

Other caregivers considered how further diagnostic assessment and treatment could ease caregiving burden as slowing the rate of cognitive deterioration could enable better management of difficult daily behaviours. Participant 3 expressed that further assessment could highlight areas in the patient's life that required more assistance, thereby facilitating ease of caregiving:

> *Because I know it will help us... It's better than we just, we try to look after her blindly and not know what's going on or what has gone wrong. It's better that we know exactly. Because this test will actually zero in right, which area and where she needs help. So we, we in fact we are happy to have such thing you see. We don't mind the inconvenience. Ultimately it will help her and it will help us as well. [Participant 3]*

4. Discussion

This study explored caregivers' experience in decision-making regarding patients' participation in further diagnostic assessment to confirm cognitive screening results for dementia. Caregivers described a process of monitoring the patient, drawing parallels, and making comparisons between the patient's cognitive difficulties and their physical ailments—this suggests an effort to process information leading up to a decision. Healthcare professionals advocating further testing may therefore find it helpful to discuss cognitive impairment in relation to physical problems as a means of facilitating caregivers and patients' understanding of dementia. Caregivers appeared to worry more about patients' physical health compared to cognitive health. Furthermore, cognitive problems appeared to receive more attention when they progress to a point which markedly increases caregiver burden. Hence, psycho-education regarding how addressing cognitive impairment helps reduce caregiver burden could increase motivation for attending further diagnostic assessment.

While all caregivers considered patients' preferences, the caregivers in this sample reported that they played a bigger role in the decision-making than patients did. This could be due to patients' risk of moderate to severe cognitive impairment. While caregivers who rejected further testing highlighted that the patient's refusal significantly influenced the decision, those who overrode patients' preferences and opted for further tests considered the patient's inability to make informed and rational decisions.

There was a lack of transparency by caregivers about the purpose of testing as caregivers saw this as a way of protecting the patient from distress. This aligns with the previous research which showed that approximately 80% of a sample of caregivers (n = 100) wanted to withhold a dementia diagnosis from patients due to fear of causing distress [37]. Medical practitioners who have withheld a diagnosis of probable Alzheimer's disease from patients have similarly revealed beliefs that patients would have reduced motivation and hope if they were informed of their diagnosis [38]. Issues such as the patient's right to know and the importance of being transparent with information appeared to be less salient for caregivers. This is at odds with a humanistic perspective of dementia that promotes the concept of personhood which states that recognition of the needs and rights of a patient with dementia enhances their well-being [39, 40].

Confucianism is a school of philosophy that has shaped family structures and behaviours in East Asia [41]. Values such as filial piety and interdependence that stem from the Confucian tradition [41] likely explain caregivers' keen interest in protecting the patient's well-being. Protecting a patient from distress by not providing full information could be an unspoken norm for caregivers in Singapore. Research has also shown that people from Asia use less open communication styles compared to European Americans [42]. It could then be that decision-making was further affected by a cultural norm where caregivers used less open communication styles and were less active in eliciting patient's preferences. Interestingly, the lack of open communication between caregivers and patients in the current study seems to have made decision-making easier for some participants because they were able to make decisions independently without the need to represent all views equally.

Caregivers' understanding of dementia influenced their protective stance over the patient. Therapeutic nihilism, or the belief that there is no available intervention for dementia, has been reported by doctors in primary healthcare [43, 44]. This perhaps contributed to some caregivers' desires to shield patients from psychological distress associated with the stigma and hopelessness of a diagnosis of dementia and the perceived futility of intervention.

Patients with dementia and their caregivers often focused on quality of life. While past research has discussed quality of life in end-of-life care decisions and assumed that there is a shared understanding of the meaning of quality of life [45], the current findings highlight that the definition of quality of life can vary among caregivers, thereby shaping decisions that lead to different outcomes. In our study, caregivers either strove to preserve quality of life by protecting from the distress of obtaining a diagnosis or strove to preserve quality of life by protecting from further decline through access to diagnosis and treatment. This is a central feature of the current results that highlights the need for healthcare professionals to facilitate caregivers' reflection on their understanding of quality of life, which would in turn influence caregiver involvement in further diagnostic assessment and treatment options.

Decision-making was made more difficult for these caregivers because of the guilt and sadness they experienced in this process. Efforts to minimize caregiving burden could contribute to caregiver guilt. Patients were resistant to diagnostic assessment as they associated dementia with going "crazy" and being abandoned. Patients' fears of being abandoned likely elicited guilt from caregivers. This is consistent with research on decisions about nursing home placements and end-of-life care being marked by caregivers' struggles with guilt and sadness [46, 47]. Additionally, the decision to accept diagnostic assessment draws caregivers closer to other difficult decisions such as residential care placement, which could exacerbate feelings of guilt and sadness.

The current findings support a recommendation for psychoeducation targeted at caregivers and patients to destigmatize dementia and provide accurate information on which to base decisions. Content might include information about the behavioural, psychological, and social changes that can occur as the disease progresses and how treatment might impact these changes. Psychoeducation might also address common negative perceptions of dementia to provide a more balanced and less condemnatory framework for understanding the disease. Caregivers and patients would also benefit from additional support from healthcare professionals during the decision-making process. Individualized meetings with a healthcare professional could help facilitate the expression of caregiver and patient views regarding further testing.

A limitation of the current study is that the current participants were all female within a limited age range and all in parent-daughter/daughter-in-law dyads; thus, no exploration of gender, age, or relationship differences in the decision-making process was possible. It is also important to note that this is a study of caregivers' decision-making: direct accounts of patients' experiences were not obtained. Future research could examine the experience of decision-making of a wider variety of caregiver demographics as well as older adults who are less cognitively impaired and able to provide reliable data.

5. Conclusions

Low rates of participation in diagnostic assessment following screening for cognitive impairment among older adults are a key concern. This study shows that caregivers played a significant role in determining uptake of further testing. Caregivers found this decision-making process difficult because of the guilt and sadness they experienced. Their decision was informed by their understanding of dementia and the disease trajectory, as well as their values and beliefs regarding quality of life. Important implications of these findings include the need for psychoeducation, individualized meetings with healthcare professionals, and specialist memory clinics to liaise with services that can provide socioemotional support for patients and their caregivers.

Conflicts of Interest

The authors declare that there are no conflicts of interest regarding the publication of this paper.

Acknowledgments

This work was supported by James Cook University Singapore Research Publication Fund.

References

[1] Alzheimer's Disease International, *World Alzheimer Report 2015: The global Impact of Dementia. An Analysis of Prevalence, Incidence, Cost and Trend*, Alzheimer's Disease International, London, UK, 2015, https://www.alz.co.uk/research/WorldAlzheimerReport2015.pdf.

[2] Researchers at Institute of Mental Health Detail Findings in Dementia, *Prevalence of Dementia in People Aged 60 Yearsand above: Results from the WiSE Study*, Vol. 147, Mental Health Weekly Digest, Atlanta, GA, USA, 2016.

[3] A. Connolly, E. Gaehl, H. Martin, J. Morris, and N. Purandare, "Underdiagnosis of dementia in primary care: variations in the observed prevalence and comparisons to the expected prevalence," *Aging and Mental Health*, vol. 15, no. 8, pp. 978–984, 2011.

[4] L. Lang, A. Clifford, L. Wei et al., "Prevalence and determinants of undetected dementia in the community: a systematic literature review and a meta-analysis," *BMJ Open*, vol. 7, no. 2, article e011146, 2017.

[5] C. Bamford, S. Lamont, M. Eccles, L. Robinson, C. May, and J. Bond, "Disclosing a diagnosis of dementia: a systematic review," *International Journal of Geriatric Psychiatry*, vol. 19, no. 2, pp. 151–169, 2004.

[6] V. A. Moyer, "Screening for cognitive impairment in older adults: U.S. preventive services task force recommendation statement," *Annals of Internal Medicine*, vol. 160, no. 11, pp. 791–797, 2014.

[7] L. Robinson, A. Gemski, C. Abley et al., "The transition to dementia - individual and family experiences of receiving a diagnosis: a review," *International Psychogeriatrics*, vol. 23, no. 7, pp. 1026–1043, 2011.

[8] H. H. Feldman, C. Jacova, A. Robillard et al., "Diagnosis and treatment of dementia: 2. Diagnosis," *Canadian Medical Association Journal*, vol. 178, no. 7, pp. 825–836, 2008.

[9] P. K. Panegyres, R. Berry, and J. Burchell, "Early dementia screening," *Diagnostics*, vol. 6, no. 1, p. 6, 2016.
[10] M. Boustani, A. J. Perkins, C. Fox et al., "Who refuses the diagnostic assessment for dementia in primary care?," *International Journal of Geriatric Psychiatry*, vol. 21, no. 6, pp. 556–563, 2006.
[11] F. W. Unverzagt, S. Gao, O. Baiyewu et al., "Prevalence of cognitive impairment: data from the Indianapolis study of health and aging," *Neurology*, vol. 57, no. 9, pp. 1655–1662, 2001.
[12] M. Boustani, A. J. Perkins, P. Monahan et al., "Measuring primary care patients' attitudes about dementia screening," *International Journal of Geriatric Psychiatry*, vol. 23, no. 8, pp. 812–820, 2008.
[13] C. Van Doorn, A. L. Gruber-Baldini, S. Zimmerman et al., "Dementia as a risk factor for falls and fall injuries among nursing home residents," *Journal of the American Geriatrics Society*, vol. 51, no. 9, pp. 1213–1218, 2003.
[14] M. A. Shaik, X. Xu, Q. L. Chan et al., "The reliability and validity of the informant ad8 by comparison with a series of cognitive assessment tools in primary healthcare," *International Psychogeriatrics*, vol. 28, no. 3, pp. 443–452, 2015.
[15] S. Y. Kim, J. H. Karlawish, and E. D. Caine, "Current state of research on decision-making competence of cognitively impaired elderly persons," *American Journal of Geriatric Psychiatry*, vol. 10, no. 2, pp. 151–165, 2002.
[16] N. R. Barbas and E. A. Wilde, "Competency issues in dementia: medical decision making, driving, and independent living," *Journal of Geriatric Psychiatry and Neurology*, vol. 14, no. 4, pp. 199–212, 2001.
[17] J. Hamann, K. Bronner, J. Margull et al., "Patient participation in medical and social decisions in Alzheimer's disease," *Journal of the American Geriatric Society*, vol. 59, no. 11, pp. 2045–2052, 2011.
[18] K. B. Hirschman, C. M. Joyce, B. D. James, S. X. Xie, and J. H. Karlawish, "Do Alzheimer's disease patients want to participate in a treatment decision, and would their caregivers let them?," *Gerontologist*, vol. 45, no. 3, pp. 381–388, 2005.
[19] M. J. Karel, J. Moye, A. Bank, and A. R. Azar, "Three methods of assessing values for advance care planning: comparing persons with and without dementia," *Journal of Aging and Health*, vol. 19, no. 1, pp. 123–151, 2007.
[20] M. E. de Boer, R. M. Dröes, C. Jonker, J. A. Eefsting, and C. M. Hertogh, "Thoughts on the future: the perspectives of elderly people with early-stage Alzheimer's disease and the implications for advance care planning," *AJOB Primary Research*, vol. 3, no. 1, pp. 14–22, 2012.
[21] C. R. MacQuarrie, "Experiences in early stage Alzheimer's disease: understanding the paradox of acceptance and denial," *Aging and Mental Health*, vol. 9, no. 5, pp. 430–441, 2005.
[22] K. Samsi and J. Manthorpe, "Everyday decision-making in dementia: findings from a longitudinal interview study of people with dementia and family carers," *International Psychogeriatrics*, vol. 25, no. 6, pp. 949–961, 2013.
[23] H. Wilkinson and A. J. Milne, "Sharing a diagnosis of dementia – learning from the patient perspective," *Aging and Mental Health*, vol. 7, no. 4, pp. 300–307, 2003.
[24] R. T. Woods, "Discovering the person with Alzheimer's disease: cognitive, emotional and behavioural aspects," *Aging and Mental Health*, vol. 5, no. 1, pp. 7–16, 2001.
[25] N. R. Fowler, A. J. Perkins, H. A. Turchan et al., "Older primary care patients' attitudes and willingness to screen for dementia," *Journal of Aging Research*, vol. 2015, Article ID 423265, 7 pages, 2015.
[26] R. Pratt and H. Wilkinson, *Tell Me the Truth: The Effect of Being Told the Diagnosis of Dementia from the Perspective of the Person with Dementia*, Mental Health Foundation, London, UK, 2001.
[27] N. R. Fowler, M. A. Boustani, A. Frame et al., "Effect of patient perceptions on dementia screening in primary care," *Journal of the American Geriatrics Society*, vol. 60, no. 6, pp. 1037–1043, 2012.
[28] T. Holsinger, M. Boustani, D. Abbot, and J. W. Williams, "Acceptability of dementia screening in primary care patients," *International Journal of Geriatric Psychiatry*, vol. 26, no. 4, pp. 373–379, 2011.
[29] M. A. Boustani, M. D. Justiss, A. Frame et al., "Caregiver and noncaregiver attitudes toward dementia screening," *Journal of the American Geriatrics Society*, vol. 59, no. 4, pp. 681–686, 2011.
[30] G. Pinner and W. P. Bouman, "Attitudes of patients with mild dementia and their carers towards disclosure of the diagnosis," *International Psychogeriatrics*, vol. 15, no. 3, pp. 279–288, 2003.
[31] N. R. Fowler, A. Frame, A. J. Perkins et al., "Traits of patients who screen positive for dementia and refuse diagnostic assessment. Alzheimer's and dementia: diagnosis," *Assessment and Disease Monitoring*, vol. 1, no. 2, pp. 236–241, 2015.
[32] S. M. Benbow and D. Jolley, "Dementia: stigma and its effects," *Neurodegenerative Disease Management*, vol. 2, no. 2, pp. 165–172, 2012.
[33] M. Vernooij-Dassen, E. Moniz-Cook, R. T. Woods et al., "Factors affecting timely recognition and diagnosis of dementia across Europe: from awareness to stigma," *International Journal of Geriatric Psychiatry*, vol. 20, no. 4, pp. 377–386, 2005.
[34] J. J. Y. Lee, C. L. Thompson, M. A. Shaik, E. Wan, C. L. Chen, and Y. H. Dong, "Service use, advance planning and lifestyle changes following cognitive screening in primary healthcare in Singapore," *International Psychogeriatrics*, vol. 30, no. 1, pp. 139–145, 2017.
[35] J. A. Smith, P. Flower, and M. Larkin, *Interpretative Phenomenological Analysis: Theory, Method and Research*, Sage, Los Angeles, LA, USA, 2009.
[36] I. Pietkiewicz and J. A. Smith, "A practical guide to using interpretative phenomenological analysis in qualitative research psychology," *Czasopismo Psychologiczne Psychological Journal*, vol. 20, no. 1, pp. 7–14, 2014.
[37] C. P. Maguire, M. Kirby, R. Coen, D. Coakley, B. A. Lawlor, and D. O'Neill, "Family members' attitudes toward telling the patient with Alzheimer's disease their diagnosis," *BMJ*, vol. 313, no. 7056, pp. 529-530, 1996.
[38] H. Johnson, W. P. Bouman, and G. Pinner, "On telling the truth in Alzheimer's disease: a pilot study of current practice and attitudes," *International Psychogeriatrics*, vol. 12, no. 2, pp. 221–229, 2000.
[39] R. Bartlett and D. O'Connor, "From personhood to citizenship: broadening the lens for dementia practice and research," *Journal of Aging Studies*, vol. 21, no. 2, pp. 107–118, 2007.
[40] G. Mitchell and J. Agnelli, "Person-centred care for people with dementia: kitwood reconsidered," *Nursing Standard*, vol. 30, no. 7, pp. 46–50, 2015.
[41] M. Park and C. Chesla, "Revisiting confucianism as a conceptual framework for Asian family study," *Journal of Family Nursing*, vol. 13, no. 3, pp. 293–311, 2007.
[42] Y. S. Park and B. S. Kim, "Asian and European American cultural values and communication styles among Asian American and European American college students," *Cultural*

Diversity and Ethnic Minority Psychology, vol. 14, no. 1, pp. 47–56, 2008.

[43] S. Cahill, M. Clark, H. O'Connell, B. Lawlor, R. F. Coen, and C. Walsh, "The attitudes and practices of general practitioners regarding dementia diagnosis in Ireland," *International Journal of Geriatric Psychiatry*, vol. 23, no. 7, pp. 663–669, 2008.

[44] S. Iliffe, J. Wilcock, and D. Haworth, "Obstacles to shared care for patients with dementia: a qualitative study," *Family Practice*, vol. 23, no. 3, pp. 353–362, 2006.

[45] C. D. Caron, J. Griffith, and M. Arcand, "End-of-life decision making in dementia: the perspective of family caregivers," *Dementia: The International Journal of Social Research and Practice*, vol. 4, no. 1, pp. 113–136, 2005.

[46] C. E. Gessert, S. Forbes, and M. Bern-Klug, "Planning end-of-life care for patients with dementia: roles of families and health professionals," *OMEGA - Journal of Death and Dying*, vol. 42, no. 4, pp. 273-291, 2000.

[47] U. H. Graneheim, A. Johansson, and B. M. Lindgren, "Family caregivers' experiences of relinquishing the care of a person with dementia to a nursing home: insights from a meta-ethnographic study," *Scandinavian Journal of Caring Sciences*, vol. 28, no. 2, pp. 215–224, 2014.

24

HIV Infection in the Elderly: Arising Challenges

Bonaventura C. T. Mpondo

Department of Internal Medicine, School of Medicine, College of Health Sciences, The University of Dodoma, Dodoma, Tanzania

Correspondence should be addressed to Bonaventura C. T. Mpondo; boniempondo@gmail.com

Academic Editor: Arshad Jahangir

Globally there is an increase in the number of people living with HIV at an advanced age (50 years and above). This is mainly due to prolonged survival following the use of highly active antiretroviral therapy. Living with HIV at an advanced age has been shown to be associated with a number of challenges, both clinical and immunological. This minireview aims at discussing the challenges encountered by elderly HIV-infected patients.

1. Introduction

Globally the number of elderly HIV-infected patients is increasing [1]. Estimates show that the percentage of people living with HIV aged 50 years and above had increased to more than 17% over the past decade [2]. In sub-Saharan Africa (SSA), estimates show that the percentage will triple by the year 2040 [3]. Previous data showed that HIV associated morbidity and mortality was higher in elderly patients as compared to their younger counterparts [4, 5]. More recent studies have also found that old age is associated with rapid progression to AIDS [6, 7]. Treatment response may also differ between elderly patients and younger patients. Several reports have demonstrated impaired immune recovery in elderly patients [8, 9]. Toxicities to antiretroviral drugs are more likely in elderly patients than in younger ones. Elderly patients are also more likely to have comorbidities including cardiovascular disease, renal disease, and diabetes.

2. Epidemiology

Since its discovery in 1980s, HIV has largely been considered as the disease of young people. However, recent reports indicate that the epidemiology of the infected population is fast changing, with significant increase in the number of elderly patients [1]. The number of people living with HIV has been shown to be on the rise in both developed countries as well as developing countries [3, 10]. Projections indicate that the number will continue to rise in the coming decades [3]. In 2007, it was estimated that approximately 15% of all HIV-infected individuals were aged 50 years and above in Tanzania [11]. The proportion remained stable in another report in 2014 [12]. In HIV/AIDS, the age of 50 years and above is considered to be old age because it was much older when compared to the lower mean age of HIV-infected patients early in the epidemic [13].

One of the reasons for the epidemiological change in the population living with HIV is the longevity of life following the use of highly active antiretroviral therapy (HAART). With the use of HAART, HIV has become a chronic manageable disease [14]. The causes of morbidity and mortality are no longer AIDS related, but rather complications from cancers, renal diseases, liver diseases, and the like [15]. There are also reports that show increased risk of acquiring HIV in elderly individuals [16, 17].

When compared to younger patients, elderly patients are usually diagnosed at an advanced stage of HIV [18, 19]. Several factors have been associated with late or missed diagnosis in this population. These factors include lack of awareness of HIV risk factors in this population, failure of health care providers to suspect HIV in this population, absence of routine HIV screening in this population, and overriding of HIV symptoms with symptoms of other common conditions associated with aging [16, 20].

3. Effects of Aging and HIV Infection on the Immune System

3.1. Effects on T Cell Function. As a person gets old (45 years and above), involution of the thymus occurs which results to a decrease in thymic volume [21]. The thymus is an organ that is involved in the development of human immune system and takes part in T lymphocyte maturation. Apart from the contraction of thymic volume, the production of naïve T cells decreases with increasing age [22]. There is also an association between increasing age reduced T cell functionality, decreased population of memory T cells, and reduced number of functional cytotoxic T cells [23].

HIV may also directly affect the immune system. HIV infection may inhibit the function of thymus and the production of naïve T cells [24]. Therefore HIV compounds the effect of aging on the immune system. This explains why the progression of HIV in elderly patients is usually more pronounced. In one case control study, it was found that both HIV-infected and noninfected elderly individuals had significantly lower proportions of functional cytotoxic T cells when compared to younger patients; the lowest proportions being in HIV-infected elderly patients [21]. Since cytotoxic T cells are involved in inhibiting HIV replication, reduction in the number and functionality of these cells coupled with the loss of CD4 cells leads to accelerated progression of HIV in elderly patients. Several studies have found that age is a predictor of HIV progression [25].

3.2. Effects on B Cells and Antibody Function. HIV infection and aging affect not only T cell function, but also the B cell functions [26]. There is evidence of impaired B cell functioning in both HIV-infected and older adults. With old age or HIV infection, evidence shows that there is a decrease in naïve B cell reserve. There is also evidence of depletion of memory B cells from peripheral blood in HIV-infected individuals [27]. In HIV-infected patients, studies have shown that there is abnormal B cell activation and immunoregulation [26, 28]. The effect of age on B cell activation remains unclear [29]. In both HIV-infected patients and older adults, the ability of antigens to activate B cells and generate effective antibody response is impaired [30].

4. Response to HAART

Data regarding the clinical, immunological, and virological benefits of HAART in elderly HIV-infected patients have been conflicting. Early in the HAART era, data suggested that age was inversely proportional to the rate of immune system recovery [9, 31]. This means that the immune recovery in older patients was lower than that in younger patients. This was hypothesized to be related to the reduction in thymic size and function [32–34].

Studies comparing immunological and virological responses among elderly and younger patients have come up with mixed results. Some studies concluded that CD4 response in elderly patients was lower compared to younger patients [8, 9, 35]; however other studies did not find any significant difference [36, 37]. A study done in Tanzania found a significant difference in absolute CD4 gain between elderly and younger patients with a lower gain among elderly patients [38]. Controversy also remains regarding virological response when the two populations are compared. Some studies indicated better response in elderly patients [37, 39]; another study showed better response in younger patients [40]; some studies did not find any significant difference between the two populations [31, 41]. Results from the largest cohort study comparing virological and immunological response found that virological response was better in elderly patients; however the immunological response was poor in this population [42]. The study also found poor clinical outcomes in elderly patients as compared to younger patients. Several studies have concluded that mortality rates are higher in elderly patients than in young patients [42, 43]. The causes of death were noted to be non-HIV-related complications. Studies evaluating immunological and clinical responses to HAART are summarized in Table 1.

5. Functional and Metabolic Complications of Aging with HIV Infection

5.1. HAART Metabolism and Toxicity. Data on the toxicities of antiretrovirals in elderly patients is very limited. This is due to the fact that most studies on antiretroviral metabolism exclude patients with advanced age with comorbid conditions. The pathophysiology of HAART toxicity is believed to be multifactorial; however, metabolic abnormalities and metabolic and endocrinological disorders are believed to be the main mechanisms.

Physiologically, there is a decline in creatinine clearance with increasing age. This reduction can potentially affect the metabolism of renally excreted drugs. There is also a challenge in estimating renal function in elderly patients. Both old age and HIV can lead to reduction in muscle mass making estimation of renal function using serum creatinine very difficult and unreliable [47]. Drugs such as nucleoside reverse transcriptase inhibitors (NRTIs) which are the backbone of HIV treatment regimen in Africa are eliminated by the kidneys through both tubular secretion and glomerular filtration; these need dose adjustments in patients with renal insufficiency.

Drug pharmacokinetics can also be influenced by the age related changes in body composition. The decrease in body weight and in total body water leads to change in drug volume of distribution which in turn leads to increased concentration of drugs in blood and other tissues [48]. There is also a possibility of delayed onset of drug effects due to slower gastrointestinal absorption rate in elderly patients [49]. Protein bound drugs usually have enhanced effects in elderly patients who have decline in protein concentrations as they age.

Tenofovir, which constitutes the first-line regime in most African countries, is nephrotoxic and may exacerbate renal insufficiency in elderly patients especially when used in combination with protease inhibitors (PIs) [50]. Most of the PIs and nonnucleoside reverse transcriptase inhibitors

TABLE 1: Studies evaluating immunological and clinical responses to HAART.

Study, year	Aspect studied	Main findings
Semeere et al., 2014 [44]	Immunological recovery by age	Adults younger than 50 years had on average a higher CD4 increase of 45 cells per cubic millimeter (95% confidence interval: 17 to 72; $P = 0.001$) compared with counterparts aged 60 years and older; mortality was highest among older adults compared with younger counterparts
Grabar et al., 2004 [8]	Immunologic and clinical responses to HAART in patients over 50 years old	CD4 mean increase during the first 6 months on HAART was $+42.9 \times 10^6$ cells/L per month in patients under 50 years and $+36.9 \times 10^6$ cells/L per month in patients over 50 years ($P < 0.0001$) Older patients had a significantly higher risk of clinical progression (hazard ratio (HR) = 1.52 [95% confidence interval (CI), 1.15–2.00])
Mutevedzi et al., 2011 [45]	To assess whether treatment outcomes vary with age for adults receiving antiretroviral therapy	Older adults had 32% excess mortality ($P = 0.004$) CD4 count reconstitution was lower, despite better virological response in the older adults
Maskew et al., 2012 [46]	Differences in treatment outcomes by age category	The adjusted hazard ratios (HRs) for all-cause mortality increased with increasing age Older patients were less likely to increase their CD4 count by ≥50 cells/mm

(NNRTIs) can potentially exacerbate hepatic insufficiency especially in patients with preexisting liver disease [51].

5.2. Comorbid Disease States. With the use of HAART, HIV has become a chronic and manageable condition. Rates of opportunistic infections (OIs) have declined significantly; however the non-HIV-related complications have been noted to be on the rise especially in elderly patients [14]. Conditions such as diabetes, cerebrovascular diseases, ischemic heart diseases, liver diseases, renal diseases, and cognitive abnormalities have been on the rise in elderly HIV-infected patients. Compared with HIV-negative elderly patients, HIV-infected elderly patients show accelerated aging [52, 53]. Age related complications are more common and present earlier in HIV-infected than in HIV-negative elderly patients as a result [54].

5.2.1. Metabolic Changes and the Risk of Cardiovascular Disorders. HIV infection and some of the antiretroviral drugs have been associated with fat and metabolic changes which increase the risk of cardiovascular disorders (CVDs) [55, 56]. Both nucleoside reverse transcriptase inhibitors, specifically stavudine that has been phased out and the protease inhibitors, have been associated with lipodystrophy [57, 58]. Some studies found association between lipodystrophy and age [58]. There is also evidence of increasing prevalence of CVDs with increasing age among HIV-infected individuals [59].

Evidence suggests that age is an independent predictor for cardiovascular diseases. Studies have shown that there is accumulation of atherosclerosis which predicts the chances of future development of cardiovascular disease [60]. The role of HAART in causing cardiovascular disorders remains unclear. While other studies have concluded that there is an association between the use of HAART and cardiovascular events [61, 62], others have not found an association [63, 64]. In one study, rates of hypertension were higher in ART naïve HIV-infected patients 1 year after starting HAART [65].

5.2.2. Kidney and Liver Diseases. With aging, there is physiological decline in renal and liver functions. Hepatic and renal insufficiencies are therefore common in HIV-infected elderly patients. With the increasing prevalence of diabetes, hypertension, and hepatitis C viral infection, the prevalence of renal insufficiency will further increase in this population. Old age, hepatitis C coinfection, black race, and advanced HIV have been associated with kidney disease [66]. The prevalence of kidney diseases increases with both age of the HIV-infected individuals and the type of HAART used [67, 68]. Both old age and HIV can lead to reduction in muscle mass making estimation of renal function using serum creatinine very difficult and unreliable [47].

HIV-infected elderly patients are predisposed to hepatic insufficiency. With aging, the size of the liver decreases; the blood flow to the liver decreases as well [69]. Coinfection between HIV and viral hepatitis is common. Studies show that between 10% and 20% of HIV-infected individuals are coinfected with hepatitis B [70, 71]. One global meta-analysis found consistently higher hepatitis C virus prevalence in HIV-infected individuals than HIV-negative individuals across all risk groups and regions [72].

Even in the HAART era, morbidity and mortality associated with liver disease among HIV-infected people remain high [73]. Liver related morbidity and mortality among HIV-infected people are four times higher in elderly patients than younger ones [74]. The risk of liver cirrhosis is higher in patients coinfected with HIV and viral hepatitis [75]. In one study both HIV infection and old age were associated with progression to end stage liver disease in patients with hepatitis C [76]. There is no evidence on the best ways to manage viral hepatitis in HIV-infected people. Hepatic insufficiency is common in HIV-infected elderly patients; screening for liver function and viral hepatitis is important in this population.

5.2.3. Non-AIDS-Defining Cancers. Prior to the use of HAART, the prevalence of AIDS-defining malignancies (ADMs) (e.g., non-Hodgkin's lymphoma, Kaposi's sarcoma, and invasive cervical carcinoma) was high and was directly correlated with the degree of immunosuppression. With the rapid scale up of HAART, however, the prevalence of ADM has significantly declined [77]. In the HAART era, the incidence of non-AIDS-defining malignancies (NADMs) has been on the rise [77, 78]. These include lung, liver, brain, and anal cancers which have been found to be more common in HIV-infected than in HIV-negative individuals [79, 80]. Most of the NADMs unlike ADMs are not correlated with the degree of immunosuppression [77]. Although the rate of ADMs continues to decline in the HAART era, the rate of NADMs continues to rise and now accounts for the majority of cancers in HIV-infected persons [81]. The development of NADMs is associated with increasing age among HIV patients [81]. HAART use is therefore protective for ADMs, but does not seem to significantly impact the incidence of NADMs.

5.2.4. Neuropsychiatric Manifestations. There is also an issue of neuropsychiatric manifestations of HIV [82]. HIV infection is considered the most common cause of preventable neurocognitive abnormalities [83]. It is estimated that between 30% and 50% of HIV-infected individuals will experience some form of neurocognitive decline [84] ranging from mild decline in motor and information processing decline to severe dysfunction impairing activities of daily living (ADLs) [85].

Neurocognitive abnormalities have been found to be more common in HIV-infected elderly patients than in age matched HIV-negative patients. Studies show that elderly patients are at an increased risk of developing cognitive impairment as compared to younger patients [86]. In elderly patients, depressive symptoms and low CD4 count have been found to be the risk factors for cognitive impairment [87]. Besides the higher prevalence of dementia in older versus younger adults, differences also have been found in milder cognitive diagnoses, with 44.7% of the older group and 26.3% of the younger group meeting formal criteria for minor cognitive motor disorder (MCMD).

5.3. Polypharmacy and Potential Drug to Drug Interactions. Studies have shown an increase in comorbid and multimorbid non-AIDS conditions such as diabetes mellitus, hypertension, osteoporosis, and cardiovascular diseases among elderly patients living with HIV [88]. Elderly HIV patients are faced with the challenge of consuming multiple drugs for the treatment of both HIV and the comorbid conditions. Combination antiretroviral therapy, which consists of at least three medications, together with medications needed to treat comorbidities makes this population at high risk for polypharmacy [89–91] which is defined as the concomitant use of multiple drugs commonly ≥5 different drugs [92, 93]. One review found that the prevalence of polypharmacy is increasing in elderly patients and is associated with increased morbidity and mortality [94].

Patients taking multiple drugs have an increased risk for falls, drug to drug interactions (DDI), adverse drug effects (ADE), increased hospitalization, and poor drug adherence [92]. Studies have shown that HIV elderly patients with multiple medication are at an increased risk of having DDI than the younger patients [91]. Because of the physiological changes that alter drug metabolism, drug toxicities are also exacerbated in these patients when they use several types of drugs concomitantly. Health care providers should therefore be aware of the risks and fully evaluate all medications at each patient visit to prevent polypharmacy from occurring in HIV-infected elderly patients who are at increased risk.

5.4. Frailty, Functional Impairment, and Disability

5.4.1. Frailty. Frailty is defined as a state of increased vulnerability in old age due to diminished physical reserve [95, 96]. Its phenotype is defined by presence of three of the following features: exhaustion, low activity level, weakness, weight loss, or slowed walking speed [97]. Studies have shown that frailty is associated with poor health outcomes including hospitalization, morbidity, and mortality among affected individuals [98]. The exact mechanism for frailty remains unclear; however there is association with increased free radical levels, mitochondrial dysfunction, and cytokines that might activate inflammatory pathways. In older individuals with frailty phenotype, the levels of C-reactive protein, D-dimer, fibrinogen, and IL-6 have been found to be elevated [99].

Overlap between HIV and frailty has been reported since early in the AIDS epidemic. Frailty continues to be most frequently recognized among HIV-infected persons not on ART, with low CD4 T cell count, or high HIV-1 RNA [100]. The prevalence of frailty in routine HIV care has been reported to be between 5% and 33%. It was also observed in one study that frailty occurs earlier in HIV-infected than in HIV-negative individuals [97]. Old age has been found to be one of the factors associated with frailty [100–102]. A study done in South Africa found significantly higher rates of frailty among HIV-infected adults than in HIV seronegative ones; in this study old age was a significant predictor of frailty [100].

5.4.2. Functional Impairment. Functional impairments in HIV/AIDS were initially reported in patients with advanced HIV. Tools used to assess functional impairment are used to identify differences in exercise tolerance, grip strength, balance, gait speed, and chair rise time in HIV-infected individuals. Previous studies assessing functional impairment in HIV-infected patients showed that middle-aged, HIV-infected men on HAART have reductions in exercise capacity, functional performance, physical activity, and grip strength [103]. HIV-infected elderly patients usually present with comorbid conditions, sometimes multimorbid, related to aging and the serostatus. One cohort study found that age-associated comorbidity affects physical function in HIV-infected patients and may modify the effect of aging [104].

5.4.3. Disability. Increased risk of disability among HIV-infected patients was described early in the epidemic. Disability describes the difficulty or dependency in carrying out activities in the environment. Reports on disability exist both from pre-ART and in the era of effective ART. One of the largest studies assessing disability in pre-ART era found that 14% of study participants reported difficulties in independent activities of daily living (IADLs) only and 4% in both activities of daily living (ADLs) and IADLs [105]. In the era of ART, several studies have also found higher rates of disability in HIV-infected patients [106, 107]. In these studies, age and HIV status had synergistic effects in causing disability [108].

6. Aging with HIV in Africa

With the rapid scale up of ART, the number of HIV-related deaths has declined significantly in SSA [109]. As a result, the number of people living with HIV at an advanced age has been projected to increase significantly in the coming years [110]. Despite the increasing number of elderly HIV-infected patients, very little data has been published over the subject. Studies addressing the challenges of living with HIV at an advanced age in Africa are scarce [111].

One of the challenges of aging with HIV in Africa is the increase in the burden of noncommunicable diseases that was previously hidden by the high HIV-related deaths [112]. Countries in SSA already experience an increasing burden of noncommunicable diseases [113]. This will in the long run overwhelm the health care services in SSA. The risks of noncommunicable diseases have been documented to be high in SSA [114], while the prevention efforts are limited. The lifestyle has been largely westernized in SSA; the meals contain high levels of calories and smoking habit is high and still increasing.

The rates of chronic comorbid conditions have been found to be high in elderly HIV-infected patients in SSA [115]. Mortality is higher in elderly than younger HIV-infected patients [12]; immune recovery has been found to be poor [38, 116]. In addition, malnutrition has been found to be more common in elderly than younger individuals in SSA [117]. In most SSA countries, the elderly are not a priority in health care services. The priority has always been given to children under five, pregnant women, and young men living with HIV. More studies are required in SSA to better understand the challenges in this population and their needs. Studies evaluating HIV and aging in sub-Saharan Africa are summarized in Table 2.

7. Areas for Future Research

As a response to the change in epidemiology of HIV infection and the increase in the number of elderly HIV-infected individuals, office of AIDS Research of the National Institutes of Health (NIH) assembled a working group with the goal of assessing what is known and unknown, and what the priorities should be for research at the interface of HIV, aging, and multimorbidity. The team met face to face in 2011 and came up with several themes and areas of critical need for research. Key identified themes by the group included multimorbidity, polypharmacy, and the need to emphasize maintenance of function; the complexity of assessing HIV versus treatment effects versus aging versus concurrent disease; the interrelated mechanisms of immune senescence, inflammation, and hypercoagulability; the utility of multivariable indices for predicting outcomes; a need to emphasize human studies to account for complexity; and a required focus on issues of community support, caregivers, and systems infrastructure [119]. Future research in this population should therefore be focused on these themes, trying to fill research gaps that exist.

8. Conclusions and Recommendations

The number of elderly people living with HIV is on the rise globally. This increase is attributed to the effectiveness of ART that increase longevity of life but also to the increased risk of acquiring HIV in this population. Living with HIV at an advanced age is associated with a number of challenges in the range of physical, clinical, and immunological. Late presentation is common; treatment outcomes are relatively poor. Comorbidities are more common as a result of aging and HIV status. Physiological changes associated with aging alter drug metabolism in these patients who in most cases experience polypharmacy exposing them to drug toxicities and drug to drug interactions. Special designed preventive measures and screening programmes should be designed to target elderly individuals. Clinicians should also suspect HIV early in these patients to minimize late presentation. Clinicians should also pay attention to the principles of geriatric prescribing in order to minimize complications from multiple medication use. More research is needed in this population especially in sub-Saharan Africa to better understand the special needs of this population of HIV-infected individuals.

Competing Interests

The author declares that they have no competing interests.

TABLE 2: Studies evaluating aging with HIV in sub-Saharan Africa.

Study, year	Aspect studied	Main findings
Negin and Cumming, 2010 [11]	Prevalence of HIV among elderly patients	Of the approximately 21 million people in sub-Saharan Africa aged ≥15 years that were HIV+, 14.3% were ≥50 years old
Negin et al., 2012 [115]	Prevalence of HIV and chronic comorbidities among those aged 50 years and older	Rates of chronic disease were higher among all older adults compared with those aged 18–49; of those aged 50 years and older, 29.6% had two or more of the seven chronic conditions compared with 8.8% of those aged 18–49 years
Greig et al., 2012 [118]	Associations between older age and adverse outcomes in HIV/AIDS antiretroviral programmes across 17 programmes in sub-Saharan Africa	Median gain in CD4 cell count at 6 and 12 months was significantly higher in patients less than 50 years old compared with those who are at least 50 years (134 versus 112 cells/μL at 6 months; 170 versus 139 cells/μL at 12 months; both $P < 0.001$); in multivariate analysis, there was a significant increased risk of mortality beyond 3 months after ART initiation in all age groups of at least 40 years of age compared with less than 40 years

References

[1] M. Mahy, C. S. Autenrieth, K. Stanecki, and S. Wynd, "Increasing trends in HIV prevalence among people aged 50 years and older: evidence from estimates and survey data," *AIDS*, vol. 28, supplement 4, pp. S453–S459, 2014.

[2] Centers for Disease Control and Prevention, *HIV/AIDS Surveillance Report*, CDC, Atlanta, Ga, USA, 2006, http://www.cdc.gov/hiv/topics/surveillance/resources/reports.

[3] J. A. C. Hontelez, S. J. de Vlas, R. Baltussen et al., "The impact of antiretroviral treatment on the age composition of the HIV epidemic in sub-Saharan Africa," *AIDS*, vol. 26, supplement 1, pp. S19–S30, 2012.

[4] A. N. Phillips, C. A. Lee, J. Elford et al., "More rapid progression to AIDS in older HIV-infected people: the role of CD4+ T-cell counts," *Journal of Acquired Immune Deficiency Syndromes*, vol. 4, no. 10, pp. 970–975, 1991.

[5] U. Balslev, A. D. Monforte, G. Stergiou et al., "Influence of age on rates of new AIDS-defining diseases and survival in 6546 AIDS patients," *Scandinavian Journal of Infectious Diseases*, vol. 29, no. 4, pp. 337–343, 1997.

[6] H. Jiang, N. Xie, B. Cao et al., "Determinants of progression to AIDS and death following HIV diagnosis: a retrospective cohort study in Wuhan, China," *PLoS ONE*, vol. 8, no. 12, Article ID e83078, 2013.

[7] F. Bonnet, R. Thiébaut, G. Chêne et al., "Determinants of clinical progression in antiretroviral-naive HIV-infected patients starting highly active antiretroviral therapy. Aquitaine Cohort, France, 1996–2002," *HIV Medicine*, vol. 6, no. 3, pp. 198–205, 2005.

[8] S. Grabar, I. Kousignian, A. Sobel et al., "Immunologic and clinical responses to highly active antiretroviral therapy over 50 years of age. Results from the French Hospital Database on HIV," *AIDS*, vol. 18, no. 15, pp. 2029–2038, 2004.

[9] J.-P. Viard, A. Mocroft, A. Chiesi et al., "Influence of age on CD4 cell recovery in human immunodeficiency virus-infected patients receiving highly active antiretroviral therapy: evidence from the EuroSIDA study," *The Journal of Infectious Diseases*, vol. 183, no. 8, pp. 1290–1294, 2001.

[10] D. Costagliola, "Demographics of HIV and aging," *Current Opinion in HIV & AIDS*, vol. 9, no. 4, pp. 294–301, 2014.

[11] J. Negin and R. G. Cumming, "HIV infection in older adults in sub-Saharan Africa: extrapolating prevalence from existing data," *Bulletin of the World Health Organization*, vol. 88, no. 11, pp. 847–853, 2010.

[12] E. Eduardo, M. R. Lamb, S. Kandula et al., "Characteristics and outcomes among older HIV-positive adults enrolled in HIV programs in four Sub-Saharan African countries," *PLoS ONE*, vol. 9, no. 7, Article ID e103864, 2014.

[13] Centers for Disease Control and Prevention, "1993 Revised classification system for HIV infection and expanded surveillance case definition for AIDS among adolescents and adults," *Morbidity and Mortality Weekly Report*, vol. 41, no. 17, pp. 1–19, 1992.

[14] F. J. Palella, K. M. Delaney, A. C. Moorman et al., "Declining morbidity and mortality among patients with advanced human immunodeficiency virus infection. HIV Outpatient Study Investigators," *The New England Journal of Medicine*, vol. 338, no. 13, pp. 853–860, 1998.

[15] C. Lewden, T. May, E. Rosenthal et al., "Changes in causes of death among adults infected by HIV between 2000 and 2005: the 'Mortalité 2000 and 2005' surveys (ANRS EN19 and Mortavic)," *Journal of Acquired Immune Deficiency Syndromes*, vol. 48, no. 5, pp. 590–598, 2000.

[16] K. A. Mack and M. G. Ory, "AIDS and older Americans at the end of the twentieth century," *Journal of Acquired Immune Deficiency Syndromes*, vol. 33, supplement 2, pp. S68–S75, 2016.

[17] D. Zablotsky and M. Kennedy, "Risk factors and HIV transmission to midlife and older women: knowledge, options, and the initiation of safer sexual practices," *Journal of Acquired Immune Deficiency Syndromes*, vol. 33, supplement 2, pp. S122–S130, 2003.

[18] G. Orlando, P. Meraviglia, L. Cordier et al., "Antiretroviral treatment and age-related comorbidities in a cohort of older HIV-infected patients," *HIV Medicine*, vol. 7, no. 8, pp. 549–557, 2006.

[19] S. Mensforth, L. Goodall, N. Bodasing, and J. Coultas, "Late diagnosis among our ageing HIV population: a cohort study," *Journal of the International AIDS Society*, vol. 17, no. 4, supplement 3, Article ID 19692, 2014.

[20] S. Grabar, L. Weiss, and D. Costagliola, "HIV infection in older patients in the HAART era," *Journal of Antimicrobial Chemotherapy*, vol. 57, no. 1, pp. 4–7, 2006.

[21] R. C. Kalayjian, A. Landay, R. B. Pollard et al., "Age-related immune dysfunction in health and in human immunodeficiency virus (HIV) disease: association of age and HIV infection with naive $CD8^+$ cell depletion, reduced expression of CD28 on $CD8^+$ cells, and reduced thymic volumes," *The Journal of Infectious Diseases*, vol. 187, no. 12, pp. 1924–1933, 2003.

[22] K. Naylor, G. Li, A. N. Vallejo et al., "The influence of age on T cell generation and TCR diversity," *The Journal of Immunology*, vol. 174, no. 11, pp. 7446–7452, 2005.

[23] R. B. Effros, "T cell replicative senescence: pleiotropic effects on human aging," *Annals of the New York Academy of Sciences*, vol. 1019, pp. 123–126, 2004.

[24] D. C. Douek, M. R. Betts, B. J. Hill et al., "Evidence for increased T cell turnover and decreased thymic output in HIV infection," *Journal of Immunology*, vol. 167, no. 11, pp. 6663–6668, 2001.

[25] M. Egger, M. May, G. Chêne et al., "Prognosis of HIV-1-infected patients starting highly active antiretroviral therapy: a collaborative analysis of prospective studies," *The Lancet*, vol. 360, no. 9327, pp. 119–129, 2002.

[26] K. Titanji, F. Chiodi, R. Bellocco et al., "Primary HIV-1 infection sets the stage for important B lymphocyte dysfunctions," *AIDS*, vol. 19, no. 17, pp. 1947–1955, 2005.

[27] A. De Milito, C. Mörch, A. Anders Sönnerborg, and F. Chiodi, "Loss of memory (CD27) B lymphocytes in HIV-1 infection," *AIDS*, vol. 15, no. 8, pp. 957–964, 2001.

[28] H. C. Lane, H. Masur, L. C. Edgar, G. Whalen, A. H. Rook, and A. S. Fauci, "Abnormalities of B-cell activation and immunoregulation in patients with the acquired immunodeficiency syndrome," *The New England Journal of Medicine*, vol. 309, no. 8, pp. 453–458, 1983.

[29] P. J. Linton and K. Dorshkind, "Age-related changes in lymphocyte development and function," *Nature Immunology*, vol. 5, pp. 133–139, 2004.

[30] L. A. Jackson, K. M. Neuzil, O. Yu et al., "Effectiveness of pneumococcal polysaccharide vaccine in older adults," *The New England Journal of Medicine*, vol. 348, no. 18, pp. 1747–1755, 2003.

[31] R. Manfredi and F. Chiodo, "A case-control study of virological and immunological effects of highly active antiretroviral therapy in HIV-infected patients with advanced age," *AIDS*, vol. 14, no. 10, pp. 1475–1477, 2000.

[32] D. C. Douek, R. D. McFarland, P. H. Keiser et al., "Changes in thymic function with age and during the treatment of HIV infection," *Nature*, vol. 396, no. 6712, pp. 690–695, 1998.

[33] B. F. Haynes, M. L. Markert, G. D. Sempowski, D. D. Patel, and L. P. Hale, "The role of the thymus in immune reconstitution in aging, bone marrow transplantation, and HIV-1 infection," *Annual Review of Immunology*, vol. 18, pp. 529–560, 2000.

[34] A. L. Gruver, L. I. Hudson, and G. D. Sempowski, "Immunosenescence of ageing," *The Journal of Pathology*, vol. 211, no. 2, pp. 144–156, 2007.

[35] G. R. Kaufmann, H. Furrer, B. Ledergerber et al., "Characteristics, determinants, and clinical relevance of CD4 T cell recovery to <500 cells/μL in HIV type 1—infected individuals receiving potent antiretroviral therapy," *Clinical Infectious Diseases*, vol. 41, no. 3, pp. 361–372, 2005.

[36] L. Cuzin, C. Delpierre, S. Gerard, P. Massip, and B. Marchou, "Immunologic and clinical responses to highly active antiretroviral therapy in patients with HIV infection aged > 50 years," *Clinical Infectious Diseases*, vol. 45, no. 5, pp. 654–657, 2007.

[37] M. Tumbarello, R. Rabagliati, K. de Gaetano Donati et al., "Older age does not influence CD4 cell recovery in HIV-1 infected patients receiving highly active antiretroviral therapy," *BMC Infectious Diseases*, vol. 4, article 46, 2004.

[38] B. C. T. Mpondo, D. W. Gunda, S. B. Kilonzo, and E. Mgina, "Immunological and clinical responses following the use of antiretroviral therapy among elderly HIV-infected individuals attending care and treatment clinic in Northwestern Tanzania: a retrospective cohort study," *Journal of Sexually Transmitted Diseases*, vol. 2016, Article ID 5235269, 4 pages, 2016.

[39] K. Goodkin, P. Shapshak, D. Asthana et al., "Older age and plasma viral load in HIV-1 infection," *AIDS*, vol. 18, supplement 1, pp. S87–S98, 2004.

[40] R. Manfredi, L. Calza, D. Cocchi, and F. Chiodo, "Antiretroviral treatment and advanced age: epidemiologic, laboratory, and clinical features in the elderly," *Journal of Acquired Immune Deficiency Syndromes*, vol. 33, no. 1, pp. 112–114, 2003.

[41] M. Tumbarello, R. Rabagliati, K. De Gaetano Donati et al., "Older HIV-positive patients in the era of highly active antiretroviral therapy: changing of a scenario," *AIDS*, vol. 17, no. 1, pp. 128–131, 2003.

[42] C. A. Sabin, C. J. Smith, A. d'Arminio Monforte et al., "Response to combination antiretroviral therapy: variation by age," *AIDS*, vol. 22, no. 12, pp. 1463–1473, 2008.

[43] A. H. Greenbaum, L. E. Wilson, J. C. Keruly, R. D. Moore, and K. A. Gebo, "Effect of age and HAART regimen on clinical response in an urban cohort of HIV-infected individuals," *AIDS*, vol. 22, no. 17, pp. 2331–2339, 2008.

[44] A. S. Semeere, I. Lwanga, J. Sempa et al., "Mortality and immunological recovery among older adults on antiretroviral therapy at a large urban HIV clinic in Kampala, Uganda," *Journal of Acquired Immune Deficiency Syndromes*, vol. 67, no. 4, pp. 382–389, 2014.

[45] P. C. Mutevedzi, R. J. Lessells, A. J. Rodger, M. Newell, and L. Myer, "Association of age with mortality and virological and immunological response to antiretroviral therapy in rural South African adults," *PLoS ONE*, vol. 6, no. 7, Article ID e21795, 2011.

[46] M. Maskew, A. T. Brennan, A. P. MacPhail, I. M. Sanne, and M. P. Fox, "Poorer ART outcomes with increasing age at a large public sector HIV clinic in Johannesburg, South Africa," *Journal of the International Association of Providers of AIDS Care*, vol. 11, no. 1, pp. 57–65, 2012.

[47] M. S. Rhee and D. J. Greenblatt, "Pharmacologic consideration for the use of antiretroviral agents in the elderly," *Journal of Clinical Pharmacology*, vol. 48, no. 10, pp. 1212–1225, 2008.

[48] R. Bressler and J. J. Bahl, "Principles of drug therapy for the elderly patient," *Mayo Clinic Proceedings*, vol. 78, no. 12, pp. 1564–1577, 2003.

[49] A. A. Mangoni and S. H. D. Jackson, "Age-related changes in pharmacokinetics and pharmacodynamics: basic principles and practical applications," *British Journal of Clinical Pharmacology*, vol. 57, no. 1, pp. 6–14, 2004.

[50] M. Goicoechea, S. Liu, B. Best et al., "Greater tenofovir-associated renal function decline with protease inhibitor-based versus nonnucleoside reverse-transcriptase inhibitor-based therapy," *The Journal of Infectious Diseases*, vol. 197, no. 1, pp. 102–108, 2008.

[51] A. O. Ogedegbe and M. S. Sulkowski, "Antiretroviral-associated liver injury," *Clinical Liver Disease*, vol. 7, no. 2, pp. 475–499, 2003.

[52] R. Bhatia, P. Ryscavage, and B. Taiwo, "Accelerated aging and human immunodeficiency virus infection: emerging challenges of growing older in the era of successful antiretroviral therapy," *Journal of NeuroVirology*, vol. 18, no. 4, pp. 247–255, 2012.

[53] K. Meir-Shafrir and S. Pollack, "Accelerated aging in HIV patients," *Rambam Maimonides Medical Journal*, vol. 3, no. 4, Article ID e0025, 2012.

[54] G. Guaraldi, G. Orlando, S. Zona et al., "Premature age-related comorbidities among HIV-infected persons compared with the general population," *Clinical Infectious Diseases*, vol. 53, no. 11, pp. 1120–1126, 2011.

[55] Study of Fat Redistribution and Metabolic Change in HIV Infection (FRAM), "Fat distribution in women with HIV infection," *Journal of Acquired Immune Deficiency Syndromes*, vol. 42, no. 5, pp. 562–571, 2006.

[56] P. Bacchetti, B. Gripshover, C. Grunfeld et al., "Fat distribution in men with HIV infection," *Journal of Acquired Immune Deficiency Syndromes*, vol. 40, no. 2, pp. 121–131, 2005.

[57] D. Nolan and S. Mallal, "The role of nucleoside reverse transcriptase inhibitors in the fat redistribution syndrome," *Journal of HIV Therapy*, vol. 9, no. 2, pp. 34–40, 2004.

[58] E. Martínez, A. Mocroft, M. A. García-Viejo et al., "Risk of lipodystrophy in HIV-1-infected patients treated with protease inhibitors: a prospective cohort study," *The Lancet*, vol. 357, no. 9256, pp. 592–598, 2001.

[59] S. A. Riddler, E. Smit, S. R. Cole et al., "Impact of HIV infection and HAART on serum lipids in men," *Journal of the American Medical Association*, vol. 289, no. 22, pp. 2978–2982, 2003.

[60] S. C. Smith, R. Jackson, T. A. Pearson et al., "Principles for national and regional guidelines on cardiovascular disease prevention: a scientific statement from the World Heart and Stroke Forum," *Circulation*, vol. 109, no. 25, pp. 3112–3121, 2004.

[61] S. D. Holmberg, A. C. Moorman, J. M. Williamson et al., "Protease inhibitors and cardiovascular outcomes in patients with HIV-1," *The Lancet*, vol. 360, no. 9347, pp. 1747–1748, 2002.

[62] S. D. Holmberg, A. C. Moorman, and A. E. Greenberg, "Trends in rates of myocardial infarction among patients with HIV," *The New England Journal of Medicine*, vol. 350, no. 7, pp. 370–372, 2004.

[63] P. M. Coplan, A. Nikas, A. Japour et al., "Incidence of myocardial infarction in randomized clinical trials of protease inhibitor-based antiretroviral therapy: an analysis of four different protease inhibitors," *AIDS Research and Human Retroviruses*, vol. 19, no. 6, pp. 449–455, 2003.

[64] S. A. Bozzette, C. F. Ake, H. K. Tam, S. W. Chang, and T. A. Louis, "Cardiovascular and cerebrovascular events in patients treated for human immunodeficiency virus infection," *The New England Journal of Medicine*, vol. 348, pp. 702–710, 2003.

[65] R. Palacios Muñoz, J. Santos, A. García et al., "Impact of highly active antiretroviral therapy on blood pressure in HIV-infected patients. A prospective study in a cohort of naive patients," *HIV Medicine*, vol. 7, no. 1, pp. 10–15, 2006.

[66] C. M. Wyatt, J. A. Winston, C. D. Malvestutto et al., "Chronic kidney disease in HIV infection: an urban epidemic," *AIDS*, vol. 21, no. 15, pp. 2101–2103, 2007.

[67] A. Mocroft, O. Kirk, J. Gatell et al., "Chronic renal failure among HIV-1-infected patients," *AIDS*, vol. 21, no. 9, pp. 1119–1127, 2007.

[68] G. M. Lucas, S. H. Mehta, M. G. Atta et al., "End-stage renal disease and chronic kidney disease in a cohort of African-American HIV-infected and at-risk HIV-seronegative participants followed between 1988 and 2004," *AIDS*, vol. 21, no. 18, pp. 2435–2443, 2007.

[69] K. Tajiri and Y. Shimizu, "Liver physiology and liver diseases in the elderly," *World Journal of Gastroenterology*, vol. 19, no. 46, pp. 8459–8467, 2013.

[70] A. Risbud, S. Mehendale, S. Basu et al., "Prevalence and incidence of hepatitis B virus infection in STD clinic attendees in Pune, India," *Sexually Transmitted Infections*, vol. 78, no. 3, pp. 169–173, 2002.

[71] C. J. Uneke, O. Ogbu, P. U. Inyama, G. I. Anyanwu, M. O. Njoku, and J. H. Idoko, "Prevalence of hepatitis-B surface antigen among blood donors and human immunodeficiency virus-infected patients in Jos, Nigeria," *Memórias do Instituto Oswaldo Cruz*, vol. 100, no. 1, pp. 13–16, 2005.

[72] L. Platt, P. Easterbrook, E. Gower et al., "Prevalence and burden of HCV co-infection in people living with HIV: a global systematic review and meta-analysis," *The Lancet Infectious Diseases*, vol. 16, no. 7, pp. 797–808, 2016.

[73] R. Weber, C. A. Sabin, N. Friis-Møller et al., "Liver-related deaths in persons infected with the human immunodeficiency virus: the D:A:D study," *Archives of Internal Medicine*, vol. 166, no. 15, pp. 1632–1641, 2006.

[74] D. L. Schmucker, "Age-related changes in liver structure and function: implications for disease?" *Experimental Gerontology*, vol. 40, no. 8-9, pp. 650–659, 2005.

[75] J. J. Goedert, M. E. Eyster, M. M. Lederman et al., "End-stage liver disease in persons with hemophilia and transfusion-associated infections," *Blood*, vol. 100, no. 5, pp. 1584–1589, 2002.

[76] D. Posthouwer, M. Makris, T. T. Yee et al., "Progression to end-stage liver disease in patients with inherited bleeding disorders and hepatitis C: an international, multicenter cohort study," *Blood*, vol. 109, no. 9, pp. 3667–3671, 2007.

[77] R. Bedimo, R. Y. Chen, N. A. Accortt et al., "Trends in AIDS-defining and non-AIDS-defining malignancies among HIV-infected patients: 1989–2002," *Clinical Infectious Diseases*, vol. 39, no. 9, pp. 1380–1384, 2004.

[78] R. J. Bedimo, K. A. McGinnis, M. Dunlap, M. C. Rodriguez-Barradas, and A. C. Justice, "Incidence of non-AIDS-defining malignancies in HIV-infected versus noninfected patients in the HAART Era: impact of immunosuppression," *Journal of Acquired Immune Deficiency Syndromes*, vol. 52, no. 2, pp. 203–208, 2009.

[79] G. M. Clifford, J. Polesel, M. Rickenbach et al., "Cancer risk in the swiss HIV Cohort Study: associations with immunodeficiency, smoking, and highly active antiretroviral therapy," *JNCI*

Journal of the National Cancer Institute, vol. 97, no. 6, pp. 425–432, 2005.

[80] E. A. Engels and J. J. Goedert, "Human immunodeficiency virus/acquired immunodeficiency syndrome and cancer: past, present, and future," *JNCI Journal of the National Cancer Institute*, vol. 97, no. 6, pp. 407–409, 2005.

[81] N. Crum-Cianflone, K. H. Hullsiek, V. Marconi et al., "Trends in the incidence of cancers among HIV-infected persons and the impact of antiretroviral therapy: a 20-year cohort study," *AIDS*, vol. 23, no. 1, pp. 41–50, 2009.

[82] C. C. Watkins and G. J. Treisman, "Cognitive impairment in patients with AIDS—prevalence and severity," *HIV/AIDS*, vol. 7, pp. 35–47, 2015.

[83] B. M. Ances and R. J. Ellis, "Dementia and neurocognitive disorders due to HIV-1 infection," *Seminars in Neurology*, vol. 27, no. 1, pp. 86–92, 2007.

[84] R. K. Heaton, I. Grant, N. Butters et al., "The HNRC 500—neuropsychology of HIV infection at different disease stages. HIV Neurobehavioral Research Center," *Journal of the International Neuropsychological Society*, vol. 1, no. 3, pp. 231–251, 1995.

[85] R. K. Heaton, T. D. Marcotte, M. R. Mindt et al., "The impact of HIV-associated neuropsychological impairment on everyday functioning," *Journal of the International Neuropsychological Society*, vol. 10, no. 3, pp. 317–331, 2004.

[86] V. Valcour, C. Shikuma, B. Shiramizu et al., "Higher frequency of dementia in older HIV-1 individuals: the Hawaii aging with HIV-1 Cohort," *Neurology*, vol. 63, no. 5, pp. 822–827, 2004.

[87] N. Sacktor, M. P. McDermott, K. Marder et al., "HIV-associated cognitive impairment before and after the advent of combination therapy," *Journal of Neurovirology*, vol. 8, no. 2, pp. 136–142, 2002.

[88] B. Hasse, B. Ledergerber, H. Furrer et al., "Morbidity and aging in HIV-infected persons: the Swiss HIV cohort study," *Clinical Infectious Diseases*, vol. 53, no. 11, pp. 1130–1139, 2011.

[89] C. Holtzman, C. Armon, E. Tedaldi et al., "Polypharmacy and risk of antiretroviral drug interactions among the aging HIV-infected population," *Journal of General Internal Medicine*, vol. 28, no. 10, pp. 1302–1310, 2013.

[90] C. Marzolini, L. Elzi, S. Gibbons et al., "Prevalence of comedications and effect of potential drug-drug interactions in the Swiss HIV Cohort study," *Antiviral Therapy*, vol. 15, no. 3, pp. 413–423, 2010.

[91] A. Tseng, L. Szadkowski, S. Walmsley, I. Salit, and J. Raboud, "Association of age with polypharmacy and risk of drug interactions with antiretroviral medications in HIV-positive patients," *Annals of Pharmacotherapy*, vol. 47, no. 11, pp. 1429–1439, 2013.

[92] L. J. Gleason, A. E. Luque, and K. Shah, "Polypharmacy in the HIV-infected older adult population," *Journal of Clinical Interventions in Aging*, vol. 8, pp. 749–763, 2013.

[93] E. J. Edelman, K. S. Gordon, J. Glover, I. R. McNicholl, D. A. Fiellin, and A. C. Justice, "The next therapeutic challenge in HIV: polypharmacy," *Drugs & Aging*, vol. 30, no. 8, pp. 613–628, 2013.

[94] E. R. Hajjar, A. C. Cafiero, and J. T. Hanlon, "Polypharmacy in elderly patients," *The American Journal of Geriatric Pharmacotherapy*, vol. 5, no. 4, pp. 345–351, 2007.

[95] R. E. Pel-Littel, M. J. Schuurmans, M. H. Emmelot-Vonk, and H. J. Verhaar, "Frailty: defining and measuring of a concept," *The Journal of Nutrition, Health and Aging*, vol. 13, no. 4, pp. 390–394, 2009.

[96] L. P. Fried, Q.-L. Xue, A. R. Cappola et al., "Nonlinear multisystem physiological dysregulation associated with frailty in older women: implications for etiology and treatment," *The Journals of Gerontology Series A: Biological Sciences and Medical Sciences*, vol. 64, no. 10, pp. 1049–1057, 2009.

[97] L. P. Fried, C. M. Tangen, J. Walston et al., "Frailty in older adults: evidence for a phenotype," *Journals of Gerontology A: Biological Sciences and Medical Sciences*, vol. 56, no. 3, pp. M146–M156, 2001.

[98] L. P. Fried, L. Ferrucci, J. Darer, J. D. Williamson, and G. Anderson, "Untangling the concepts of disability, frailty, and comorbidity: implications for improved targeting and care," *The Journals of Gerontology. Series A, Biological Sciences and Medical Sciences*, vol. 59, no. 3, pp. 255–263, 2004.

[99] N. F. Önen and E. T. Overton, "A review of premature frailty in HIV-infected persons; another manifestation of HIV-related accelerated aging," *Current Aging Science*, vol. 4, no. 1, pp. 33–41, 2011.

[100] S. Pathai, C. Gilbert, H. A. Weiss, C. Cook, R. Wood, L.-G. Bekker et al., "Frailty in HIV-infected adults in South Africa," *JAIDS Journal of Acquired Immune Deficiency Syndromes*, vol. 62, no. 1, pp. 43–51, 2013.

[101] N. F. Onen, A. Agbebi, E. Shacham, K. E. Stamm, A. R. Onen, and E. T. Overton, "Frailty among HIV-infected persons in an urban outpatient care setting," *The Journal of Infection*, vol. 59, no. 5, pp. 346–352, 2009.

[102] U. Sandkovsky, K. R. Robertson, J. L. Meza et al., "Pilot study of younger and older HIV-infected adults using traditional and novel functional assessments," *HIV Clinical Trials*, vol. 14, no. 4, pp. 165–174, 2014.

[103] K. K. Oursler, J. D. Sorkin, B. A. Smith, and L. I. Katzel, "Reduced aerobic capacity and physical functioning in older HIV-infected men," *AIDS Research and Human Retroviruses*, vol. 22, no. 11, pp. 1113–1121, 2006.

[104] K. K. Oursler, J. L. Goulet, S. Crystal et al., "Association of age and comorbidity with physical function in HIV-infected and uninfected patients: results from the Veterans Aging Cohort Study," *AIDS Patient Care and STDs*, vol. 25, no. 1, pp. 13–20, 2011.

[105] D. L. Stanton, A. W. Wu, R. D. Moore et al., "Functional status of persons with HIV infection in an ambulatory setting," *Journal of Acquired Immune Deficiency Syndromes*, vol. 7, no. 10, pp. 1050–1056, 1994.

[106] R. Harding, C. Clucas, F. C. Lampe et al., "What factors are associated with patient self-reported health status among HIV outpatients? A multi-centre UK study of biomedical and psychosocial factors," *AIDS Care*, vol. 24, no. 8, pp. 963–971, 2012.

[107] J. S. Merlin, A. O. Westfall, E. Chamot et al., "Pain is independently associated with impaired physical function in HIV-infected patients," *Pain Medicine*, vol. 14, no. 12, pp. 1985–1993, 2013.

[108] E. E. Morgan, J. E. Iudicello, E. Weber et al., "Synergistic effects of HIV infection and older age on daily functioning," *Journal of Acquired Immune Deficiency Syndromes*, vol. 61, no. 3, pp. 341–348, 2012.

[109] UNAIDS, "Global HIV/AIDS epidemic," Fact Sheet 2015, 2015.

[110] J. A. C. Hontelez, M. N. Lurie, M.-L. Newell et al., "Ageing with HIV in South Africa," *AIDS*, vol. 25, no. 13, pp. 1665–1667, 2011.

[111] J. Negin, T. Bärnighausen, J. D. Lundgren, and E. J. Mills, "Aging with HIV in Africa," *AIDS*, vol. 26, pp. S1–S5, 2012.

[112] T. Bärnighausen, T. Welz, V. Hosegood et al., "Hiding in the shadows of the HIV epidemic: obesity and hypertension in a rural population with very high HIV prevalence in South Africa," *Journal of Human Hypertension*, vol. 22, no. 3, pp. 236–239, 2008.

[113] S. Dalal, J. J. Beunza, J. Volmink et al., "Non-communicable diseases in sub-Saharan Africa: what we know now," *International Journal of Epidemiology*, vol. 40, no. 4, pp. 885–901, 2011.

[114] M. Thorogood, M. Connor, S. Tollman, G. Lewando Hundt, G. Fowkes, and J. Marsh, "A cross-sectional study of vascular risk factors in a rural South African population: data from the Southern African Stroke Prevention Initiative (SASPI)," *BMC Public Health*, vol. 7, article 326, 2007.

[115] J. Negin, A. Martiniuk, R. G. Cumming et al., "Prevalence of HIV and chronic comorbidities among older adults," *AIDS*, vol. 26, supplement 1, pp. S55–S63, 2012.

[116] G. Fatti, E. Mothibi, G. Meintjes, A. Grimwood, and R. V. Barnabas, "Antiretroviral treatment outcomes amongst older adults in a large multicentre cohort in South Africa," *PLoS ONE*, vol. 9, no. 6, article e100273, 2014.

[117] R. W. Kimokoti and D. H. Hamer, "Nutrition, health, and aging in sub-Saharan Africa," *Nutrition Reviews*, vol. 66, pp. 611–623, 2008.

[118] J. Greig, E. C. Casas, D. P. O'Brien, E. J. Mills, and N. Ford, "Association between older age and adverse outcomes on antiretroviral therapy: a cohort analysis of programme data from nine countries," *AIDS*, vol. 26, supplement 1, pp. S31–S37, 2012.

[119] K. P. High, M. Brennan-Ing, D. B. Clifford et al., "HIV and aging: state of knowledge and areas of critical need for research. A report to the NIH Office of AIDS Research by the HIV and Aging Working Group," *Journal of Acquired Immune Deficiency Syndromes*, vol. 60, supplement 1, pp. S1–S18, 2012.

25

Effects of Strength Training on Muscle Properties, Physical Function, and Physical Activity among Frail Older People

Atle Hole Saeterbakken, Hilde Bremseth Bårdstu, Anine Brudeseth, and Vidar Andersen

Faculty of Teacher Education, Culture and Sport, Western Norway University of Applied Sciences, Bergen, Norway

Correspondence should be addressed to Atle Hole Saeterbakken; atle.saeterbakken@hvl.no

Academic Editor: Jean-Francois Grosset

The aim of this study was to determine the effects of a 10-week strength training intervention on isometric strength, rate of force development (RFD), physical function (stair climbing, rising from a chair, and preferred and maximal walking speed), and physical activity among frail elderly people receiving home-care services. Thirty participants were randomly assigned (by sex) to a control group (CON) or a strength training group (ST) performing a supervised training programme using elastic bands, box-lifting, and body weight exercises twice per week. Twenty-three participants were selected to complete the study (age 84.9 ± 6.1 years). For the ST, only improvement in muscle properties was the peak RFD in leg extension ($p = 0.04$). No significant differences were observed in muscle properties for the control group (CON) ($p = 0.16$–1.00) or between groups ($p = 0.39$–1.00). There were no changes within and between the groups in physical function ($p = 0.12$–0.19) or physical activity levels ($p = 0.06$–0.73). The results of this pilot study did not demonstrate greater improvements in muscle properties and physical function and improved physical activity after attending a home-based resistance program compared to physical activity advise; however, larger population studies should examine these findings. This trial is registered with ISRCTN10967873.

1. Introduction

With increasing age, human skeletal muscle undergoes both structural and functional changes, with a reduction in muscle mass and muscle strength [1, 2]. In addition, ageing atrophy is associated with a notable decrease in maximum muscle strength, power, and rate of force development (RFD) [3, 4]. Reduced muscle mass and muscle strength is associated with loss of function during typical daily living activities such as rising from a chair, stair climbing, and in postural balance [5].

Strength training has improved muscle strength, muscle mass, and physical function among older adults [6–10]. Traditional strength training studies with elderly people are conducted in fitness centres with multiple training machines [6–10]. However, fitness centres may exclude frail older adults to participate due to their functional level, discomfort, lack of confidence, or inability to travel to another place. Further, very few nurse-care centres have well equipped strength training facilities. Recently, the interest in low-cost home-based intervention studies examining the older adults has grown in popularity [11, 12]. A home-based exercise programme may contribute to increased participations, especially among frail older adults who might not have the opportunity to use gym or fitness facilities [13]. However, the isolated effects of home-based strength training programs are not conclusive and have not examined frail older adults [11, 14–17]. Therefore, pilot studies with frail older adults examining training programs (i.e., equipment, volume, frequency, intensity, and ability to participate) need to be conducted before starting large-scale studies.

However, typical equipment used in home-based interventions studies is elastic bands, body weight exercises, and other undersized training devices [13], and the equipment is cheap, portable, and saves space compared to a training centre. Intervention studies for the older adults using this training equipment have found improvements in muscle strength [16, 17]. However, the transferability of the improved strength to physical function (i.e., rising from a chair, stair climbing, and postural balance) is not clear. While traditional and explosive strength training improved RFD by 12–50% among 60–89-year-old participants [18–20], none of the studies examining home-based programs have trained explosive strength or included measurement of RFD.

It is well documented that physical activity (PA) can reduce the risks of chronic diseases and contribute to the enhancement of physical function and maintenance of independence for older adults [21–23]. Overall, the PA level decreases with ageing, and only 12% of the 80–85-year-old age group fulfilled the current PA recommendation of 30 minutes of moderate daily activity [24, 25]. However, there is a lack of knowledge about the effects of low-cost home-based strength training and PA levels among frail older adults. Further, the effects of home-based strength training programs among community-dwelling older adults receiving health-care services have not been properly examined as a rehabilitation strategy to prevent the age-related changes in muscle properties and physical function. With a rapid increasing numbers of older adults in the next centuries, low-cost and home-based rehabilitation programs need to be examined to decrease the factors associated with needy elderly being able to live independent and self-reliant of health-care services. Therefore, the aim of this study was to conduct a pilot study to determine the possible harms or benefits of a home-based strength training programme on physical function tests and level of physical activity in addition to muscle strength and RFD among frail old adults. Accordingly, we hypothesized that a 10-week intervention could be beneficial for frail older adults by improving muscle strength, peak RFD, and physical function, but not the PA due to the short intervention period.

2. Materials and Methods

2.1. Study Design. The pilot study was parallel group design where 30 community-dwelling older adults receiving health-care services were randomly assigned to either a strength-training group (ST) or a control group (CON). The ST group performed a progressive strength-training programme twice a week with 10–12 repetitions for 10 weeks. The CON was instructed and encouraged to continue their normal activities during the intervention. Pre- and postintervention, all participants were tested in maximal and explosive strength and physical function tests (walking speed (preferred and maximal), stair climbing, and rising from a chair) and wore an accelerometer for six days to determine the physical activity.

2.2. Participants. Due to low founding, only one municipality was invited to participate in this pilot study. The health-care services in a municipality (7000 residents) informed all elderly people meeting the inclusion criteria (45 potential participants) to participate in this pilot study. 2/3 of them volunteered, and 30 community-dwelling older adults (6 male and 24 female) were recruited. The participants were stratified randomly by sex. The name of each participant was written on a patch and divided into two heaps—one for each sex. The patches were thoroughly mixed before drawing first the male and then the female to either a strength-training group (ST) (n = 16) or a control group (CON) (n = 14). The first, third, fifth, and more patches from each heaps were assigned to the ST group and remaining to the CON group. Seven participants dropped out during the intervention (five from the ST and two from the CON) with reason not related to the study. Twenty-three participants (6 male and 17 female) aged 71–97 years completed the study (Figure 1). Due to the nature of the intervention, neither participants nor staff were blinded to the group allocation or the outcome assessors. Anthropometric measurements for the two groups are shown in Table 1.

To participate in the study, the following inclusion criteria had to be fulfilled: (1) >70 years of age living at home and (2) in need of home care due to functional disabilities and/or medication. The exclusion criteria were older adults diagnosed with chronic mental disorders, for example, Alzheimer's disease or injuries and/or diagnoses not justifiable to execute testing or training. Explanation of the purpose, procedures, potential risks, and benefits of the study was given orally and in writing to all participants. A written consent was provided prior to testing. The study was approved by the local ethics committee (REK sør-øst B, 2014/1147).

2.3. Measures

2.3.1. Maximal Strength and Rate of Force Development (RFD). To test the maximal isometric force output in leg extension and elbow flexion, a nonelectric sling (ROPES A/S, Asgardstrand, Norway) was placed around the dominant ankle or hand and attached to a force cell (Ergotest A/S, Porsgrunn, Norway). The knee and elbow angles were measured for each participant with a paragraph protractor. Both tests were performed with a 90° angle flexion in the knee or elbow joint. Performing the leg extension test, the participants were seated with a hip angle of 90° which had to be maintained during testing [15]. The participants' dominant hand was used to holda semisupinated grip [26], and the elbow was held closed to the body. Each participant had three attempts with a contraction duration of five seconds and a 60-second rest between each attempt [27]. Participants were carefully instructed to contract "as fast and forcefully as possible." The highest force output over a three seconds window was used in the analysis. The rate of force development (RDF) was calculated over a 200-millisecond sampling window where the steepest vertical generation occurred [19].

2.3.2. Physical Performance Tests. Four physical performance tests, designed to replicate daily living activities, were

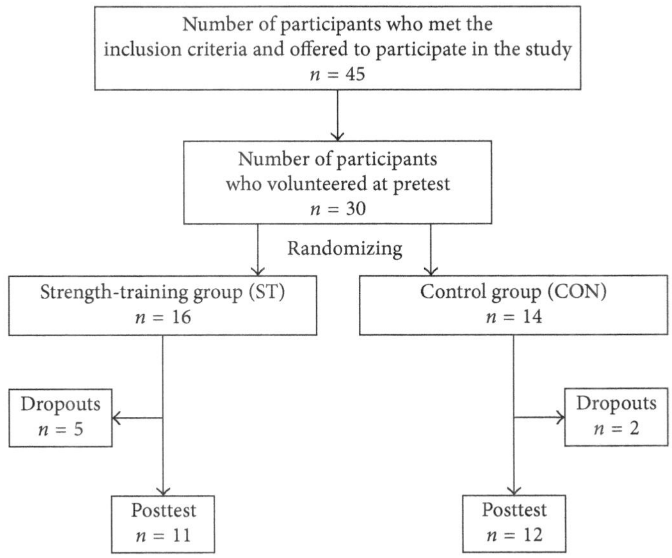

FIGURE 1: An overview of the study design.

TABLE 1: Age, height, and BMI for both groups.

	ST (n = 11)	CON (n = 12)	p value between groups
Age (years)	86.5 ± 6.4	83.5 ± 5.7	0.26
Height (cm)	163.1 ± 9.5	165.4 ± 11.2	0.73
Weight (kg)	64.3 ± 21.2	66.6 ± 8.7	0.60
BMI (kg/m^2)	23.9 ± 6.2	24.3 ± 1.6	0.81

ST = strength-training group; CON = control group; cm = centimetres; kg = kilograms; BMI = body mass index; all values are presented as mean ± standard deviation.

conducted [14, 28, 29]. All tests were performed minimum twice and maximum three times based on the physical capacity of the participants. The best attempt was used for further analysis. Participants who had problems executing the tests used necessary support, that is, an aid for walking such as a stick or crutches during the walking test, handrails for stair climbing, or armrests for rising from a chair. The use of support and number of attempts by each participant were noted for similar execution at posttest. 72% and 49% of the participants in the ST and the CON, respectively, needed support to perform one or more tests.

Two measurements of walking speed were carried out: preferred walking speed, in which the participants were instructed to walk at a pace similar to daily walking speed, and maximal speed, where the participants walked as fast as they could without running. The time was assessed by photocells (Ergotest A/S, Porsgrunn, Norway) placed 20 meters apart along a corridor. The first photocell was placed 2 metres in front of the start line for proper acceleration.

In the stair climbing test, the participants were instructed to ascend a staircase consisting of 16 steps with an 8 cm rise per step as fast as possible. Time was assessed using photocells (Ergotest A/S, Porsgrunn, Norway) placed at the beginning and end of the staircase. The staircase had a handrail on each side, and the participants were instructed to perform the test in the same way as they normally ascended a staircase.

In the rising from a chair test, the participants were seated in a hard-backed chair (seat height 44 cm from the floor) with their arms folded across their chest. The participants were instructed to rise to a full-standing position and return to a full-sitting position five times as fast as possible. The time was assessed using a stopwatch. The participants who were not able to rise without the use of aids (walker or armrests) were allowed to use the aids.

2.3.3. Physical Activity. Physical activity (PA) was measured using an accelerometer (ActiGraph GT1M, ActiGraph, LLC, Pensacola, Florida, USA) before and after the intervention. The measures were carried out over three weekdays and the weekend (Wednesday to Sunday). Valid registrations had to represent a minimum of eight hours of valid registration per day with three approved days to be included in the analysis [30]. The participants were instructed to wear the accelerometer on the right hip while awake and to remove the accelerometer only during night time and during water activities. All registrations between 12:00 am and 06:00 am were excluded [25]. Nonwear time was defined by an interval of at least 60 consecutive minutes of zero activity intensity counts, with allowances of 1-2 minutes of counts between 1 and 100 [30]. Based on previous studies, a 10-second epoch period was used [31]. Adult standard was used for overall physical activity level (counts per minute) in addition to limits for three different intensity zones. The intensity threshold criteria were 100–2019 counts for low intensity, 2020–5999 for moderate intensity, and over 5999 counts for vigorous intensity. Activity under 100 counts per minute was registered as inactivity [30]. The number of steps per day was registered using an embedded pedometer function [25]. The software program Actilife v 6.10.1 (Actigraph, LLC, Pensacola, Florida, USA) was used for options and analyses.

2.3.4. Intervention. The CON group was encouraged and instructed to continue their normal activities, to stay physically active, and to make physically active choices. An individual conversation between the participants and a health professional regarding the importance of staying physically active, make physically active choices, and the benefits of physical activity was conducted for the CON group. The session was conducted at the beginning of the intervention period. The conversation took place in the residence of each participant in the CON group and lasted between 30 and 45 minutes. In addition, they received a folder from the health ministry with information, benefits, and recommendations of physical activity.

The participants in the strength-training group performed a progressive strength-training programme twice a week for 10 weeks. The participants were instructed to perform 10–12 repetitions maximum at a controlled tempo but concentrating on a fast explosive concentric phase and a slow eccentric phase [29]. A professional training instructor was present in every training session to make sure of the correct technique, intensity, and numbers of sets. The training load gradually increased in numbers of sets and resistance level. The participants were instructed to add greater resistance when they could easily perform 10–12 repetitions of a movement in the last set without significant fatigue (i.e., perform 5 extra repetitions). One–four weeks of training consisted of two sets per exercise. The number of sets was increased to three sets from week five and throughout the intervention. The training sessions were performed with a training instructor present. The participants had to attend minimum 80% of the sessions for a valid training quantity. The mean training attendance was 84%.

The programme consisted of five minutes of general warmup and 40–55 minutes of strength training depending on the number of sets. Five exercises were conducted: squats, box lifts, seated row, chest press, and biceps curl. Squats were performed using the body weight as resistance (Figures 2(a) and 2(b)). Box lifts were performed with a soda crate as resistance (Figures 2(c) and 2(d)). The external weight was gradually increased by placing 0.5 or 1 litre bottles of water in the crate. Elastic bands were used as resistance in the exercises seated row, chest press, and biceps curl. The training instructor held the elastic band for the chest and rowing exercises (Figures 2(e)–2(h)). Biceps curls were performed seated by placing the elastic band underneath the feet of the training instructor with an equal length in each hand (Figures 2(i) and 2(j)). Further, three different elastic bands of assorted colours were used, with each colour denoting a different resistance level [32]. The bands required a force of approximately 79, 181, and 283 Newton, respectively, to stretch the bands to double their length.

2.3.5. Data Analysis. To assess differences in physical function, muscle strength, and physical activity, we used a two-way (groups × time) within-between analysis of variance (ANOVA) with repeated measures. When a significant interaction was detected by ANOVA, paired t-tests with Bonferroni post hoc correction were applied to locate where the differences lay. Tests were analysed using the SPSS (SPSS 23; SPSS Inc., Chicago, IL USA) statistical software package and were analysed per protocol. All results are presented as mean ± SD unless otherwise noted, and significant results are presented with a Cohen's d effect size (ES) of 0.2 considered small, 0.5 medium, and 0.8 large [33]. A p level of 0.05 was used for statistical significance.

3. Results

3.1. Maximal Strength and Rate of Force Development (RFD). For the maximal strength and RFD, there was no interaction for the ($F = 0.714$–4.114, $p = 0.0.3$–0.409) or a main effect for groups ($F = 0.032$–0.269, $p = 0.390$–0.861). With exceptions for maximal strength in the arm ($F = 1.162$, $p = 0.294$), there was a main effect for time ($F = 4.473$–10.043, $p = 0.005$–0.047). After the post hoc tests, the ST group had a 15.3% nonsignificant improvement in the leg extension test ($p = 0.10$, ES $= 0.31$) and a 53.1% increase for peak RFD ($p = 0.04$, ES $= 0.69$). In the elbow flexion test, a nonsignificant 51.3% improvement for peak RFD ($p = 0.08$, ES $= 0.60$) was observed. No significant differences were observed for the CON ($p = 0.16$–1.00) (Figures 3 and 4).

3.2. Physical Function. For the physical function tests, there was no interaction ($F = 0.087$–2.519, $p = 0.130$–0.770) or a main effect for groups ($F = 1.888$–2.696, $p = 0.115$–0.186) or time ($F = 0.55$–2.223, $p = 0.151$–0.817) with one exception. The stair climbing test had significant main effect for time ($F = 4.659$, $p = 0.044$). Despite an overall improvement in stair climbing of 26.6%, the improvement was not significant for the ST ($p = 0.22$). Furthermore, no significant difference was observed for the CON ($p = 0.22$). All details are presented in Table 2.

3.3. Physical Activity (PA). For PA, there was no interaction ($F = 0.009$–0.939, $p = 0.341$–0.927), main effects for time (0.001–0.223, $p = 0.644$–0.980) or group ($F = 0.120$–4.178, $p = 0.059$–0.734) for the variables overall PA, inactivity, moderate intensity, high intensity, and numbers of steps per day. However, an interaction was observed for the variable low intensity ($F = 5.008$, $p = 0.041$). Post hoc tests demonstrated no differences between the groups ($p = 0.480$–1.000) or differences between pre- and posttest ($p = 0.133$–0.698). All details are presented in Table 3.

4. Discussion

The home-based strength-training intervention among frail older adults did not increase the strength but improved RFD in the lower body for the strength-training group. Furthermore, there were no significant changes in physical function, and the physical activity level was unaltered after the intervention. No differences were observed in the CON group or between the groups in any of the tests.

Leg extension strength increased by 15.3% in the ST but only tended towards statistical significant ($p = 0.100$).

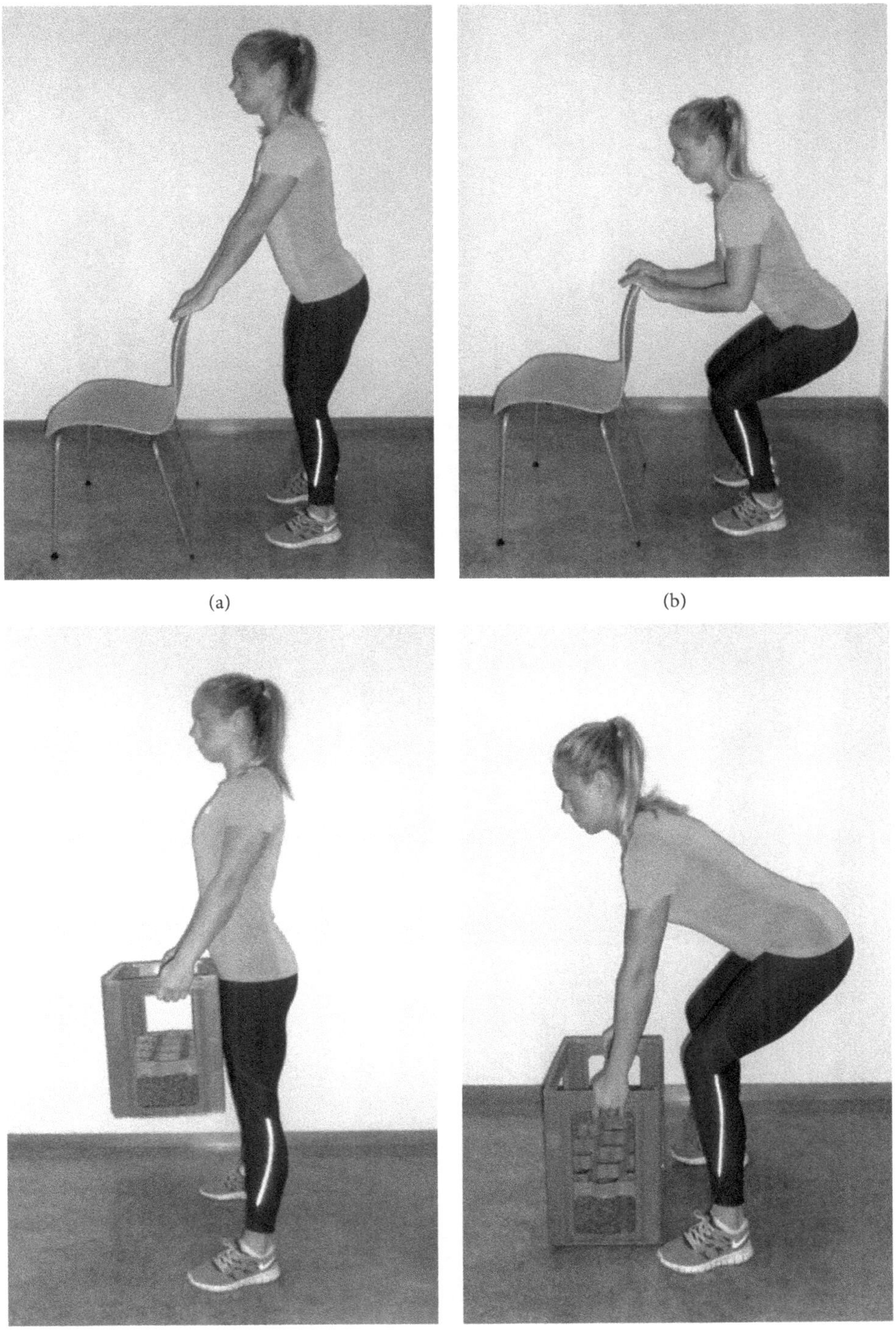

(a) (b)

(c) (d)

Figure 2: Continued.

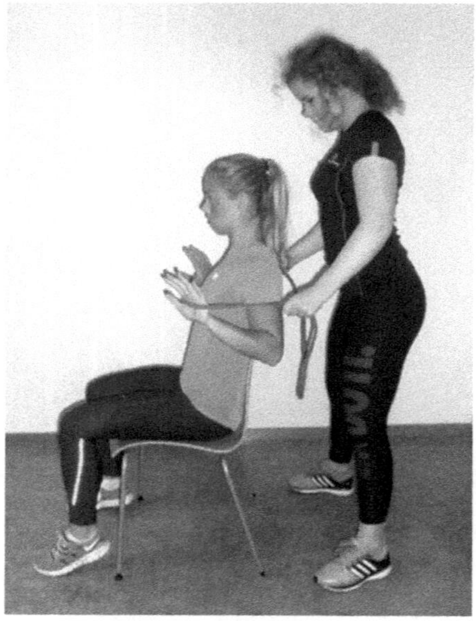

(e)

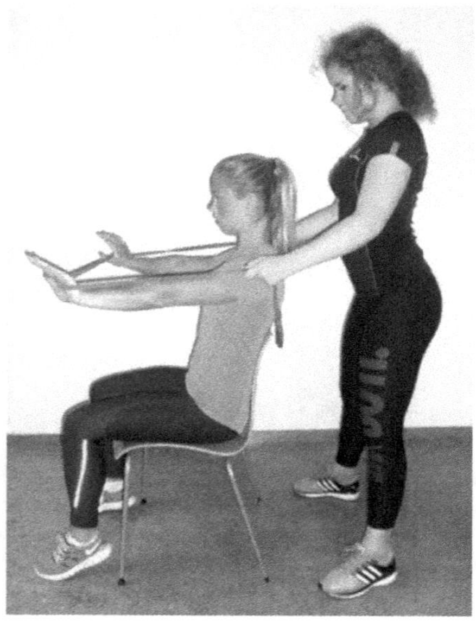

(f)

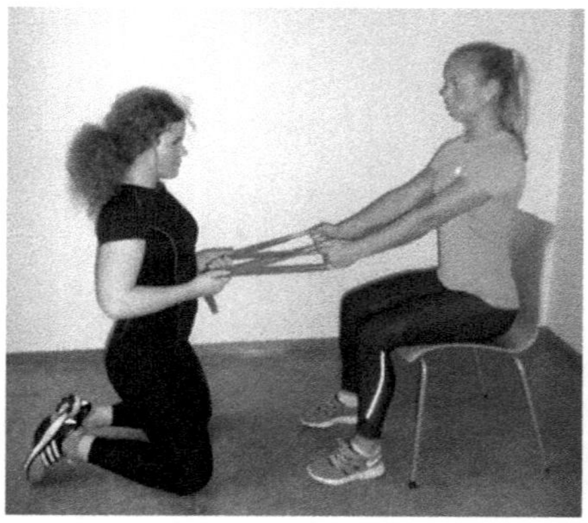

(g)

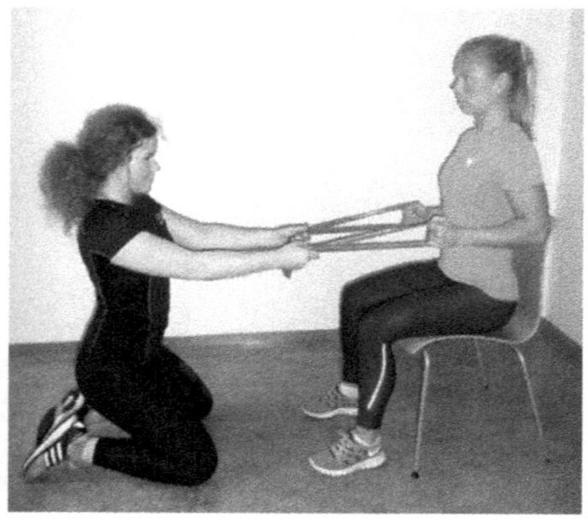

(h)

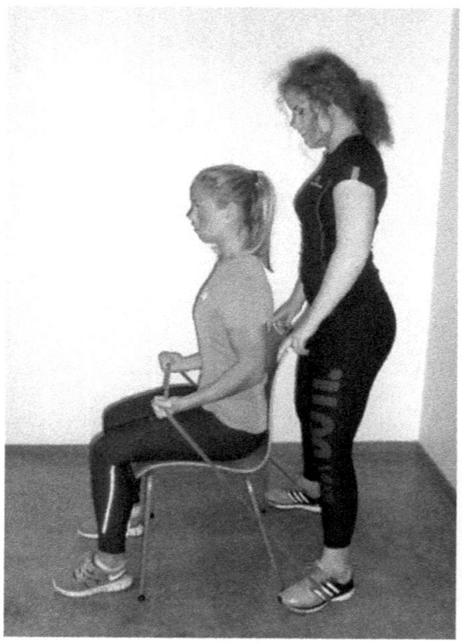

(i)

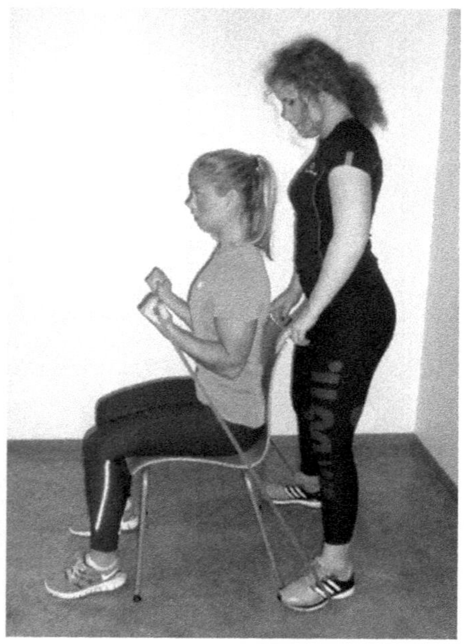

(j)

FIGURE 2: (a–j) An overview of the five training exercises.

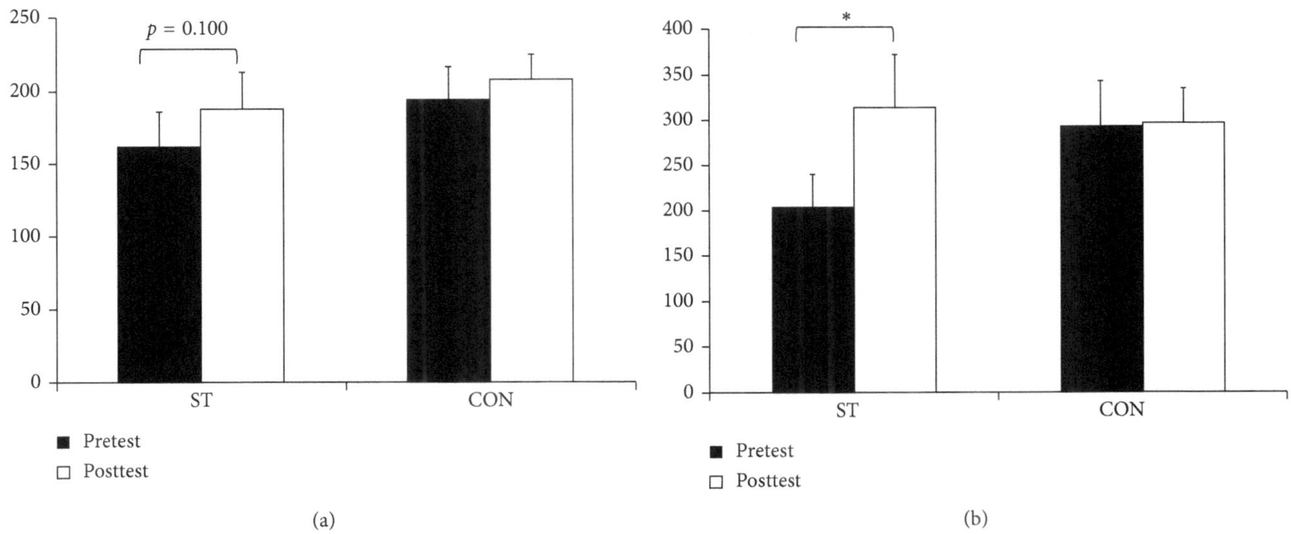

FIGURE 3: The pre- and posttest results of the (a) maximal strength and (b) RFD in leg extension for the strength-training group (ST) and control group (CON). All values are presented as mean ± SE. *Within-group differences, $p < 0.05$.

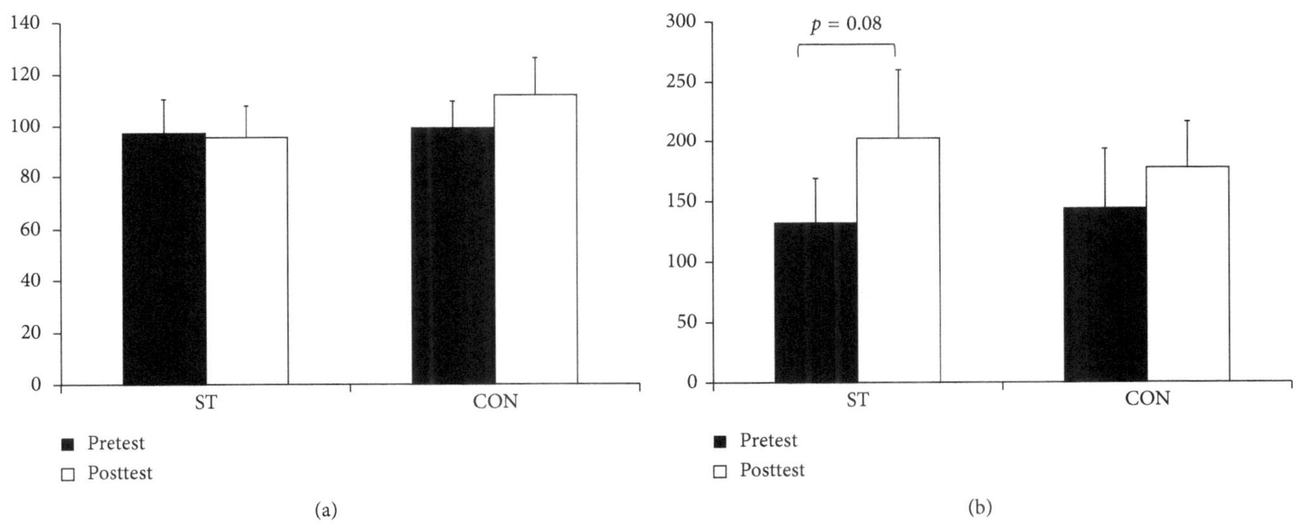

FIGURE 4: The pre- and posttest results of the (a) maximal strength and (b) RFD in arm flexion for the strength-training group (ST) and control group (CON). All values are presented as mean ± SE. *Within-group differences, $p < 0.05$.

None of the participants trained strength before the intervention. The numbers of exercises and sets were therefore low. Additionally, the strength-training group only trained twice per week. The lack of improvement was most likely a result of low training volume, low statistical power, and large standard deviation. The result supports not our hypotheses nor previous studies despite similar improvements as comparable studies [16, 17, 34]. For example, Capodaglio et al. demonstrated a 14.9% improvement in maximal isometric leg extension after five months of strength training performed at home using elastic bands [34]. In addition, Frontera et al. observed an 11.9% increase in the right quadriceps cross-section area in addition to an 8.5% improvement in dynamic muscle strength after attending a 12 wk strength training program [35].

The arm flexion strength was unaltered for the ST. Despite the participants' effort to perform the exercises with proper execution until failure, the limited training load on the biceps (only one isolating exercise) may explain the lack of strength improvement. Furthermore, the moderate training load using an elastic band and the choice of 10–12 repetitions in the present study may have contributed to the lack of improvement in upper-body strength. However, the number of repetitions is recommended for novice individuals [36]. Still, the same findings were presented by Skelton and McLaughlin, who failed to observe an improvement in isometric elbow flexion despite a 20% improvement in leg extension after an eight-week supervised training period among 80-year-olds [5]. Furthermore, Zion et al. used a similar training protocol as the present study

Table 2: Pre- and posttest results of physical function for the ST and CON.

Tests	Group	Pretest	Posttest
Stair climbing (sec)	ST	26.0 ± 6.0	19.3 ± 3.4
	CON	18.3 ± 3.6	17.1 ± 3.3
Preferred walking speed (km/h)	ST	2.3 ± 0.3	2.3 ± 0.2
	CON	3.0 ± 0.3	2.9 ± 0.3
Maximal walking speed (km/h)	ST	3.5 ± 0.3	3.8 ± 0.4
	CON	4.5 ± 0.4	4.3 ± 0.4
Rising from a chair (sec)	ST	27.6 ± 4.6	25.5 ± 4.1
	CON	20.6 ± 2.2	19.1 ± 2.3

ST = strength-training group; CON = control group; sec = seconds; km/h = kilometres per hour; all values are presented as mean ± standard error.

Table 3: Pre- and posttest results of physical activity for the ST and CON.

Tests	Group	Pretest	Posttest
Overall PA (cpm)	ST	57.6 ± 8.4	67.7 ± 12.5
	CON	129.5 ± 25.5	120.5 ± 24.7
Inactivity (min/day)	ST	673.4 ± 16.3	688.0 ± 32.6
	CON	663.1 ± 28.4	621.7 ± 31.2
Low intensity (min/day)	ST	83.8 ± 12.8	91.1 ± 13.0
	CON	120.4 ± 21.5	101.6 ± 16.4
Moderate intensity (min/day)	ST	2.9 ± 0.5	2.8 ± 0.7
	CON	11.1 ± 2.8	10.7 ± 3.7
High intensity (min/day)	ST	0.2 ± 0.1	0.2 ± 0.1
	CON	0.2 ± 0.1	0.2 ± 0.1
Steps (per day)	ST	1360 ± 322	1262 ± 312
	CON	2868 ± 547	2396 ± 501

ST = strength-training group; CON = control group; s = seconds; km/h = kilometres per hour; cpm = counts per minute; min/day = minutes per day; all values are presented as mean ± standard error.

with only one isolating exercise for biceps and observed no changes in isometric handgrip [12]. Importantly, the training in the present study was performed dynamically while the tests were isometric. Previous studies have reported substantially lower improvement in isometric than dynamic strength after a dynamic strength-training program [37–39].

Our findings demonstrate that the execution of the exercises, performed in a fast explosive concentric phase, contributed to the improvements in RFD. These results support our hypotheses and previous studies [18–20, 40]. The increase in RFD in the present study may be the result of neurological adaptations as RFD is highly influenced by the magnitude of neuromuscular activity irrespective of age [41, 42]. To our knowledge, no previous studies have carried out RFD tests after home-based strength training using low costs portable training equipment. Previous studies have used traditional strength training equipment (training machines or free weights), but the need of such facilities may exclude several frail older adults. Comparing the strength and RFD results, the substantially lower strength improvement is supported by previous studies. The improvement in RFD has shown to increase greater than isometric strength [40], and accordingly, there is evidence that the decline in muscle power is greater than the decline in muscle strength in the older adults [3, 43]. Older adults may therefore have a larger potential to improve the RFD compared to muscle strength.

This study did not demonstrate a significant effect of the resistance training programme on functional outcome measures. However, there was a consistent trend towards nonsignificant improvements in physical function by 3.5–25.6% for the ST. Although the training programme trained the same muscles/muscles groups as the physical tests target, the exercises might not have been specific enough to give significant changes in the physical functional tests [38]. Moreover, the absence of significant changes in physical function may be explained by variability in performance, age (78–97 years), and physical characteristics at baseline. For example, differences in execution of the tests due to frailty and the need for support (i.e., walking aids and the use of handrails and armrests) may have influenced the variation in the test results within and between groups. However, the older adults with assistive devices (3 in the ST and 4 in the CON) were not significant differences in the physical function tests compared to the one without.

Comparable studies have usually carried out the tests with identical execution for all participants [11, 29, 44], and this might contribute to less variation in the test results, mainly because the participants in these studies were younger and healthier, resulting in more homogeneity compared to the participants in our study. Despite the differences in execution among the participants, the test protocol was carefully standardized and the use of support was noted for similar execution at pre- and posttest. The training volume was quite low (2x per week and only 2 sets in the first weeks) due to the lack of experience with resistance training and relative low physical function (all participants received health-care services). We cannot exclude that a higher volume may have resulted in greater benefits.

Our findings are supported by a previous study who reported no significant changes, but a tendency for improvements in rising from a chair (10 times) and the time-up and go among frail older adults after resistance training intervention [45].

The physical activity level concerning inactivity and low, moderate, and high intensity was unaltered for both groups after the intervention. However, the overall PA (counts per minute) increased with 17.4% for the ST, but not significantly. Importantly, the ST maintained their physical activity attending strength training twice per week. A systematic review demonstrated a compensation of physical activity in over 50% of the studies attending different training interventions [46]. Despite having benefits of participation in the strength-training program, the physical activity level of the ST was not increased. The physical activity results supported our hypothesis that due the short intervention period, the PA level did not increase. Importantly and most likely, our findings may have been affected by the variation of the season, with pretesting being performed in late summer and posttesting during the late autumn. In addition, the weather conditions may have influenced the activity level due to dry weather at pretest and precipitation/snow at posttest and might explain the nonsignificant changes. Lemmer et al. demonstrated no significant changes in PA for younger (20–30 years) or older adult (65–75 years) individuals after 24 weeks of strength training supporting the PA results of the present study [47].

With a small sample size, there is a risk of conducting type II errors and the additional moderate dropout rate of five participants in the ST and two in the CON. The results should therefore be interpreted with caution. Importantly, the participants were frail older adults, but we experienced no harms of unintended effects. The only harms observed were delayed onset of muscle soreness but only in the first weeks. Furthermore, several of the participants in the strength-training group reported different and often several muscle-skeletal disorders. Still, none reported greater pain after the intervention, but rather the opposite. There are some limitations to the current study that need to be addressed. There was a large variation in physical performance, age, and physical characteristics (i.e., need of walking aid). The large variation may therefore influence the statistical analyses. To reduce a possible learning effect, we intended to complete two testing sessions as part of the baseline measures. Unfortunately, only one session of testing was performed at baseline due to a time limitation for the intervention. Moreover, the lack of statistically significant findings in physical function and the PA level may be related to the high variability of the results and the differences in weather conditions.

Further studies should include a more homogeneous population (i.e., not need of walking aid), decrease the variation in age (and thereby the age related loss of muscle mass), and recruit more participants. Still, a larger population may detect differences among older adults with need of walking aids and those without as well as differences between age groups (i.e., 70–80 years versus 80–90 years). Including older adults with receiving health-care services, it is important to gradually increase intensity, sets, and training frequency. Long-lasting intervention studies should therefore try to increase the training volume to a greater extent than the present. Finally, further studies should include factor analyses with age and assistive devices as two important factors, as well as analyses of the ability to live self-reliant and independent of further health-care services.

5. Conclusion

The results of this pilot study did not demonstrate greater improvement in muscle properties and physical function and improved physical activity after attending a home-based resistance program compared to physical activity advice. However, the strength-training group improved explosive strength. Hopefully, further trails would benefit from this pilot study and make rehabilitation strategies with older adults a research priority.

Conflicts of Interest

The authors declare that there are no conflicts of interest regarding the publication of this paper.

Acknowledgments

The authors wish to thank all the individuals who took part in this intervention study.

References

[1] M. M. Porter, A. A. Vandervoort, and J. Lexell, "Aging of human muscle: structure, function and adaptability," *Scandinavian Journal of Medicine and Science in Sports*, vol. 5, no. 3, pp. 129–142, 2007.

[2] A. A. Vandervoort and A. J. McComas, "Contractile changes in opposing muscles of the human ankle joint with aging," *Journal of Applied Physiology*, vol. 61, no. 1, pp. 361–367, 1986.

[3] P. Aagaard, C. Suetta, P. Caserotti, S. P. Magnusson, and M. Kjaer, "Role of the nervous system in sarcopenia and muscle atrophy with aging: strength training as a countermeasure," *Scandinavian Journal of Medicine and Science in Sports*, vol. 20, no. 1, pp. 49–64, 2010.

[4] K. Hakkinen, R. U. Newton, S. E. Gordon et al., "Changes in muscle morphology, electromyographic activity, and force production characteristics during progressive strength training in young and older men," *Journals of Gerontology Series A: Biological Sciences and Medical Sciences*, vol. 53, no. 6, pp. B415–B423, 1998.

[5] D. A. Skelton and A. W. McLaughlin, "Training functional ability in old age," *Physiotherapy*, vol. 82, no. 3, pp. 159–167, 1996.

[6] M. A. Fiatarone, E. C. Marks, N. D. Ryan, C. N. Meredith, L. A. Lipsitz, and W. J. Evans, "High-intensity strength training in nonagenarians. Effects on skeletal muscle," *JAMA*, vol. 263, no. 22, pp. 3029–3034, 1990.

[7] G. R. Hunter, C. J. Wetzstein, D. A. Fields, A. Brown, and M. M. Bamman, "Resistance training increases total energy expenditure and free-living physical activity in older adults," *Journal of Applied Physiology*, vol. 89, no. 3, pp. 977–984, 2000.

[8] A. I. Kryger and J. L. Andersen, "Resistance training in the oldest old: consequences for muscle strength, fiber types, fiber size, and MHC isoforms," *Scandinavian Journal of Medicine and Science in Sports*, vol. 17, no. 4, pp. 422–430, 2007.

[9] H. Lohne-Seiler, M. K. Torstveit, and S. A. Anderssen, "Traditional versus functional strength training: effects on muscle strength and power in the elderly," *Journal of Aging and Physical Activity*, vol. 21, no. 1, pp. 51–70, 2013.

[10] M. E. Nelson, M. A. Fiatarone, C. M. Morganti, I. Trice, R. A. Greenberg, and W. J. Evans, "Effects of high-intensity strength training on multiple risk factors for osteoporotic fractures. A randomized controlled trial," *JAMA*, vol. 272, no. 24, pp. 1909–1914, 1994.

[11] E. V. Cyarto, W. J. Brown, A. L. Marshall, and S. G. Trost, "Comparison of the effects of a home-based and group-based resistance training program on functional ability in older adults," *American Journal of Health Promotion*, vol. 23, no. 1, pp. 13–17, 2008.

[12] A. S. Zion, R. De Meersman, B. E. Diamond, and D. M. Bloomfield, "A home-based resistance-training program using elastic bands for elderly patients with orthostatic hypotension," *Clinical Autonomic Research*, vol. 13, no. 4, pp. 286–292, 2003.

[13] R. S. Thiebaud, M. D. Funk, and T. Abe, "Home-based resistance training for older adults: a systematic review," *Geriatrics and Gerontology International*, vol. 14, no. 4, pp. 750–757, 2014.

[14] H. C. Boshuizen, L. Stemmerik, M. H. Westhoff, and M. Hopman-Rock, "The effects of physical therapists' guidance on improvement in a strength-training program for the frail elderly," *Journal of Aging and Physical Activity*, vol. 13, no. 1, pp. 5–22, 2005.

[15] J. L. Helbostad, O. Sletvold, and R. Moe-Nilssen, "Home training with and without additional group training in physically frail old people living at home: effect on health-related quality of life and ambulation," *Clinical Rehabilitation*, vol. 18, no. 5, pp. 498–508, 2004.

[16] A. M. Jette, M. Lachman, M. M. Giorgetti et al., "Exercise–it's never too late: the strong-for-life program," *American Journal of Public Health*, vol. 89, no. 1, pp. 66–72, 1999.

[17] T. Suzuki, H. Kim, H. Yoshida, and T. Ishizaki, "Randomized controlled trial of exercise intervention for the prevention of falls in community-dwelling elderly Japanese women," *Journal of Bone and Mineral Metabolism*, vol. 22, no. 6, pp. 602–611, 2004.

[18] P. Caserotti, P. Aagaard, J. B. Larsen, and L. Puggaard, "Explosive heavy-resistance training in old and very old adults: changes in rapid muscle force, strength and power," *Scandinavian Journal of Medicine and Science*, vol. 18, no. 6, pp. 773–782, 2008.

[19] A. L. Gurjao, L. T. Gobbi, N. H. Carneiro et al., "Effect of strength training on rate of force development in older women," *Research Quarterly for Exercise and Sport*, vol. 83, no. 2, pp. 268–275, 2012.

[20] D. I. Lovell, R. Cuneo, and G. C. Gass, "The effect of strength training and short-term detraining on maximum force and the rate of force development of older men," *European Journal of Applied Physiology*, vol. 109, no. 3, pp. 429–435, 2010.

[21] S. N. Blair, "C. H. McCloy research lecture: physical activity, physical fitness, and health," *Research Quarterly for Exercise and Sport*, vol. 64, no. 4, pp. 365–376, 1993.

[22] W. W. Spirduso and D. L. Cronin, "Exercise dose-response effects on quality of life and independent living in older adults,"*Medicine and Science in Sports and Exercise*, Vol. 33, pp. S598–S608, discussion S609-S510, 2001.

[23] A. H. Taylor, N. T. Cable, G. Faulkner, M. Hillsdon, M. Narici, and A. K. Van Der Bij, "Physical activity and older adults: a review of health benefits and the effectiveness of interventions," *Journal of Sports Sciences*, vol. 22, no. 8, pp. 703–725, 2004.

[24] N. Y. Arnardottir, A. Koster, D. R. Van Domelen et al., "Objective measurements of daily physical activity patterns and sedentary behaviour in older adults: age, gene/environment susceptibility-Reykjavik study," *Age and Ageing*, vol. 42, no. 2, pp. 222–229, 2013.

[25] H. Lohne-Seiler, B. H. Hansen, E. Kolle, and S. A. Anderssen, "Accelerometer-determined physical activity and self-reported health in a population of older adults (65–85 years): a cross-sectional study," *BMC Public Health*, vol. 14, no. 1, p. 284, 2014.

[26] S. Vestergaard, C. Kronborg, and L. Puggaard, "Home-based video exercise intervention for community-dwelling frail older women: a randomized controlled trial," *Aging Clinical and Experimental Research*, vol. 20, no. 5, pp. 479–486, 2008.

[27] V. Andersen, M. S. Fimland, M. K. Kolnes, and A. H. Saeterbakken, "Elastic bands in combination with free weights in strength training: neuromuscular effects," *Journal of Strength and Conditioning Research*, vol. 29, no. 10, pp. 2932–2940, 2015.

[28] M. A. Fiatarone, E. F. O'Neill, N. D. Ryan et al., "Exercise training and nutritional supplementation for physical frailty in very elderly people," *New England Journal of Medicine*, vol. 330, no. 25, pp. 1769–1775, 1994.

[29] T. R. Henwood and D. R. Taaffe, "Short-term resistance training and the older adult: the effect of varied programmes for the enhancement of muscle strength and functional performance," *Clinical Physiology and Functional Imaging*, vol. 26, no. 5, pp. 305–313, 2006.

[30] R. P. Troiano, D. Berrigan, K. W. Dodd, L. C. Masse, T. Tilert, and M. McDowell, "Physical activity in the United States measured by accelerometer," *Medicine & Science in Sports & Exercise*, vol. 40, no. 1, pp. 181–188, 2008.

[31] B. H. Hansen, E. Kolle, S. M. Dyrstad, I. Holme, and S. A. Anderssen, "Accelerometer-determined physical activity in adults and older people," *Medicine & Science in Sports & Exercise*, vol. 44, no. 2, pp. 266–272, 2012.

[32] M. E. Rogers, H. S. Sherwood, N. L. Rogers, and R. M. Bohlken, "Effects of dumbbell and elastic band training on physical function in older inner-city African-American women," *Women Health*, vol. 36, no. 4, pp. 33–41, 2002.

[33] J. Cohen, *Statistical Power for the Behavioral Sciences*, Lawrence Erlbaum Associates Inc., Hillsdale, NJ, USA, 1988.

[34] P. Capodaglio, M. Facioli, E. Burroni, A. Giordano, A. Ferri, and G. Scaglioni, "Effectiveness of a home-based strengthening program for elderly males in Italy. A preliminary study," *Aging Clinical and Experimental Research*, vol. 14, no. 1, pp. 28–34, 2002.

[35] W. R. Frontera, C. N. Meredith, K. P. O'Reilly, H. G. Knuttgen, and W. J. Evans, "Strength conditioning in older men: skeletal muscle hypertrophy and improved function," *Journal of Applied Physiology*, vol. 64, no. 3, pp. 1038–1044, 1988.

[36] ACSM, "American College of Sports Medicine position stand. Progression models in resistance training for healthy adults," *Medicine and Science in Sports and Exercise*, vol. 41, no. 3, pp. 687–708, 2009.

[37] O. M. Rutherford and D. A. Jones, "The role of learning and coordination in strength training," *European Journal of Applied Physiology and Occupational Physiology*, vol. 55, no. 1, pp. 100–105, 1986.

[38] D. Sale and D. MacDougall, "Specificity in strength training: a review for the coach and athlete," *Canadian Journal of Applied Sport Sciences*, vol. 6, no. 2, pp. 87–92, 1981.

[39] A. Thorstensson, B. Hulten, W. Von Dobeln, and J. Karlsson, "Effect of strength training on enzyme activities and fiber characteristics in human skeletal muscle," *Acta Physiologica Scandinavica*, vol. 96, no. 3, pp. 392–398, 1976.

[40] C. Suetta, P. Aagaard, A. Rosted et al., "Training-induced changes in muscle CSA, muscle strength, EMG, and rate of force development in elderly subjects after long-term unilateral disuse," *Journal of Applied Physiology*, vol. 97, no. 5, pp. 1954–1961, 2004.

[41] C. Del Balso and E. Cafarelli, "Adaptations in the activation of human skeletal muscle induced by short-term isometric resistance training," *Journal of Applied Physiology*, vol. 103, no. 1, pp. 402–411, 2007.

[42] M. Klass, S. Baudry, and J. Duchateau, "Age-related decline in rate of torque development is accompanied by lower maximal motor unit discharge frequency during fast contractions," *Journal of Applied Physiology*, vol. 104, no. 3, pp. 739–746, 2008.

[43] E. J. Metter, R. Conwit, J. Tobin, and J. L. Fozard, "Age-associated loss of power and strength in the upper extremities in women and men," *Journals of Gerontology Series A: Biological Sciences and Medical Sciences*, vol. 52, no. 5, pp. B267–B276, 1997.

[44] J. L. Helbostad, O. Sletvold, and R. Moe-Nilssen, "Effects of home exercises and group training on functional abilities in home-dwelling older persons with mobility and balance problems. A randomized study," *Aging Clinical and Experimental Research*, vol. 16, no. 2, pp. 113–121, 2004.
[45] M. E. McMurdo and R. Johnstone, "A randomized controlled trial of a home exercise programme for elderly people with poor mobility," *Age and Ageing*, vol. 24, no. 5, pp. 425–428, 1995.
[46] S. R. Gomersall, A. V. Rowlands, C. English, C. Maher, and T. S. Olds, "The ActivityStat hypothesis: the concept, the evidence and the methodologies," *Sports Medicine*, vol. 43, no. 2, pp. 135–149, 2013.
[47] J. T. Lemmer, F. M. Ivey, A. S. Ryan et al., "Effect of strength training on resting metabolic rate and physical activity: age and gender comparisons," *Medicine and Science in Sports and Exercise*, vol. 33, pp. 532–541, 2001.

The Cooccurrence of Obesity, Osteoporosis, and Sarcopenia in the Ovariectomized Rat: A Study for Modeling Osteosarcopenic Obesity in Rodents

Zahra Ezzat-Zadeh,[1] Jeong-Su Kim,[1,2] P. Bryant Chase,[3] and Bahram H. Arjmandi[1,2]

[1] *Department of Nutrition, Food, and Exercise Sciences, Florida State University, Tallahassee, FL, USA*
[2] *Center for Advancing Exercise and Nutrition Research on Aging (CAENRA), College of Human Sciences, Florida State University, Tallahassee, FL 32306, USA*
[3] *Department of Biological Science, Florida State University, Tallahassee, FL, USA*

Correspondence should be addressed to Bahram H. Arjmandi; barjmandi@fsu.edu

Academic Editor: Arshad Jahangir

Background. Obesity, osteoporosis, and sarcopenia may individually occur due to age-related gradual alterations in body composition. This study investigates the cooccurrence of these age-related diseases in female animals with low levels of ovarian hormone in the absence of complex multifactorial process of chronological aging. *Methods.* Thirty-six 5- and 10-month-old female rats were chosen to model pre- and postmenopausal women, respectively. Rats were divided into three treatment groups in each age category—sham, ovariectomized (ovx), and ovx + E_2 (17β-estradiol, 10 μg/kg)—and were pair-fed. Volunteer wheel running activity, body composition, bone microstructure, serum C-telopeptides of type I collagen, bone specific alkaline phosphatase, E_2, and gastrocnemius and soleus muscles were analyzed. *Results.* The cooccurrence of osteoporosis, sarcopenia, and obesity was observed in the older ovx rats associated with a significant ($p < 0.05$) increased fat mass (30%), bone loss (9.6%), decreased normalized muscle mass-to-body-weight ratio (10.5%), and a significant decrease in physical activity (57%). The ratio of tibial bone mineral density to combined muscle mass was significantly decreased in both ovx age categories. *Conclusion.* Ovariectomized rat could be used as an experimental model to examine the effect of loss of ovarian hormones, while controlling for energy intake and expenditure, to conduct obesity and body composition translational research in females without the confounding effect of genetic background.

1. Introduction

Obesity, osteoporosis, and sarcopenia are three disease conditions that may occur due to age-related gradual alterations in body composition [1, 2]. Excess fat mass has been suggested as a risk factor for the gradual decline in muscle mass and the combination of both conditions has termed sarcopenic obesity [1]. Interestingly, in spite of the traditional belief that obesity was protective against osteoporosis, a more recent, growing body of evidence indicates that fat mass is negatively correlated with bone mass, suggesting that excess body fat has deleterious effects on bone [3, 4].

In women and certain animal models such as rat, estrogen is considered a major regulator of adipose tissue development and its deposition [5–9]. In addition to the direct role of estrogen on adipose tissue [6–8], it may also indirectly affect adiposity via regulation of food intake and energy expenditure by affecting hypothalamus functions [5, 9]. Moreover, ovarian hormone deficiency often not only is associated with an increase in fat mass, but also is linked to an accelerated loss of bone mass and development of osteoporosis [2, 3].

While the effect of estrogen on bone is better understood, its effect on other tissues including skeletal muscle is poorly understood and needs further investigation. Available findings suggest both direct and indirect roles for estrogen in muscle protein synthesis or maintaining lean tissues in both human and rodents [10, 11]. However, there is disagreement in available literature related to the effects of estrogen on skeletal muscle mass. Declined, increased, and maintained skeletal muscle mass has been reported following ovarian hormone deficiency and administration of estrogen, making it difficult to interpret the role of estrogen in the progressive decline of muscle mass which is clinically known as sarcopenia [12–15]. Differences in energy intake and expenditure—two main factors that affect body weight and that vary as a consequence of ovarian hormone deficiency—may partially explain discrepancies among previous findings. Additionally, the effects of ovarian hormone may be age specific and impact the role of estrogen manipulation on lean mass in growing versus mature animals [13, 14]. The duration of the estrogen deficiency [16] and specific metabolic alterations following ovariectomy in mice and rats could also be reasons of these inconstancies in the available literature [17]. It is likely that ovarian hormone deficiency results in an increased adiposity in the face of bone and muscle loss due to the adverse effect on osteoblastogenesis and myogenesis [11, 18]. These unfavorable changes in body composition may interact negatively to predispose women with low levels of ovarian hormone to impaired physical function and age-related chronic disease.

The cooccurrence of obesity, osteoporosis, and sarcopenia—three diseases that occur with advancing age and which may be affected by fluctuations in ovarian hormone production or its deficiency—has not been investigated in females while controlling for energy intake and expenditure. This study addresses two important questions: (1) do these three age-related disease conditions cooccur in females with low levels of ovarian hormone? (2) How the presence or absence of estradiol (E_2), the most biologically active form of estrogen, affects muscle, bone, and fat mass in an experimental model without the confounding effects of chronological aging or genetic background?

To investigate these issues, we used Sprague-Dawley (SD) rats that were 5 or 10 months old at the beginning of the study to model pre- and postmenopausal women, respectively. Using these two age groups, we were able to compare the impact of estrogen deficiency along with advancing age without any sign and complexity of chronological aging that negatively affects body composition. We hypothesized that ovarian hormone deficiency slows resting metabolic rate and energy expenditure resulting in an increased adiposity and a body weight (BW) gain while exerting catabolic effects on lean mass, including bone mass, in both young and old experimental categories. Furthermore, we postulated that this hypothesis was independent of age. To test this hypothesis, we controlled the effects of ovarian hormone deficiency on food intake by pair-feeding all of our ovariectomized (ovx) animals to the mean food intake of sham-operated rats. We also measured changes in physical activity in response to the interventions. The study was concluded once significant loss of whole body bone mineral density (BMD) was observed. We also measured bone mineral content (BMC) of whole body, tibia, and 4th lumbar vertebra and their microstructural properties. We examined sarcopenia by measuring lean and skeletal muscle mass and adjusting the values of skeletal muscle mass by weight as the most recommended diagnostic approach to determine presarcopenia, according to the European Working Group on Sarcopenia in Older People (EWGSOP). For our investigation we selected two hindlimb skeletal muscles: the soleus (SOL) that is mostly comprised of slow-twitch muscle fibers (type I) and the gastrocnemius (GAS) that is mostly comprised of fast-twitch muscle fibers (type II). The combined muscle mass of these two skeletal muscles that either are attached (SOL) or span the tibia (GAS) was used in computing the ratio of tibial BMC to muscle mass (MM). Although there are a number of studies that have evaluated the effects of ovarian hormone deficiency on body weight, fat, muscle, and bone status, to our knowledge this is the first study that addresses osteosarcopenic obesity in experimental model and evaluates the effects of the presence or absence of estradiol on these components of body composition, while simultaneously controlling the food intake and measuring physical activity in two different aged cohorts of rats.

2. Methods

2.1. Animals and Diet. Animal protocol was approved by the Institutional Animal Care and Use Committee at Florida State University. A total of thirty-six ($n = 36$) 5- and 10-month-old female SD rats were divided into sham, ovariectomized (ovx), and ovx + E_2 (immediately after surgery 10 μg/kg BW 17β-estradiol was injected subcutaneously twice per week) in each age group ($n = 6$ per treatment group). During the study period animals were pair-fed to the mean food intake of the sham with a semipurified control diet (AIN-93M) and weighed weekly until the occurrence of significant bone loss in ovx rats, which was after 3.5 months (age 8.5 months) for young and after 5 months (age 15 months) for older animals. Younger and older ovx + E_2 groups received estradiol for the full duration of the study (3.5 months or 5 months, resp.). Rats were provided with free access to continuous voluntary running wheels in their individual cages for 24 hours, within 24 to 48 hours after E_2 injection, one week before sacrifice. These running wheels were connected to a distance counter to measure animals' voluntary running activity.

2.2. Tissue Collection. At the termination of the study, animals were anesthetized with ketamine/xylazine (100 mg/5 mg/kg BW) and bled from their abdominal aortas. Tissues, including bone, muscle, liver, heart, and uterus, were harvested. An incision through the skin from the medial side of the thigh to the abdomen was made. The skin was then reflected to expose the muscles of the lower leg. An incision was made along the white facial line demarcating lateral aspects of the lower leg, from the ankle to 3–5 mm proximal to the ankle. GAS and SOL muscles from hindlimb were isolated from the distal end using forceps and scissors and weighted. Bone specimens including vertebrae and tibiae were collected, cleaned of adhering tissues, and stored at −20°C for further analysis. Additionally, in order to confirm the success of ovariectomy, atrophied uterus was removed, nicked, and weighed.

2.3. Body Composition and Bone Microstructural Properties. Lean mass and fat mass, whole body, and vertebral and tibial BMD and BMC were assessed using dual-energy X-ray absorptiometry (DXA) (Hologic Inc., Bedford, MA, USA) one week prior to removal of the ovaries (baseline) and again two weeks prior to the end of study (final) after rats were anesthetized with ketamine/xylazine (100 mg/5 mg/kg BW). Microarchitectural properties of the right tibia and 4th lumbar vertebra were assessed using a μCT 35 scanner (Scanco Medical, Brüttisellen, Switzerland). Bone and muscle specimens were frozen at −20°C for further examination in a blind manner. Tibia was scanned at the volume of interest (VOI) that was twenty-five slices away from the proximal growth plate in the distal direction (16 μm/slice) to 125 slices. The VOI for lumbar vertebra was twenty-five slices away from the growth plate at each end of the vertebral body and was scanned from the cephalic to the caudal growth plate, resulting in a total of slices. Both bone specimens were scanned at an isotropic voxel resolution of 22 μm3 using a 1024 × 1024 matrix. The integration time per projection was 70 ms and rotational step was 0.36° with a total acquisition time of 150 min per sample. The scanned VOI resulted in a total of 350 and 530 images for tibia and lumbar vertebra, respectively. Morphometric parameters calculated by scanning the VOI included bone volume over total volume (BV/TV), trabecular number (Tb. N), separation (Tb. Sp.), thickness (Tb. Th.), structure model index (SMI), and connectivity density (Conn. D). The obtained 3D microarchitecture allowed visualization of these morphometric measurements.

2.4. Blood Parameters. Blood samples were centrifuged (4°C) at 1500g for 15 minutes. Serum samples were separated, aliquoted, and stored at −20°C for analyses of 17β-estradiol and two of the most widely accepted markers of bone turnover for rats, namely, C-telopeptides of type I collagen (CTX) and bone specific alkaline phosphatase (B-ALP) [19]. These measurements were performed using enzyme linked immunoassay (ELISA) kits from TSZ ELISA (Framingham, MA, USA) and Immunodiagnostic Systems Inc. (Fountain Hills, AZ, USA), respectively, following the manufacturer's protocols.

2.5. Statistics. Power calculation: powers for detecting differences were calculated based on a range of possible decreases in BMD of ovx rats when compared to sham-operated rats. The range of possible increases was set beginning at 1% and increased by 1.0% increments to 8%. The power was calculated as follows: probability (rejecting mean (i) = mean (j) given difference = x).

A two-tailed significance level of 0.05 was used. The difference stated in the above probability statement was expressed as a percentage of a reported standard deviation. Thus, 5% increase was one standard deviation, and the square of this value was what was assumed to estimate the pooled variance estimate calculated in the analysis of variance. Six rats per treatment group provided us with a power of more than 0.80 at $\alpha = 0.05$ to detect a difference in BMD of one standard deviation.

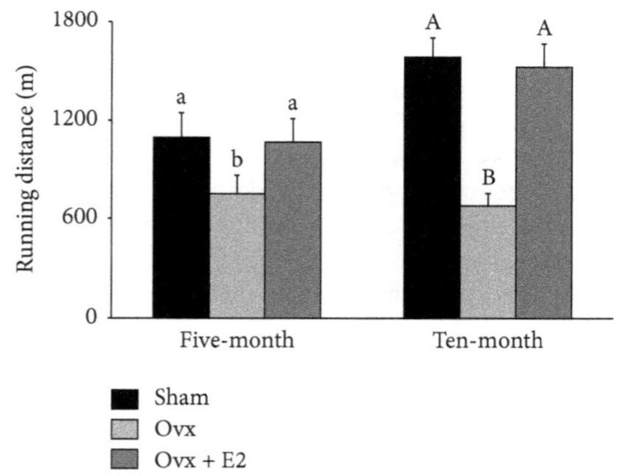

FIGURE 1: The effects of ovariectomy (ovx) and 17β-estradiol (ovx + E_2) on 24-hour voluntary running distance in rats from the cohorts of initial ages of five months (A) and ten months (B). Values are means ± SEM. Bars that do not share the same superscript letters are significantly ($p < 0.05$) different from each other ($n = 6$ per treatment group). Voluntary running activity measured by activity wheel and distance counter in individual cages for 24 hours between one and two weeks before sacrifice was significantly decreased in older ovx rats (younger ovx rats tended to have a lower activity). E_2 administration prevented the lower activity level.

Data Analysis. For each age group (initial age of 5 months or 10 months), a 3-way randomized design (ovx, ovx + E_2, and sham) was utilized. SigmaStat 3.5 (Systat Software Inc., San Jose, CA) was used to analyze the data and when a one-way ANOVA indicated any significant differences among the means, Tukey's post hoc test was performed. Statistical significance was set at the $p < 0.05$ level for all analyses. Study was designed to detect the significant cooccurrence of obesity, osteoporosis, and sarcopenia and was terminated upon DXA measurements that provided significant changes in these body tissues. Therefore, the duration of ovarian hormone deficiency was different between the two age groups; three and half months for young animals and five months for older group. To avoid the impact of time differences in duration of ovarian hormone deficiency and estradiol exposure on body composition, the comparison was made among sham and ovx and sham and ovx + E_2 in each age group only, using one-way ANOVA.

3. Results

3.1. Food Intake, Physical Activity, and Body and Organ Weights. Even though ovx rats were pair-fed with the mean food intake of sham animals, the final BWs of ovx rats in both age groups were significantly higher than sham rats (Table 1). E_2 administration prevented the ovariectomy-induced weight gain. Success of the surgical procedure was evident by atrophy of the uterus that was prevented by E_2. No significant differences were found between mean heart and liver weights (Table 1). Older ovx rats significantly decreased 24-hour voluntary wheel running activity by 57% compared with sham animals and younger ovx rats tended ($p = 0.08$) to have a lower activity (Figure 1).

TABLE 1: The effects of ovariectomy (ovx) and 17β-estradiol (ovx + E_2) on food intake, body, and organ weight in rats with initial ages of five and ten months. Despite pair-feeding the animals, ovariectomy significantly increased body weight and caused atrophy of uterine tissue without any effects on heart or liver weights.

Parameter	5-month-old			10-month-old		
	Sham	Ovx	Ovx + E_2	Sham	Ovx	Ovx + E_2
Food intake (g/day)	16.38 ± 9.1	16.39 ± 9.8	16.05 ± 9.4	15.65 ± 9.1	15.68 ± 9.8	15.01 ± 9.4
Body weight (g)						
Initial	294.00 ± 6.96	293.33 ± 6.65	293.67 ± 4.99	369.40 ± 6.96	370.00 ± 6.65	361.98 ± 4.99
Final	366.40 ± 9.8^a	400.40 ± 9.8^b	350.33 ± 13.38^a	421.80 ± 9.8^A	474.00 ± 10.35^B	404.00 ± 6.91^A
Organ weight (mg)						
Uterus	0.618 ± 0.05^a	0.098 ± 0.01^b	0.287 ± 0.03^c	0.733 ± 0.05^A	0.140 ± 0.02^B	0.232 ± 0.01^C
Liver	10.640 ± 0.653	9.362 ± 0.236	8.750 ± 0.617	12.98 ± 1.33	13.22 ± 2.03	10.66 ± 0.06
Heart	1.050 ± 0.057	0.965 ± 0.0293	0.950 ± 0.029	1.186 ± 0.029	1.167 ± 0.035	1.125 ± 0.027

Values are means ± SEM. Values that do not share the same superscript letters in each age category are significantly ($p < 0.05$) different from each other ($n = 6$ per treatment group).

TABLE 2: The effects of ovariectomy (ovx) and 17β-estradiol (ovx + E_2) on body composition in rats with initial ages of five and ten months. Ovariectomy induced a significant increase in total fat mass and a decrease in bone mineral density in both age groups and a decrease in lean mass in the older group. E_2 administration prevented ovx-induced alterations in body composition.

Parameters	5-month-old			10-month-old		
	Sham	Ovx	Ovx + E_2	Sham	Ovx	Ovx + E_2
Total fat mass (g/cm^2)						
Baseline	69.4 ± 6.5	70.5 ± 5.9	73.2 ± 5.5	102.6 ± 14.9	100.3 ± 12.8	101.3 ± 10.0
Final	172.0 ± 10.5^a	226.0 ± 8.7^b	170.2 ± 13.2^a	218.6 ± 11.5^A	284.0 ± 7.5^B	217.7 ± 7.7^A
Total lean mass (g)						
Baseline	204.6 ± 10.6	203.8 ± 7.5	203.0 ± 7.1	221.4 ± 9.3	231.2 ± 8.3	219.8 ± 6.6
Final	167.0 ± 11.0^a	146.2 ± 9.1^b	160.2 ± 9.6^a	168.2 ± 10.5	152.2 ± 11.1	160.2 ± 4.6
Total BMD (g/cm^2)						
Baseline	0.159 ± 0.0008	0.160 ± 0.004	0.161 ± 0.002	0.186 ± 0.007	0.187 ± 0.003	0.181 ± 0.003
Final	0.173 ± 0.003^a	0.158 ± 11.96^b	0.172 ± 0.004^a	0.181 ± 0.008^A	0.169 ± 0.002^B	0.179 ± 0.006^A
Total BMC (g)						
Baseline	8.940 ± 0.108	8.800 ± 0.144	9.100 ± 0.224	11.460 ± 0.93	11.350 ± 0.19	10.517 ± 0.53
Final	11.54 ± 0.42	11.60 ± 0.004	11.18 ± 0.004	13.60 ± 0.80	13.73 ± 0.34	13.17 ± 0.38

Values are means ± SEM. Values that do not share the same superscript letters in each age category are significantly ($p < 0.05$) different from each other. BMD, bone mineral density; BMC, bone mineral content ($n = 6$ per treatment group).

3.2. Body Composition. The excess BW gain in ovx rats of both age groups was mainly due to a 30% increase of fat mass ($p = 0.006$ and $p = 0.02$, resp., for young and old animals) that was completely prevented by E_2 (Table 2).

In both age groups ovariectomy significantly reduced whole body BMD, in comparison with sham animals, without affecting BMC due to the simultaneous increases in bone areas (Table 2). Furthermore, the whole body BMD was 9% lower in older animals, reflecting the impact of aging in addition to ovariectomy. E_2 prevented these alterations in both age groups.

Ovariectomy induced a significant loss of tibial and vertebral BMD in both age groups which was more pronounced in older rats (22% and 16% loss, resp., for tibiae and vertebrae in older animals). The loss of BMC was observed in both tibiae and vertebrae in older ovx rats and only in vertebrae of younger ovx animals. E_2 prevented the loss of BMD and BMC only in younger animals (Table 3).

3.3. Microcomputed Tomography (μCT) Analysis. Representative images of the 3D trabecular microstructures of proximal tibiae of the three groups in the older (initial age of 10 months) cohort are presented in Figure 2. Ovariectomy significantly decreased trabecular BV/TV in tibiae (73% and 86%, resp., in young and old rats) and lumbar (46% and 49%, resp., for young and old rats), compared with their corresponding sham animals (Figures 3(a) and 3(b)). E_2 only prevented the vertebral trabecular bone loss in younger animals.

The mean proximal tibial values for Tb. N were significantly reduced in both age groups (65% and 73%, resp., in young and old rats) that were prevented by E_2. Only older

TABLE 3: The effects of ovariectomy (ovx) and 17β-estradiol (ovx + E_2) on bone mineral density and bone mineral content of the 4th lumbar and right tibia in rats with initial ages of five and ten months. The mean tibial and vertebral bone mineral density and bone mineral content of ovx rats were significantly lower in comparison with sham rats in both age groups and E_2 administration prevented the bone loss.

Parameters	5-month-old			10-month-old		
	Sham	Ovx	Ovx + E_2	Sham	Ovx	Ovx + E_2
4th lumbar						
BMD (g/cm^2)	0.246 ± 0.005^a	0.195 ± 0.002^b	0.240 ± 0.005^a	0.266 ± 0.016^A	0.207 ± 0.004^B	0.230 ± 0.004^C
BMC (g)	0.130 ± 0.007^a	0.089 ± 0.005^b	0.128 ± 0.006^a	0.162 ± 0.017^A	0.115 ± 0.003^B	0.127 ± 0.005^C
Right tibia						
BMD (g/cm^2)	0.211 ± 0.003^a	0.183 ± 0.004^b	0.209 ± 0.002^a	0.240 ± 0.009^A	0.204 ± 0.004^B	0.218 ± 0.004^C
BMC (g)	0.314 ± 0.003	0.292 ± 0.007	0.309 ± 0.007	0.375 ± 0.002^A	0.331 ± 0.009^B	0.338 ± 0.006^C

Values are means ± SEM. Values that do not share the same superscript letters in each age category are significantly ($p < 0.05$) different from each other. BMD, bone mineral density; BMC, bone mineral content ($n = 6$ per treatment group).

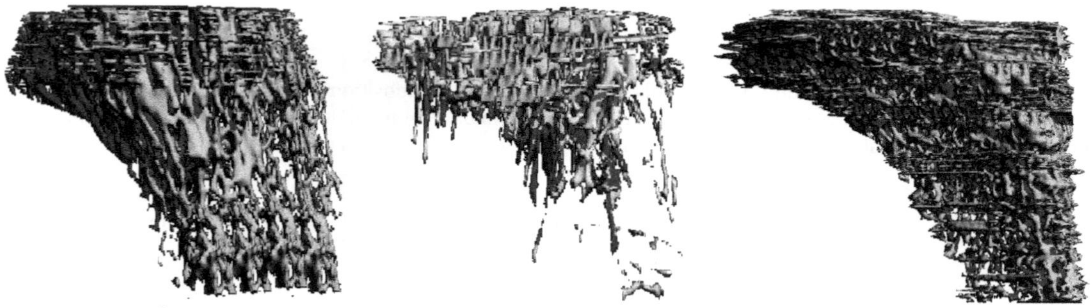

Sham (a) Ovx (b) Ovx + E2 (c)

FIGURE 2: 3D trabecular images representative of proximal right tibia of sham (a), ovariectomy (ovx) (b), and 17β-estradiol (ovx + E_2) (c). The images were acquired using μCT (Methods). Ovariectomy decreased trabecular bone structure when compared to sham in rats from the cohort of initial age of ten months. This effect was prevented by E_2 administration. Similar effects were observed in younger animals ($n = 6$ per treatment group).

ovx rats experienced a significant loss (45%) of vertebral Tb. N (Figures 3(c) and 3(d)).

Tb. Sp. significantly increased in both tibiae and vertebrae of the older ovx rats (74% and 46%, resp.) and tibiae of the younger ovx group; only the latter was prevented by E_2 (Figures 3(e) and 3(f)).

Both ovx age groups experienced a reduced Tb. Th. that reached a significant level only in the tibiae of the older ovx animals which was not prevented by E_2 (Figures 3(g) and 3(h)).

A significant reduction of Conn. D was observed in tibiae of both ovx age groups and vertebrae of the older animals. The latter was prevented by E_2 (Figures 3(i) and 3(j)).

SMI, which quantifies the pattern of trabeculae as either more rod- or plate-like, was 1.69 and 0.572 in tibiae and vertebrae of younger sham rats, respectively (Figure 3(k)). SMI values for both bones increased in ovx rats; that is, SMI = 2.753 and 1.18 in tibiae and vertebrae, respectively, indicating a shift to less favorable rod-like trabecular bone. Similarly in older animals SMI values for tibiae and vertebrae were both increased compared to those of sham values, that is, 2.78 versus 1.49 and 1.07 versus 0.41 (Figure 3(l)). The higher SMI values in ovx rats indicated that ovariectomy made the remaining bone inferior. E_2 prevented the vertebral increase in SMI (Figure 3(l)).

3.4. Muscle Mass and Ratios. Muscle mass was not significantly affected by ovariectomy. However, when SOL and GAS values were normalized to BW, mean GAS value in the younger ovx + E_2 group tended ($p = 0.09$) to increase compared with that of sham group (Table 4).

In older ovx rats, normalized SOL value tended ($p = 0.094$) to decrease and GAS value was significantly lower than that of the sham and/or ovx + E_2 groups. E_2 prevented the loss of SOL and GAS by 50% and 100%, respectively. In both age groups the ratio of tibial BMC to combined GAS and SOL values of ovx group was significantly lower (12% and 21%, resp., for young and old animals) than that of sham and/or ovx + E_2 groups which was prevented by estrogen (Table 4).

3.5. Blood Parameters. Ovariectomy significantly lowered serum E_2 levels and increased B-ALP (28% and 26% resp., for ovx young and old rats) and CTX (31% and 34% resp., for ovx young and old animals) in both age groups. Although E_2 administration in both age groups lowered B-ALP and CTX levels, they were higher than that of sham animals (Table 5).

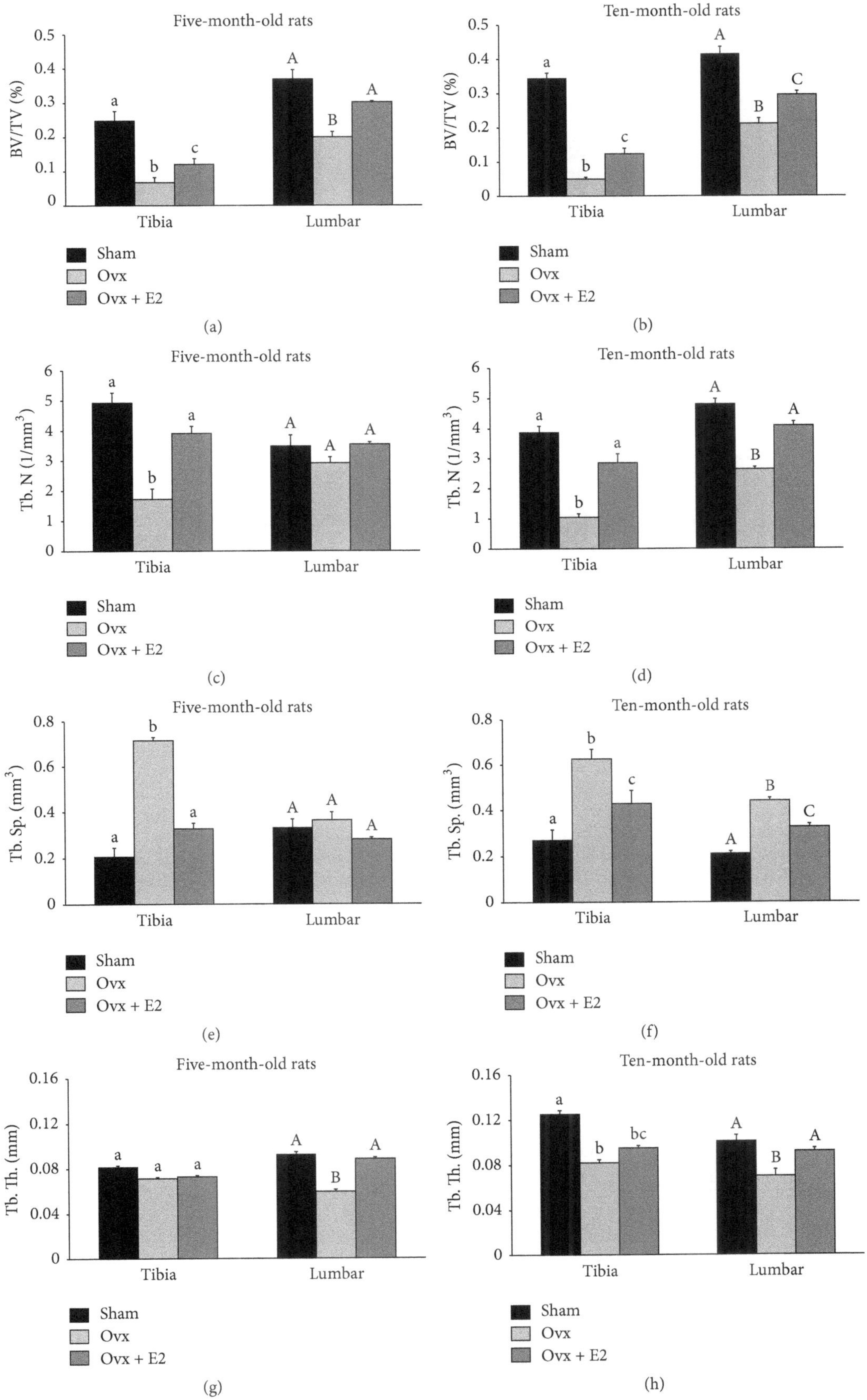

Figure 3: Continued.

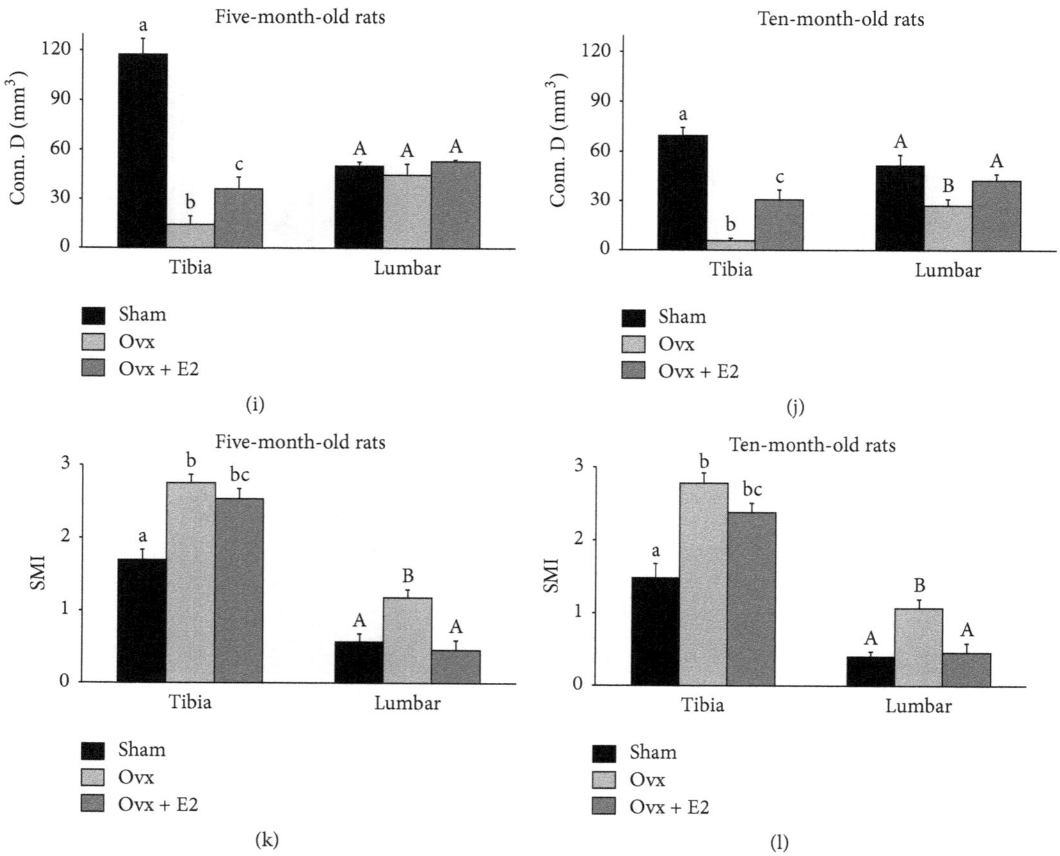

FIGURE 3: The effects of ovariectomy (ovx) and 17β-estradiol (ovx + E_2) on BV/TV, bone volume/total volume (a and b); Tb. N, trabecular number (c and d); Tb. Sp., trabecular separation (e and f); Tb. Th., trabecular thickness (g and h); Conn. D, connectivity density (i and j); SMI, structure model index (k and l) of right tibiae and 4th lumbar vertebrae in rats from the cohorts of initial ages of five (a, c, e, g, i, and k) and ten months (b, d, f, h, j, and l). Values are means ± SEM. Bars that do not share the same superscript letters are significantly ($p < 0.05$) different from each other. Small and large letters represent tibia and lumbar, respectively ($n = 6$ per treatment group). Ovariectomy significantly decreased tibia and lumbar trabecular BV/TV, bone volume/total volume, in both age groups that was only prevented by estrogen, in the vertebral bone of younger animals (a and b). In both age groups the mean proximal tibial values for Tb. N were significantly reduced following ovariectomy that was prevented by E_2. However, a significant loss of vertebral Tb. N only was observed in ovx rats (c and d). Tb. Sp. significantly increased in both tibiae and vertebrae of the older ovx rats and tibiae of the younger ovx group; only the latter was prevented by E_2 (e and f). Reduced levels of Tb. Th. reached a significant level only in the tibiae of the older ovx animals which was not prevented by E_2 (g and h). Conn. D was reduced in tibiae of both ovx age groups and vertebrae of the older animals. The latter was prevented by estrogen (i and j). SMI values for both bones increased in both ovx age groups which was prevented by E_2 only in vertebral bones (l).

TABLE 4: The effects of ovariectomy (ovx) and 17β-estradiol (ovx + E_2) on muscle mass and normalized muscle mass in rats with initial ages of five and ten months. Ovariectomy did not affect the muscle mass but decreased ratio of tibial bone mineral content to combined muscle mass in both age groups and lowered normalized values of gastrocnemius muscle to body weight in older rats that were prevented by E_2 administration.

Parameters	5-month-old			10-month-old		
	Sham	Ovx	Ovx + E_2	Sham	Ovx	Ovx + E_2
Muscle mass						
Gastrocnemius (g)	1.7814 ± 5.886	2.0763 ± 4.442	1.8828 ± 5.747	2.228 ± 1.09	2.242 ± 0.004	2.129 ± 0.054
Soleus (mg)	135 ± 9.2	163 ± 9.1	139 ± 12	150 ± 7.0	151 ± 9.1	140 ± 5.1
MM/BW (mg/g)						
Gastrocnemius	4.881 ± 0.0231	5.191 ± 0.0118	5.458 ± 0.0197	5.28 ± 0.005^A	4.73 ± 0.011^B	5.28 ± 0.015^A
Soleus	0.401 ± 0.029	0.408 ± 0.024	0.402 ± 0.034	0.37 ± 0.001	0.31 ± 0.02	0.34 ± 0.003
BMC/CMM (μg/mg)	16.483 ± 0.596^a	13.042 ± 0.125^b	14.872 ± 0.400^a	15.728 ± 0.795^A	13.879 ± 0.304^B	14.541 ± 0.439^A

Values are means ± SEM. Values that do not share the same superscript letters in each age category are significantly ($p < 0.05$) different from each other. MM, muscle mass; BW, body weight, BMC, right tibia bone mineral content; CMM, combined muscle mass ($n = 6$ per treatment group).

TABLE 5: The effects of ovariectomy (ovx) and 17β-estradiol (ovx + E_2) on blood parameters in rats with initial ages of five and ten months. Ovariectomy significantly lowered serum E_2 and increased B-ALP and CTX in both age groups.

Parameter	5-month-old			10-month-old		
	Sham	Ovx	Ovx + E_2	Sham	Ovx	Ovx + E_2
E_2 (ng/mL)	18.50 ± 4.5^a	7.89 ± 3.8^b	24.19 ± 3.1^c	21.07 ± 7.1^A	8.45 ± 2.1^B	28.10 ± 4.5^C
B -ALP (U/L)	24.16 ± 13.51^a	29.77 ± 8.81^b	25.10 ± 11.43^a	20.56 ± 7.75^A	27.35 ± 9.02^B	24.01 ± 8.8^C
CTX (ng/ml)	84.25 ± 9.05^a	110.22 ± 11.01^b	90.03 ± 10.03^c	77.50 ± 9.05^A	103.95 ± 11.02^B	82.32 ± 8.01^C

Values are means ± SEM. Values that do not share the same superscript letters in each age category are significantly ($p < 0.05$) different from each other. CTX, C-telopeptides of type I collagen; B-ALP, bone specific alkaline phosphatase; and E_2, estrogen ($n = 6$ per treatment group).

4. Discussion

Our data suggest that ovarian hormone deficiency underlies pathophysiologic obesity followed by osteoporosis that also extended to sarcopenia. Since pair-feeding the animals ruled out the confounding factor of energy intake, excess fat mass suggests a significant decrease in energy expenditure in both age groups. This was partially reflected by decreased 24-hour voluntary wheel running activity that was prevented by E_2. Estradiol administration prevented both ovariectomy-induced increase in fat mass and decrease in lean mass including bone mass. Therefore, these alterations in body composition and in physical activity can be attributed to estradiol, the main ovarian hormone. Advancing age in these younger age ovarian deficient animal models negatively affects body composition, years before traditional diagnosis of these age-related diseases. We also observed a site specific, age independent protective effect of E_2 on muscle mass. Moreover, our data suggest an anticatabolic role for E_2 in younger rats, reflected by higher ratio of normalized mean GAS value in the ovx + E_2 group compared with that of corresponding mean sham value.

Ovarian hormones may have a direct role on adiposity by increasing hormone-sensitive lipase activity, lipolytic effects of epinephrine, and beta oxidation of fatty acids [6–8]. In addition to the direct effect of ovarian hormone on adipose tissue, it may indirectly affect adiposity via regulation of food intake and energy expenditure through the hypothalamus, the key regulator of food intake and energy homeostasis in the brain [5, 9]. In the present study, BW was greater for ovx animals in both age groups despite similar food consumption compared with those of sham-operated rats. The observed increase in BW was associated with increased fat mass suggesting a shift in energy metabolism. Reduced voluntary physical activity may, in part, explain these unfavorable ovariectomy-induced body compositional changes. Similar results have been reported from ovx animals, displaying an increase in food consumption and a decrease in voluntary physical activity [20, 21]. Consistent with animal findings, human studies have also demonstrated that women, particularly a few years after the onset of menopause, gain weight because of increased fat mass and that postmenopausal women have greater appetite with less desire for physical activity [22].

In addition to the interrelationship between E_2 and adiposity, it is known to be positively associated with bone mass. Despite the commonly held belief that obesity is beneficial to maintain bone health [23], recent findings show an inverse relationship between fat mass and bone mass in both humans and laboratory animals [3, 4]. In the present study, our obese ovx rats lost bone mass and quality. We observed a significant loss of BMD and BMC in whole body and regional bones in the ovx groups, and this loss was more pronounced in our older ovx animals. The microarchitectural properties of the trabecular bone in both tibiae and lumbar vertebrae, in contrast to the effects of ovariectomy and ovx + E_2 with those of sham values in each age group, clearly demonstrate the importance of ovarian hormones. Our results also confirmed that ovariectomy caused loss of tibial BV/TV, Tb. N, and Conn. D and increased Tb. Sp. although the degree of loss was greater in older rats than in younger animals. These findings indicate that advancing age, aside from other factors, such as ovarian hormone deficiency that deleteriously affect bone microstructure, can be an independent factor affecting bone loss. This could be related in part to age-dependent changes in bone mesenchymal stem cells [24] and the role of estrogen in directing their differentiation into either adipocytes or osteoblasts [25]. Our results are consistent with findings of other investigators reporting that in addition to BMD bone microarchitecture deteriorates because of ovarian hormone deficiency in both women and in ovx animals [26, 27].

Unlike the observations made in postmenopausal women and osteoporotic men [28] who often experience increases in trabecular thickness as a result of reduced trabeculae, our results showed a decrease in Tb. Th. following ovariectomy. This, in part, can be explained by the morphological differences between the two species in bone and in muscle structures. Because of their structural physiology, rats do not experience fractures even when severe bone loss is evident [29]. Alternatively, the skeletal system in humans compensates for the loss of trabeculae through an increase in the thickness of the remaining trabeculae [30]. Although this may postpone fracture, continued bone loss in humans eventually leads to fracture because of increased stress associated with thinning and perforation of trabeculae [30]. In the present study, μCT analysis indicated that E_2 treatment partially prevented the loss of trabecular structures, findings which concur with observations by Lark et al. [31, 32]. Administration of E_2 also had a more pronounced modulating effect in younger rats than in older rats.

In addition to the structural parameters, other morphological parameters, such as SMI, reflect bone quality and strength. The SMI value is based on surface density and thickness of a 3-dimensional structure. Its value is multiplied by a factor to yield more practical numbers, 0 for ideal plates, 3 for ideal rods, and 4 for true spheres [33]. A plate-like structure is generally stronger than a rod-like structure [33]. The SMI values in both age categories were higher in ovx rats compared to corresponding sham animals, indicating that ovarian hormone deficiency not only causes bone loss, but also, at the same time, decreases the quality of the remaining bone.

In humans and rodents, both estrogen receptors (ERs), ERα and ERβ, are expressed in skeletal muscle, making it a target tissue of estrogen action [10]. Although a number of studies support a link between muscle mass and estrogen [34, 35], not all results from human and animal studies are in agreement about the relationship between estrogen and skeletal muscle. Results of human studies are inconsistent because of the variety of study designs (e.g., cross-sectional versus longitudinal) and because of age and gender differences of the samples examined [34]. Other contributing factors adding to these inconsistencies among animal studies include variations in animal models used, the duration of experiments, and the age of the animals [13, 14]. In the present study, we were able to demonstrate the coexistence of obesity with sarcopenia in the older osteopenic ovx rats. Our findings are consistent with several reports by other investigators [13, 14] which have reported that ovarian hormone deficiency delays recovery of the skeletal muscle mass from disuse-induced muscle atrophy in rats. ERα interacts with nuclear troponin I in fast skeletal muscle [36]. Interestingly, nuclear localization of troponin I has also been identified in cardiac muscle [37] and could be associated with some forms of cardiomyopathy that alter myocyte size [38]. In addition, nuclear localization of troponin T, which is a binding partner of troponin I in striated muscles, has been shown to vary with age, and this may be associated with some aspects of sarcopenia [39–41]. Interestingly, we observed a greater response to E_2 manipulation in GAS skeletal muscle compared with SOL that may in part be explained by higher proportion of ERα on fast-twitch muscle fibers. Also, in cross-sectional studies, a positive relationship between muscle mass and plasma levels of estrogen, estrone, and estradiol in women has been reported suggesting a faster decline of muscle mass in premenopausal women [35]. Furthermore, consistent with Frost's hypothesis and data from postmenopausal women [42, 43], we observed a significant decline in the ratio of tibial BMC to skeletal muscle mass in our ovx rats in both age groups, an effect that was prevented by E_2. These findings suggest that E_2 may lower the required load to prevent bone loss or promote bone formation.

Consistent with available literature we observed a site specific protective effect of E_2 on skeletal muscle [43]. Our estrogen administered rats maintained muscle weights, irrespective of age. Furthermore, our findings revealed an apparent anticatabolic effect of E_2 in five-month-old animals, as the mean normalized GAS and SOL weights of E_2 treated rats were higher than both sham and ovx groups. The potential anticatabolic effect of E_2 on skeletal muscle has been reported using young ovx rats and human studies with younger subjects; however, there may be less of an effect of E_2 with advancing age, but the strength of evidence to support this contention is minimal.

Ovx rat is the most commonly used model demonstrating bone loss [19]. Similar to menopause, the ovx rats experience increased rates of bone resorption and bone formation with the rate of resorption exceeding that of formation [19] which results in a net loss of bone mass. In our study, the bone resorption marker CTX was significantly elevated in both obese ovx rats and exceeded that of bone formation marker B-ALP in these animals compared to corresponding sham rats of both age groups. E_2 deficiency in the ovx rat model appears to be the most appropriate method available for modeling excess resorption not accompanied by formation deficit [19]. In addition to loss of bone mass, ovx rats increase fat mass along with a gradual decline in muscle mass. Therefore, the ovx rat could be used as an experimental model to conduct obesity translational research without the confounding effects of diet or genetic background.

Our findings suggested that the cooccurrence of obesity and sarcopenia along with osteoporosis may be found in ovarian hormone deficient women as a result of several factors which work together and exacerbate mobility disability. First, the gradual reduction in female sex hormones by advancing age can affect energy intake and expenditure and potentially contribute to added fat accumulation and obesity. Low levels of ovarian hormones are linked to decreased spontaneous physical activity and to decreased energy expenditure, leading to an increase in fat mass even without additional energy intake. Second, excess adiposity may impair bone and muscle mass and function on a physiological basis through certain mechanisms affected by systemic inflammation and impaired metabolic function. Third, the excess weight, along with bone and muscle loss, may result in an impaired functionality that accounts for a higher rate of obesity and obesity related medical complications. All of these factors may contribute to frailty and to increased risk of mortality in women with low levels of ovarian hormones.

5. Conclusion

In summary, using five- and ten-month-old ovx rats (initial age of five or ten months) enabled us to disentangle the effect of ovarian hormone deficiency from the complex multifactorial process of chronological aging in the female body while controlling for energy intake and measuring physical inactivity. Our findings in these two age cohorts ovx SD rats suggested that removal of ovaries alters BC similar to what can be manifested as osteosarcopenic obesity in postmenopausal women. While previous studies have investigated these age-related disease conditions in isolation, in older animals that mimic the same age as of menopausal women, to the best of our knowledge, the cooccurrence of all of these three conditions has not yet been examined. To understand the mechanistic relationship between these diseases, our study demonstrates the utility of ovx rat as a proper model for future translational research. Future studies are needed to examine the effects of ovarian hormone deficiency on changes that occur in energy metabolism in fat and fat-free mass and the roles that E_2 plays in promoting homeostasis and the mechanistic crossroads that lead to divergent outcomes following E_2 exposure. Also, the related clinical dimensions and interactions of obesity, sarcopenia, and osteoporosis need to be investigated.

Conflicts of Interest

Zahra Ezzat-Zadeh, Jeong-Su Kim, P. Bryant Chase, and Bahram H. Arjmandi have no conflicts of interest.

References

[1] J. A. Batsis, T. A. Mackenzie, F. Lopez-Jimenez, and S. J. Bartels, "Sarcopenia, sarcopenic obesity, and functional impairments in older adults: National Health and Nutrition Examination Surveys 1999–2004," *Nutrition Research*, vol. 35, no. 12, pp. 1031–1039, 2015.

[2] E. M. Lewiecki, J. P. Bilezikian, L. Bonewald et al., "Osteoporosis update: proceedings of the 2013 santa fe bone symposium," *Journal of Clinical Densitometry*, vol. 17, no. 3, pp. 330–343, 2014.

[3] S. Migliaccio, E. A. Greco, R. Fornari, L. M. Donini, L. Di Luigi, and A. Lenzi, "Skeletal alterations in women affected by obesity," *Aging Clinical and Experimental Research*, vol. 25, supplement 1, pp. S35–S37, 2013.

[4] G. V. Halade, M. M. Rahman, P. J. Williams, and G. Fernandes, "High fat diet-induced animal model of age-associated obesity and osteoporosis," *The Journal of Nutritional Biochemistry*, vol. 21, no. 12, pp. 1162–1169, 2010.

[5] P. S. Cooke and A. Naaz, "Role of estrogens in adipocyte development and function," *Experimental Biology and Medicine*, vol. 229, pp. 1127–1135, 2004.

[6] S. B. Pedersen, K. Kristensen, P. A. Hermann, J. A. Katzenellenbogen, and B. Richelsen, "Estrogen controls lipolysis by up-regulating α2A-adrenergic receptors directly in human adipose tissue through the estrogen receptor α. Implications for the female fat distribution," *Journal of Clinical Endocrinology and Metabolism*, vol. 89, no. 4, pp. 1869–1878, 2004.

[7] S. L. Palin, P. G. McTernan, L. A. Anderson, D. W. Sturdee, A. H. Barnett, and S. Kumar, "17β-Estradiol and anti-estrogen ICI:compound 182,780 regulate expression of lipoprotein lipase and hormone-sensitive lipase in isolated subcutaneous abdominal adipocytes," *Metabolism: Clinical and Experimental*, vol. 52, no. 4, pp. 383–388, 2003.

[8] M. L. Misso, Y. Murata, W. C. Boon, M. E. E. Jones, K. L. Britt, and E. R. Simpson, "Cellular and molecular characterization of the adipose phenotype of the aromatase-deficient mouse," *Endocrinology*, vol. 144, no. 4, pp. 1474–1480, 2003.

[9] R. Meli, M. Pacilio, G. M. Raso et al., "Estrogen and raloxifene modulate leptin and its receptor in hypothalamus and adipose tissue from ovariectomized rats," *Endocrinology*, vol. 145, no. 7, pp. 3115–3121, 2004.

[10] A. Wiik, M. Ekman, O. Johansson, E. Jansson, and M. Esbjörnsson, "Expression of both oestrogen receptor alpha and beta in human skeletal muscle tissue," *Histochemistry and Cell Biology*, vol. 131, no. 2, pp. 181–189, 2009.

[11] D. J. Glass, "Signalling pathways that mediate skeletal muscle hypertrophy and atrophy," *Nature Cell Biology*, vol. 5, no. 2, pp. 87–90, 2003.

[12] A. L. Moran, G. L. Warren, and D. A. Lowe, "Removal of ovarian hormones from mature mice detrimentally affects muscle contractile function and myosin structural distribution," *Journal of Applied Physiology*, vol. 100, no. 2, pp. 548–554, 2006.

[13] J. M. McClung, J. M. Davis, M. A. Wilson, E. C. Goldsmith, and J. A. Carson, "Estrogen status and skeletal muscle recovery from disuse atrophy," *Journal of Applied Physiology*, vol. 100, no. 6, pp. 2012–2023, 2006.

[14] A. M. Moran, S. A. Nelson, R. M. Landisch, G. L. Warren, and D. A. Lowe, "Estradiol replacement reverses ovariectomy-induced muscle contractile and myosin dysfunction in mature female mice," *Journal of Applied Physiology*, vol. 102, no. 4, pp. 1387–1393, 2007.

[15] M. Brown, A. Foley, and J. A. Ferreria, "Ovariectomy, hindlimb unweighting, and recovery effects on skeletal muscle in adult rats," *Aviation Space and Environmental Medicine*, vol. 76, no. 11, pp. 1012–1018, 2005.

[16] D. L. Enns and P. M. Tiidus, "The influence of estrogen on skeletal muscle: sex matters," *Sports Medicine*, vol. 40, no. 1, pp. 41–58, 2010.

[17] J. J. Sciote, M. J. Horton, Y. Zyman, and G. Pascoe, "Differential effects of diminished oestrogen and androgen levels on development of skeletal muscle fibres in hypogonadal mice," *Acta Physiologica Scandinavica*, vol. 172, no. 3, pp. 179–187, 2001.

[18] M. Kassem, "Cellular and molecular effects of growth hormone and estrogen on human bone cells," *APMIS*, vol. 105, supplement 71, pp. 7–30, 1997.

[19] D. N. Kalu, "The ovariectomized rat model of postmenopausal bone loss," *Bone and Mineral*, vol. 15, no. 3, pp. 175–191, 1991.

[20] E. J. Roy and G. N. Wade, "Role of food intake in estradiol-induced body weight changes in female rats," *Hormones and Behavior*, vol. 8, no. 3, pp. 265–274, 1977.

[21] H. Fonseca, S. K. Powers, D. Gonalves, A. Santos, M. P. Mota, and J. A. Duarte, "Physical inactivity is a major contributor to ovariectomy-induced sarcopenia," *International Journal of Sports Medicine*, vol. 33, no. 4, pp. 268–278, 2012.

[22] J. C. Lovejoy, C. M. Champagne, L. de Jonge, H. Xie, and S. R. Smith, "Increased visceral fat and decreased energy expenditure during the menopausal transition," *International Journal of Obesity*, vol. 32, no. 6, pp. 949–958, 2008.

[23] I. R. Reid, R. Ames, M. C. Evans et al., "Determinants of total body and regional bone mineral density in normal postmenopausal women—a key role for fat mass," *The Journal of Clinical Endocrinology & Metabolism*, vol. 75, no. 1, pp. 45–51, 1992.

[24] F. Z. Asumda and P. B. Chase, "Age-related changes in rat bone-marrow mesenchymal stem cell plasticity," *BMC Cell Biology*, vol. 12, article 44, 2011.

[25] J.-W. Zhao, Z.-L. Gao, H. Mei, Y.-L. Li, and Y. Wang, "Differentiation of human mesenchymal stem cells: the potential mechanism for estrogen-induced preferential osteoblast versus adipocyte differentiation," *American Journal of the Medical Sciences*, vol. 341, no. 6, pp. 460–468, 2011.

[26] M. D. Walker, X. S. Liu, B. Zhou et al., "Premenopausal and postmenopausal differences in bone microstructure and mechanical competence in Chinese-American and white women," *Journal of Bone and Mineral Research*, vol. 28, no. 6, pp. 1308–1318, 2013.

[27] Å. Tivesten, S. Movérare-Skrtic, A. Chagin et al., "Additive protective effects of estrogen and androgen treatment on trabecular bone in ovariectomized rats," *Journal of Bone and Mineral Research*, vol. 19, no. 11, pp. 1833–1839, 2004.

[28] J. S. Thomsen, M. V. Jensen, A. S. Niklassen, E. N. Ebbesen, and A. Brüel, "Age-related changes in vertebral and iliac crest 3D bone microstructure—differences and similarities," *Osteoporosis International*, vol. 26, no. 1, pp. 219–228, 2014.

[29] T. Mawatari, H. Miura, H. Higaki et al., "Quantitative analysis of three-dimensional complexity and connectivity changes in trabecular microarchitecture in relation to aging, menopause, and inflammation," *Journal of Orthopaedic Science*, vol. 4, no. 6, pp. 431–438, 1999.

[30] V. Pattijn, T. Van Cleynenbreugel, J. V. Sloten, R. Van Audekercke, G. Van Der Perre, and M. Wevers, "Structural and radiological parameters for the nondestructive characterization of trabecular bone," *Annals of Biomedical Engineering*, vol. 29, no. 12, pp. 1064–1073, 2001.

[31] M. W. Lark, G. B. Stroup, R. A. Dodds et al., "Antagonism of the osteoclast vitronectin receptor with an orally active nonpeptide inhibitor prevents cancellous bone loss in the ovariectomized rat," *Journal of Bone and Mineral Research*, vol. 16, no. 2, pp. 319–327, 2001.

[32] M. W. Lark, G. B. Stroup, I. E. James et al., "A potent small molecule, nonpeptide inhibitor of cathepsin K (SB 331750) prevents bone matrix resorption in the ovariectomized rat," *Bone*, vol. 30, no. 5, pp. 746–753, 2002.

[33] T. Hildebrand and P. Rüegsegger, "Quantification of bone microarchitecture with the structure model index," *Computer Methods in Biomechanics and Biomedical Engineering*, vol. 1, no. 1, pp. 15–23, 1997.

[34] V. Messier, R. Rabasa-Lhoret, S. Barbat-Artigas, B. Elisha, A. D. Karelis, and M. Aubertin-Leheudre, "Menopause and sarcopenia: a potential role for sex hormones," *Maturitas*, vol. 68, no. 4, pp. 331–336, 2011.

[35] T. A. C. M. van Geel, P. P. Geusen, B. Winkens, J.-P. J. E. Sels, and G.-J. Dinant, "Measures of bioavailable serum testosterone and estradiol and their relationships with muscle mass, muscle strength and bone mineral density in postmenopausal women: a cross-sectional study," *European Journal of Endocrinology*, vol. 160, no. 4, pp. 681–687, 2009.

[36] Y. Li, B. Chen, J. Chen, G. Lou, S. Chen, and D. Zhou, "Fast skeletal muscle troponin I is a co-activator of estrogen receptor-related receptor α," *Biochemical and Biophysical Research Communications*, vol. 369, no. 4, pp. 1034–1040, 2008.

[37] F. Z. Asumda and P. B. Chase, "Nuclear cardiac troponin and tropomyosin are expressed early in cardiac differentiation of rat mesenchymal stem cells," *Differentiation*, vol. 83, no. 3, pp. 106–115, 2012.

[38] P. B. Chase, M. P. Szczypinski, and E. P. Soto, "Nuclear tropomyosin and troponin in striated muscle: new roles in a new locale?" *Journal of Muscle Research and Cell Motility*, vol. 34, no. 3-4, pp. 275–284, 2013.

[39] T. Zhang, A. Birbrair, Z.-M. Wang, J. Taylor, M. L. Messi, and O. Delbono, "Troponin T nuclear localization and its role in aging skeletal muscle," *Age*, vol. 35, no. 2, pp. 353–370, 2013.

[40] T. Zhang, A. S. Pereyra, Z.-M. Wang et al., "Calpain inhibition rescues troponin T3 fragmentation, increases Cav1.1, and enhances skeletal muscle force in aging sedentary mice," *Aging Cell*, vol. 15, no. 3, pp. 488–498, 2016.

[41] J. R. Pinto, J. Muller-Delp, and P. B. Chase, "Will you still need me (Ca2+, TnT, and DHPR), will you still cleave me (calpain), when I'm 64?" *Aging Cell*, vol. 16, no. 2, pp. 202–204, 2017.

[42] H. M. Frost, "The role of changes in mechanical usage set points in the pathogenesis of osteoporosis," *Journal of Bone and Mineral Research*, vol. 7, no. 3, pp. 253–261, 1992.

[43] W. M. Kohrt, D. B. Snead, E. Slatopolsky, and S. J. Birge Jr., "Additive effects of weight-bearing exercise and estrogen on bone mineral density in older women," *Journal of Bone and Mineral Research*, vol. 10, no. 9, pp. 1303–1311, 1995.

Permissions

All chapters in this book were first published in JAR, by Hindawi Publishing Corporation; hereby published with permission under the Creative Commons Attribution License or equivalent. Every chapter published in this book has been scrutinized by our experts. Their significance has been extensively debated. The topics covered herein carry significant findings which will fuel the growth of the discipline. They may even be implemented as practical applications or may be referred to as a beginning point for another development.

The contributors of this book come from diverse backgrounds, making this book a truly international effort. This book will bring forth new frontiers with its revolutionizing research information and detailed analysis of the nascent developments around the world.

We would like to thank all the contributing authors for lending their expertise to make the book truly unique. They have played a crucial role in the development of this book. Without their invaluable contributions this book wouldn't have been possible. They have made vital efforts to compile up to date information on the varied aspects of this subject to make this book a valuable addition to the collection of many professionals and students.

This book was conceptualized with the vision of imparting up-to-date information and advanced data in this field. To ensure the same, a matchless editorial board was set up. Every individual on the board went through rigorous rounds of assessment to prove their worth. After which they invested a large part of their time researching and compiling the most relevant data for our readers.

The editorial board has been involved in producing this book since its inception. They have spent rigorous hours researching and exploring the diverse topics which have resulted in the successful publishing of this book. They have passed on their knowledge of decades through this book. To expedite this challenging task, the publisher supported the team at every step. A small team of assistant editors was also appointed to further simplify the editing procedure and attain best results for the readers.

Apart from the editorial board, the designing team has also invested a significant amount of their time in understanding the subject and creating the most relevant covers. They scrutinized every image to scout for the most suitable representation of the subject and create an appropriate cover for the book.

The publishing team has been an ardent support to the editorial, designing and production team. Their endless efforts to recruit the best for this project, has resulted in the accomplishment of this book. They are a veteran in the field of academics and their pool of knowledge is as vast as their experience in printing. Their expertise and guidance has proved useful at every step. Their uncompromising quality standards have made this book an exceptional effort. Their encouragement from time to time has been an inspiration for everyone.

The publisher and the editorial board hope that this book will prove to be a valuable piece of knowledge for researchers, students, practitioners and scholars across the globe.

List of Contributors

Gurtej Grewal and David G. Armstrong
Southern Arizona Limb Salvage Alliance (SALSA), University of Arizona College of Medicine, Tucson, AZ, USA

Bijan Najafi
Southern Arizona Limb Salvage Alliance (SALSA), University of Arizona College of Medicine, Tucson, AZ, USA
Arizona Center on Aging, University of Arizona, Tucson, AZ, USA

James S. Wrobel
University of Michigan, Medical School, Ann Arbor, MI, USA

Robert A. Menzies, Talal K. Talal and Mahmoud Zirie
Diabetic Foot and Wound Center, Department of Medicine, Hamad Medical Corporation, Doha, Qatar

Margaret Markiewicz and Anna Ludwicka-Bradley
Division of Rheumatology and Immunology, Medical University of South Carolina, 114 Doughty Street, STB, Charleston, SC 29425, USA

Erin Richard
Department of Biology, College of Charleston, Rita Liddy Hollings Science Center, Charleston, SC 29424, USA

Natalia Marks
Department of Radiology, Maimonides Medical Center, Brooklyn, NY 11219, USA

Myuri Ruthirakuhan, Angela C. Luedke, Angela Tam, Ankita Goel, Ayaz Kurji and Angeles Garcia
Department of Medicine (Geriatrics) and Centre for Neuroscience, Queen's University, Kingston, ON, Canada K7L 5A2

Kai Sun and Richard D. Semba
Department of Ophthalmology, Johns Hopkins University School of Medicine, Baltimore, MD 21287, USA

Linda P. Fried
Mailman School of Public Health, Columbia University, New York, NY 10032, USA

Debra A. Schaumberg
Division of Preventive Medicine, Department of Medicine, Brigham and Women's Hospital, Harvard Medical School, Boston, MA 02215, USA

Luigi Ferrucci
Longitudinal Studies Section, Clinical Research Branch, National Institute on Aging, Baltimore, MD 21225, USA

Ravi Varadhan
Department of Medicine, Johns Hopkins University School of Medicine, Baltimore, MD 21287, USA

Enrica Menditto, Francesca Guerriero and Valentina Orlando
Center of Pharmacoeconomics (CIRFF), Federico II University, 80131 Naples, Italy

Maddalena Illario and Catherine Crola
Research and Development Board, Federico II University Hospital, 80131 Naples, Italy
Translational Medical Sciences (DISMET), Federico II University, 80131 Naples, Italy

Carolina Di Somma
IRCCS SDN, 80131Naples, Italy

Donald E. Morisky
Department of Community Health Sciences, UCLA Fielding School of Public Health, Los Angeles, CA 90095-1772, USA

Annamaria Colao
Department of Clinical Medicine and Surgery, Federico II University, 80131 Naples, Italy

Philip A. De Fina and Jonathan Fellus
International Brain Research Foundation Inc., 227 Route 206 North, Building 2, Suite 101, Flanders, NJ 07836, USA

Jonathan D. Lichtenstein, Rosemarie Scolaro Moser and Megan Glenn
RSM Psychology Center, LLC 3131 Princeton Pike, Building 5, Suite 110, Lawrenceville, NJ 08648, USA

Marie-Louise Bird, Iain Robertson, Madeleine J. Ball, Jane K. Pittaway and Andrew D. Williams
School of Human Life Sciences, University of Tasmania, Launceston, TAS 7250, Australia

Keith D. Hill
School of Physiotherapy, Curtin University, Perth, WA 6845, Australia

Ann M. Albertson
General Mills: Bell Institute of Health and Nutrition, James Ford Bell Technical Center, 9000 Plymouth Avenue North, Minneapolis, MN 55427, USA

A. Christine Wold
General Mills: Quality & Regulatory Operations, 1 General Mills Boulevand, BT 10-D-1, Minneapolis, MN 55426, USA

Nandan Joshi
General Mills India Pvt. Ltd., 601-Prudential, Hiranandani Business Park, Powai, Mumbai 400076, India

Ping Kwan
ST013a, Department of Rehabilitation Sciences, Hong Kong Polytechnic University, Hong Kong

Anthony J. Perkins, Hilary A. Turchan and Amie Frame
Indiana University Center for Aging Research, Indianapolis, IN 46202, USA
Regenstrief Institute, Inc., Indianapolis, IN 46202, USA

Nicole R. Fowler and Malaz A. Boustani
Indiana University Center for Aging Research, Indianapolis, IN 46202, USA
Regenstrief Institute, Inc., Indianapolis, IN 46202, USA
Indiana University School of Medicine, Indianapolis, IN 46202, USA

Patrick Monahan and Sujuan Gao
Indiana University School of Medicine, Indianapolis, IN 46202, USA
Indiana University Department of Biostatistics, Indianapolis, IN 46202, USA
Erik Olsson, Niklas Klasson, Josef Berge, Carl Eckerström, Åke Edman and

Anders Wallin
Department of Neuroscience and Physiology, Institute of Psychiatry and Neurochemistry, The Sahlgrenska Academy, University of Gothenburg, 40530 Gothenburg, Sweden

Helge Malmgren
Department of Neuroscience and Physiology, Institute of Psychiatry and Neurochemistry, The Sahlgrenska Academy, University of Gothenburg, 40530 Gothenburg, Sweden
Department of Philosophy, Linguistics and Theory of Science, University of Gothenburg, 40530 Gothenburg, Sweden

Kevin D. Ballard, Amanda L. Zaleski, Donna M. Polk, Paul D. Thompson and Francis J. Kiernan
Division of Cardiology, Hartford Hospital, 80 Seymour Street, Hartford, CT 06102, USA

Michael E. Tschakovsky
School of Kinesiology and Health Studies, Queen's University, 28 Division Street, Kingston, ON, Canada K7L 3N6

Beth A. Parker
Division of Cardiology, Hartford Hospital, 80 Seymour Street, Hartford, CT 06102, USA
Department of Health Sciences, University of Hartford, 200 Bloomfield Avenue, West Hartford, CT 06117, USA

Seyed Ahmad Raeissadat, Leyla Sedighipour, Safura Pournajaf and Shahram Sadeghi
Department of Physical Medicine & Rehabilitation, Clinical Research Development Center of Shahid Modares Hospital, Shahid Beheshti University of Medical Sciences, Tehran, Iran

Reza Vahab Kashani
Department of Orthotics and Prosthetics, University of SocialWelfare and Rehabilitation Science, Kodakyar street, Daneshjo Boulevard, Evin, Tehran 1985713834, Iran

Lex van Velsen, Stephanie Jansen-Kosterink and Miriam Vollenbroek-Hutten
Roessingh Research and Development, Telemedicine Cluster, 7500 AH Enschede, Netherlands
University of Twente, Biomedical Signals and Systems Group, AE Enschede, Netherlands

Maddalena Illario and Catherine Crola
Federico II University, Department of Translational Medical Sciences, Largo S. Marcellino 10, 80138 Naples, Italy
Federico II University Hospital, Research & Development, Largo S. Marcellino 10, 80138 Naples, Italy

Carolina Di Somma and Annamaria Colao
Federico II University Hospital, Department of Clinical Medicine and Surgery, Largo S. Marcellino 10, 80138 Naples, Italy
Federico II University Hospital, Department of Gastroenterology, Endocrinology and Surgery, Largo S. Marcellino 10, 80138 Naples, Italy

Hongliang Li, Benjamin J. Scherlag, David C. Kem, Caitlin Zillner, Shailesh Male, Sorkko Thirunavukkarasu, Xiaohua Shen, Alexandria Benbrook, Ralph Lazzara and Xichun Yu
Heart Rhythm Institute, Department of Medicine, University of Oklahoma Health Sciences Center and Veterans Affairs Medical Center, Oklahoma City, OK 73104, USA

Jan V. Pitha
Department of Pathology, University of Oklahoma Health Sciences Center and Veterans Affairs Medical Center, Oklahoma City, OK 73104, USA

C. D. Reimers
Klinik für Neurologie, Zentralklinik Bad Berka, Robert-Koch-Allee 9, 99438 Bad Berka, Germany

G. Knapp
Fakultät Statistik, Technische Universit¨at Dortmund, 44221 Dortmund, Germany

A. K. Reimers
Sport wissenschaft, Universität Konstanz, Universitätsstraße 10, 78457 Konstanz, Germany

Carla Vande Weerd
The Harrell Center for The Study of Family Violence, Department of Community and Family Health, College of Public Health, University of South Florida, 13301 Bruce B. Downs Boulevard, MDC 56, Tampa, FL 33612, USA

Gregory J. Paveza
School of Health and Human Services, Southern Connecticut State University, 501 Crescent Street, Lang House, New Haven, CT 06515, USA

Margaret Walsh
Department of Community and Family Health, College of Public Health, University of South Florida, 13301 Bruce B. Downs Boulevard, MDC 56, Tampa, FL 33612, USA

Jaime Corvin
Department of Global Health, College of Public Health, University of South Florida, 13301 Bruce B. Downs Boulevard, MDC 56, Tampa, FL 33612, USA

Varsha Shetty, Mukta N. Chowta, Nithyananda Chowta K, Ashok Shenoy, Ashwin Kamath and Priyanka Kamath
Department of Medicine and Pharmacology, Kasturba Medical College, Mangalore, Manipal Academy of Higher Education, Mangalore, India

Matthew Lee Smith
The University of Georgia, College of Public Health, Department of Health Promotion and Behavior, 330 River Road, 315 Ramsey Center Athens, GA 30602, USA
Texas A&M Health Science Center, School of Rural Public Health, Department of Health Promotion and Community Health Sciences, TAMU 1266, College Station, TX 77843, USA

Marcia G. Ory
Texas A&M Health Science Center, School of Rural Public Health, Department of Health Promotion and Community Health Sciences, TAMU 1266, College Station, TX 77843, USA

Sang Nam Ahn
The University of Memphis, School of Public Health, Division of Health Systems Management and Policy, Robison Hall 133, Memphis, TN 38152-3530, USA

Toni P. Miles
The University of Georgia, College of Public Health, Department of Epidemiology and Biostatistics, 255 E. Hancock Avenue, Athens, GA 30602, USA

Sarah Stott-Eveneshen and Megan McAllister
Centre for Hip Health and Mobility, Robert H.N. Ho Research Centre, 2635 Laurel Street, Vancouver, BC, Canada V5Z 1M9

Joanie Sims-Gould and Maureen C. Ashe
Centre for Hip Health and Mobility, Robert H.N. Ho Research Centre, 2635 Laurel Street, Vancouver, BC, Canada V5Z 1M9
Department of Family Practice, University of British Columbia, Vancouver, BC, Canada

Lena Fleig
3Freie Universität Berlin, AB Gesundheits psychologie, Habelsch werdter Allee 45, PF 10, 14195 Berlin, Germany

Michael Hoerger
Departments of Psychology, Psychiatry and Medicine, Tulane Cancer Center, 3070 Stern Hall, New Orleans, LA 70118, USA

Maria Coletta
Main Line Health, Newtown Square, PA 19073, USA

Silvia Sörensen, Benjamin P. Chapman and Paul R. Duberstein
Department of Psychiatry, University of Rochester Medical Center, 300 Crittenden Boulevard, Rochester, NY 14642, USA

Kim Kaukeinen and Xin Tu
Department of Biostatistics, University of Rochester Medical Center, 300 Crittenden Boulevard, Rochester, NY 14642, USA

Regina L. Leckie and Jennifer C. Hodzic
Department of Psychology, University of Pittsburgh, Sennott Square 3417, 210 S. Bouquet Street, Pittsburgh, PA 15260, USA

Andrea M. Weinstein and Kirk I. Erickson
Department of Psychology, University of Pittsburgh, Sennott Square 3417, 210 S. Bouquet Street, Pittsburgh, PA 15260, USA
Center for the Neural Basis of Cognition, Department of Psychology, University of Pittsburgh, Sennott Square 3417, 210 S. Bouquet Street, Pittsburgh, PA 15213, USA

Jamie J. Y. Lee and Joanna Barlas
School of Psychology, James Cook University, Singapore

Claire L. Thompson
School of Psychology, Central Queensland University, Rockhampton, Australia

Yan Hong Dong
Centre for Healthy Brain Ageing (CHeBA) and Dementia Collaborative Research Centre—Assessment and Better Care, School of Psychiatry, UNSW Medicine, The University of New South Wales, Sydney, Australia

Bonaventura C. T. Mpondo
Department of Internal Medicine, School of Medicine, College of Health Sciences, The University of Dodoma, Dodoma, Tanzania

Atle Hole Saeterbakken, Hilde Bremseth Bårdstu, Anine Brudeseth and Vidar Andersen
Faculty of Teacher Education, Culture and Sport, Western Norway University of Applied Sciences, Bergen, Norway

Zahra Ezzat-Zadeh
Department of Nutrition, Food and Exercise Sciences, Florida State University, Tallahassee, FL, USA

Jeong-Su Kim and Bahram H. Arjmandi
Department of Nutrition, Food and Exercise Sciences, Florida State University, Tallahassee, FL, USA
Center for Advancing Exercise and Nutrition Research on Aging (CAENRA), College of Human Sciences, Florida State University, Tallahassee, FL 32306, USA

P. Bryant Chase
Department of Biological Science, Florida State University, Tallahassee, FL, USA

Index

CPSIA information can be obtained
at www.ICGtesting.com
Printed in the USA
LVHW062009100122
708212LV00002B/134

9 781639 27002